Kaplan's Essentials of Cardiac Anesthesia for Noncardiac Surgery

Kaplan's Essentials of Cardiac Anesthesia for Noncardiac Surgery

Editor

Joel A. Kaplan, MD, CPE, FACC

Professor of Anesthesiology
University of California, San Diego
La Jolla, California;
Dean Emeritus, School of Medicine
Former Chancellor, Health Sciences Center
University of Louisville
Louisville, Kentucky

Associate Editors

Brett Cronin, MD

Assistant Clinical Professor
Department of Anesthesiology
University of California, San Diego
La Jolla, California

Timothy M. Maus, MD, FASE

Associate Clinical Professor
Director, Cardiac Anesthesia
Department of Anesthesiology
University of California, San Diego
La Jolla, California

ELSEVIER

ELSEVIER

1600 John F. Kennedy Blvd.
Ste 1600
Philadelphia, PA 19103-2899

KAPLAN'S ESSENTIALS OF CARDIAC ANESTHESIA FOR NONCARDIAC SURGERY

ISBN: 978-0-323-56716-9

Senior Content Strategist: Sarah Barth
Senior Content Development Specialist: Ann Anderson
Publishing Services Manager: Catherine Jackson
Senior Project Manager/Specialist: Carrie Stetz
Design Direction: Ryan Cook

Printed in China

Last digit is the print number: 9 8 7 6 5 4 3 2 1

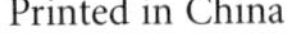

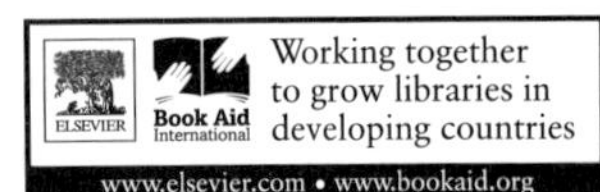

Dedication

To all of the residents and fellows in cardiac anesthesia with whom we have been fortunate to work over the past decades, and to Norma, my loving wife of more than 50 years.

JAK

To my two girls, Hayley and Berkeley.

BC

To my wife, Molly, and my children, William, Owen, Winston, and Porter, for all of your love and support.

TMM

Contributors

Dalia Banks, MD, FASE

Clinical Professor of Anesthesiology
Vice-Chair, Cardiac Anesthesia
University of California San Diego
La Jolla, California

Ron Barak, MD

Assistant Clinical Professor
Department of Anesthesiology
University of California, San Diego
La Jolla, California

Victor C. Baum, MD

U.S. Food and Drug Administration
Silver Spring, MD;
Adjunct Professor
Departments of Anesthesiology &
  Critical Care Medicine and
  Pediatrics
George Washington University
Washington, DC

Matthew G. Bean, DO

Senior Fellow
Cardiac Anesthesia and Critical Care
Department of Anesthesiology
Duke University School of Medicine
Durham, North Carolina

Yaakov Beilin, MD

Professor of Anesthesiology and
  OB/GYN
Vice-Chair for Quality
Department of Anesthesiology
Director, Obstetric Anesthesiology
Icahn School of Medicine at Mount
  Sinai;
Chair, Clinical Review Committee
Mount Sinai Hospital
New York, New York

Dean Bowker, MD

Cardiothoracic Anesthesia Fellow
Department of Anesthesiology
University of California, San Diego
La Jolla, California

Edmond Cohen, MD

Professor of Anesthesiology and
  Thoracic Surgery
Director of Thoracic Anesthesia
Icahn School of Medicine at Mount
  Sinai
New York, New York

Brett Cronin, MD

Assistant Clinical Professor of
  Anesthesiology
University of California, San Diego
La Jolla, California

Lev Deriy, MD

Associate Professor of Anesthesiology
Department of Anesthesiology and
  Critical Care
University of New Mexico
Albuquerque, New Mexico

Duncan G. de Souza, MD, FRCPC

Clinical Assistant Professor of
  Anesthesiology
University of British Columbia
Vancouver, British Columbia, Canada;
Director
Cardiac Anesthesia
Kelowna General Hospital
Kelowna, British Columbia, Canada

Byron Fergerson, MD

Associate Clinical Professor
Associate Director of Resident
  Education
Department of Anesthesiology
University of California, San Diego
La Jolla, California;
Staff Physician
Departments of Anesthesiology and
  Cardiology
VA San Diego
San Diego, California

Brian Frugoni, MD

Assistant Professor of Anesthesiology
University of California, San Diego
La Jolla, California

Neal S. Gerstein, MD, FASE

Professor
Director, UNM Cardiac Anesthesia
University of New Mexico
Albuquerque, New Mexico

Kamrouz Ghadimi, MD

Assistant Professor
Anesthesiology and Critical Care
  Medicine
Duke University School of Medicine
Durham, North Carolina

Steven B. Greenberg, MD

Director of Critical Care Services
Evanston Hospital
Department of Anesthesiology
NorthShore University Health System
Evanston, Illinois

Joshua Hamburger, MD

Assistant Professor of Anesthesiology
Icahn School of Medicine at Mount
  Sinai
New York, New York

Alexander Huang, MD, FRCPC

Lecturer
University of Toronto;
Staff Anesthesiologist
Toronto General Hospital
Toronto, Ontario, Canada

Peter M. Jessel, MD, FHRS

Knight Cardiovascular Institute
VA Portland Health Care System
Portland, Oregon

Joel A. Kaplan, MD

Professor of Anesthesiology
University of California, San Diego
La Jolla, California;
Dean Emeritus, School of Medicine
Former Chancellor, Health Sciences
University of Louisville
Louisville, Kentucky

Jeffrey Katz, MD

Attending Anesthesiologist and
  Critical Care Medicine
NorthShore University Health System
Evanston, Illinois

Swapnil Khoche, MBBS, DNB

Assistant Clinical Professor of
  Anesthesiology
University of California, San Diego
La Jolla, California

Giovanni Landoni, MD

Associate Professor of Anesthesia and
  Intensive Care
IRCCS San Raffaele Scientific Institute
Vita-Salute San Raffaele University
Milan, Italy

Marshall K. Lee, MD

Assistant Professor of Anesthesiology
  and Perioperative Medicine
Oregon Health and Science University
Portland, Oregon

Emilio B. Lobato, MD

Staff Anesthesiologist
North Florida/South Georgia VHA
Gainesville, Florida

Gerard R. Manecke Jr, MD

Professor
Department of Anesthesiology
UC San Deigo Health
San Diego, California

Timothy M. Maus, MD

Associate Clinical Professor of
   Anesthesiology
Director, Cardiac Anesthesia
Department of Anesthesiology
University of California, San Diego
La Jolla, California

K. Annette Mizuguchi, MD, PhD, MMSc

Assistant Professor
Department of Anesthesiology
Harvard Medical School
Brigham and Women's Hospital
Boston, Massachusetts

Steven M. Neustein, MD

Professor of Anesthesiology
Icahn School of Medicine at Mount
   Sinai
New York, New York

Albert P. Nguyen, MD

Assistant Clinical Professor
Department of Anesthesiology
University of California, San Diego
La Jolla, California

Liem Nguyen, MD

Associate Clinical Professor of
   Anesthesiology
UCSD Medical Center
San Diego, California

E. Orestes O'Brien, MD

Associate Professor of Anesthesiology
University of California, San Diego
La Jolla, California

E. Andrew Ochroch, MD, MSCE

Professor of Anesthesiology, Critical
   Care, & Surgery
University of Pennsylvania
Philadelphia, Pennsylvania

Michele Oppizzi, MD

Director, Coronary Care Unit
Department of Cardiology
San Raffaele Hospital
Milan, Italy

Pramod Panikkath, MD

Associate Professor of Anesthesiology
Director, Perioperative
   Echocardiography
Department of Anesthesiology and
   Critical Care
University of New Mexico
Albuquerque, New Mexico

Antonio Pisano, MD

Staff Cardiac Anesthesiologist and
   Intensivist
Department of Critical Care
Azienda Ospedaliera Dei Colli
Monaldi Hospital
Naples, Italy

Harish Ram, MD, FASE, FACC

Assistant Professor
Department of Anesthesiology
Division of Cardiothoracic Anesthesia
University of Kentucky
Lexington, Kentucky

Marc A. Rozner, PhD, MD

Professor of Anesthesiology and
   Perioperative Medicine
Professor of Cardiology
University of Texas MD Anderson
   Cancer Center
Houston, Texas

Engy T. Said, MD

Assistant Clinical Professor
Division of Regional Anesthesia and
   Acute Pain
University of California, San Diego
La Jolla, California

Ulrich H. Schmidt, MD, PhD, MBA

Professor
Department of Anesthesia
University of California, San Diego
La Jolla, California

Peter M. Schulman, MD

Associate Professor of Anesthesiology
   and Perioperative Medicine
Oregon Health and Science University
Portland, Oregon

Torin Shear, MD

Clinical Associate Professor of
   Anesthesia
NorthShore University Health System
Evanston, Illinois

Peter D. Slinger, MD, FRCPC

Professor of Anesthesia
University of Toronto;
Staff Anesthesiologist
Toronto General Hospital
Toronto, Ontario, Canada

Brian Starr, MD

Associate Professor of Anesthesiology
Department of Anesthesiology and
   Critical Care
University of New Mexico
Albuquerque, New Mexico

Marc E. Stone, MD

Professor of Anesthesiology
Program Director, Fellowship in
   Cardiothoracic Anesthesiology
Icahn School of Medicine at Mount
   Sinai
New York, New York

Annemarie Thompson, MD

Professor of Anesthesiology and
   Medicine
Duke University School of Medicine
Durham, North Carolina

Stefano Turi, MD

Department of Anesthesia and
   Intensive Care
IRCCS San Raffaele
Milan, Italy

Elizabeth A. Valentine, MD

Assistant Professor
Director, Vascular Anesthesia
Department of Anesthesiology and
   Critical Care
University of Pennsylvania
Philadelphia, Pennsylvania

Ruth S. Waterman, MD

Associate Professor and Interim Chair
Department of Anesthesiology
University of California, San Diego
La Jolla, California

Menachem M. Weiner, MD

Associate Professor of Anesthesiology
Director of Cardiac Anesthesiology
Icahn School of Medicine at Mount
   Sinai
New York, New York

Joshua Zimmerman, MD, FASE

Associate Professor
Director, Preoperative Medicine
Director, Perioperative
   Echocardiography
Department of Anesthesiology
University of Utah
Salt Lake City, Utah

Preface

This is the first edition of the *Essentials of Cardiac Anesthesia for Noncardiac Surgery*. It serves as a companion to the *Essentials of Cardiac Anesthesia for Cardiac Surgery*, Second Edition, published in 2017. This new volume incorporates some of the clinically relevant material from the large textbook, *Kaplan's Cardiac Anesthesia*, Seventh Edition; the 10 chapters in the section "The Cardiac Patient for Noncardiac Surgery" have been updated and expanded, along with 12 additional chapters covering key areas in our specialty.

Patients with cardiac conditions routinely present for noncardiac surgery, which requires special knowledge and techniques for successful perioperative assessment, anesthetic management, and postoperative care. This books deals with these cardiac patients undergoing surgery or interventional procedures and provides current, easily accessible information on these increasingly complex patients undergoing either routine or sophisticated procedures. The book is intended for all providers of anesthesia and perioperative clinical care, including general anesthesiologists, certified registered nurse anesthetists, anesthesia assistants, residents and fellows, surgeons, critical care medicine specialists, referring physicians, and other practitioners involved in perioperative medicine.

In the first edition of *Cardiac Anesthesia,* published in 1979, J. Willis Hurst, MD, Professor of Cardiology and Chairman of the Department of Medicine at Emory University School of Medicine, stated in his preface to the book that "this cardiologist views the modern cardiac anesthesiologist with awe for what they do for our patients." Today, those skills are needed by all anesthesia providers caring for surgical patients who are older, sicker, and have more complicated cardiovascular problems than even Dr. Hurst could have imagined almost 40 years ago. These high-risk patients undergo diagnostic and therapeutic procedures in outpatient settings, non–operating room settings in hospitals, modern operating rooms, and hybrid operating rooms. In all of these locations, cardiac anesthesia–related information on specific diseases (e.g., structural heart disease), complex equipment (e.g., left ventricular assist devices, automatic internal defibrillators), and advanced pharmacologic management (e.g., pulmonary vasodilators) is critical to producing good outcomes. This book is designed to help improve the care of these high-risk patients.

The chapters in *Essentials of Cardiac Anesthesia for Noncardiac Surgery* have been written by acknowledged experts in each specific area, and the material has been coordinated to maximize its clinical value. Recent information has been integrated from anesthesiology, surgery, cardiology, critical care medicine, and clinical pharmacology to present a complete clinical picture. This "essential" information will assist the clinician in understanding the basic principles of each subject and facilitate their application in practice. Because of the large volume of information presented, several teaching aids have been included to help highlight the most important clinical information. Teaching boxes include many of the key take-home messages. In addition, the Key Points at the start of each chapter highlight the major areas covered. Finally, each chapter includes a list of Suggested Reading for additional information, rather than an extensive list of references. For further information, the reader can refer to *Kaplan's Cardiac Anesthesia,* Seventh Edition.

This book has been organized into three main sections:

Section I: Perioperative Medicine includes the clinical approach to complex cardiac patients with coronary stents and scaffolds, new cardiac internal electrical devices, mechanical support devices, prior heart transplants, pulmonary hypertension, or adult congenital heart disease.

Section II: Anesthesia for Noncardiac Surgery includes chapters on cardiovascular monitoring, the role of echocardiography outside the cardiac operating room, cardiovascular pharmacology, and anesthetic management for vascular and thoracic surgery, electrophysiologic procedures, emergency operations, or pregnant cardiac patients.

Section III: Critical Care Medicine covers cardiovascular problems in postanesthesia care and intensive care units, as well as an overview for reducing major adverse cardiac events.

This material should further facilitate the application of the knowledge and skills that have been learned in cardiac surgical operating rooms to the larger number of cardiac patients undergoing other surgical procedures. These patients are often just as sick as those having cardiac surgery, but their heart will not be repaired during surgery, and their cardiovascular system will be highly stressed, leading to a high incidence of complications. It requires at least as high, and sometimes even a higher, level of skill to guide these patients to a safe outcome.

The editors acknowledge the contributions made by the authors of all the chapters. They are the clinical experts who have advanced perioperative medicine to its highly respected place at the present time. In addition, they are the teachers of our residents and students who will further improve the care of our progressively older and sicker patients in the future.

Joel A. Kaplan, MD, CPE, FACC

Contents

Section II
ANESTHESIA FOR NONCARDIAC SURGERY

Section III
CRITICAL CARE MEDICINE

Section I
Perioperative Medicine

Chapter 1

Perioperative Cardiovascular Evaluation and Management for Noncardiac Surgery

Matthew G. Bean, DO • Annemarie Thompson, MD • Kamrouz Ghadimi, MD

> **Key Points**
>
> 1. Preoperative assessment of the cardiac patient undergoing noncardiac surgery includes risk assessment for major adverse cardiac events (MACEs).
> 2. Categorizing risk for MACEs is dependent on patient risk factors, including the noncardiac procedure, patient age, emergent status of the procedure, preexisting organ dysfunction, and independence in daily activities.
> 3. Cardiac risk model calculators exist to facilitate quantification of risk and aid the perioperative physician with optimizing patient care.
> 4. The 2014 American College of Cardiology (ACC)/American Heart Association (AHA) guideline document of perioperative cardiovascular evaluation and management of patients undergoing noncardiac surgery provides a valuable stepwise approach to the care of the patient with cardiovascular disease presenting for noncardiac surgery.
> 5. Within the 2014 ACC/AHA guideline document are important updates related to the perioperative administration of various cardiac-related medications.
> 6. Antiplatelet therapy and the temporal relationship between percutaneous coronary interventions (PCIs) and scheduled surgery determine timing of and perioperative management during noncardiac surgery.
> 7. The 2016 ACC/AHA guideline focused update on duration of dual antiplatelet therapy (DAPT) in patients with coronary artery disease provides important updates related to the timing of surgery and management of DAPT after PCI.
> 8. No specific recommendations are available regarding transfusion and the decision to transfuse; the hemoglobin goal is decided by the perioperative team.
> 9. Pulmonary arterial hypertension and subsequent right ventricular dysfunction are a major cause of poor perioperative outcomes, and the perioperative team should optimize ventilation/perfusion matching and reduce pulmonary vascular resistance.

Patients undergoing surgery experience a well-described stress response of sympathetic nervous system activation, insulin resistance, cytokine production, leukocyte demargination, and pituitary hormone secretion. These physiologic changes, in addition to preexisting patient comorbidities, surgical complexity, and postoperative complications, may contribute to the occurrence of adverse perioperative cardiovascular events in patients undergoing noncardiac surgery. Every patient should undergo an individualized risk assessment to delineate the risks, benefits, and alternatives of surgical intervention as part of a perioperative team approach. In the absence of a net benefit, interventions for optimizing cardiovascular health or consideration of alternative approaches should be performed to ensure the maximum potential benefit at a minimum risk to the patient.

This chapter reviews preoperative cardiac evaluation, including a discussion of common risk calculators, to assist perioperative clinicians with risk assessment and surgical planning. The American College of Cardiology (ACC) and American Heart Association (AHA) clinical practice guideline on perioperative cardiovascular evaluation and management of patients undergoing noncardiac surgery is also reviewed. Recommendations regarding specific and frequently encountered perioperative challenges are discussed, such as medical therapy with β-blockers, angiotensin-converting enzyme (ACE) inhibitors and angiotensin receptor blockers (ARBs), α_2-agonists, aspirin (including dual antiplatelet therapy [DAPT]), vitamin K antagonists (VKAs), and new oral anticoagulants (NOACs) are addressed. Perioperative management of anemia, pulmonary vascular disease, and right ventricular (RV) dysfunction is also discussed.

PREOPERATIVE CARDIAC ASSESSMENT: CATEGORIZING RISK

Compared with their healthier counterparts, patients with underlying cardiovascular disease have an increased risk of perioperative cardiac complications. This is in part due to the presence of coronary artery disease (CAD), leading to impaired left ventricular ejection fraction (LVEF) and in part due to the physiologic factors associated with surgery that predispose patients to myocardial ischemia. Oxygen supply and demand mismatch may occur secondary to blood loss and hemodynamic changes related to anesthetic administration and surgical stimulation.

Validated algorithms have been developed to determine the cardiovascular risk of mortality and morbidity encountered per patient for each noncardiac operation. Stratification is performed to objectively determine and categorize patients as low, intermediate, or high risk. High-risk patients include those with recent myocardial infarction (MI) or unstable angina, decompensated heart failure (HF), high-grade arrhythmias, or hemodynamically significant valvular heart disease, such as aortic stenosis. These patients are at increased risk for perioperative major adverse cardiac events (MACE), including MI, HF, cardiac arrest, conduction abnormalities, and sudden cardiac death. Certainly, the emergent or urgent status of some surgery plays a large role in estimating risk due to the absence of time for risk assessment and modification. Patients with the high-risk conditions listed are at increased risk of a perioperative cardiovascular event compared with normal, age-matched control participants; however, in most emergent cases, the benefit of proceeding with surgery outweighs the risk of delay to perform additional testing.

The initial preoperative evaluation is typically performed by either a primary care physician or an anesthesiologist, and referral to a cardiologist is warranted if specialized procedures are indicated for life-threatening conditions. Intermediate- or high-risk patients may have angina, dyspnea, syncope, and palpitations, as well as history of heart disease (ischemic, valvular, structural myocardial disease), hypertension, diabetes, chronic kidney disease, and cerebrovascular or peripheral arterial disease. Cardiac functional status may be expressed in metabolic equivalents (METs), as initially determined by the Duke Activity Status Index (Table 1.1). One MET is equivalent to the adult resting oxygen utilization, and an important indicator for MACE after major noncardiac surgery is the preoperative inability to achieve 4 METs or greater, such

Table 1.1 **Duke Activity Status Index**	
Can You...	**Weight (in METs)**
1. Take care of yourself, i.e., eating, dressing, bathing, or using the toilet?	2.75
2. Walk indoors, such as around your house?	1.75
3. Walk a block or two on level ground?	2.75
4. Climb a flight of stairs or walk up a hill?	5.50
5. Run a short distance?	8.00
6. Do light work around the house such as dusting or washing dishes?	2.70
7. Do moderate work around the house such as vacuuming, sweeping floors, or carrying groceries?	3.50
8. Do heavy work around the house such as scrubbing floors or lifting or moving heavy furniture?	8.00
9. Do yardwork such as raking leaves, weeding, or pushing a power mower?	4.50
10. Have sexual relations?	5.25
11. Participate in moderate recreational activities such as golf, bowling, dancing, doubles tennis, or throwing a baseball or football?	6.00
12. Participate in strenuous sports such as swimming, singles tennis, football, basketball, or skiing?	7.50

MET, Metabolic equivalents where 1 MET is the equivalent of resting oxygen consumption. From Hlatky MA, Boineau RE, Higginbotham MB, et al. A brief self-administered questionnaire to determine functional capacity (the Duke Activity Status Index). *Am J Cardiol.* 1989;64:651–654.

as by climbing two flights of stairs or walking four city blocks. The decision to pursue cardiovascular or pulmonary testing should be considered only if the results would impact surgical decision making or would likely identify an immediately life-threatening condition requiring timely management.

PREOPERATIVE CARDIAC ASSESSMENT USING RISK MODELING CALCULATORS

Risk model calculators estimate the probability of a perioperative event based on information obtained from the history, physical examination, and surgery type. These models are more applicable for patients at intermediate or high perioperative cardiac risk during noncardiac surgery. Patients at low risk for MACEs should proceed to surgery without further evaluation.

Specific information pertaining to both the patient and the surgery must be provided to appropriately identify individualized risk using a risk calculator. Perioperative information is entered into one or both of two commonly used perioperative risk indices: the Revised Cardiac Risk Index (RCRI) (Fig. 1.1) (http://www.mdcalc.com/revised-cardiac-risk-index-for-pre-operative-risk) or the American College of Surgeons' National Surgical Quality Improvement Program (ACS-NSQIP) (Fig. 1.2) surgical risk calculators (http://site.acsnsqip.org). The RCRI determines preoperative risk based on risk of surgery, history of ischemic heart disease, congestive heart failure (CHF), cerebrovascular disease, preoperative use of insulin, and creatinine greater than 2.0 mg/dL. The ACS-NSQIP calculator incorporates 20 patient risk factors in addition to the

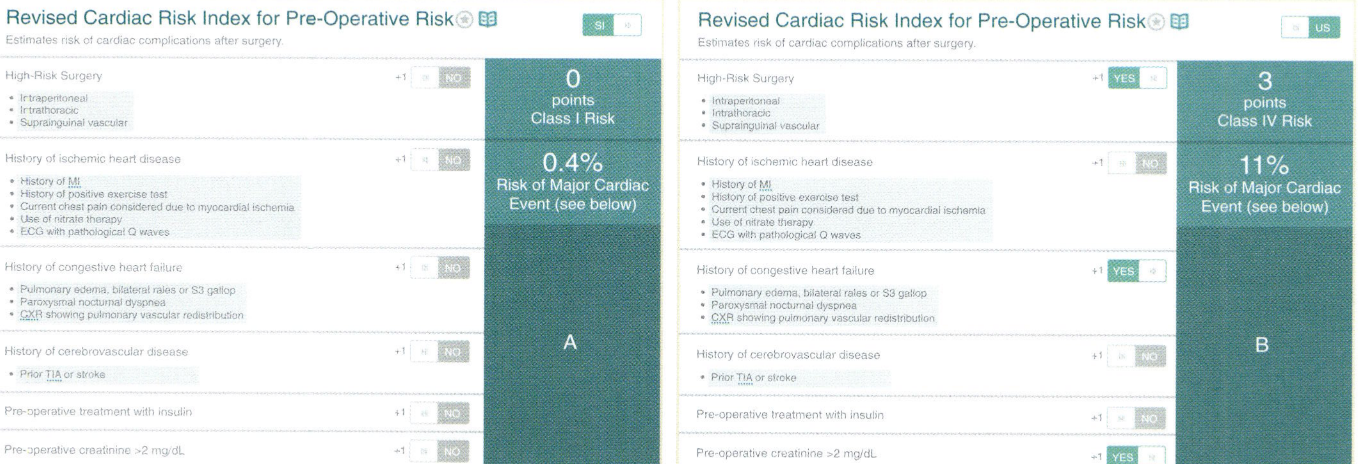

Fig. 1.1 Revised Cardiac Risk Index calculator depicted for two patients entered into the risk calculator. Patient A has no risk factors and a calculated risk for major cardiac event equal to 0.4%. Patient B has several risk factors and a calculated risk for major cardiac event equal to 11%. (From http://www.mdcalc.com/revised-cardiac-risk-index-for-pre-operative-risk/.)

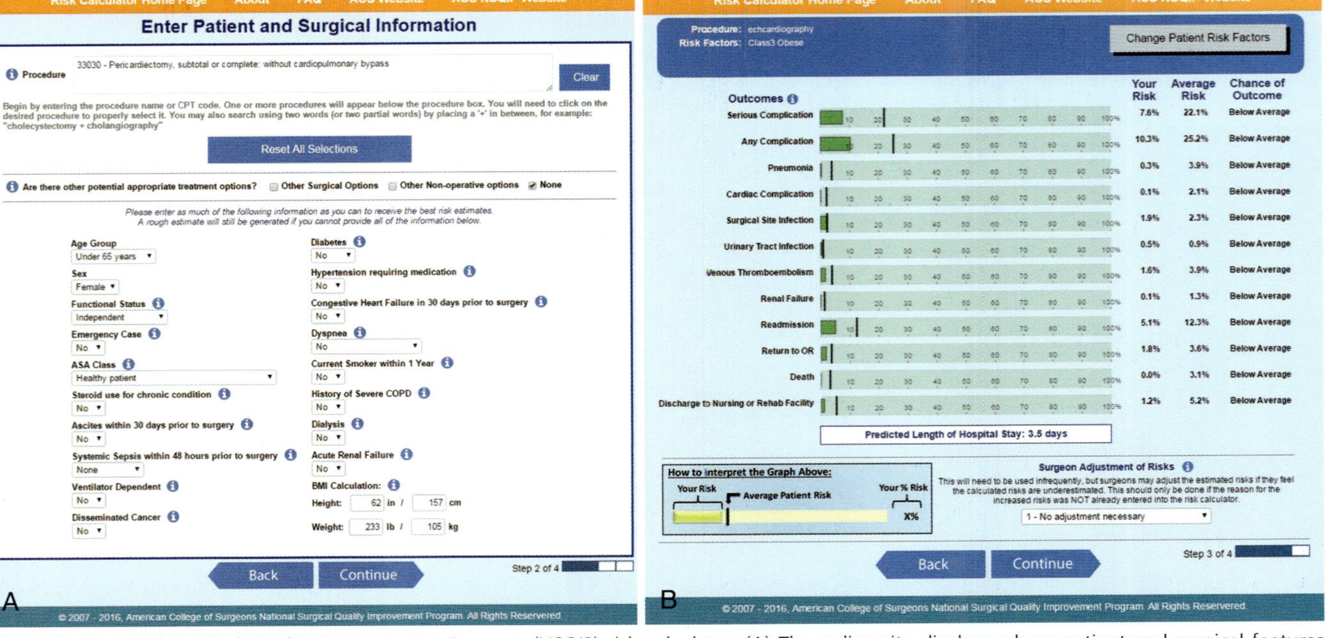

Fig. 1.2 National Surgical Quality Improvement Program (NSQIP) risk calculator. (A) The online site displays where patient and surgical features may be input into the data calculator. (B) As an example, the surgical risk calculation has been performed for a patient undergoing echocardiography with specific risk factors. The resulting surgical risk calculation, including negative outcomes, percent risk of these outcomes occurring, and the chance of the outcome (e.g., average, above average) are displayed. Note in the lower right corner that the surgeon may adjust this risk calculation. In this example, no adjustment has been made. (From http://site.acsnsqip.org.)

surgical procedure. Surgery-specific risk calculation using RCRI or ACS-NSQIP report the rate of cardiac death or nonfatal MI and are noted to be greater than 5% in high-risk procedures, 1% to 5% in intermediate-risk procedures, and less than 1% in low-risk procedures. Emergency surgery is associated with higher risk of MACEs compared with elective procedures.

After patient risk has been estimated, perioperative physicians and the patient can use the information to proceed with the planned operation, postpone, or modify the treatment plan. Options include proceeding directly with the operative plan, delaying surgery pending further diagnostic evaluation, or changing the planned surgery. This last option may involve altering the surgical plan to a lesser risk procedure, a nonsurgical alternative, or cancelling the operation so that cardiac interventions (e.g., coronary revascularization) can be performed. The risk calculation models are discussed individually in the following section.

Revised Cardiac Risk Index

In the derivation of the RCRI, 2893 patients undergoing elective major noncardiac operations were monitored for major cardiac complications (death, acute MI, pulmonary edema, ventricular fibrillation or cardiac arrest, and complete heart block) (see Fig. 1.1). The index was validated in a cohort of 1422 similar individuals. The predictive value was significant in all types of major noncardiac surgery except for abdominal aortic aneurysm surgery. The RCRI performs well in distinguishing patients at low compared with high risk for all types of noncardiac surgery but is less accurate in patients undergoing vascular, noncardiac surgery. In addition, the RCRI does not predict all-cause mortality well, which is inherent to a risk predictor that does not capture risk factors for noncardiac causes of perioperative mortality.

ACS-NSQIP Universal Surgical Risk Calculator

A universal surgical risk calculator model was developed using a web-based tool consisting of 20 patient factors plus the surgical procedure (see Fig. 1.2) and has excellent performance for predicting mortality and morbidity. The ACS-NSQIP has not been validated through external studies, but it remains more comprehensive than the other risk calculators.

After a patient is deemed as being at intermediate or high risk, the ACC/AHA guidelines may then be used to guide further preoperative optimization and perioperative management.

ALGORITHMIC APPROACH TO PERIOPERATIVE CARDIAC ASSESSMENT

The 2014 ACC/AHA Perioperative Guideline proposed a stepwise approach to perioperative cardiac assessment, incorporating both the physician's role in managing risk and providing informed consent while also involving the patient's perspective in weighing risk, benefit, and alternatives to invasive testing or preventive therapies. The emphasis on sharing information contextually with other perioperative physicians and the patient highlights the importance of patient-centered care while minimizing risk for each intervention. The algorithmic flow chart begins with determination of surgical urgency followed by assessment of the presence or absence of a preoperative unstable cardiac condition (Box 1.1) and concludes with a perioperative risk calculation

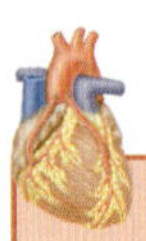

BOX 1.1	*Unstable Cardiac Conditions*

Acute coronary event
Recent myocardial infarction with residual myocardial ischemia
Acute heart failure
Significant cardiac arrhythmias
Symptomatic valvular heart disease

for MACEs (Fig. 1.3). For patients at low risk of MACE, no further testing is needed, and the patient may proceed to surgery without further evaluation. For patients at high risk for MACE, an objective determination of the functional capacity of the patient is recommended. If a patient at high risk for MACE has 4 METs or greater as determined by objective testing, no further evaluation is required (Fig. 1.3). For high-risk patients who exert less than 4 METs without symptoms or have an indeterminate functional capacity, the perioperative clinician should consult with the perioperative team to determine whether or not further testing will impact the decision to undergo the current surgery or delay surgery for cardiac evaluation and possible intervention (e.g., pharmacologic stress testing, coronary revascularization). If further testing will not impact the surgical plan or perioperative care, then the high-risk patient should either proceed directly to surgery or noninvasive treatment, and palliation strategies should be considered.

The 2014 ACC/AHA guideline update features important information extracted from the critical analysis of nearly 500 referenced articles, which are summarized and appended to the document. Important updates in the evaluation of myocardial ischemia, perioperative management of medical therapy in patients with risk factors for cardiovascular disease, and management of established disease after percutaneous coronary intervention (PCI) and stent implantation are discussed in the subsequent sections. Perioperative medical therapy recommendations have undergone major changes, and management of β-blockers, ACE inhibitors, and α$_2$-agonists (e.g., clonidine) are discussed. Many patients with established cardiovascular disease and a history of coronary stents are on antiplatelet therapy, and management of antiplatelet therapy and timing of surgery are addressed.

CLASSIFICATION OF RECOMMENDATIONS

The development of recommendations occurs as a result of literature searches that focus on randomized controlled trials, registries, nonrandomized comparative, and descriptive studies, case series, cohort studies, systematic reviews, and expert opinion. Each recommendation is assigned a class, and level of evidence (LOE) is determined by the guideline writing committee to provide information to the clinician regarding the likelihood that the recommendations are well-supported by the evidence (Fig. 1.4). Understanding the classification and LOE of a particular recommendation is important when considering implementing or foregoing a particular treatment intervention. Class I suggests that benefit clearly outweigh the risks of a particular intervention and that the particular procedure or treatment *should* be performed or administered. Class IIa suggests that it is reasonable to perform a particular intervention, class IIb

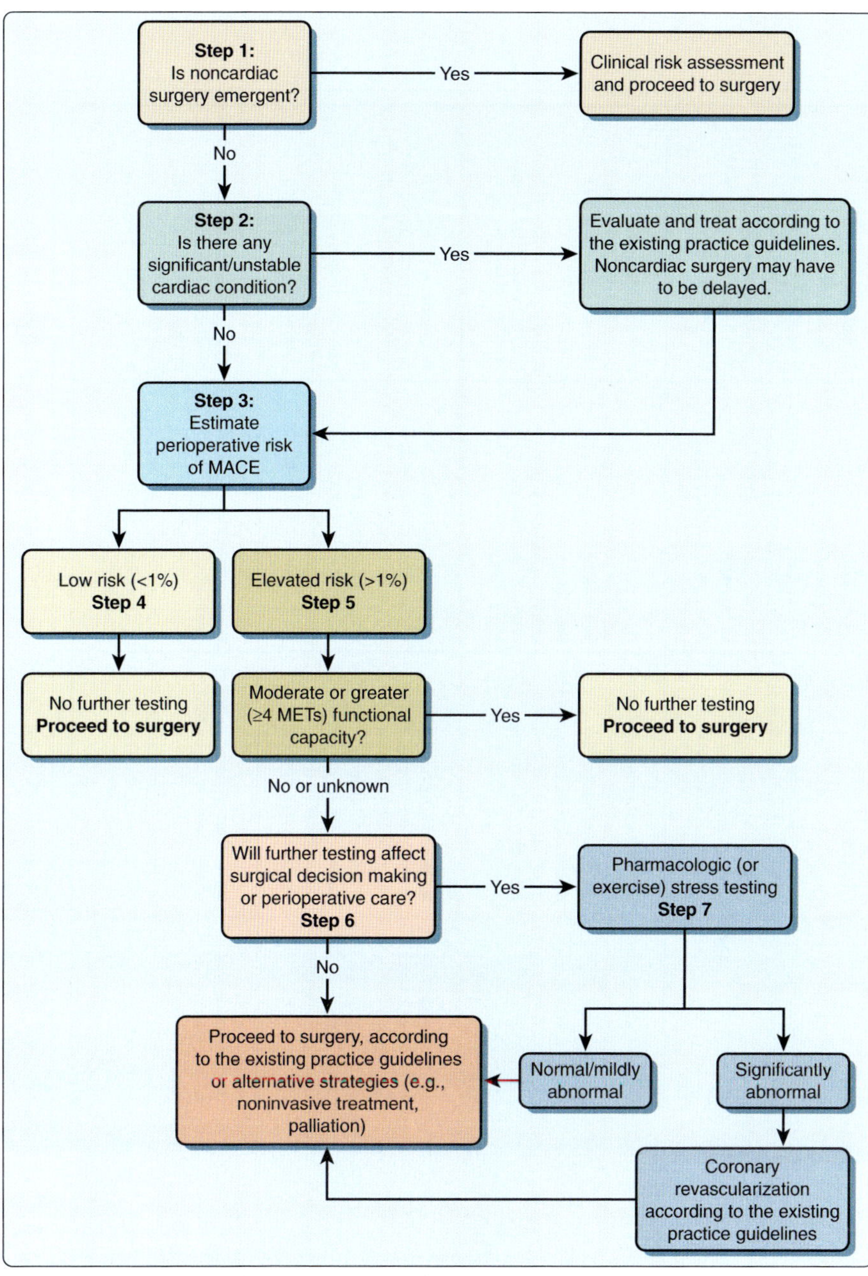

Fig. 1.3 Stepwise approach to perioperative cardiac risk assessment in patients undergoing noncardiac surgery. *MACE,* Major adverse cardiovascular event; *MET,* metabolic equivalent. (Modified from Fleisher LA, Fleischmann KE, Auerbach AD, et al. 2014 ACC/AHA guideline on perioperative cardiovascular evaluation and management of patients undergoing noncardiac surgery: a report of the American College of Cardiology/American Heart Association Task Force on practice guidelines. *J Am Coll Cardiol.* 2014;64:e77–e137; Kristensen SD, Knuuti J, Saraste A, et al. 2014 ESC/ESA guidelines on non-cardiac surgery: cardiovascular assessment and management. The Joint Task Force on Non-cardiac Surgery: Cardiovascular Assessment and Management of the European Society of Cardiology (ESC) and the European Society of Anaesthesiology (ESA). *Eur Heart J.* 2014;35:2383–2431.)

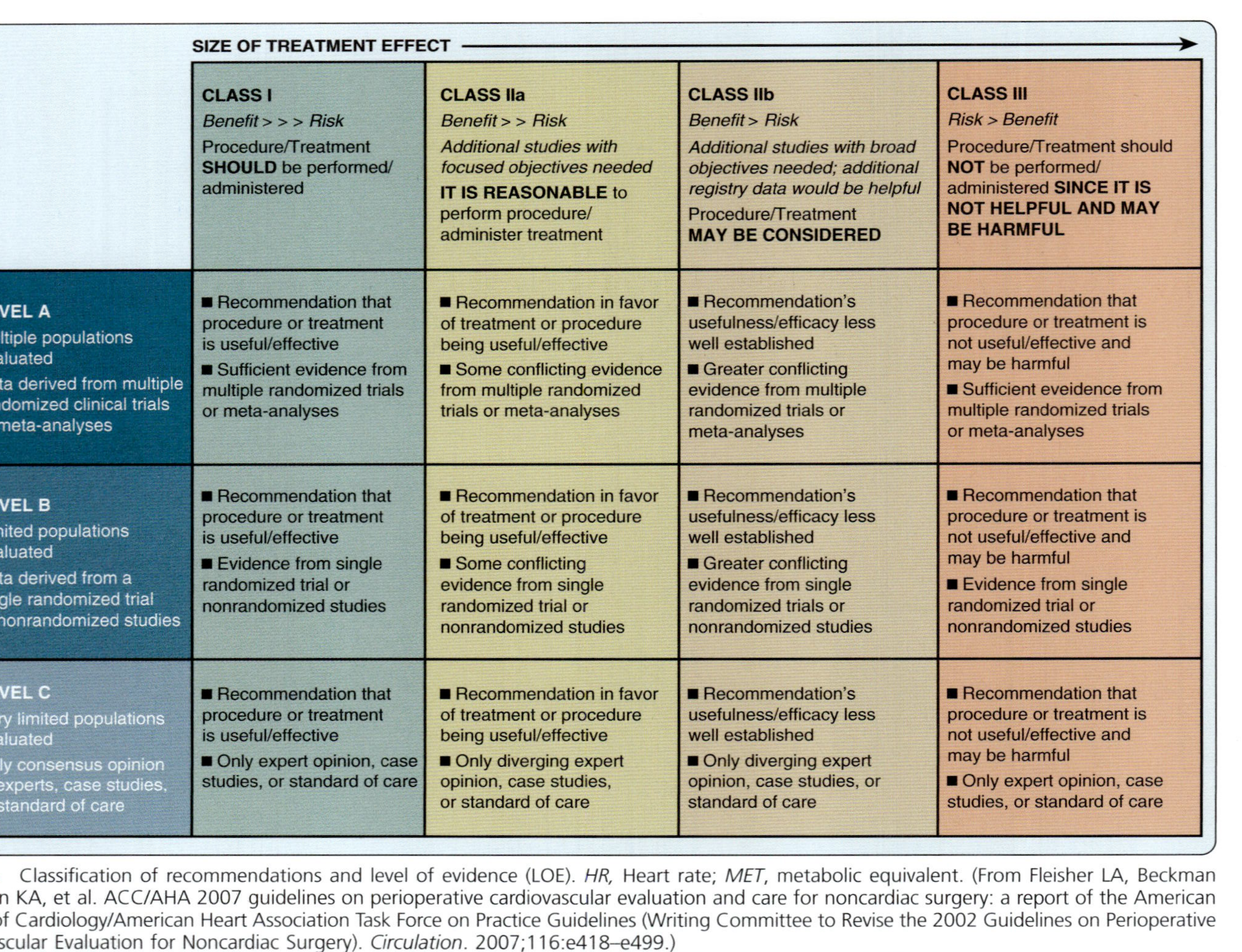

	CLASS I *Benefit > > > Risk* Procedure/Treatment **SHOULD** be performed/administered	CLASS IIa *Benefit > > Risk* *Additional studies with focused objectives needed* **IT IS REASONABLE** to perform procedure/administer treatment	CLASS IIb *Benefit > Risk* *Additional studies with broad objectives needed; additional registry data would be helpful* Procedure/Treatment **MAY BE CONSIDERED**	CLASS III *Risk > Benefit* Procedure/Treatment should **NOT** be performed/administered **SINCE IT IS NOT HELPFUL AND MAY BE HARMFUL**
LEVEL A Multiple populations evaluated Data derived from multiple randomized clinical trials or meta-analyses	■ Recommendation that procedure or treatment is useful/effective ■ Sufficient evidence from multiple randomized trials or meta-analyses	■ Recommendation in favor of treatment or procedure being useful/effective ■ Some conflicting evidence from multiple randomized trials or meta-analyses	■ Recommendation's usefulness/efficacy less well established ■ Greater conflicting evidence from multiple randomized trials or meta-analyses	■ Recommendation that procedure or treatment is not useful/effective and may be harmful ■ Sufficient eveidence from multiple randomized trials or meta-analyses
LEVEL B Limited populations evaluated Data derived from a single randomized trial or nonrandomized studies	■ Recommendation that procedure or treatment is useful/effective ■ Evidence from single randomized trial or nonrandomized studies	■ Recommendation in favor of treatment or procedure being useful/effective ■ Some conflicting evidence from single randomized trial or nonrandomized studies	■ Recommendation's usefulness/efficacy less well established ■ Greater conflicting evidence from single randomized trials or nonrandomized studies	■ Recommendation that procedure or treatment is not useful/effective and may be harmful ■ Evidence from single randomized trial or nonrandomized studies
LEVEL C Very limited populations evaluated Only consensus opinion of experts, case studies, or standard of care	■ Recommendation that procedure or treatment is useful/effective ■ Only expert opinion, case studies, or standard of care	■ Recommendation in favor of treatment or procedure being useful/effective ■ Only diverging expert opinion, case studies, or standard of care	■ Recommendation's usefulness/efficacy less well established ■ Only diverging expert opinion, case studies, or standard of care	■ Recommendation that procedure or treatment is not useful/effective and may be harmful ■ Only expert opinion, case studies, or standard of care

Fig. 1.4 Classification of recommendations and level of evidence (LOE). *HR,* Heart rate; *MET,* metabolic equivalent. (From Fleisher LA, Beckman JA, Brown KA, et al. ACC/AHA 2007 guidelines on perioperative cardiovascular evaluation and care for noncardiac surgery: a report of the American College of Cardiology/American Heart Association Task Force on Practice Guidelines (Writing Committee to Revise the 2002 Guidelines on Perioperative Cardiovascular Evaluation for Noncardiac Surgery). *Circulation.* 2007;116:e418–e499.)

indicates that an intervention may be considered, and class III indicates that the intervention will be of no benefit and may even be harmful. The LOE encompasses the extent to which populations have been evaluated regarding a certain intervention. For example, LOE A implies that multiple populations have been evaluated and that data have been derived from multiple randomized clinical trials or meta-analyses. On the other hand, LOE C suggests that a very limited population of patients have been evaluated regarding a particular intervention and may include expert opinion or case studies (Fig. 1.4).

PRINCIPLES OF MANAGEMENT AND CARDIAC MEDICATIONS

Electrocardiograms

The 2014 ACC/AHA guideline on preoperative evaluation and management of the cardiac patient undergoing noncardiac surgery recommends a 12-lead electrocardiogram (ECG) for patients with CAD, arrhythmias, peripheral artery disease, cerebrovascular disease, and structural cardiac disease unless they are undergoing low-risk procedures (class IIa recommendation, LOE B). Routine preoperative ECG is not helpful in managing patients undergoing low-risk surgery regardless of cardiovascular disease burden or risk factors. Postoperative ECG is recommended for patients with a clinical suspicion for myocardial ischemia, infarction, or arrhythmia after noncardiac surgery; however, routine postoperative ECGs in asymptomatic patients is not useful regardless of the presence of patient risk factors. The decision to perform a postoperative ECG should be guided based on patient symptoms and clinical evaluation.

Cardiac Enzymes

The measurement of laboratory markers of myocardial injury (e.g., troponins) is recommended in patients at high risk for MACE who may benefit from an intervention (class II, LOE B). Routine measurement is not recommended without patient selection (class II, LOE B). The usefulness of postoperative screening with troponin levels for perioperative MI in patients without signs or symptoms suggestive of myocardial ischemia or infarction is uncertain in the absence of established risks and benefits of a defined management strategy. Furthermore, routine screening with troponin provides a nonspecific assessment of risk, does not specify a particular course of therapy, and is not clinically useful outside of the patient with signs or symptoms of myocardial ischemia or MI.

β-Receptor Antagonists

The 2014 ACC/AHA guideline provides recommendations for perioperative β-blockade based on multiple research articles, including a recent meta-analysis by Wijeysundera and colleagues. There are two recommendations of particular interest. First, β-blockade should be continued in patients undergoing noncardiac surgery who have been prescribed these medications chronically (class I, LOE B). This recommendation emphasizes the importance of continuing chronic β-blockade in patients with certain conditions, such as myocardial ischemia or infarction or CHF, in whom long-term survival benefit from β-blockade administration has been demonstrated. Second, it is recommended that β-blockers not be initiated within 1 day of noncardiac surgery. The benefit of MI prevention is offset by the increase in stroke, hypertension, and death, although β-blocker immediately before surgery may prevent nonfatal MI (class III, LOE B).

Angiotensin-Converting Enzyme Inhibitors or Angiotensin Receptor Blockers

Angiotensin-converting enzyme inhibitors and ARBs are among the most commonly prescribed antihypertensives. Both ACE inhibitors and ARBs have cardiovascular and metabolic effects beyond their antihypertensive properties, and their prescription frequency partially relates to their demonstrated outcome and mortality benefit in patients with MI with residual left ventricular dysfunction, HF, and diabetic kidney disease with respect to prevention of the progression to end-stage renal disease. There is increased transient intraoperative hypotension among patients taking ACE inhibitors, but no differences in outcomes have been illustrated in patients receiving ACE inhibitors compared with those who did not. Of note, clinical practice guidelines recommend continuing ACE inhibitors in the setting of acute HF treatment or hypertension, and it is reasonable to continue ACE inhibitors or ARBs perioperatively (class IIa, LOE B). Nevertheless, some practitioners prefer to hold these drugs for 24 hours before surgery to reduce the incidence of intraoperative hypotension. However, if ACE inhibitors or ARBs are held before surgery, it is recommended that they be restarted as soon as clinically feasible in the postoperative period (class IIa, LOE C).

Aspirin Therapy in Patients Without Coronary Stent Implantation

The 2014 ACC/AHA guidelines strongly recommend against routine aspirin therapy without previous coronary stent implantation (class III, LOE B). The effects of aspirin have also been evaluated by the PeriOperative Ischemia Evaluation (POISE-2) investigators in patients undergoing noncardiac surgery without recent history of coronary stent placement. Patients at risk for MACE were separated into whether or not they were taking preoperative aspirin. Patients who were not previously taking aspirin ($n = 5628$) were randomized to receive aspirin (initial dose 200 mg followed by 100 mg/day) or placebo on day of surgery for 30 days after surgery. Patients previously on aspirin ($n = 4382$) were also randomized to receive aspirin (similar dosing as above) or placebo beginning on day of surgery for 7 days postoperatively and then asked to resume preoperative dosing regimen. Aspirin administration did not decrease the incidence of death or nonfatal MI at 30 days after surgery (hazards ratio, 0.99; 95% confidence interval, 0.86–1.15; $P = .92$), but exposure to aspirin resulted in increased risk of clinically significant bleeding.

Aspirin administration, however, is recommended when risks of myocardial ischemia exceed the risk of surgical bleeding (class III recommendation, LOE C). The guidelines, therefore, recommend only that consideration be given to the administration of aspirin for elective noncardiac surgery in patients with CAD without history of PCI and stenting (class IIb, LOE B).

Dual Antiplatelet Therapy After Coronary Stent Implantation

Patients with a history of coronary stent implantation require special attention to management of DAPT with aspirin and a $P2Y_{12}$ inhibitor (e.g., clopidogrel, prasugrel,

Table 1.2 Percutaneous Coronary Intervention and Recommendations for Timing of Noncardiac Surgery	
Percutaneous Coronary Intervention	**Recommended Delay of Elective Noncardiac Surgery[a]**
Angioplasty	14 days
Bare-metal stent	30 days
Drug-eluting stent	180 days[b]

[a]In surgical procedures that mandate discontinuation of dual antiplatelet therapy, aspirin should be continued if possible perioperatively, and $P2Y_{12}$ inhibitor therapy should be restarted as soon as possible after surgery.

[b]May be considered after 3 months if the risk of further delay of surgery is greater than the expected risks of stent thrombosis, especially in patients with one of the newer generation stents.

Modified from Levine GN, Bates ER, Bittl JA, et al. 2016 ACC/AHA guideline focused update on duration of dual antiplatelet therapy in patients with coronary artery disease: a report of the American College of Cardiology/American Heart Association Task Force on Clinical Practice Guidelines. *J Thorac Cardiovasc Surg.* 2016;152:1243–1275.

ticagrelor) to maximize the chances of maintaining stent patency and minimize the risk of perioperative stent thrombosis. In a recent 2016 ACC/AHA guideline–focused update on duration of DAPT in patients with CAD, the acceptable interval from drug-eluting stent (DES) implantation to surgery requiring discontinuation of DAPT has been shortened from 12 months to 6 months (class I, LOE B) for most patients with stable ischemic heart disease. In patients with variable disease, prior STEMI, or a coronary scaffold, the recommendation is still 12 months. If the risk of further delay of surgery is greater than the expected risks of stent thrombosis, discontinuation of DAPT for surgery may be considered 3 months after DES placement (class IIb, LOE C). Surgery should be delayed and DAPT continued for at least 30 days after bare-metal stent placement (class I, LOE B). Perioperatively, aspirin should be continued if possible, and $P2Y_{12}$ should be restarted as soon as possible after surgery (class I, LOE C). Preoperative planning should include discussion among clinicians caring for the patient and should address the balance between risk of perioperative coagulopathy from continuation of antiplatelet agents and the risk of stent thrombosis as a result of discontinuation in complex clinical situations, bridging with the short-acting $P2Y_{12}$ inhibitor cangrelor may be considered.

A summary of the recommendations related to the timing of elective noncardiac surgery after PCI are provided in Table 1.2 and Chapter 3.

Anticoagulants: Vitamin K Antagonists and New Oral Anticoagulants

Vitamin K antagonists, such as warfarin (Coumadin), are prescribed for stroke prevention in patients with atrial fibrillation, prevention of thrombotic or thromboembolic complications in patients with prosthetic valves, and in patients requiring deep venous thrombosis prophylaxis and treatment. Dabigatran and factor Xa inhibitors are prescribed for prevention of stroke in the management of atrial fibrillation, but are not recommended for long-term anticoagulation of prosthetic valves because of an increased risk of thrombosis compared with warfarin. The risk of bleeding for any surgical procedure must be weighed against the benefit of remaining on anticoagulants. For example, an office-based procedure for minor dermatologic surgery may not require cessation or reversal of the anticoagulant. Prothrombin complex concentrates (PCCs) have been used in the acute reversal of patients taking VKAs requiring surgery. Discontinuation of NOACs for 48 hours or longer is recommended for elective surgery. New reversal agents are now available for urgent surgery with extensive bleeding for patients taking dabigatran (Idarucizumab) or factor Xa inhibitors (e.g., andexanet alfa).

Perioperative Anemia Management

Anemia is an important topic of discussion, especially because it may contribute to myocardial ischemia. Hemoglobin is a potent oxygen carrier, and ischemia may be triggered by both lack of oxygen delivery to poststenotic myocardium and a demand for increased cardiac output to supply oxygen to other vascular beds. Although blood transfusion may improve anemia, there is association with increased morbidity and mortality in addition to increased healthcare costs. Therefore hemoglobin transfusion thresholds remain a moving target to appropriately balance risk and benefit. Patients undergoing hip surgery with either CAD or known risk factors for CAD with hemoglobin of less than 10 g/dL treated with either a liberal transfusion strategy or a conservative transfusion strategy less than 8 g/dL have been studied. There were no differences in the 60-day endpoints of death or inability to walk between groups but that the study was not sufficiently powered to show a difference in the aforementioned areas if a difference did indeed exist. The 2012 American Association of Blood Banks recommended a restricted transfusion strategy (hemoglobin <7–8 g/dL) in asymptomatic, hemodynamically stable patients without CAD, a relative restricted transfusion strategy in hospitalized patients with cardiovascular disease, and consideration of transfusion for patients with symptoms or hemoglobin less than 8 g/dL. In postoperative patients, the recommended maintenance hemoglobin concentration is 8 g/dL or greater unless the patient is symptomatic (e.g., angina pectoris, orthostasis, CHF). There are no specific recommendations for hemodynamically stable patients with acute coronary syndrome because of the lack of high-quality evidence for either liberal or a restrictive transfusion strategy in these patients. The consensus of experts recommended a symptom-guided approach to evaluating hemoglobin level to determine whether to transfuse an anemic patient.

Pulmonary Vascular Disease and Right Ventricular Dysfunction

The evidence for management of patients with pulmonary hypertension is limited to those with pulmonary arterial hypertension. Perioperative events including, but not limited to hypoxia, hypercarbia, hypertension or hypotension, and positive-pressure ventilation may worsen pulmonary hypertension and RV systolic function. In addition to the urgency of the surgery and the surgical risk category, risk factors for perioperative adverse events in patients with pulmonary hypertension include the severity of symptoms related to pulmonary hypertension, the degree of RV dysfunction, and the absence of a specialized center in the treatment of patients with pulmonary hypertension. Patients with pulmonary arterial hypertension, particularly with features of increased perioperative risk, should undergo a thorough preoperative risk assessment including determination of functional capacity, hemodynamics, and echocardiography that includes evaluation of RV function. Right heart catheterization may be particularly useful to confirm the severity of illness and determine secondary causes of elevated pulmonary arterial pressures (e.g., pulmonary venous hypertension secondary to reduced LVEF, mitral regurgitation, mitral stenosis). Optimization of pulmonary hypertension and RV function are necessary to minimize perioperative cardiovascular risk.

SUGGESTED READING

Bilimoria KY, Liu Y, Paruch JL, et al. Development and evaluation of the universal ACS NSQIP surgical risk calculator: a decision aid and informed consent tool for patients and surgeons. *J Am Coll Surg.* 2013;217:833–842, e1–e3.

Carson JL, Terrin ML, Noveck H, et al. Liberal or restrictive transfusion in high-risk patients after hip surgery. *N Engl J Med.* 2011;365:2453–2462.

Connolly SJ, Milling TJ Jr, Eikelboom JW, et al. ANNEXA-4 Investigators. Andexanet alfa for acute major bleeding associated with factor Xa inhibitors. *N Engl J Med.* 2016;375(12):1131–1141.

Devereaux PJ, Mrkobrada M, Sessler DI, et al. Aspirin in patients undergoing noncardiac surgery. *N Engl J Med.* 2014;370:1494–1503.

Devereaux PJ, Yang H, et al. Effects of extended-release metoprolol succinate in patients undergoing noncardiac surgery (POISE trial): a randomised controlled trial. *Lancet.* 2008;371:1839–1847.

Drenger B, Weissman C. Failure to resume cardiac medications postoperatively negatively impacts patient outcome. *J Cardiothorac Vasc Anesth.* 2017;31:14–18.

Fleisher LA, Fleischmann KE, Auerbach AD, et al. 2014 ACC/AHA guideline on perioperative cardiovascular evaluation and management of patients undergoing noncardiac surgery: a report of the American College of Cardiology/American Heart Association Task Force on practice guidelines. *J Am Coll Cardiol.* 2014;64:e77–e137.

Ford MK, Beattie WS, Wijeysundera DN. Systematic review: prediction of perioperative cardiac complications and mortality by the revised cardiac risk index. *Ann Intern Med.* 2010;152:26–35.

Ghadimi K, Thompson A. Update on perioperative care of the cardiac patient for noncardiac surgery. *Curr Opin Anaesthesiol.* 2015;28:342–348.

Hawn MT, Graham LA, Richman JS, et al. Risk of major adverse cardiac events following noncardiac surgery in patients with coronary stents. *JAMA.* 2013;310:1462–1472.

Hosscinian L. Pulmonary hypertension and noncardiac surgery: implications for the anesthesiologist. *J Cardiothorac Vasc Anesth.* 2014;28:1064–1074.

Lee TH, Marcantonio ER, Mangione CM, et al. Derivation and prospective validation of a simple index for prediction of cardiac risk of major noncardiac surgery. *Circulation.* 1999;100:1043–1049.

Levine GN, Bates ER, Bittl JA, et al. 2016 ACC/AHA guideline focused update on duration of dual antiplatelet therapy in patients with coronary artery disease: a report of the American College of Cardiology/American Heart Association Task Force on Clinical Practice Guidelines. *J Thorac Cardiovasc Surg.* 2016;152:1243–1275.

Pollack CV Jr, Reilly PA, van Ryn J, et al. Idarucizumab for dabigatran reversal—full cohort analysis. *N Engl J Med.* 2017;377(5):431–441.

Torrado J, Buckley L, Duran A, et al. Restenosis, stent thrombosis, and bleeding complications. *J Am Coll Cardiol.* 2018;71:1676–1695.

Valgimigli M, Bueno H, Collett JP, et al. 2017 ESC focused update on dual antiplatelet therapy in coronary artery disease. *Eur Heart J.* 2018;39:213–260.

Wijeysundera DN, Duncan D, Nkonde-Price C, et al. Perioperative beta blockade in noncardiac surgery: a systematic review for the 2014 ACC/AHA Guideline on Perioperative Cardiovascular Evaluation and Management of Patients Undergoing Noncardiac Surgery: a report of the American College of Cardiology/American Heart Association Task Force on Practice Guidelines. *Circulation.* 2014;130:2246–2264.

Yancy CW, Jessup M, Bozkurt B, Mafoudi F, et al. 2017 ACCF/AHA focused update of the guideline for the management of heart failure: a report of the American College of Cardiology Foundation/American Heart Association Task Force on Practice Guidelines. *J Am Coll Cardiol.* 2017;70:776–803.

Chapter 2

Perioperative Approach to the High-Risk Cardiac Patient

Torin Shear, MD • Jeffrey Katz, MD •
Steven B. Greenberg, MD • Joel A. Kaplan, MD

Key Points

1. Perioperative triage should determine whether cardiac patients receive outpatient surgery, routine inpatient care, or critical care services.
2. Advanced hemodynamic monitoring may be required in high-risk patients with cardiac disease undergoing noncardiac surgery, including direct arterial pressure measurements, filling pressures, echocardiography, and cardiac outputs.
3. Patients with stable or unstable coronary artery disease (CAD) are commonly seen for noncardiac surgery. The unstable patients present a very high risk and have an increased mortality rate. Perioperative myocardial infarctions are difficult to diagnose and have a poor outcome.
4. The new 2017 guidelines for hypertension have markedly increased the number of patients with this disorder. Many more patients will be seen on antihypertensive therapy when coming for noncardiac surgery. In general, their therapies should be continued throughout surgery, with the possible exception of those drugs that block the renin-angiotensin system.
5. The outcome of patients with heart failure (HF) is worse than that of patients with isolated CAD in the perioperative period. Thus complete evaluation and maximum therapy should be used to reduce morbidity and mortality.
6. Takotsubo cardiomyopathy is a syndrome related to excessive catecholamines and must be differentiated in the surgical patient from acute coronary syndromes or HF. Usually the distinction can be made with echocardiography, and the outcome is often good.
7. The most common types of valvular heart disease seen in noncardiac surgical patients are aortic stenosis and mitral regurgitation. The therapeutic goals and principles used to manage these patients should be similar to those used during cardiac surgery.
8. Atrial fibrillation is the most common arrhythmia seen in older adult patients. Many of these patients are taking anticoagulants to reduce the incidence of stroke. These drugs must be managed well in surgical patients.
9. The new oral anticoagulants consist of a direct thrombin inhibitor, dabigatran, and three factor Xa inhibitors. These drugs have marked advantages over the older warfarin-type anticoagulants. However, experience with them in the perioperative period is still developing, especially regarding the use of regional anesthetic techniques.

Approximately 230 million surgical procedures are performed worldwide each year. Perioperative mortality rates are relatively low, but this may be a misleading fact because complications continue to be significant. In fact, high-risk patients may have a postoperative complication rate as high as 50%. This subset of patients accounts for only 13% of all surgical procedures but more than 80% of postoperative deaths. The management of these high-risk patients in the perioperative period presents a unique challenge for perioperative physicians. This chapter focuses on the perioperative management of "high-risk" complex cardiac patients for noncardiac surgery, with additional discussion of common diseases.

PERIOPERATIVE TRIAGE

Defining which patients are appropriate for various perioperative care areas, whether it is outpatient surgery, routine inpatient care, or critical care services, is vital. *Triage* can be defined as the process of deciding which patients should be treated first based on degree of sickness or severity of injury. In the present value-based health care system, placing the "right" patients in the "right" places is a difficult but crucial task.

Ambulatory Surgery

A challenging triage decision is identifying which surgical patients are best cared for in hospital-based versus ambulatory settings. Adequate preoperative patient assessment is important in determining the appropriate surgical environment. Criteria associated with increased hospital admission after outpatient surgery include age 65 years or older, cardiac diagnoses, peripheral vascular disease, surgery lasting more than 2 hours, cerebrovascular disease, malignancy, HIV diagnosis, and general anesthesia. Data evaluating 5 years of common ambulatory-eligible surgical procedures (≈250,000 procedures) suggest the following risk factors are associated with an increase in morbidity and mortality: previous cardiac surgical intervention (percutaneous coronary intervention [PCI] or cardiac surgery), overweight or obese body mass index, chronic obstructive pulmonary disease, prior transient ischemic attack or stroke, hypertension, and prolonged surgical time (Table 2.1). Patients with stable coronary artery disease (CAD) may not be at higher risk for perioperative complications after ambulatory surgery. Additionally, patients with cardiac pacemakers or implantable cardioverter-defibrillators can be evaluated for ambulatory surgical cases. Important information includes the type and function of these devices before proceeding with surgery. Similarly, it is appropriate to develop a definitive perioperative plan for the management of these devices (in terms of electromagnetic interference and follow-up) (see Chapter 4).

Critical Care Services

Triaging healthy and moribund patients away from critical care services (excluding palliative services and services to those who are brain dead) seems to be relatively straightforward. However, healthcare providers are challenged by a scarcity of intensive care unit (ICU) beds and an inherent cost in determining which patients will truly benefit from intensive care. Improving preoperative evidence-based strategies to identify which patients are at highest risk for postoperative complications may aid in determining patient need. Similarly, reducing hospital variability in managing these patients when they develop postoperative complications is also paramount to

Table 2.1 Factors Associated With Triage Decisions[a]

Factors Associated With ICU Admission	Factors Associated With Increased Hospital Admission After Outpatient Surgery	Factor Associated With Increased Risk of Morbidity or Mortality After Day Case–Eligible Procedures
Surgical patients (vs. medical patients)	Age >65 y	Previous cardiac surgical intervention (PCI or cardiac surgery)
Absence of comorbidities	Cardiac diagnoses	Overweight or obese BMI
Presence of hematologic malignancy	Peripheral vascular disease	COPD
Acute clinical condition	Malignancy	History of TIA or CVA
Need for active intensive care therapies	HIV	Hypertension
Trauma	General anesthesia	Prolonged surgical time
Vascular involvement	Surgery >2 h	
Hepatic involvement		
Acute severity of illness		
Lowest surgical Apgar score		

[a]Depicts the factors associated with ICU admission, increased hospital admission after outpatient surgery, and factors associated with heightened risk for morbidity and mortality after outpatient procedures.

BMI, Body mass index; *COPD*, chronic obstructive pulmonary disease; *CVA*, cerebrovascular accident; *ICU*, intensive care unit; *PCI*, percutaneous coronary intervention; *TIA*, transient ischemic attack.

reducing morbidity and mortality. Approximately 30% of patients accepted for ICU services have cardiac diseases.

Observational studies also outline the potential benefit of ICU admission for older adult patients, suggesting a greater mortality reduction in older adult patients admitted to ICUs compared with younger patients. Based on these findings, intensivists may consider accepting even older adults who appear "well."

Studies evaluating intraoperative events such as blood loss have shown a reduction in mortality rate with ICU admission. Intraoperative hemodynamics and blood loss should indeed influence ICU triage.

Triaging Patients With Coronary Stents for Noncardiac Surgery

One of the largest observational studies to date reported an approximately 23% rate of noncardiac surgery 1 year after PCI. Multiple guidelines report that elective surgery should be delayed for at least 4 to 6 weeks after bare-metal stent (BMS) placement and 6 to 12 months after drug-eluting stent (DES) placement, depending on the type of stent. The major challenge is determining the risk of perioperative surgical hemorrhage versus dual antiplatelet therapy (DAPT) interruption, and its relation to subsequent coronary stent thrombosis (see Chapter 3).

A safe time period for antiplatelet therapy interruption has yet to be clearly defined. Still, the continuation of aspirin is often recommended throughout the perioperative period. In the absence of guidelines supported by strong evidence, it may be important for the care team (primary care doctor, cardiologist, perioperative physicians) to collaborate and develop a definitive perioperative plan regarding continuation of DAPT, type and timing of stent placement, and disposition. Risk factors such as those mentioned may lead the perioperative team to suggest hospital-based surgery with the potential for an overnight stay and monitoring.

CARDIOVASCULAR SYSTEM

Cardiac issues remain a significant contributor to perioperative morbidity and mortality. The intraoperative management of cardiac complications in noncardiac surgery is discussed below with a focus on CAD, hypertension, heart failure (HF), valvular heart disease, and rhythm disturbances.

Patients with underlying cardiac disease may require advanced monitoring throughout the perioperative period. However, there is limited evidence to establish clear guidelines, and clinical discretion is advised. Invasive arterial pressure monitoring may be considered in patients requiring pharmacologic therapy to stabilize blood pressure (BP) or cardiac function. Central venous access may be needed for drug or fluid administration, but central venous pressure monitoring may not reliably reflect intravascular volume status or fluid responsiveness. The role of pulmonary artery catheters in noncardiac surgical and critically ill patients continues to be controversial and depends on local practice patterns. Transesophageal echocardiography (TEE) or focused transthoracic echocardiography (TTE) may serve as an important monitor in the operating room to evaluate cardiac function and fluid status. An understanding of common cardiac diseases will help perioperative clinicians gauge the level of monitoring and care that is appropriate for each unique scenario.

Coronary Artery Disease

Patients with or at risk for CAD present significant challenges to anesthesiologists in the perioperative period. As many as 5% of patients with CAD undergoing noncardiac surgery may develop cardiac complications. Risk factors include a history of ischemic heart disease, HF, stroke, diabetes mellitus, or renal insufficiency. Preoperative risk stratification is discussed in detail in Chapter 1. Perioperative acute coronary events may range from myocardial ischemia or myocardial injury to myocardial infarction (MI). MI is universally defined as an elevation of cardiac biomarkers such as troponin, electrocardiographic (ECG) changes, new regional wall motion abnormalities seen on echocardiography, or coronary catheterization findings consistent with acute blockages.

The perioperative management of acute coronary syndrome (ACS), unstable angina, or acute MI presents a unique challenge because these patients under anesthesia or sedated postoperatively may not have the same signs and symptoms often seen in nonoperative patients. In fact, one large study found that 65% of patients with perioperative MI did not have symptoms. Thus the diagnosis is often confirmed only when clinical suspicion leads to further laboratory testing or investigation. When patients do complain of symptoms or clinical suspicion exists, clinicians should obtain a 12-lead ECG and serial cardiac biomarkers (e.g., troponin). Cardiology consultation for risk stratification, further testing, and therapy may be warranted.

Unlike nonsurgical patients with ACS or MI, care pathways for perioperative patients are not well studied. Unique concerns such as bleeding risk, surgical stressors, and perioperative physiologic changes make protocols for therapy very challenging.

Management must be considered in context for each patient and the relative risk-to-benefit ratio of therapies applied uniquely.

Patients with ACS preoperatively must first be clinically stabilized. Therapies to augment cardiac output may be needed. Administration of β-adrenergic agonists (e.g., dobutamine [2.5–5 µg/kg per minute] or epinephrine [1–2 µg/min]) can be effective. Mechanical augmentation with devices such as an intraaortic balloon pump or axial-flow pumps may be considered in severe cases. Arrhythmias may occur and should be managed, but prophylactic lidocaine is not indicated.

Medical therapy with aspirin (162–325 mg) should be initiated if not contraindicated. Additional antiplatelet therapy with a $P2Y_{12}$ receptor blocker is indicated in ACS, but may not be safe in the perioperative period. In patients with non–ST segment elevation ACS or MI (non-STEMI), systemic anticoagulation (i.e., heparin infusion) may be indicated, but the risk of surgical bleeding must be weighed against the risk of advancing ACS. Oxygen should be administered to all hypoxemic patients in concentrations needed to achieve normoxia. There are no data to support the use of oxygen in patients with MIs and normal oxygen saturation. Nitroglycerin may be administered to patients with angina, but should be avoided in patients with severe aortic stenosis (AS), right ventricular infarction, hypotension, or a history of phosphodiesterase inhibitor use in the previous 24 hours. Caution should also be used with this vasodilator in patients under neuraxial anesthesia because this could precipitate hypotension. Pain control with opioid analgesics may be considered; however, evidence suggests that morphine may be detrimental in patients with ACS. Proposed mechanisms include a morphine-induced impaired absorption or effectiveness of certain antiplatelet therapies. Statin therapy is indicated as soon as possible (Box 2.1).

β-Blocker therapy is perhaps the most controversial perioperative cardiac therapy. Although several studies have shown improved cardiac morbidity and mortality with the administration of perioperative β-blockers, concern for increased stroke risk and all-cause mortality has been noted. Current guidelines recommend that patients on chronic β-blocker therapy continue this perioperatively. In the setting of perioperative ACS, β-blocker therapy may decrease demand ischemia by improving oxygen supply and demand imbalance and is indicated in stable patients with ACS. The use of β-blockers in unstable patients or patients with acute cocaine intoxication should be cautioned.

Angiotensin-converting enzyme (ACE) inhibitor therapy should be considered in ACS after patients are stabilized. Angiotensin receptor blockers (ARBs) may be substituted in patients with HF with a left ventricular ejection fraction (LVEF) less than 40% or significant kidney dysfunction (creatinine >2.5 mg/dL for men or >2.0 mg/dL for women).

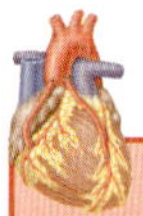

> **BOX 2.1   *Management of Acute Myocardial Infarction/Acute Coronary Syndrome***
>
> - Oxygen to maintain normoxia
> - Aspirin 162–325 mg
> - $P2Y_{12}$ antiplatelet therapy
> - Systemic anticoagulation (if no contraindication)
> - Nitroglycerin for pain (if no contraindication)
> - Opioid analgesics as needed
> - β-Blockers if stable
> - Statin therapy as soon as possible

The optimum hemoglobin level in patients with perioperative ACS or MI is not known. Routine red blood cell transfusion in stable, nonbleeding patients may not be indicated when the hemoglobin is above 8 g/dL.

More aggressive interventional therapy with cardiac catheterization or fibrinolytics is dependent on the type of myocardial injury and risk of surgical bleeding. STEMI presents a high mortality rate if left untreated. In the nonsurgical setting, patient outcome is clearly related to time to reperfusion with a recommended "door to reperfusion time" of less than 90 minutes. The mainstays of reperfusion therapy include (1) cardiac catheterization and angioplasty or stent placement or (2) fibrinolytic therapy. Multiple studies have shown an improved survival rate, fewer bleeding complications, and reduced recurrent MI with catheterization and PCI. These interventions present significant concerns in the perioperative period because of an increased risk of bleeding.

Fibrinolytic therapy is often reserved for centers without PCI capabilities. It is recommended when symptom onset is less than 12 hours before presentation and PCI would not be available within 120 minutes. However, in the perioperative setting, fibrinolytics are almost universally contraindicated because of bleeding risk. PCI may be better suited for the treatment of perioperative STEMI. This is not without risk, however, because angioplasty or stent placement often requires DAPT and anticoagulation. Finally, emergent coronary artery bypass graft (CABG) surgery is an option, although this is associated with increased mortality rate when performed in the first 7 days after STEMI. Close consultation with cardiology and surgery is needed to weigh the risks and benefits of therapeutic options in perioperative STEMI patients.

Patients with NSTEMI may be managed more conservatively. However, in patients with a low cardiac output syndrome or arrhythmias, emergent PCI and reperfusion may be warranted. In stable NSTEMI patients, noninvasive studies may be the first approach. Again, close consultation with cardiology will aid in risk stratification and management.

Patients with significant chronic stable CAD also can present for noncardiac surgery. These patients may have either severe multivessel disease or left main CAD. Both portend an increased risk in the perioperative period. Significant left main disease or its equivalent is an indication for CABG. Occasionally, however, emergency noncardiac surgery may be needed before definitive CAD treatment. The risks and benefits of noncardiac surgery in these patients should be considered carefully in consultation with a cardiologist or cardiac surgeon.

Anesthetic management in these patients should be geared toward preventing, monitoring, and detecting myocardial ischemia. Careful monitoring of the ECG and hemodynamic status is important. Hemodynamic goals include a low-normal heart rate, normal to high BP, and normothermia. Left ventricular distention caused by fluid overload should be avoided because increased wall tension may increase myocardial oxygen demand and decrease myocardial perfusion. Additional monitoring may be considered, including perioperative TEE. Medications with more favorable hemodynamic profiles (e.g., etomidate) should be considered for anesthetic induction and maintenance. Pharmacologic therapy in the form of inotropic support may be needed. Mechanical support of the heart with an aortic balloon pump or axial flow devices may help maintain coronary perfusion in the setting of severe disease. Additional anesthetic considerations must be based on patient- and procedure-specific needs.

Hypertension

Hypertension is a common perioperative illness that has included roughly one third of all noncardiac surgery patients in the past. The new 2017 guidelines on hypertension define a normal BP as less than 120/80 mm Hg. Elevated BP is systolic BP between 120 and 129 mm Hg and diastolic BP less than 80 mm Hg. Stage I hypertension is now a systolic BP between 130 and 139 or diastolic BP between 80 and 89 mm Hg. Stage II hypertension is systolic BP greater than 140 and diastolic BP greater than 90 mm Hg. These new guidelines state that BP should be treated earlier to avoid complications, and with these new definitions, nearly half of the U.S. population will be considered to be hypertensive. Chronic hypertension is associated with an increased risk of stroke, heart disease, and renal failure.

Patients presenting on the day of surgery with high BP represent a clinical challenge. Safe systolic BP cutoffs for elective surgery are not well established. Uncontrolled hypertension is listed as a "minor" risk factor by the American College of Cardiology/American Heart Association (ACC/AHA), and it remains unclear if postponing surgery for uncontrolled hypertension improves patient outcome. Diastolic BP is better studied, with the preponderance of evidence suggesting safely proceeding with elective surgery if the diastolic BP is below 110 mm Hg. The relative risks and benefits of surgery in the setting of hypertension should be considered by the care team on a patient-by-patient basis.

Most preoperative antihypertensive medication can be continued in the perioperative period. Renin–angiotensin system blockers are associated with intraoperative hypotension and vasoplegia. Therefore many centers hold ACE inhibitors or ARBs for 24 hours before surgery, although this practice is controversial. A decrease in intraoperative hypotension is noted when these medications are held. On the other hand, failure to restart ACE inhibitor or ARBs has been associated with an increased 30-day mortality rate. The initiation of new medications immediately before surgery, such as β-blockade, may increase the risk of stroke or death. These medications should not be started preoperatively unless there is sufficient time for the patient to acclimate to the new medication before surgery. Patients taking β-blocker or sympatholytic agents should continue these medications perioperatively because acute withdrawal symptoms can occur if these agents are stopped.

Appropriate BP monitoring must be considered on a case-by-case basis with patient and surgical considerations in mind. Patients with chronic hypertension are at increased risk for hemodynamic lability. Anesthetic goals, therefore, include maintenance of hemodynamic stability within a range of BP. A reasonable goal is to maintain the BP within 20% of a patient's baseline. In addition, blunting of the sympathetic response to anesthetic (laryngoscopy) and surgical stimuli should be attempted with anesthetic agents or adjunct medications. Relative hypotension can be treated with vasopressors with the goal of maintaining BP within a predefined range.

Severe hypertension must be managed expeditiously if end-organ complications are to be avoided (i.e., neurologic, cardiac, renal). First-line therapy with intravenous antihypertensive medications (e.g., calcium channel blocker, nitrates, β-blockers) is recommended. Postoperative complications related to elevated BP, such as surgical bleeding, must also be considered when determining the level of urgency in BP therapy.

Hypotension unresponsive to standard therapy may require further investigation. Surgical bleeding or manipulation of the vasculature may induce low BP and communication with the surgical team is vital. Myocardial ischemia or arrhythmias should be considered. Less common, but an important consideration, is the vasoplegic syndrome (VS), which is defined as severe hypotension refractory to catecholamine therapy without clear cause. The incidence of VS is highest in cardiac surgical patients, but it may be seen in noncardiac surgery as well. Exogenous vasopressin (dose of 1–2 units) may improve hypotension when conventional therapy has failed (i.e., decreasing anesthetic agent, volume expansion, and routine vasopressors). Alternatively, methylene blue (MB) is a well-described treatment. It is believed to interfere with the nitric oxide–cyclic guanylate monophosphate pathway, decreasing its vasorelaxant effect on smooth muscle. A bolus dose of 1 to 2 mg/kg over 10 to 20 minutes followed by an infusion of 0.25 mg/kg per hour for 48 to 72 hours is typical. Recently, the use of hydroxocobalamin (vitamin B_{12a}; dose of 125–250 mg) has been recommended in the occasional complex patient who does not respond to the above treatments.

Heart Failure

Heart failure represents a significant perioperative complication presenting in up to 10% of patients after major noncardiac surgery. A preoperative history of HF may increase cardiac risk substantially, especially in the presence of risk factors such as CAD and diabetes. HF is broadly defined as a syndrome of impaired cardiac function and is often categorized into systolic failure associated with reduced ejection fraction (HFrEF) and diastolic failure with preserved ejection fraction (HFpEF).

Similar to perioperative ACS, care pathways for the perioperative management of patients with HF are ill defined and poorly studied. Retrospective cohort studies using data from large national databases have helped elucidate risk factors, but it remains unclear how specific therapies may affect outcomes in the perioperative period. Patients may present with dyspnea, orthopnea, tachypnea, or clinical signs such as crackles or decreased oxygen saturation. Signs of right-sided HF may also be present, including nausea and vomiting, lower extremity edema, and hepatic congestion. This may present a confusing clinical picture because many of the signs and symptoms of HF may be seen in the perioperative period because of other causes such as surgical insult, pain, and medication side effects.

Clinical suspicion of HF should prompt further investigation that includes an ECG, chest radiography, and cardiac biomarkers. Elevated brain natriuretic peptide (BNP) is supportive of the diagnosis of HF. Some patients with chronic HF may have a baseline abnormal level of BNP, and further elevation of BNP from baseline may be diagnostic of an acute exacerbation. Initial laboratory evaluation also should include electrolytes, renal and liver function tests, hemoglobin, and echocardiography.

Therapies may be tailored to specific causes. Treatment must be directed at managing concomitant respiratory failure; adequate oxygenation and ventilation are paramount to normalizing cardiac function. Electrolyte imbalances and acid-base disturbances should be corrected to minimize potential detrimental effects on ventricular contractility, pulmonary arterial pressure, and cardiac rhythm. Preload, contractility, and afterload must also be optimized.

In patients with signs of volume overload, diuretic therapy and fluid restriction are mainstays of therapy. Patients with HFrEF with clinical signs and symptoms of low cardiac output may benefit from inotropic therapy (e.g., dobutamine). In the setting of failed pharmacotherapy, mechanical devices may be used to treat severe HF (e.g., intraaortic balloon pump, ventricular assist devices).

In patients with stable hemodynamics, ACE inhibitor and β-blocker therapy is recommended by the ACC/AHA. Additionally, in patients with reduced ejection fractions, newer therapies such as combinations of valsartan and sacubitril (Entresto) are recommended to improve outcome. Readers are referred to the clinical guidelines from the ACC/AHA for more detailed information.

Takotsubo Cardiomyopathy

Approximately 2% to 3% of patients presenting with ACS meet diagnostic criteria for takotsubo cardiomyopathy (TCM). It is important to distinguish patients with

TCM from those with ACS or HF because the etiology and treatment of each differ substantially.

Current data point towards a high level of circulating catecholamines as the predominant factor leading to TCM. Mammalian hearts have been found to have higher levels of β-adrenergic receptors in the apical ventricular myocardium. This phenomenon is believed to mediate an increased sensitivity to catecholamine surges in the apex of the heart. Clinically, the resultant myocardial dysfunction occurs disproportionately in the apex of the left ventricle, resulting in pathognomonic apical ballooning seen on echocardiography or ventriculography. Estrogen helps regulate the sympathetic response to catecholamines, blunting this response in reproductive years. This may explain why a predominance of TCM is seen in postmenopausal women.

Clinically, TCM often presents with a preceding physical or positive or negative emotional stressor ("happy heart syndrome" or "broken heart syndrome"). Certain diseases have been associated with TCM, including sepsis, pheochromocytoma, cerebral hemorrhage, respiratory failure, and thyrotoxicosis. Acutely, a hypertensive response to catecholamines may be noted followed by cardiomyopathy, hypotension, and HF.

Differentiating TCM from ACS is crucial. ECG findings play an important role, and abnormal findings are typically present. ST-segment elevation in lead aVR is found to have a high positive predictive value for TCM. In contrast, ST-segment depression in leads V_2 to V_4 makes ACS more likely. Non–ST segment elevation TCM is commonly associated with T-wave inversions in leads I, aVL, V_5, and V_6. However, NSTEMI is associated with ST-segment depression in V_2 and V_3 (anterior wall MI). Laboratory findings classically depict a mild elevation in cardiac biomarkers with TCM. The degree of wall motion abnormality is often disproportionately large compared with the degree of biomarker elevation in TCM. Echocardiogram findings often reveal circumferential wall motion abnormalities with the classic finding of apical ballooning occurring in 80% of cases. Other variants such as basal (see later) and midventricular types have been described. Regional wall motion abnormalities outside of a single coronary artery's distribution can help distinguish TCM from acute MI. In addition, coronary angiography typically reveals nonobstructive or absent disease (Box 2.2).

The treatment of patients with TCM may vary depending on the clinical scenario. Serious cardiac complications can occur in up to 20% of patients with TCM. Apical hypokinesis coupled with a hyperkinetic basal region can lead to left ventricular outflow obstruction. This should be managed with the cessation of inotropes and fluid administration to decrease turbulent flow through the outflow tract.

Delaying elective surgery should be considered in the setting of TCM. In cases in which surgery is deemed necessary, care must be taken given possible cardiogenic shock,

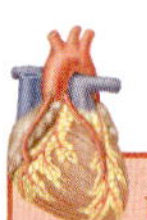

BOX 2.2   *Diagnostic Features of Takotsubo Cardiomyopathy*

- Precedent physical or emotional stressor
- Signs or symptoms of heart failure
- Mild elevation in cardiac biomarkers with disproportionately large wall motion abnormality seen on echocardiography; classically, apical ballooning
- Ventricular involvement extending beyond one vascular territory
- Normal or nonobstructed coronary arteries on angiogram

HF, or hemodynamic instability. Invasive monitoring with an arterial catheter, TEE, or both should be considered. Inotropic support should be used judiciously because catecholamines are associated with precipitating TCM. Mechanical support may be considered in low-output states. In patients with HF, standard therapies previously described are applicable, including diuretics and fluid restriction. Recovery usually occurs over days to weeks. Longer term, therapeutic blockade of the renin–angiotensin system and adrenergic system may be useful in preventing recurrences of TCM and reducing the longer term structural, functional, and metabolic changes that may follow episodes of TCM.

Reverse takotsubo syndrome (rTTS) is a more recently described variant of TCM characterized by basal hypokinesis and apical hyperkinesis. Diagnostic criteria remain similar to TCM, with hallmark echocardiographic findings of wall motion abnormalities in the basal region extending beyond a single coronary vascular territory. Similar to TCM, rTTS is thought to be caused by a relative increase in catecholamines and subsequent myocardial toxicity. Patients with rTTS often present at a younger age than those with TCM. This is thought to be due to an age-related increase in apical adrenergic receptors compared with a more basilar distribution in young people.

rTTS has a lower risk of cardiogenic shock than TCM but may have higher biomarkers than the more common apical variant. This is thought to be due to a larger area of myocardial involvement. Treatment is mainly supportive, and the long-term prognosis is good.

Valvular Heart Disease

Concomitant valvular heart disease may be common in the perioperative period. Depending on the severity of valvular disease, surgery and anesthesia may present a significant physiologic challenge. An understanding of the type and severity of valvular disease can help the clinician tailor care appropriately. Preoperative echocardiographic evaluation may help guide perioperative management. A clinical suspicion of undiagnosed valvular disease or recent changes in clinical history should prompt preoperative echocardiographic testing if none has been performed in the previous 12 months. A broad overview is discussed below, but a much greater degree of detail can be found in *Kaplan's Cardiac Anesthesia*, 7th edition.

Aortic Stenosis

Aortic stenosis is the most common form of valvular heart disease and a major predictor of morbidity in noncardiac surgery. In patients 75 years of age or older, AS is a common finding, with an incidence of 3% to 8%. Decreased cardiac reserve blunts the ability to respond to the physiologic stressors of surgery and anesthesia, likely accounting for an increased perioperative morbidity and mortality. In addition, AS may be associated with an increased risk of bleeding caused by an acquired form of von Willebrand disease. Perioperative management of patients with AS may require invasive hemodynamic monitoring, especially in major noncardiac surgery, to assure proper loading conditions and avoid potentially catastrophic decreases in preload and afterload that may lead to ischemia, left ventricular failure, and cardiac arrest.

Therapeutic goals are similar both intraoperatively and postoperatively. Hypovolemia and tachycardia should be avoided because the left ventricle is often hypertrophied and noncompliant and thus more dependent on adequate filling time and elevated filling pressures to maintain preload. Sinus rhythm should be maintained because left ventricular filling is also increasingly dependent on atrial contraction in the setting of AS. Systemic vascular resistance (SVR) should be maintained, and significant decreases in BP should be avoided because they may cause dangerous reductions in

Table 2.2	Hemodynamic Goals of Valvulopathy	
	Heart Rate	**Blood Pressure**
Aortic stenosis	Slow normal	High normal
Aortic regurgitation	Fast normal	Low normal
Mitral regurgitation	Fast normal	Low normal
Mitral stenosis	Slow normal	Normal

coronary perfusion (Table 2.2). Neuraxial anesthesia may cause a decrease in SVR and preload and should be considered with great caution in patients with AS. Phenylephrine or norepinephrine are effective medications for maintaining SVR in the perioperative period.

Aortic Regurgitation

The risk of noncardiac surgery in patients with aortic regurgitation (AR) relates directly to the severity of valvular disease, the cause of AR, and the surgical risk. Moderate to severe AR and intermediate- to high-risk surgery are risk factors for increased pulmonary edema, prolonged intubation, and in-hospital death.

Understanding the degree of AR preoperatively is key when caring for these patients. In patients with severe AR and poor LVEF (<50%), valve repair or replacement may be considered before elective noncardiac surgery.

Many anesthetic agents cause a decrease in SVR, reducing regurgitant fraction and improving AR. Nevertheless, careful management is necessary. To maintain forward cardiac output, avoidance of bradycardia is important because it may increase regurgitation due to increased diastolic time. Similarly, hypertension and volume overload should be avoided. The use of diuretics and afterload reduction medications may be helpful.

Mitral Stenosis

Patients with moderate to severe mitral stenosis (MS) undergoing noncardiac surgery present a significant challenge to clinicians. LV filling is impaired because of obstructed flow across the stenotic mitral valve. Supraventricular arrhythmias may develop because of structural changes in the left atrium (LA). Pulmonary hypertension can develop because high LA pressures are transmitted backward to the pulmonary vasculature. Eventually, patients with severe MS can develop pulmonary edema and right ventricular (RV) failure.

Caring for patients with MS in the perioperative period involves maintaining LV filling pressures and optimizing conditions for right heart function. Care must be taken to avoid hypercarbia, hypoxemia, and acidosis, all of which can increase pulmonary vascular resistance and impair RV function. Inotropic support of the RV may be needed. Dobutamine is a reasonable choice, with phosphodiesterase inhibitors such as milrinone reserved for more critical scenarios.

Medications that cause tachycardia such as ketamine and anticholinergics are best avoided. A slow heart rate allows for improved LV filling across the stenotic mitral valve; β-blockers such as esmolol should be available. Anxiolysis to avoid tachycardia is important, but care must be taken to avoid hypercarbia or hypoxemia with sedation. Avoidance of hypotension may be achieved with "hemodynamically stable medications" such as etomidate. Regional and neuraxial anesthesia may be used, but clinicians should attempt to avoid hypotension. Epidural anesthesia with gradual dosing of medication may reduce the risk of sudden hypotension.

Mitral Regurgitation

Patients with moderate to severe mitral regurgitation (MR) undergoing surgery are at increased risk of perioperative morbidity and mortality. Those with chronic MR have long-standing volume overload of the LV, which leads to dilation of the ventricle and left atrium. Because of compensatory mechanisms, chronic MR is often well tolerated by patients. Acute MR, however, is not well tolerated and is often complicated by overt HF, pulmonary hypertension, and pulmonary edema. The most common cause of acute MR is ischemia causing papillary muscle dysfunction. Addressing the underlying cause of acute MR is the mainstay of management.

Key management principles for patients with chronic MR undergoing noncardiac surgery include maintaining sinus rhythm and avoiding bradycardia, hypertension, and volume overload. Sinus rhythm is crucial because atrial contraction may account for 30% to 40% of LV end-diastolic volume. Atrial fibrillation (AF) significantly decreases LV filling and can lead to HF and shock. Most anesthetic agents improve MR by decreasing afterload and thus decreasing LV systolic pressure. Regional or neuraxial anesthesia may be reasonable in the absence of contraindications for placement such as chronic anticoagulation for AF. Diuretics and afterload reduction should be considered if volume overload or hypertension is encountered.

Arrhythmias

Atrial Fibrillation

Atrial fibrillation can be defined as the lack of coordinated contraction of the atria. The ECG reveals an irregular R-R interval and absent P waves. Perioperatively, a multitude of factors can precipitate AF, including direct surgical irritation of the atria or pulmonary veins, fluid shifts and electrolyte imbalance, or catecholamine surges related to pain or the stress of surgery. AF is associated with an increased risk of stroke because slow blood flow through the atria can lead to thrombus formation, particularly in the left atrial appendage.

In patients with AF, the decision of when to stop oral anticoagulants preoperatively is a source of continued concern. Patients at particular risk of stroke may be "bridged" from the time of cessation of oral anticoagulants to surgery with low-molecular-weight heparin (LMWH) or unfractionated heparin. The duration of cessation and timing of bridging therapy are decided on an individual basis based on surgical risk of bleeding and patient risk of thromboembolism. The management of anticoagulation therapy should be coordinated with the managing physician (e.g., primary care doctor or cardiologist).

The new non–vitamin K oral anticoagulants (NOACs; see the NOAC section for more detail) such as the direct thrombin inhibitors (DTIs) and factor Xa inhibitors pose a significant concern in surgical patients. There is far less experience regarding the safe timing of cessation; 3 days is usually adequate with normal renal and hepatic function. Furthermore, reversal with antidotes has recently become available, but there is little clinical experience with these drugs. The American Society of Regional Anesthesia has published guidelines on the timing of regional or neuraxial anesthesia in the setting of oral anticoagulants.

Perioperatively, the hemodynamic consequences of AF are of particular concern, especially in the setting of preexisting cardiac conditions. The loss of atrial contraction coupled with beat-to-beat changes in ventricular filling can lead to suboptimal ventricular preload and decreases in cardiac output and BP. Irregular electrical transmission through the atrioventricular (AV) node can lead to a rapid ventricular response.

Patients with AF in the operative or critical care setting should initially be evaluated for signs of hemodynamic compromise and categorized as stable or unstable. Unstable patients should undergo immediate cardioversion. It should be recognized that cardioversion might increase the risk of stroke, especially in patients with a history of AF and not on anticoagulation. If possible, evaluation for existing intracardiac thrombus with TEE should be considered. In stable patients, rate control with medications and anticoagulation are the mainstays of therapy.

Several different classes of medication can be used for rate control. The most common medications are calcium channel blockers, β-blockers, amiodarone, and digoxin. Therapy must be individualized to the patient and clinical scenario.

Supraventricular Tachyarrhythmia

The term *supraventricular tachyarrhythmia* (SVT) refers to any arrhythmia originating above the AV node. It can be subdivided into irregular and regular rhythms. Regular SVT includes AV nodal reentry, AV tachycardia in both orthodromic and antidromic forms, AV junctional tachycardia, and other less common types.

In the perioperative period, several pathophysiologic mechanisms may precipitate SVT. Common causes include acidosis, hypercarbia, hypoxemia, electrolyte disturbances, hypotension, mechanical irritation of the atria or pulmonary veins, medications, and myocardial ischemia. Investigation into the precipitating factor is a key component in the management of SVT and includes laboratory analysis and ECG.

Treatment is determined by the stability of the patient. Unstable patients require synchronized cardioversion and should be managed with Advanced Cardiac Life Support (ACLS) guidelines in mind. In stable patients, vagal maneuvers (e.g., Valsalva maneuver) may be attempted first. Although carotid massage is a known vagal stimulant, caution should be used because inadvertent carotid injury and stroke have been described. Adenosine temporarily slows conduction through the sinoatrial node and renders the AV node refractory to depolarization. This transient effect makes adenosine a reasonable choice for the treatment of patients with narrow-complex SVT. In the absence of underlying structural heart disease (e.g., AS, MS), SVT is often stable, and rate control with β-blockade, calcium channel blockers, or amiodarone is reasonable.

The treatment of wide-complex SVT and reentrant tachycardia may be more complex. Disorders with accessory pathways, such as Wolff-Parkinson-White syndrome, may respond paradoxically when conduction through the AV node is slowed. Amiodarone may be considered in these situations along with cardiology consultation.

Ventricular Arrhythmias

Ventricular arrhythmias arise below the AV node and are typically a wide-complex rhythm. These most commonly originate in scarred or damaged ventricular muscle, creating a conduction pathway outside the normal His-Purkinje system. Wide-complex ventricular rhythms should be differentiated from SVT with aberrancy because the treatment may differ.

Ventricular tachycardia (VT) can be subdivided into nonsustained (NSVT) and sustained VT. NSVT is defined as three or more premature ventricular contractions with a rate of 120 beats/min or more, lasting less than 30 seconds. In the absence of underlying disease (e.g., MI), aggressive therapy is likely not indicated. In patients with myocardial injury and poor ventricular function, more aggressive therapy may be indicated, and consultation with cardiology is recommended.

Sustained VT can be subdivided based on morphology into monomorphic and polymorphic types. Monomorphic VT demonstrates a consistent QRS amplitude and is often related to a reentrant pathway within scarred myocardium. Urgent synchronized cardioversion (50–100 J, biphasic) is often required. As with other arrhythmias, treatment of the underlying cause should be established. Continued therapy with amiodarone or lidocaine by infusion may be indicated in the perioperative period.

Polymorphic VT may be associated with normal or long QT intervals, and causes may vary. Normal QT polymorphic VT is often associated with myocardial ischemia. Prolonged QT forms may be related to medications such as sotalol (torsades de pointes), precipitated by underlying genetic predisposition (long QT syndrome), or both. Treatment includes correction of underlying electrolyte disturbances, intravenous magnesium (2–4 g), and asynchronous cardioversion. Consultation with cardiology is likely warranted.

Brugada syndrome is an autosomal dominant hereditary disease characterized by ST-segment elevation in the right precordial leads on the ECG, which predisposes to sudden cardiac death caused by polymorphic VT or ventricular fibrillation in the absence of structural heart disease. The disease affects young and active individuals with a life expectancy of more than 30 years. Life-threatening ventricular arrhythmias occur without obvious causes in about 20% of patients. Multiple therapies have been tried with variable success. The present therapy is to insert automatic internal defibrillators in these patients. However, if a surgical patient does not have one, an external defibrillator with pads should be in place for noncardiac surgery.

PERIOPERATIVE MANAGEMENT OF ANTICOAGULATION

The perioperative management of patients taking anticoagulants for venous thromboembolism (VTE) or pulmonary embolism prophylaxis, AF and stroke avoidance, artificial mechanical valves, or other indications can be challenging. Balancing the disease risk with the risk of surgical bleeding presents an ongoing clinical challenge. Strategies are discussed in the next sections. Risk factors for bleeding in chronically anticoagulated patients include mechanical mitral valve prosthesis (requires higher level of anticoagulation), cancer, history of bleeding complications from anticoagulation, restarting heparin anticoagulation within 24 hours of surgery, and heparin bridging. The decision to stop, continue, or bridge anticoagulant therapy must be considered in the context of patient- and procedure-related risk factors, such as a high risk of stroke from AF or low surgical bleeding risk (e.g., cataract surgery). This section provides a brief review of the anticoagulants, the suggested timing of cessation before elective surgery, and anticoagulation reversal agents for emergent surgery or bleeding complications. Alterations in these medications are best coordinated with the managing physician.

Warfarin

Warfarin (Coumadin) impairs the coagulation cascade by interrupting the carboxylation of factors II, VII, IX, and X, as well as the synthesis of proteins C and S. The resultant anticoagulated state can be monitored with the prothrombin time (PT) or international normalized ratio (INR). Cessation of warfarin 5 days before surgery is a recognized strategy. Postoperatively, warfarin can be reinitiated when the risk of thromboembolic disease outweighs the risk of bleeding. Patients may require bridging therapy with LMWH. The continuation of warfarin throughout the perioperative procedure may be acceptable in certain situations (e.g., cataract surgery), and warfarin may be beneficial in some procedures such as catheter ablation of AF in which the perioperative stroke risk is high and surgical bleeding risk is low.

Several modalities of warfarin reversal exist, including vitamin K, fresh-frozen plasma, and prothrombin complex concentrates (PCCs). Activated factor VII may be considered as well. Reversal agents should be chosen based on the relative level of urgency, pharmacologic properties, and their associated side effect profiles.

New Oral Anticoagulants

New pharmacologic agents have been developed with more specific inhibition of the coagulation cascade than warfarin. Several potential advantages over warfarin have been described: no requirement for serial laboratory testing, decreased dietary restrictions, and few drug interactions. These include DTIs (e.g., dabigatran) and direct factor Xa inhibitors (e.g., rivaroxaban, apixaban, and edoxaban). Notably, these medications have been shown to have a decreased risk of intracranial hemorrhage versus warfarin. Until recently, the newest factor Xa inhibitors have had a decisive disadvantage to warfarin in the perioperative period since no specific antidotes existed, and the treatment of serious and life-threatening bleeding could be difficult. Four-factor PCCs are nonspecific but potentially useful reversal agents for the NOACs when hemorrhagic complications occur. In 2018, the Food and Drug Administration approved andexanet alfa as a reversal agent for the factor Xa inhibitors.

Direct Thrombin Inhibitors

There are several DTIs, including hirudin, argatroban, and bivalirudin. The most commonly used intravenous agent is argatroban, which is often used in patients who develop heparin-induced thrombocytopenia. Argatroban undergoes hepatic metabolism, and its elimination is independent of the kidneys, making it ideal for critically ill patients at risk for kidney injury. The anticoagulation effect can be measured by the partial thromboplastin time (PTT) with a goal 1.5 to 3 times the patient's baseline. Argatroban infusions should be stopped 2 to 4 hours before an intervention or surgery. Confirmation of normal coagulation can be made by a normalization of the PTT.

Dabigatran (Pradaxa) is an oral, reversible DTI that is indicated for treatment of AF and VTE prophylaxis or treatment. Dabigatran use with artificial mechanical valves is unproven and not indicated at present. Caution should be used in patients with renal impairment because the half-life of dabigatran may be increased from 12 to 24 hours. Routine coagulation tests such as the PT and PTT may be altered with dabigatran; however, the degree of alteration and the presence of a normal test result do not exclude impaired coagulation. A normal dilute thrombin time suggests that the anticoagulation activity of dabigatran has resolved; this is the most specific and clinically useful measurement of this drug's activity. The AHA/ACC suggests that dabigatran should be held for at least 2 days before surgery and a dilute thrombin time obtained to confirm normalization. It is recommended that patients with renal dysfunction should have surgery delayed at least 5 days. The timing of neuraxial anesthesia in patients who have stopped dabigatran is not well defined. Dabigatran should be restarted after surgery when the risk of thrombosis outweighs the risk of bleeding because the onset of anticoagulation is very rapid.

In the past, treatment of serious and life-threatening bleeding was difficult with dabigatran because there was no specific antidote. Key steps included cessation of the drug and supportive care. In life-threatening bleeding, dialysis could facilitate faster removal of dabigatran from plasma. Four-factor PCCs and activated factor VII were considered in life-threatening bleeding from dabigatran, but these were of unproven efficacy. Consultation with a hematologist was warranted.

In 2016, the Food and Drug Administration approved use of idarucizumab (Praxbind) to reverse dabigatran in patients with severe bleeding or requiring an urgent procedure or surgery. This drug is a monoclonal antibody fragment developed specifically to reverse the anticoagulation produced by dabigatran. In a study of 500 patients (RE-VERSE AD study) with a prolonged dilute thrombin time, a single dose of 5 g was adequate in 98% of patients and lasted for 24 hours. No other therapy was needed in the surgical patients.

Factor Xa Inhibitors

Factor X is produced in the liver by a vitamin K–dependent process, and the activated form converts prothrombin to thrombin. Oral inhibitors of activated factor X, rivaroxaban (Xarelto), apixaban (Eliquis), and edoxaban (Savaysa), have been shown to be effective in the prevention of stroke in patients with nonvalvular AF. In addition, there is a decreased rate of major bleeding when compared with warfarin. Factor Xa inhibitors are indicated for VTE treatment and prophylaxis, including in postsurgical patients after major joint arthroplasty. Factor Xa inhibitors are associated with a decreased incidence of bleeding versus LMWH. Similar to dabigatran, they are not indicated for treatment of artificial heart valves. Specific laboratory assays of factor Xa inhibitors are available; however, routine monitoring of anticoagulation is not required. The safety of these three drugs with neuraxial anesthesia does not have a large database, but the American Society for Regional Anesthesia says that it can be used after 3 days of drug withdrawal. Bridging for procedures is not necessary for oral factor Xa inhibitors because they have short half-lives. Discontinuation of these factor Xa inhibitors for 3 days is considered appropriate for most elective surgical procedures.

A specific reversal agent for oral factor Xa inhibitors has recently been approved in the United States. Andexanet alfa has been designed specifically to reverse factor Xa inhibitors. It is a recombinant, modified human factor Xa decoy protein that binds to factor Xa inhibitors. The administration of an andexanct alfa bolus and 2-hour infusion results in rapid and substantial reversal of anti–factor Xa activity for 12 hours.

SUGGESTED READING

Agarwal S, Bean MG, Hata JS, Castresana MR. Perioperative takotsubo cardiomyopathy: a systemic review of published cases. *Semin Cardiothorac Vasc Anesth*. 2017;21:277–290.

Amsterdam EA, Wenger NK, Brindis RG, et al. 2014 AHA/ACC Guideline for the management of patients with non-st-elevation acute coronary syndromes: a report of the American College of Cardiology/American Heart Association Task Force on Practice Guidelines. *J Am Coll Cardiol*. 2014;64:e139–e228.

Anderson JL, Morrow DA. Acute myocardial infarction. *NEJM*. 2017;376:2053–2064.

Beattie WS, Wijeysundera DN. The growing burden of perioperative heart failure. *Anesth Analg*. 2014;119:506–508.

Biykem B, Butler J, et al. 2013 ACCF/AHA guideline for the management of heart failure. *JACC*. 2013;62:e147–e239.

Connolly SJ, Milling TJ, Eikelboom JW, et al. Andexanet alfa for acute major bleeding associated with Factor Xa Inhibitors. *NEJM*. 2016;375:1131–1141.

Devereaux PJ, Yang H, Yusuf S, et al. Effects of extended-release metoprolol succinate in patients undergoing noncardiac surgery (POISE trial): a randomised controlled trial. *Lancet*. 2008;371:1839–1847.

Fleisher LA, Fleischmann KE, Auerbach AD, et al. 2014 ACC/AHA guideline on perioperative cardiovascular evaluation and management of patients undergoing noncardiac surgery: a report of the American College of Cardiology/American Heart Association Task Force on Practice Guidelines. *Circulation*. 2014;130:e278–e333.

Grottke O, Levy JH. Prothrombin complex concentrates in trauma and perioperative bleeding. *Anesthesiology*. 2015;122:923–931.

Hawn MT, Graham LA, Richman JS, et al. Risk of major adverse cardiac events following noncardiac surgery in patients with coronary stents. *JAMA*. 2013;310:1462–1472.

Helwani M, Amin A, Lavigne P, et al. Etiology of acute coronary syndrome after noncardiac surgery. *Anesthesiology*. 2018;128:1084–1091.

Hernandez-Ojeda J, Arbelo E, Borras R, et al. Patients with Brugada syndrome and implanted cardioverter-defibrillators. *JACC*. 2017;70:1991–2002.

Horlocker TT, Wedel DJ, Rowlingson JC, et al. Regional anesthesia in the patient receiving antithrombotic or thrombolytic therapy: American Society of Regional Anesthesia and Pain Medicine Evidence-Based Guidelines (Third Edition). *Reg Anesth Pain Med*. 2010;35:64–101.

January CT, Wann LS, Alpert JS, et al, ACC/AHA Task Force Members. 2014 AHA/ACC/HRS guideline for the management of patients with atrial fibrillation: a report of the American College of Cardiology/American Heart Association Task Force on practice guidelines and the Heart Rhythm Society. *Circulation*. 2014;130:e199–e267.

Kato K, Lyon AR, Ghadri JR, Templin C. Takotsubo syndrome: etiology, presentation and treatment. *Heart*. 2017;103:1461–1469.

London M. Type 2 perioperative myocardial infarction. *Anesthesiology*. 2018;128:1055–1059.

Mathis MR, Naughton NN, Shanks AM, et al. Patient selection for day case-eligible surgery: identifying those at high risk for major complications. *Anesthesiology*. 2013;119:1310–1321.

Nishimura RA, Otto CM, Bonow RO, et al, ACC/AHA Task Force Members. 2014 AHA/ACC guideline for the management of patients with valvular heart disease: a report of the American College of Cardiology/American Heart Association Task Force on Practice Guidelines. *Circulation*. 2014;129: pe521–pe643.

Nishimura RA, Otto CM, Bonow RO, et al. 2017 AHA/ACC Focused update of the 2014 guideline for management of valvular heart disease. *JACC*. 2017;70(2):252–289.

O'Gara PT, Kushner FG, Ascheim DD, et al. 2013 ACCF/AHA guideline for the management of ST-elevation myocardial infarction: a report of the American College of Cardiology Foundation/American Heart Association Task Force on Practice Guidelines. *Circulation*. 2013;127:e362–e425.

Pollack CV, Reilly PA, van Ryn J, et al. Idarucizumab for dabigatran reversal–full cohort analysis. *NEJM*. 2017;377:431–441.

Roshanov PS, Rochwerg B, Patel A, et al. Withholding versus continuing angiotensin-converting enzyme inhibitors or angiotensin II receptor blockers before noncardiac surgery: an analysis of the vascular events in noncardiac surgery patients. *Anesthesiology*. 2017;126:16.

Whelton PK, Carey RM, Aronow WS, et al. 2017 ACC/AHA guideline for the prevention, detection, evaluation, and management of high blood pressure in adults. *JACC*. 2017.

Yancy C, Jessup M, O'Gara PT, et al. 2013 ACCF/AHA guideline for the management of ST-elevation myocardial infarction: a report of the American College of Cardiology Foundation/American Heart Association Task Force on Practice Guidelines. *Circulation*. 2013;127:e362–e425.

Yancy CW, Jessup M, Bozkurt B, et al. 2017 ACC/AHA Focused Update of the 2013 Guideline for the management of heart failure. *JACC*. 2017;70(6):776–797.

Chapter 3

Care of the Patient With Coronary Stents Undergoing Noncardiac Surgery

Emilio B. Lobato, MD

Key Points

1. Percutaneous coronary intervention (PCI) with stent placement is frequently performed, with a substantial number of patients requiring subsequent noncardiac surgery (NCS).
2. Three types of stents are currently available for clinical use: bare metal stents (BMSs), drug-eluting stents (DESs), and bioresorbable stents (BRSs).
3. The two main stent-related complications are restenosis and thrombosis.
4. The risk of restenosis peaks within the first year after PCI and is more commonly seen with BMS.
5. The risk of stent thrombosis (ST) is highest within the first 30 days regardless of stent type. It decreases subsequently. Newer generations of DESs are less thrombogenic than first-generation DESs and even BMSs. Bioabsorbable stents have the highest risk at 12 months.
6. Treatment with dual antiplatelet therapy (DAPT) is necessary to prevent ST. The optimal duration with any stent must balance the risk of thrombosis versus bleeding.
7. There are several recognized clinical, procedural, and angiographic risk factors of ST. The most important is premature discontinuation of DAPT, yet many cases of ST still occur in the presence of platelet inhibitors.
8. The standard combination for long-term DAPT consists of aspirin (ASA) and clopidogrel; however, there is significant variability in patients' response to each drug. The more potent drugs prasugrel and ticagrelor exhibit more predictable antiplatelet effects but are associated with higher bleeding risk.
9. The use of platelet function tests to individualize antiplatelet therapy (APT) has not proven superior in medical patients, yet it has shown effectiveness before cardiac surgery and may hold promise for NCS.
10. The incidence of perioperative ST is low, but it is associated with major morbidity and mortality.
11. The two most important decisions for patients undergoing NCS are the timing of the procedure and management of DAPT.
12. Most recommendations are not very well defined and are based on low-quality evidence and expert opinion. Management should balance each patient's specific thrombotic risk against a particular surgery's specific hemorrhagic risk.
13. For patients with stable ischemic heart disease (SIDH) and low thrombotic risk, elective surgery should be delayed at least 6 weeks after BMS placement and 3 months with DESs, with ASA continued for most procedures. For patients with PCI during acute coronary syndrome or at high risk for thrombosis, the waiting period should be at least

> 6 months or perhaps longer regardless of stent type. For patients with current BRSs, the waiting period appears to be at least 12 months regardless of the indication for PCI. If surgery cannot be postponed, decisions on DAPT should be based on the patient's individual thrombotic or hemorrhagic risk.
> 14. Selected patients may benefit from bridging therapy with intravenous platelet inhibitors, but such an approach is not without risks and is associated with increased hospitalization and cost.
> 15. The frequency and complexity of this important topic require an interdisciplinary structured approach with input from the different specialties involved in the care of these patients

Percutaneous coronary intervention (PCI) is one of the most common procedures worldwide, with approximately 600,000 performed annually in the United States alone. The term includes balloon angioplasty as well as coronary stent placement, with the overwhelming majority of individuals undergoing the latter because of superior results in preserving vessel patency.

Despite the obvious advantages over balloon angioplasty, the long-term care of patients with coronary stents is haunted by the risk of restenosis and stent thrombosis (ST). Refinements in stent technology, implantation technique, and antiplatelet therapy (APT) have increased stent safety profiles; however, long-term management still faces significant challenges aiming to achieve an optimal balance of maintaining vascular integrity while minimizing thrombotic and bleeding risks.

The reported incidence of noncardiac surgery (NCS) after PCI ranges from 4% to 11% at 12 months, and 7% to 34% by 2 years. One of the greatest causes for clinical concern is how to best manage these patients because the presence of coronary artery stents is a recognized risk for perioperative cardiac morbidity and mortality.

The issue is further complicated by a frequent lack of consensus among perioperative providers, either because of unawareness or personal preferences; as a result, patients may remain uninformed of potential risks. Because of the magnitude of the problem, professional societies have provided guidelines for perioperative physicians to assist in their evaluation and management, but these are mostly based on low-quality evidence and expert opinion, including recent focused updates or consensus-driven documents. Furthermore, rapid improvements in stent technology (e.g., bioresorbable stents [BRSs]) and new pharmacologic agents find their way into clinical use before long-term outcomes from clinical trials are published, adding to the confusion about the best way to manage these patients in the perioperative period.

As part of a multidisciplinary team, anesthesiologists are in a unique position to provide important critical input because they are frequently sought by perioperative providers for their expertise. This chapter addresses the various coronary stents available for clinical use, long-term risks associated with these devices, the use of antiplatelet agents, and implications for those patients undergoing noncardiac procedures.

TYPES OF STENTS

The basic concept of a stent is that of a solid scaffold that prevents vessel closure due to elastic recoil or vessel contracture. In general, stents can be categorized according to material composition, durability, thickness of struts, and the presence of eluting drugs for local delivery (Table 3.1).

Table 3.1 Stents Available for Clinical Use

Bare Metal Stents

Name	Manufacturer	Stent Generation	Stent Platform
Veri-FLEX	Boston Scientific	First	Stainless steel
Vision	Abbott Vascular	Second	Cobalt chromium
Integrity	Medtronic	Second	Cobalt chromium
REBEL	Boston Scientific	Third	Platinum chromium

Drug-Eluting Stents

Name	Manufacturer	Stent Generation	Stent Platform	Polymer	Antirestenotic Drug	Elution Kinetics
Cypher[a]	Cordis/J&J	First	Stainless steel	PEVA/PBMA	Sirolimus	80% at 4 wk
Taxus[a]	Boston Scientific	First	Stainless steel	SIBBS	Paclitaxel	10% at 4 wk
Xience	Abbott Vascular	Second	Cobalt chromium	PBMA/PVDF-HFP	Everolimus	80% at 4 wk
Promus	Boston Scientific	Second	Cobalt chromium	PBMA/PVDF-HFP	Everolimus	80% at 4 wk
Endeavor	Medtronic	Second	Cobalt chromium	PPChol	Zotarolimus	95% at 2 wk
Resolute	Medtronic	Second	Cobalt chromium	Biolynx	Zotarolimus	85% at 8 wk
Promus Element	Boston Scientific	Third	Platinum chromium	PBMA/PVDF-HFP	Everolimus	80% at 4 wk
Taxus Ion	Boston Scientific	Third	Platinum chromium	SIBBS	Paclitaxel	10% at 2 wk
Absorb BVS	Abbott	BVS DES	PLLA	PLLA	Everolimus	75% at 4 wk
DESolve[b]	Elixir	BVS DES	PLLA	Bioresorbable polymer	Novolimus	85% at wk
ART Pure[b]	ART	BVS	PDLLA	None	None	3–6 mo
Magmaris[b]	Biotronik	BRS DES	Magnesium alloy	PLLA	Sirolimus	3–6 mo

[a]No longer used (Cypher was discontinued in 2011).
[b]Not approved for use in the United States.
BRS, Bioresorbable stent; *BVS,* bioresorbable vascular scaffold; *PBMA,* poly n-butyl methacrylate; *PDLLA,* poly (L-lactide-CO-D,L-lactide); *PEVA,* polyethylene-co-vinyl acetate; *PLLA,* poly-L-lactide; *PPChol,* phosphorylcholine; *PVDF-HFP,* polyvinylidene fluoride–heaxafluoropropylene; *SIBBS,* styrene-b-isobutylene-b-styrene.

Bare Metal Stents

Current bare metal stents (BMSs) are made of stainless steel, cobalt chromium, or platinum chromium. Stainless steel BMSs were the first devices used for coronary stenting. They successfully reduced the incidence of abrupt vessel closure and restenosis compared with balloon angioplasty, thereby decreasing the rate of target lesion revascularization (TLR). One advantage of BMSs is that on average, endothelial stent coverage is complete in approximately 12 weeks, which decreases the risk of ST. Nevertheless, despite refinements in stent design, significant restenosis within the stented segment develops in approximately 20% to 30% of lesions.

Current accepted indications to place a BMS include patients who are likely to be noncompliant with long-term dual antiplatelet therapy (DAPT); patients at a higher risk of bleeding, including individuals taking oral anticoagulants; and patients who are scheduled for NCS requiring cessation of antiplatelet therapy beyond 6 weeks post-PCI.

Drug-Eluting Stents

Drug-eluting stents (DESs) consist of a metallic stent platform coated with a polymer carrier vehicle that stores an antiproliferative agent. The carrier releases the drug in a gradual and controlled fashion (elution), allowing local diffusion into the vascular tissue, thus preventing excessive cell growth (neointimal hyperplasia) encroachment into the lumen in response to device implantation. DESs have been shown to outperform BMSs with respect to the rates of restenosis and TLR, particularly within the first year postimplantation. Thereafter it appears that the restenosis rate is similar between DESs and BMSs.

Older DESs (so called first generation) are composed of stainless steel platforms with thick struts and durable polymers. These have been shown to produce long-term inflammatory reactions, resulting in delayed vascular healing and endothelial stent coverage. Durable DESs (second and third generation) consist of thin cobalt or platinum chromium scaffolds coated with polymers that cause less local inflammation and interference with reendothelialization (Box 3.1).

Bioabsorbable DESs consist of either a metallic or polylactate scaffold coated with polymers. After drug elution, either the polymer or the polymer and scaffold reabsorb over time, leaving a BMS or in some instances, no stent at all.

All DESs contain a reservoir of one of two classes of antiproliferative agents to prevent vascular smooth cell replication and thus stent restenosis.

1. Sirolimus and derivatives (Everolimus, Zotarolimus, Myolimus, Neolimus, and Biolimus) have potent cytostatic properties.
2. Paclitaxel is an antineoplastic agent that stabilizes cellular microtubules before cell division, thus arresting the mitotic cell cycle.

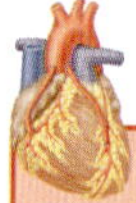

BOX 3.1   *Advantages of Second- and Third-Generation Drug-Eluting Stents*

- Improved flexibility
- Thinner struts
- Enhanced polymer biocompatibility
- Better elution kinetics

First-Generation Drug-Eluting Stents

Although widely used since first introduced in 2003, first-generation DESs are rarely used today because they have been largely replaced by safer and more refined stents. However, first-generation DESs are still represented in the majority of the existing body of literature regarding perioperative risk and management of surgical patients.

Second- and Third-Generation Drug-Eluting Stents

Second- and third-generation DESs offer numerous improvements that increase their safety profile over their first-generation counterparts. They have decreased strut thickness, improved flexibility, enhanced polymer biocompatibility and drug elution profiles, and superior reendothelialization kinetics. These devices are now the predominant coronary stents implanted worldwide.

Differences Among Drug-Eluting Stents

All DESs are superior to BMSs by reducing the incidence of restenosis and TLR, particularly at 12 months. First-generation DESs are inferior to newer DESs regarding TLR and late thrombosis. With respect to second- and third-generation DESs, very little differences in outcomes are apparent between zotarolimus and everolimus DES, although a slight decrease in ST may be associated with the cobalt chromium everolimus stents. Published data have shown that newer generation DESs are associated with lower rates of ST than BMSs.

Biodegradable Coronary Stents

Although newer generation DESs are known to be safer, the stent platform and polymer matrix are permanent. This is associated with decreased late lumen enlargement, lack of reactive vasomotion, the development of neoatherosclerosis, and the persistent risk of reintervention on the stent. A potential method to overcome these limitations would be to shorten the length of exposure to either the polymer or to the scaffold with the use of BRSs, in which either the polymer or the scaffold itself can degrade over time. The main rationale to use a bioabsorbable polymer is based on the expectation of decreased chronic inflammation and improved vascular healing. The principle behind a BRS platform is based on the fact that restenosis is uncommonly seen after 12 months after a procedure; thus the clinical need for stent scaffolding is likely to be very limited.

Some of the potential advantages of BRSs relate to restoration of normal vascular physiology of the stented segment, as well as maintaining suitability for future therapeutic options in conditions such as multivessel disease. Currently, there are four available BRSs for clinical use (see Table 3.1). Of these, only the Absorb stent has been tested in several clinical trials. Results have been somewhat concerning because of the higher incidence of complications from periprocedural myocardial infarction (MI) as well as ST during a 2-year follow-up. Earlier complications seem to be related to the fact that a different technique is required for BRS deployment compared with metallic durable DESs. The higher occurrence of long-term ST may be additionally explained by thicker struts and discontinuity of biodegradation. Table 3.2 shows the advantages and limitations of available BRSs. At present, more than 21 second-generation BRSs, with thinner struts, are being tested to overcome the drawbacks associated with first-generation BRSs.

Table 3.2	**Features of Bioabsorbable Stents**
Advantages	**Limitations**
Preservation of vessel geometry	Limited expansion during placement
Restoration of physiological vasomotion and shear stress	Risk of strut fracture
	Low tensile strength
Late luminal gain	Larger, thicker struts
Restoration of endothelial coverage	Different implantation techniques
Feasibility of noninvasive imaging	Late discontinuity
Suitability for potential future interventions	

RESPONSES TO STENT PLACEMENT

Most clinical decisions surrounding the perioperative evaluation and management of patients with coronary stents are based on the body's natural responses to the presence of a foreign body in the coronary lumen; therefore it is important to review the associated pathophysiology as well as the therapeutic interventions aimed to counteract such reactions.

Balloon dilation of an atheromatous lesion with concomitant stretching of the vascular wall initiates three sequentially distinct responses:

1. Immediate vessel recoil
2. Negative arterial remodeling
3. Neointimal hyperplasia

Elastic recoil represents the immediate shrinkage of the vessel after PCI caused by the elastic properties of the arterial wall, which usually occurs within 24 hours after the procedure. This is followed by negative remodeling, which is the process of local contraction of the arterial wall and narrowing of the lumen of the injured vascular segment. The etiology of negative remodeling is not well established but may be related to the healing process as well as interactions between the vascular endothelium and laminar flow. Neointimal hyperplasia constitutes a delayed healing response. This is represented by proliferation and migration of smooth muscle cells from the media and perhaps circulating endothelial progenitor cells from the bone marrow into the intima.

Placement of an intracoronary stent eliminates the first two processes, leaving only that of neointimal hyperplasia playing a role in normal healing as well as the exaggerated response responsible for restenosis. Additionally, unlike plain balloon angioplasty, the permanent presence of a foreign body serves as a constant stimulus for thrombus formation caused by activation of platelet function and coagulation mechanisms, which persist until complete endothelial stent coverage occurs.

STENT-RELATED COMPLICATIONS

In-Stent Restenosis

This process involves a gradual renarrowing of the stented segment or immediately proximal or distal to it because of excessive neointimal growth. Restenosis occurs because of peak neointimal thickening mostly between 4 and 12 months after stent placement.

The incidence of restenosis within the first year after PCI in patients with BMSs is approximately 20% to 30%. Thereafter, myocardial ischemia, if present, occurs mostly from progression of native vessel disease. DESs consistently reduce the incidence of in-stent restenosis and the rate of TLR by about 75%, with the benefits seen across all subgroups of patients.

Although less frequent with DES, restenosis still occurs depending on periprocedural challenges and the complexity of the initial lesions. Thus, unlike BMSs, it seems that most predictors of restenosis with DESs may relate more to lesion characteristics and technical aspects of stent deployment rather than to the clinical status of the patient.

Clinical Presentation

Stent restenosis is primarily suspected by recurrent symptoms of myocardial ischemia. The most common syndrome is that of stable or progressive angina, but up to 10% of patients present with acute MI. The diagnosis of in-stent restenosis is confirmed by coronary angiography.

Treatment

In patients who are symptomatic or fulfill anatomic criteria, repeat PCI is frequently required. Patients for whom repeat PCI is not likely to be successful should be considered candidates for surgical myocardial revascularization.

Stent Thrombosis

Definition

Thrombosis of a coronary stent is one of the most serious complications of PCI and is associated with major morbidity and mortality. It is defined as an abrupt occlusion at the site of the stent resulting from a platelet-rich thrombus, which can occur any time from the moment of stent placement to years after PCI.

Clinicians in the past have used various definitions of ST, which made interpretation of events very difficult. Since 2006, the Academic Research Consortium (ARC) has proposed criteria for the diagnosis of ST and timing of events in relation to the index procedure (Tables 3.3 and 3.4). These criteria, although imperfect, have allowed fairly consistent interpretations in comparing outcomes among different trials of DESs.

The common denominator is heightened platelet activation and aggregation by one or more of the following mechanisms (Box 3.2).

Table 3.3	Timing of Stent Thrombosis
Acute	Within 24 h of stent implantation
Subacute	From 24 h to 30 d
Late	From 30 d to 12 mo
Very late	More than 1 year

Modified from Cutlip DE, Windecker S, Mehran R, et al. Clinical end points in coronary stent trials. *Circulation.* 2007;115:2344–2351.

Table 3.4 Diagnosis of Stent Thrombosis

Definite	Angiographic evidence of stent thrombosis *and*
	Chest pain with new ECG *or* echocardiographic changes or cardiac biomarker elevation
	Pathologic evidence on autopsy
Probable	Unexplained death within 30 days of PCI
	MI in the location supplied by the stented vessel
Possible	Unexplained death >30 days after PCI

Modified from Cutlip DE, Windecker S, Mehran R, et al. Clinical end points in coronary stent trials. *Circulation* 2007;115:2344–2351.

ECG, Electrocardiogram; *MI*, myocardial infarction; *PCI*, percutaneous coronary intervention.

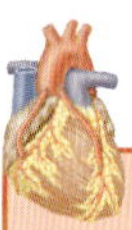

BOX 3.2 *Mechanisms of Stent Thrombosis*

- Slow blood flow around stent
- Exposure of platelets to nonendothelial surface
- Absence of or low response to platelet inhibition
- Local hypersensitivity or inflammation of the vascular wall
- Presence of neoatherosclerotic plaques

1. Persistent slow coronary flow, which may occur with wall dissection or hypoperfusion.
2. Exposure of blood elements to prothrombotic constituents in the vasculature (e.g., tissue factor, collagen) or to the stent itself before reendothelial stent coverage.
3. Failure to suppress platelet aggregation during the period of high thrombotic risk, such as premature cessation of antiplatelet therapy or drug resistance.
4. In some patients (particularly with DESs) who develop very late stent thrombosis (VLST), other factors such as hypersensitivity reactions, excessive fibrin deposits, and ruptured neoatherosclerotic plaques within the stent struts play an important role.

Timing

Most cases of ST occur within 30 days after placement irrespective of stent type, ranging from 0.5% in low-risk patients to 2.5% in high-risk patients. Episodes of ST during this period are commonly related to periprocedural complications or abrupt interruption of DAPT, such as major bleeding or emergency high-risk surgery.

Stent thrombosis with BMSs occurs much less often after 6 weeks. This observation is consistent with angioscopic studies that have shown complete reendothelialization by 3 to 6 months. VLST is even more uncommon with BMS, and it occurs most often after a repeat procedure performed in the stented segment.

Similar to BMS, most episodes of ST associated with DESs occur in the first year, with the majority of these occurring within the first 30 days after PCI. The cumulative incidence of ST with DESs at 1 year also is approximately between 0.5% and 1%. Events thereafter continue at a rate between 0.4% and 0.6% per year.

Risk Factors for Stent Thrombosis

The complex interaction among the presence of a stent, blood elements, and vascular wall is a strong stimulus for thrombus formation. Thus it is not surprising that multiple factors have been shown to predispose patients for LST and VLST (Table 3.5).

STENT TYPE

Historically, the rates of LST and VLST were highest with first-generation DESs. The risk was lowest with second- or third-generations DESs, even when compared with BMSs. Regarding BRS, the only available BRS for widespread clinical use (Absorb) has a higher thrombotic potential compared with second-generation metallic DESs.

PROCEDURE-RELATED FACTORS

Several features have been correlated with higher rates for ST such as incomplete stent apposition, persistent vessel dissection, and incomplete strut coverage. These factors highlight the importance of achieving optimal results via appropriate stent selection as well as the right technique, determined by the clinical circumstance, location, and characteristics of the lesion.

Table 3.5 Risk Factors for Stent Thrombosis

Stent Type	Procedure	Lesions	Clinical
First generation > Absorb (BRS) > BMS ≥ DES second and third generation	Stent underexpansion or malposition	Ostial, long, bifurcations, multiple stents	Premature discontinuation of DAPT
	Vessel dissection	Small vessel diameter (<2.5 mm)	Prior stent thrombosis
	Incomplete strut coverage	Overlapping stents	PCI for ACS
	Pre- or poststent vessel stenosis	Calcified lesions	Documented HTPR
	Stent deployed on necrotic plaques	Prior brachytherapy	Diabetes mellitus
		Saphenous grafts	Chronic kidney disease
			HF with low LVEF
			Cancer
			Systemic inflammatory conditions
			Cigarette smoking
			Cocaine use

ACS, Acute coronary syndrome; *BMS,* bare metal stent; *BRS,* bioresorbable stent; *DAPT,* dual antiplatelet therapy; *DES,* drug-eluting stent; *HF,* heart failure; *HTPR,* high on-treatment platelet reactivity; *LVEF,* left ventricular ejection fraction; *PCI,* percutaneous coronary intervention.

LESION-RELATED FACTORS

Lesion characteristics may present a risk for ST, for example, plaques with a necrotic-filled lipid core during acute coronary syndromes (ACSs), in which struts have demonstrated reduced neointimal coverage. Other factors include complex anatomy such as multiple lesions, small vessel size, lesions larger than 3 cm, ostial and bifurcation lesions, total occlusions, saphenous vein graft stenosis, previous ST, and prior brachytherapy.

TREATMENT-RELATED FACTORS

Undoubtedly, the single most important predictor of early and late thrombosis is premature discontinuation of DAPT (one or both drugs), presumably during the period when vascular healing is incomplete. This change is commonly related to the need to perform surgery or invasive procedures, poor patient compliance, side effects from treatment (e.g., bleeding), or economic hardship. Although the duration of such a period is still a matter of controversy, it is longer with DESs than BMSs. With any stent, the highest risk period is the first 30 days postimplantation, which correlates with the highest intensity of the inflammatory and thrombotic response within the vascular wall.

Between 1 and 6 months, the risk for ST decreases some but still remains high, particularly in patients with other risk factors. Beyond 6 months, evidence has shown no difference in the rates of ST between DES patients who underwent discontinuation of DAPT (while continuing aspirin [ASA]) compared with those who did not. With current-generation stents, it appears that discontinuation of $P2Y_{12}$ receptor blocker even after 3 to 6 months is relatively safe in selected patients, but DAPT of long duration may be indicated for those with persistent ischemic or thrombotic burden. The timing of LST or VLST during discontinuation of DAPT ranges from a few days to several months, depending on the agent discontinued and additional risk factors contributing to a prothrombotic state (e.g., surgery).

MEDICAL COMORBIDITIES

Patients shown to be at increased risk for ST include those with diabetes mellitus, particularly those with insulin deficiency, chronic kidney disease, heart failure with systolic dysfunction, malignancy, low response to platelet inhibitors, cigarette smoking, and cocaine use. The etiology is multifactorial, and mechanisms include increased platelet turnover, vascular inflammation, decreased endothelial nitric oxide production, overexpression of platelet receptors, deficient antithrombotic pathways, bypass of pathways blocked by antiplatelet agents, impaired fibrinolysis, and vascular constriction.

Management

Management of patients with ST requires the immediate recanalization of the occluded artery by aspiration of the mural thrombus and restenting the vessel. With emergency surgical intervention reserved for those in whom successful PCI may be unlikely, many practitioners will perform intravascular ultrasound-guided stent sizing and confirm complete stent apposition. Patients with ST while taking clopidogrel are at increased risk for recurrent events. Often clopidogrel is exchanged for a different agent such as prasugrel or ticagrelor.

Outcome

The consequences of ST can be devastating, thus highlighting the importance of timely intervention. Reported acute mortality of patients with coronary ST presenting as ST-segment elevation myocardial infarction (STEMI) is more than 50% and for survivors is between 20% and 25% at 6 months. Furthermore, the incidence of recurrent

ST is approximately 10% to 12%. Compared with patients with native lesions, treatment of patients with ST seems to be associated with less procedural long-term success.

ANTIPLATELET THERAPY

Numerous pathways and platelet membrane receptors play important roles in the activation phase that may lead to ST, thus providing pharmacologic targets for APT (Fig. 3.1). Currently, those available for platelet inhibition in patients with coronary stents include (1) activation of cyclooxygenase 1 (COX1) responsible for the production of thromboxane A_2 (TxA$_2$); (2) adenosine-induced activation of membrane purinergic receptors P2X$_1$, P2Y$_1$, and P2Y$_{12}$; (3) activation of protease-activated receptors (PARs) by thrombin; and (4) active expression of membrane glycoprotein (GP) IIb/IIIa receptors (Box 3.3). Agents targeting other platelet receptors or pathways have been synthesized, but they have been found to be ineffective (e.g., dipyridamole) or are at an early stage of development (e.g., picotamide, terutroban).

Currently, several platelet inhibitors are used in the management of coronary stents (Table 3.6).

Oral Antiplatelet Agents

Aspirin

Aspirin specifically and irreversibly inhibits platelet COX1, thereby blocking the production of TxA$_2$ through this pathway and thus rendering platelets incapable of

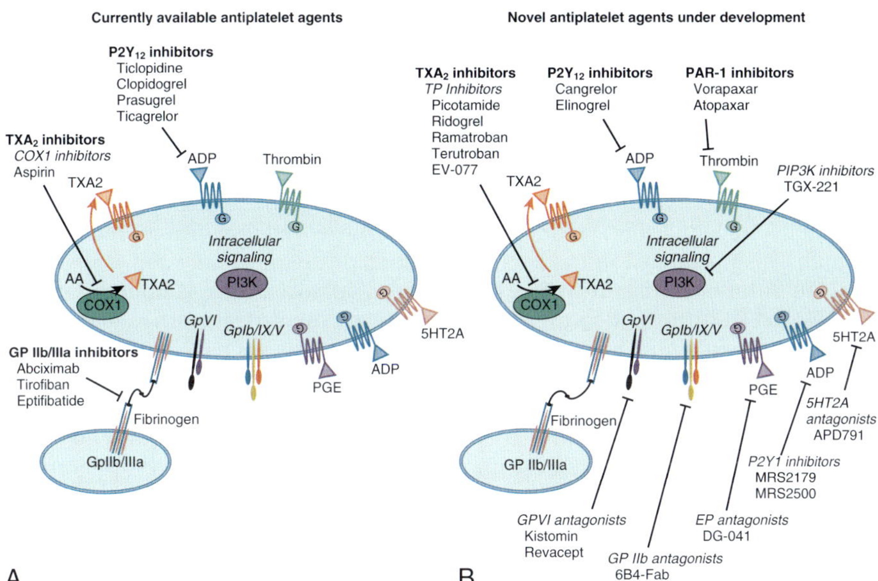

Fig. 3.1 Sites of action of antiplatelet agents. (A) Currently available agents for acute coronary syndromes or percutaneous coronary intervention. (B) Novel antiplatelet agents under development. Vorapaxar and cangrelor are now available for clinical use. *AA,* Arachidonic acid; *ADP,* adenosine diphosphate; *COX1,* cyclooxygenase-1; *EP,* prostaglandin receptor; *5HT2A,* serotonin; *G,* g-protein; *GP,* glycoprotein; *PG,* prostaglandin; *PAR-1,* platelet protease-activated receptor-1; *PGE,* prostaglandin E; *PI3K,* phosphatidylinositol 3-kinase; *TP,* thromboxane receptor; *TxA$_2$,* thromboxane A$_2$. (From Ferreiro JL, Angiolillo DM. New directions in antiplatelet therapy. *Circ Cardiovasc Interv.* 2012;5:433–435.)

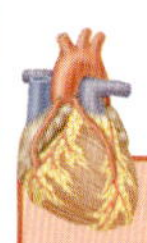

> ### BOX 3.3 *Mechanism of Action of Antiplatelet Agents Used With Coronary Stents*
>
> - ASA: irreversible inhibition of COX1
> - Clopidogrel and prasugrel: irreversible binding of $P2Y_{12}$ receptors via active metabolite
> - Ticagrelor and cangrelor: reversible binding of $P2Y_{12}$ receptors
> - Vorapaxar: reversible binding of PAR1 receptors
> - Abciximab, tirofiban, eptifibatide: reversible binding of GP IIb/IIIa receptors
>
> *ASA,* Aspirin; *COX1,* cyclooxygenase 1; *GP,* glycoprotein; *PAR1,* protease-activated receptor 1.

functioning normally. At higher doses, ASA also inhibits COX2-dependent prostacyclin synthesis in the endothelial cell. Other effects of ASA include enhanced fibrinolysis and antioxidant, antiinflammatory, and antiatherosclerotic effects on endothelial cells and leukocytes.

In normal subjects, a single dose of 30 mg of ASA is enough to produce complete and irreversible inactivation of COX1, with a ceiling effect observed on platelet activity with doses beyond 300 mg. The current recommended dose to exert a fully antithrombotic effect is between 75 and 150 mg/day.

Plain ASA is rapidly absorbed through the gastric and enteric mucosae; peak plasma levels are seen within 30 or 40 minutes with a serum half-life of 15 to 20 minutes. Because the effects of ASA are irreversible, they last for the life of the platelet ($\approx$7–10 days); thus once-a-day dosing is sufficient to sustain platelet inhibition. However, enteric-coated preparations are associated with longer absorption time, reaching peak plasma levels between 2 and 4 hours postingestion.

After a single dose of ASA, platelet production begins to recover. Approximately 10% of new platelets are released from the bone marrow each day, with full replacement of ASA free platelets within 10 days after discontinuing the drug. Such platelets tend to exhibit a "rebound effect" characterized by an exaggerated response to procoagulant stimuli. This phenomenon has been demonstrated experimentally and may in fact increase thrombotic risk in certain populations. Moreover, there is no need to wait for full platelet turnover because normal hemostasis can be seen with as few as 20% of platelets maintaining normal COX1 activity. Many subjects have 80% normalized platelet function more than 72 hours from their last ASA dose.

When compared with other platelet antagonists, ASA is comparatively weak. Nevertheless, its benefits in risk reduction against MI in patients with established coronary artery disease (CAD) are undeniable. Currently, the strongest indications for chronic ASA include secondary prevention of CAD and post-PCI patients. The latter is the cornerstone for DAPT and for lifelong monotherapy in most patients unless contraindicated.

Adenosine Receptor Antagonists

Current available drugs for clinical use are the thienopyridines, clopidogrel and prasugrel, and the nucleoside analog ticagrelor. All three share a common mechanism of action (binding to the $P2Y_{12}$ platelet receptor), yet there is major pharmacokinetic variability among them (Fig. 3.2). These differences translate into significant clinical differences regarding efficacy and bleeding risk.

Table 3.6 Antiplatelet Agents

Oral

Drug	Target	Mechanism	Loading Dose (mg)	Time to Maximum IPA (%)	Maintenance Dose	Plasma Half-Life	Time to Platelet Recovery for Adequate Hemostasis Upon Drug Cessation
ASA	COX1	Irreversible inhibition	325	30 min	80–325 mg/d	15–30 min	5–7 d
Clopidogrel	$P2Y_{12}$ receptor	Irreversible binding	300–600	6 h (37%)	75–150 mg/d	6-8 h	5 d
Prasugrel	$P2Y_{12}$ receptor	Irreversible binding	60	4 h (85%)	5–10 mg/d	7–9 h	5–7 d
Ticagrelor	$P2Y_{12}$ receptor	Reversible binding	180	2 h (88%)	90 mg twice daily	8 h	3–5 d
Vorapaxar	PAR1 receptor	Reversible binding	40	2 h (80%)	2.5 mg/d	4–13 d	Weeks

Intravenous

Drug	Target	Mechanism	Loading Dose	Time to Maximum IPA (%)	Maintenance Infusion	Plasma Half-Life	Time to Platelet Recovery for Adequate Hemostasis Upon Drug Cessation
Abciximab	GP IIb/IIIa receptor	Reversible binding	250 µg/kg	Immediate (80%)	125 µg/kg/min	10–15 min	12 h
Eptifibatide	GP IIb/IIIa receptor	Reversible binding	180 µg/kg	15 min (80%)	2 µg/kg/min	2.5 h	4–8 h
Tirofiban	GP IIb/IIIa receptor	Reversible binding	0.4 µg/kg	5 min (80%)	0.1–0.15 µg/kg/min	1.5–2.5 h	4–6 h
Cangrelor	$P2Y_{12}$ receptor	Reversible binding	30 µg/kg	<5 min (80%)	2 µg/kg/min	<5 min	60–90 min

ASA, Aspirin; *COX1,* cyclooxygenase 1; *GP,* glycoprotein; *IPA,* inhibition of platelet aggregation; *PAR1,* protease-activated receptor 1.

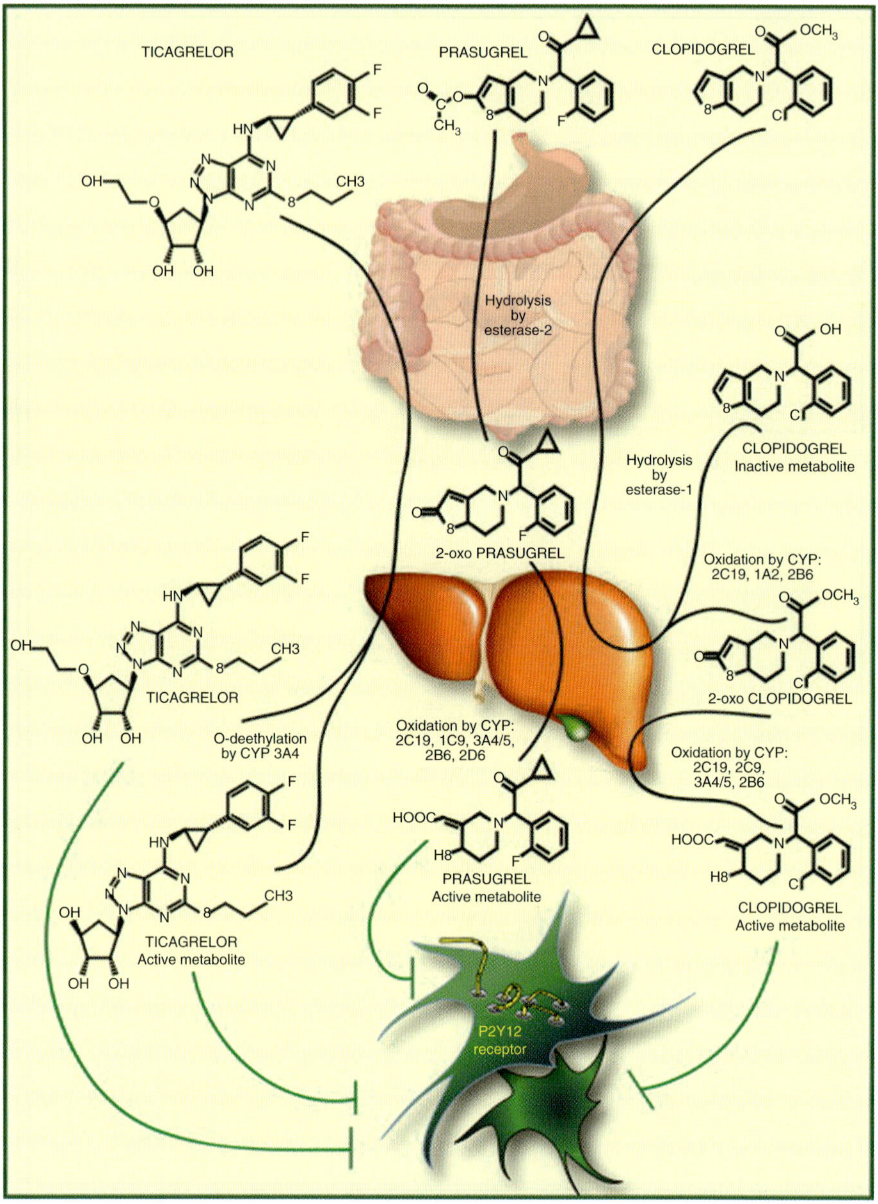

Fig. 3.2 Metabolic pathways of adenosine diphosphate receptor (ADP) blockers. The actions of clopidogrel and prasugrel depend on hepatic biotransformation to an active metabolite, which binds irreversibly to the platelet P2Y$_{12}$ receptor. In contrast, both ticagrelor and its active metabolite bind to the P2Y$_{12}$ receptor in a reversible fashion. *CYP,* Cytochrome P450. (From Siller-Matula JM, Trenk D, Schror K, et al. Response variability to P2Y12 receptor inhibitor: expectations and reality. *JACC Cardiovasc Interv.* 2013;6:1111–1128.)

CLOPIDOGREL

Clopidogrel is a second-generation thienopyridine (the first-generation thienopyridine, ticlopidine, is no longer used because of concerns of toxicity). Ingested clopidogrel acts as a prodrug whose active thiol metabolite binds permanently to the $P2Y_{12}$ platelet receptor, thus preventing adenosine diphosphate (ADP)–mediated platelet activation. Platelets blocked by clopidogrel remain so for the remainder of their 7- to 10-day lifespan.

After a loading dose of 300 to 600 mg, the time to maximum inhibition of platelet aggregation (IPA) (37% inhibition) is 6 hours. The parent compound is absorbed in the intestine, after which it is carried to the liver, where 85% is hydrolyzed to an inactive metabolite by liver esterases. The other 15% must undergo a two-step enzymatic process via the actions of several isoenzymes of cytochrome p450, predominantly by the actions of CYP 2C19 and CYP3A4. Elimination of the parent drug is in 6 hours and of the active metabolite about 30 minutes. Approximately 50% of the drug is eliminated in urine and 45% in feces.

Disadvantages of clopidogrel include the many possible interactions, which can interfere with the drug's antiplatelet ability. Different genetic polymorphisms involved in clopidogrel biotransformation or the platelet receptor's response and interactions with commonly prescribed drugs yield a certain degree of unpredictability, resulting in either an increased risk for thrombosis or bleeding. Despite its inherent limitations and modest antiplatelet effects, clopidogrel is the $P2Y_{12}$ receptor antagonist of choice in most patients because of its proven efficacy in many clinical studies. It is considered the standard component with ASA as part of DAPT.

Upon discontinuation of clopidogrel, complete platelet recovery is expected within 7 days, but appreciable platelet aggregation is already noticed by 72 hours. A phenomenon of platelet rebound has been described associated with an increased prothrombotic state. The etiology is likely multifactorial, and its clinical significance is unclear, but an increased risk for ischemic syndromes has been reported.

PRASUGREL

Prasugrel is a third-generation thienopyridine. Similar to clopidogrel, prasugrel must be biotransformed into an active metabolite to achieve its antiplatelet effect. The inhibition of the $P2Y_{12}$ receptor is also irreversible and thus lasts for the lifespan of the platelet.

Prasugrel undergoes hydrolysis in the liver, and CYP elements assist in biotransformation to the active metabolite. However, this drug is less subject to interference with other agents, and important genetic polymorphisms that seriously affect its metabolism are less frequent. The end result is a more predictable and potent antiplatelet effect. The time to maximal IPA (85% inhibition) achieved after a loading dose of 60 mg of prasugrel is approximately 4 hours. The maintenance dose is 10 mg/day. To decrease bleeding risk, certain groups of patients, such as those older than 65 years and less than 60 kg in weight, require reduced doses of 5 mg/day. Prasugrel is eliminated primarily by the kidneys. Upon discontinuation of the drug, platelets fully recover within 7 to 10 days, reflecting new platelet production.

The most common side effect is bleeding. This drug is contraindicated in patients with history of transient ischemic attack or stroke or active pathologic bleeding. Although less common than with clopidogrel, platelet hyporesponsiveness has been described in some patients receiving maintenance doses of prasugrel.

Prasugrel is superior to clopidogrel in reducing the incidence of LT and VLT; however, this improvement occurs at the expense of increased bleeding, which may necessitate discontinuation of the drug.

TICAGRELOR

This drug represents a nonthienopyridine class of ADP receptor antagonist. Ticagrelor does not require conversion to an active metabolite to produce IPA. Its effects are more potent than those exerted by thienopyridines Because of its reversible interaction with the $P2Y_{12}$ receptor, recovery of platelet function is likely with decreased serum concentrations of the drug.

After a 180-mg loading dose of ticagrelor, the time to maximum IPA (88% inhibition) is 2 hours, which may be maintained up to 8 hours. The maintenance dose is 90 mg twice a day. Less than 10% IPA is seen 5 days after discontinuation of the drug. The main route of elimination is enteric, with a lower percentage via the urine.

In clinical trials, ticagrelor has been shown to be superior to clopidogrel or prasugrel in the prevention of ST, at the expense of a higher risk for bleeding. It is also the agent of choice during PCI for STEMI. This drug is contraindicated in patients with a history of active bleeding or intracranial hemorrhage. Patients may also experience dyspnea caused by an apparent mild autoimmune response. When given in combination with ASA as part of DAPT, the dose of ASA should not exceed 100 mg because higher doses are associated with decreased effectiveness. The mechanism of this blunted response is currently unknown.

Protease-Activated Receptor-1 Receptor Antagonists

The importance of thrombin in platelet aggregation via interaction with PAR receptors has led to efforts to synthetize inhibitors to provide additional benefits over standard APT. Although multiple compounds have been synthetized, only one, vorapaxar, has been approved for clinical use. Its mechanism of action is by high-affinity yet reversible attachment to the PAR-1 platelet receptor, thus preventing granule procoagulant release without interfering with thrombin-induced fibrin formation.

Unlike thienopyridines, vorapaxar does not require biotransformation into an active metabolite. A full inhibitor effect (>80% platelet activity inhibition) is reached after a loading dose of 40 mg. When a maintenance dose of 2.5 mg is administered for several days, platelets are effectively inhibited for 4 weeks.

Vorapaxar is rapidly absorbed through the intestine and undergoes biotransformation by CYP 3A4, mainly into an inactive metabolite. However, with prolonged dosing, an active metabolite (M20) becomes relevant, representing up to 25% of the parent compound.

The drug is primarily eliminated as the inactive metabolite and has a plasma half-life of 5 to 13 days, with no significant accumulation in the presence of kidney or liver disease. When added to a preexisting regimen of ASA and clopidogrel, vorapaxar reduces the risk of thrombotic events, albeit at the risk of significant bleeding (particularly intracerebral hemorrhage) in certain populations. Its long half-life may represent a challenge in management for patients undergoing NCS because it may require discontinuing the drug several weeks before the procedure.

Intravenous Antiplatelet Agents

Glycoprotein IIb/IIIa Receptor Inhibitors

Glycoprotein IIb/IIIa inhibitors bind to the receptor, thus impairing platelet-dependent thrombogenesis caused by cross-linkage between neighboring platelets. Currently, three molecularly distinct agents are approved for clinical use as adjunctive therapy during PCI or ACS.

ABCIXIMAB

This is a monoclonal Fab molecule that binds with high affinity to the GP inhibitor receptor. When given as a bolus dose of 0.25 mg/kg or as a continuous infusion of

0.125 µg/kg per minute, maximum IPA (80% inhibition) is achieved almost immediately. The serum half-life of the drug is 10 to 15 minutes, but recovery of platelet function is not seen until 48 hours because of slow dissociation of the drug from platelets. In the presence of ADP antagonists, the effects can last up to 15 days after the drug is discontinued. Because very little free drug is present in the blood, platelet inhibition can rapidly be reversed with platelet transfusions.

EPTIFIBATIDE

A cyclic peptide, this drug produces selective inhibition. With a loading dose of 180 µg/kg and a continuous infusion of 2 µg/kg per minute, the time to maximum IPA (80% inhibition) is about 15 minutes. The serum half-life is approximately 2.5 hours, and it undergoes renal elimination. Eptifibatide dissociates rapidly from platelets; thus free drug is likely to be present for several hours after its discontinuation. Transfusion of platelets is not likely to be helpful in reversing platelet inhibition because free circulating drug will rapidly bind to the new platelets. Drug reversal in this case is achieved primarily by stopping the medication and may take several hours.

TIROFIBAN

Tirofiban is a small, nonpeptide antagonist that causes rapid (5 minutes) selective blockade of GP IIb/IIIa receptors. The usual loading dose is 0.4 µg/kg followed by a continuous infusion of 0.1 to 0.15 µg/kg per minute. The serum half-life is 1.5 to 2 hours, and the primary elimination route is by the kidney. Four hours after discontinuation, less than 20% platelet inhibition remains. Tirofiban also dissociates rapidly from platelets, so the main approach for return of platelet function is stopping the drug.

Adenosine Diphosphate Antagonists

CANGRELOR

This drug is an intravenous (IV) analog of ticagrelor and produces selective and reversible inhibition of the $P2Y_{12}$ receptor. Its major advantages are its rapid onset and short duration of action, both of which are desirable properties during acute interventions. With a loading dose of 30 µg/kg followed by a steady-state infusion of 2 to 4 µg/kg per minute, it produces 80% platelet inhibition within less than 5 minutes. Upon discontinuation, cangrelor is rapidly deactivated by serum ectonucleotidases, resulting in a serum half-life of 2 to 5 minutes. Complete platelet recovery occurs within 60 to 90 minutes. In cardiac surgical patients, preoperative use of cangrelor has shown a positive association with decreased postoperative chest tube drainage. No studies have been performed in patients undergoing NCS, although its use is theoretically appealing for bridging high-risk patients.

LONG-TERM ANTIPLATELET MANAGEMENT

Dual Antiplatelet Therapy

The majority of patients undergoing coronary stenting require DAPT to protect the stented vascular segment from ST while vascular healing occurs. Evidence shows adverse outcomes, including ST, when DAPT is discontinued during the period of time when incomplete endothelialization is likely.

Unlike the incidence of restenosis, which peaks several months after PCI, the long-term cumulative incidence of ST seems to be similar whether BMSs or DESs are used, as long as patients are treated with DAPT for the recommended duration of therapy, which is influenced by additional risk factors for ST (Fig. 3.3). In general,

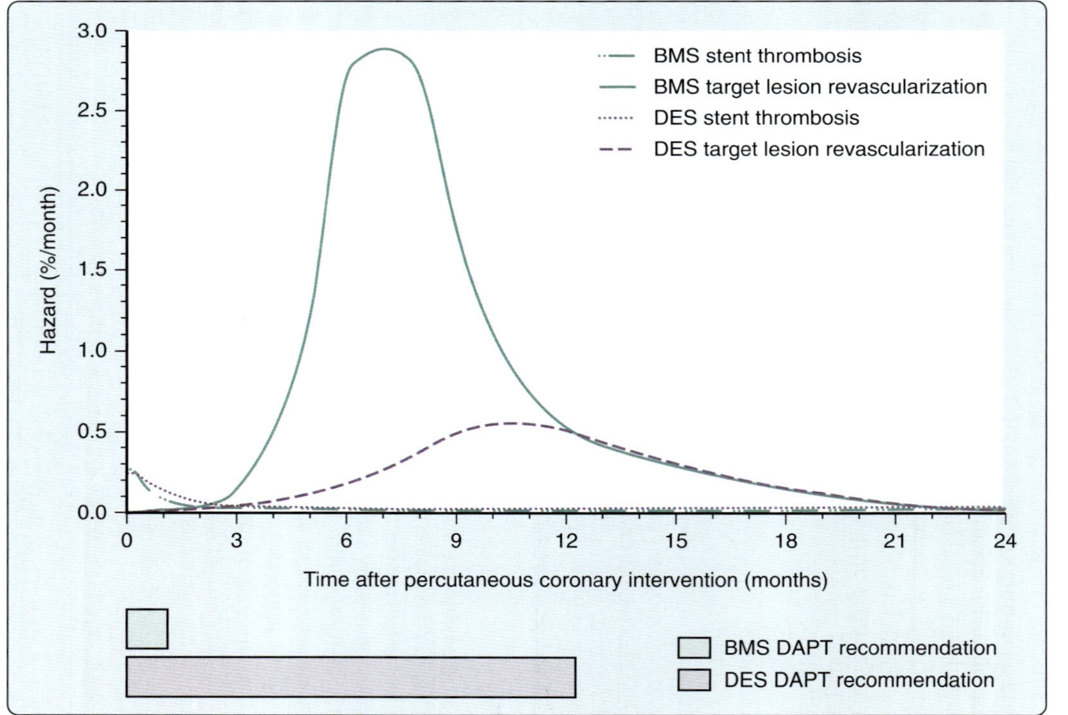

Fig. 3.3 Hazard of stent thrombosis and target lesion revascularization over time according to type of stent. *BMS,* Bare metal stent; *DAPT,* dual antiplatelet therapy; *DES,* drug-eluting stent. (From Mathew A, Mauri L. Optimal timing of noncardiac surgery after stents. *Circulation* 2012;126:1322–1324.)

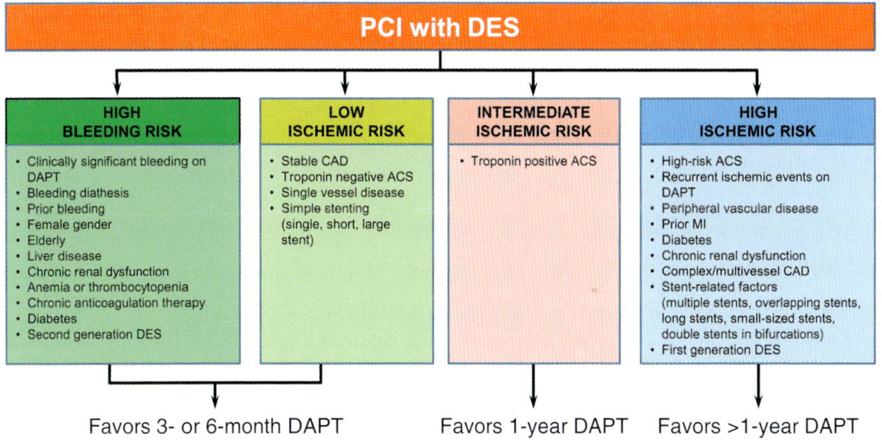

Fig. 3.4 Evaluation of bleeding and ischemic risk factors related to dual antiplatelet therapy (DAPT) after drug-eluting stent implantation. *ACS,* Acute coronary syndrome; *CAD,* coronary artery disease; *DES,* drug-eluting stent; *MI,* myocardial infarction; *PCI,* percutaneous coronary intervention. (From Palmerini T, Stone GW. Optimal duration of dual antiplatelet therapy after drug-eluting stent implantation: conceptual evolution based on emerging evidence. *Eur Heart J.* 2016;37:353–364.)

DAPT for most patients refers to the combination of ASA and clopidogrel, with ASA to be taken indefinitely after PCI regardless of stent type. Patients receiving BMSs for non-ACS indications should undergo DAPT at least for 4 to 6 weeks or even longer if tolerated. For second- and third-generation DESs, several studies have shown that in low-risk patients with SIDH, DAPT can be discontinued after 6 or even 3 months, without an increase in ischemic syndromes while minimizing bleeding complications. DAPT beyond 1 year may be indicated for those with increased ischemic burden because thrombotic risk exceeds that of bleeding-related complications. Patients after PCI for ACS must receive DAPT for 1 year regardless of the stent type, with DES patients remaining on DAPT even longer if tolerated. This approach is currently recommended by the most recent focused updates Additionally, certain groups that are more likely to benefit from prolonged DAPT include those with high-risk clinical factors for ST, patients undergoing complex PCI, and those receiving first-generation BRSs (e.g., Absorb). The decision regarding DAPT duration in an individual patient must be based on balancing thrombotic and hemorrhagic risks (Fig. 3.4). Most experts recommend clopidogrel as the initial drug in stable patients, with prasugrel and ticagrelor reserved for patients with ACS or those deemed nonresponsive to clopidogrel.

Triple Antithrombotic Therapy

Current estimates are that 5% to 10% of patients undergoing coronary stent placement are or will require oral anticoagulant therapy. The three most common indications are stroke prevention in patients with atrial fibrillation, prevention of recurrent deep vein thrombosis or pulmonary embolism, and mechanical heart valves. Management of these patients is extremely challenging and largely based on scarce evidence and expert opinion, with most preferring placement of BMSs.

Current recommendations are that for elective procedures in patients with low or intermediate risk of bleeding, triple antithrombotic therapy (DAPT plus an oral anticoagulant) is recommended for 1 month if undergoing BMS, followed by up to 12 months with single antiplatelet agent plus the oral anticoagulant. For patients with

DESs, triple antithrombotic therapy is recommended for 3 to 6 months, followed by 12 months of anticoagulant therapy with either clopidogrel or ASA. In general, oral anticoagulants plus one single antiplatelet agent with careful monitoring of international normalized ratio is preferable to DAPT. After 12 months in patients requiring lifetime oral anticoagulant therapy, low-dose ASA is preferred over an ADP antagonist.

Variability in Patients' Response to Antiplatelet Therapy

Optimal use of DAPT with ASA and clopidogrel does not ensure that the patient will not experience ST. In fact, several cases of early or subacute and LST have been known to occur while on DAPT, including throughout the perioperative period.

In these patients, it is likely that the presence of a high prothrombotic environment makes it difficult for DAPT to be fully effective. Some patients, however, may also exhibit what has been coined "high on-treatment platelet reactivity" (HTPR) caused by variable efficacy of the antiplatelet drugs, leading to clinical treatment failure (Box 3.4). There seems to be strong association between HTPR and post-PCI ischemic events such as ST. On the other hand, certain patients exhibit an exaggerated response to ADP antagonists (particularly prasugrel and ticagrelor) and are labeled to have low platelet reactivity (LPR). These patients frequently exhibit bleeding complications (perhaps excessive surgical bleeding) with standard doses of platelet inhibitors.

Response to Aspirin

Variability in the response to ASA, in which thrombotic events occur despite the use of the drug, has been known for many years. When defined by clinical events, the incidence of ASA resistance has been estimated to be approximately 13%; however, when based on laboratory tests, it ranges between 5.5% and 60%, depending on the assay used. A strict definition of "resistance" consists of the inability of ASA to inhibit platelet COX1, thus preventing TxA_2 production measured directly by laboratory methods. When analyzing ST or ischemic syndromes within a patient population, a better term is to label such individuals as nonresponsive or treatment failure.

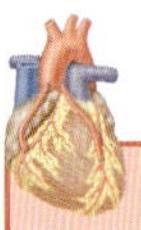

BOX 3.4   *Causes of High on-Treatment Platelet Reactivity*

- Noncompliance with antiplatelet agents
- Drug interactions (nonsteroidal antiinflammatory drugs, proton pump inhibitors)
- Pharmacokinetic variants (e.g., CYP 2C19)
- Platelet receptor and enzyme polymorphisms
- Clinical conditions
  - Diabetes mellitus
  - Obesity
  - Congestive heart failure
  - Chronic kidney dysfunction
  - Old age
  - Chronic smoking
  - Cocaine use

Evidence from real-world experience has demonstrated that the most common etiology of nonresponsiveness to ASA is poor patient compliance. Consequently, when compliance is assured, this phenomenon is significantly reduced.

In patients known to be compliant, several reasons can explain why they might be at risk for ST. The presence of multiple pathways for platelet aggregation independent of COX1-induced TxA_2 production can override the effects of ASA despite effective inhibition of COX1, particularly in a prothrombotic environment such as surgery. In addition, many chronic clinical conditions are associated with HTPR independent of ASA therapy (Box 3.4). While on ASA, failure to inhibit COX1 function can be caused by either pharmacokinetic or pharmacodynamic factors. Pharmacokinetic elements limit drug bioavailability because of poor absorption of the drug as with enteric preparations, increased inactivation by gastrointestinal esterases by proton pump inhibitors, increased volume of distribution (e.g., obesity), or interaction with other COX1 inhibitors such as ibuprofen and other nonsteroidal antiinflammatory drugs (NSAIDs) that compete with ASA for the COX1 binding site. Pharmacodynamic resistance is related to genetic polymorphisms of COX1 that decrease the inhibitory response to ASA.

The first steps in management of a patient with apparent nonresponse to ASA are to address issues of compliance, avoid PPIs if possible, and delay the intake of NSAIDs. In addition, better control of comorbidities, weight loss, and cessation of smoking decrease platelet activity. Use of nonenteric preparations and a higher dose of ASA may increase effectiveness in some patients (e.g., obesity, chronic inflammation), and twice-a-day dosing may prove more efficacious in conditions of high platelet turnover such as diabetes. Last, the addition of another antiplatelet agent may be indicated.

Response to Adenosine Antagonists

Between 25% and 50% of individuals taking clopidogrel exhibit HTPR, which has a strong association with ischemic events. This phenomenon has also been shown, although less commonly, with prasugrel and ticagrelor.

When issues of noncompliance are excluded, poor response to these agents is more often due to abnormal absorption, biotransformation, or the presence of interaction with other drugs (e.g., statins and proton pump inhibitors). As with ASA, clinical factors such as diabetes, obesity, renal failure, age, hyperlipidemia, heart failure, and the presence of ACS can trigger platelet reactivity independent of the ADP pathway.

Management of patients exhibiting thrombotic events while on clopidogrel usually consists of switching to a more potent drug such as prasugrel or ticagrelor. Some clinicians test for HTPR and decide on treatment accordingly. Hyporesponsiveness in the absence of ACS may sometimes be reversed by removing adverse drug interactions or increasing the maintenance dose of clopidogrel, although this approach seems to be effective in only some patients.

The incidence of HTPR among the three available $P2Y_{12}$ inhibitors appears to be lowest in patients taking ticagrelor followed by prasugrel, with clopidogrel being the least effective at either standard or high maintenance doses.

Platelet Function Tests

Because response to antiplatelet drugs varies from one patient to another, platelet function tests represent an attractive strategy to optimize antiplatelet therapy. A host of platelet function tests of varying specificity and sensitivity are available, each with its own advantages and disadvantages (Table 3.7).

Table 3.7 Tests to Measure Platelet Function in Patients

Test	Measurement	Advantages	Disadvantages
Light transmission aggregometry	Platelet aggregation	Gold standard	Needs plasma, time consuming, high sample volume
Impedance aggregometry	Platelet aggregation	Measures smaller platelet aggregates than with light transmission	Time consuming, high sample volume
VerifyNow	Platelet aggregation	Point of care	Limited hematocrit and platelet count range
Plateletworks	Platelet aggregation	Minimal sample prep	Not enough experience
TEG platelet mapping system	Platelet contribution to clot strength	Clot information	Limited studies
Impact cone and plate analyzer	Shear-induced platelet adhesion	Point of care	Not widely used
PFA-100	High shear blood cessation by platelet plug	Point of care	Depends on hematocrit, von Willebrand factor; lack of correlation with thienopyridines
VASP	Platelet $P2Y_{12}$ receptor activation signaling	Specific for ADP antagonists	Requires flow cytometer and experienced technician
Serum thromboxane B_2	Activation-dependent release from platelets	Relates to ASA inhibition of COX1	Indirect measure, not platelet specific
Urinary 11-dehydro-thromboxane B_2	Urinary metabolite of thromboxane B_2	Relates to ASA inhibition of COX1	Indirect measure, not platelet specific

ADP, Adenosine diphosphate; *ASA*, aspirin; *COX1*, cyclooxygenase 1; *VASP*, vasodilator-associated phosphoprotein.

Modified from Michelson AD. Methods for the measurement of Platelet Function. *Am J Cardiol.* 2009;103(suppl 2):20A–26A.

Platelet function tests more commonly used to evaluate antiplatelet agents during clinical trials of coronary stents include:

1. **VerifyNow** (Accumetrics) is a point-of-care device based on GP IIb/IIIa receptor–dependent platelet aggregation, augmented by the presence of fibrinogen-coated beads. It requires only a small sample of anticoagulated whole blood, and it can be performed rapidly. Results are expressed in platelet reactive units (PRUs). Whereas ASA response is measured with the use of a cartridge containing arachidonic acid, an ADP cartridge is used to test the effects of ADP antagonists. Values greater than 550 PRUs with ASA and greater than 208 PRUs with $P2Y_{12}$ inhibitors are considered diagnostic of HTPR. A response of less than 85 PRUs with ADP suggests LPR (Box 3.5).

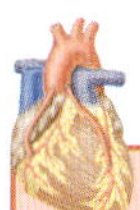

> **BOX 3.5** *Cutoff Values of High and Low Platelet Reactivity With Commonly Used Platelet Function Tests*
>
> - VerifyNow: ASA >550 PRUs; $P2Y_{12}$ inhibitors >208 PRUs or <85 PRUs
> - TEG: MA >47 mm or <30 mm
> - Multiplate analyzer: >46 AU or <19 AU
> - VASP-P: >50% PRI or <16% PRI
>
> *ASA,* Aspirin; *MA,* maximum amplitude; *PRI,* platelet reactivity index; *PRU,* platelet reactive units; *TEG,* thromboelastography; *VASP-P,* phosphorylation of vasodilator-associated phosphoprotein.

2. **Thromboelastography** (TEG; haemoscope) with platelet mapping system: Updated to a more platelet-specific test in the form of the TEG platelet mapping system, this test has been used to evaluate the effects of antiplatelet therapy and requires whole blood. A particular advantage is that it measures platelet function and the platelet contribution to clot strength. Its disadvantages are that it is not a true point-of-care instrument, and experience with it is limited. Within a TEG trace, the maximum amplitude reflects platelet function. HTPR to ADP antagonists is said to occur if the maximum amplitude ADP is greater than 47 mm and the LPR is less than 30 mm.

3. **Multiplate analyzer** (Roche Diagnostics): This is a point-of-care method that measures GP IIB/IIIA integrin-dependent platelet aggregation by changes in electrical impedance, as platelets attach to electrodes in plates containing different agonists (collagen, AA, ADP). The increase in impedance is measured by arbitrary aggregation units (AUs) plotted against time. Greater than 46 AU is associated with HTPR and less than 19 AU with LPR.

4. **Phosphorylation of vasodilator-associated phosphoprotein** (VASP-P; Biocytex) This test uses prostaglandin E, which binds to its platelet membrane receptor, thus triggering the production of cyclic adenosine monophosphate (cAMP) by activation of adenylyl cyclase, which through protein kinase A, converts VASP to phosphorylated VASP (VASP-P). Binding of ADP to the $P2Y_{12}$ receptor inhibits adenylyl cyclase, decreasing intracellular cAMP, thus preventing the formation of VASP-P. In the presence of a $P2Y_{12}$ receptor inhibitor, the level of VASP-P will increase as measured by whole-blood flow cytometry. Results are expressed in terms of platelet reactivity index (PRI). The platelet reactivity cutoff of more than 50% implies HTPR, and lower than 16% suggests LPR. The principal advantage of this test is that it is the most sensitive assay for $P2Y_{12}$ receptor signaling. The disadvantages include the number of steps involved and requirements for flow cytometry equipment and experienced technicians.

Use of Platelet Function Tests

Current recommendations are against the routine use of platelet function tests (PFTs) in post-PCI patients as a result of prospective randomized trials showing the lack of benefit of personalized therapy based on results of platelet function. However, a large number of observational studies have demonstrated that HTPR during clopidogrel treatment represents a strong and independent risk factor for ST. PFTs may be considered in selective patients thought to exhibit HTPR (e.g., patients with type 1 diabetes or history of prior ST), thus allowing a switch to more potent agents such as prasugrel or ticagrelor.

Another potential advantage for PFTs is the capability to tailor antiplatelet management in the perioperative period, thereby reducing preoperative waiting time, compared with recommended guidelines. Although currently no studies evaluating such an approach in NCS are available, preliminary data have shown that testing for platelet reactivity before coronary artery bypass surgery led to improved times to surgery and less postoperative transfusion. PFTs are currently endorsed for selected patients by the Society of Thoracic and Cardiovascular Surgeons.

Studies using receiver operating characteristic analysis to define a threshold or cutoff value largely depend on the patients studied. Reported indicators of HTPR have a very negative predictive value for thrombotic events, yet their positive predictive value is low. This observation is consistent with the fact that HTPR, although an important determinant, is not the sole factor responsible for thrombotic events. Moreover, current evidence suggests that there may be a ceiling effect in decreasing the incidence of ST, while the risk of bleeding may be heightened. Thus the focus has shifted to finding strategies that could avoid excessive bleeding while maintaining the benefit of reduced ischemic thrombotic events. A model of a therapeutic window of platelet reactivity has been suggested in which an optimal balance between the risk of bleeding and ST is achieved. This approach in theory should help to design better APT (Fig. 3.5).

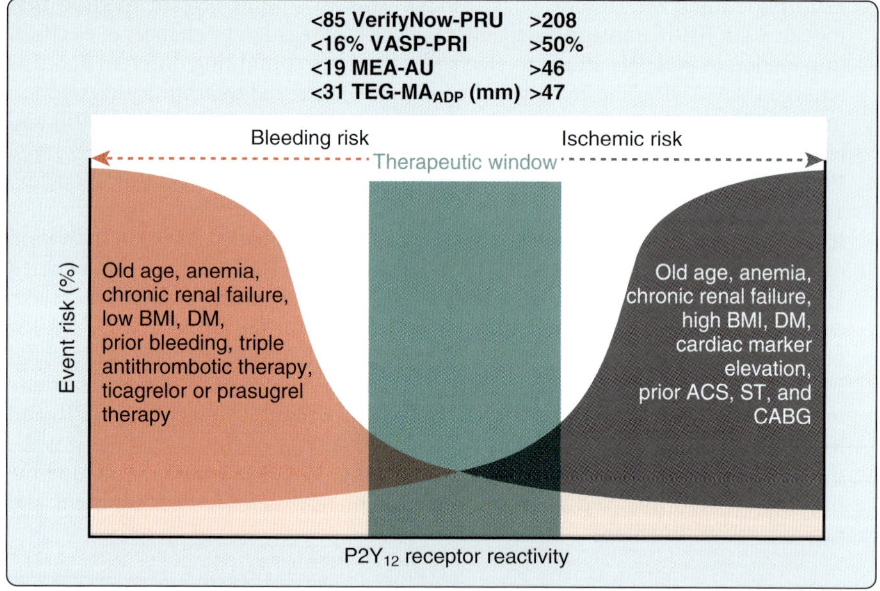

Fig. 3.5 Evidence for P2Y$_{12}$ receptor reactivity with either post–percutaneous intervention (PCI) ischemic (gray) and bleeding (red) events. Cutoff values from platelet function tests showing associations with either ischemic or bleeding events. Although yet untested, the concept of a therapeutic window for optimal on-treatment platelet reactivity to prevent either bleeding or thrombotic events is suggested. *ACS*, Acute coronary syndromes; *AU*, aggregation units; *BMI*, body mass index; *CABG*, coronary artery bypass grafting; *DM*, diabetes mellitus; *MA*, maximum amplitude; *MEA*, multiplate analyzer; *PRI*, platelet reactivity index; *PRU*, P2Y$_{12}$ reaction units; *ST*, stent thrombosis; *TEG*, thromboelastography; *VASP*, phosphorylation of vasodilator-associated phosphoprotein. (From Tantry US, Bonello L, Aradi D, et al. Consensus and update on the definition of on-treatment platelet reactivity to adenosine diphosphate associated with ischemic and bleeding. *J Am Coll Cardiol.* 2013;62:2261–2273.)

NONCARDIAC SURGERY AND CORONARY STENTS

Surgery as a Prothrombotic State

One of the major challenges in the care of patients with coronary stents are those undergoing NCS. It is well recognized that surgery constitutes a risk factor for myocardial ischemic events, including ST, which may be triggered by the physiological response to surgical stress. Enhanced sympathetic response increases catecholamines, cortisol, and renin, leading to increased myocardial stress and heightened platelet activation. These are accompanied by concomitant increases in procoagulant factors (fibrinogen and plasminogen activator inhibitor), with simultaneous inhibition of fibrinolysis. Thus the cumulative result is a prothrombotic, proinflammatory, and catabolic state, the magnitude of which correlates with the severity of surgical trauma and preexisting inflammatory state.

The risk for thrombosis in the presence of a foreign body such as a stent is enhanced, particularly in the setting of incomplete endothelial strut coverage. However, it is important to recognize that perioperative myocardial ischemic syndromes other than ST can also occur because of stent restenosis or progression of native disease elsewhere in the coronary circulation. In fact, the frequency of documented perioperative ST in published series is low, with most authors reporting major adverse cardiac events (MACEs) as a composite outcome (Box 3.6). Consequences of perioperative ST, however, can be devastating because it is associated with a 50% to 70% incidence of STEMI and up to 40% mortality rate. In addition, performing a PCI in the perioperative period is particularly challenging because of the added risk of major bleeding from the use of antithrombotic agents.

Limitations of Current Guidelines and Physician Knowledge

There is general agreement that elective PCI and stent placement should not be performed as a preoperative revascularization strategy aiming at risk reduction during NCS. This concept is largely reinforced by the results of two trials in which preoperative revascularization was ineffective when performed for the sole purpose of reducing perioperative cardiac events. In fact, several series have shown that patients with prior coronary stents have increased risk for perioperative MACE and bleeding compared with matched patients. Nevertheless, some providers view preoperative elective PCI as a beneficial strategy in some patients, when in fact it does the opposite, and at a minimum it may delay the operative procedure.

In selected high-risk surgical patients, preoperative revascularization may be indicated based on preoperative risk assessment (e.g., left main or proximal left anterior descending

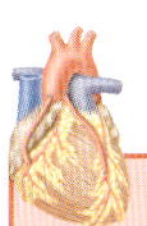

BOX 3.6 *Major Adverse Cardiac Events*

- Perioperative myocardial ischemia or infarction
- Ischemia-related acute heart failure
- Target vessel revascularization
- Stent thrombosis (uncommon)
- Death

coronary artery lesion). In this circumstance, the decision to perform PCI versus myocardial revascularization must be reached after considering the risk/benefit ratio of the cardiac procedure and the risk associated with the planned surgery.

For patients with preexisting coronary stents, guidelines are available to assist providers with decision making, but they focus primarily on timing of elective surgery and management of antiplatelet agents according to stent type. Because all are based on poor-quality evidence and expert opinion, they frequently give variable recommendations. Moreover, such recommendations address primarily the first 12 months after PCI. Very little guidance is provided beyond 1 year, although the risk of VLST and MACEs is well described up to several years after PCI.

The American College of Cardiology/American Heart Association (ACC/AHA) and European Society of Cardiology/European Society of Anaesthesiology (ESC/ESA) guidelines are limited by the lack of incorporation of specific clinical risk factors for ST (e.g., diabetes, chronic renal failure, heart failure, low ejection fraction) and a standard classification of surgical hemorrhagic risk. Instead, they provide a broad statement encouraging practitioners to gauge the risk of thrombosis vs bleeding. In addition, they offer very little guidance on the management of APT when surgery cannot be deferred or on reinstitution of DAPT in patients who discontinued it preoperatively. Recent focused updates on antiplatelet management by both ACC/AHA and ESC/European Association for Cardio-Thoracic Surgery (EACTS) provide an improvement over previous guidelines, thus making recommendations on surgical timing and perioperative DAPT for patients with stable ischemic heart disease (SIHD; defined as stable angina or MI >12 months without subsequent ischemia) versus those undergoing PCI for ACS. It is worth mentioning, however, that clinical risk factors and specific surgical risks are notoriously absent. The Surgery After Stent registry created by various Italian societies has addressed such limitations by allocating a specific hemorrhagic risk associated with each individual surgical procedure (albeit by consensus). This is plotted against the patient's thrombotic risk based on clinical and angiographic factors as well as the stent-to-surgery interval. Unfortunately, patients with later generation DESs have been relatively underrepresented, and thus thrombotic risk may be overestimated.

Despite different recommendations, variable success has been achieved when translated to local practice among individuals, in particular with the management of antiplatelet agents. The reasons are likely multifactorial, such as lack of guideline awareness, disagreement with the recommendations, emphasis on long-standing practice, and personal bias. Among specialists, surveys have demonstrated a high degree of agreement following guideline recommendations among most cardiologists and between cardiologists and anesthesiologists compared with surgeons. This observation can be largely explained by the fact that cardiologists and anesthesiologists are mainly concerned with ischemic or thrombotic phenomena, but surgeons primarily are concerned with hemorrhagic risk, having little to no experience with coronary thrombosis. Within the surgical specialties, vascular surgeons are more likely to follow current guidelines than nonvascular surgeons.

Minimizing perioperative risk requires the incorporation of several patient- and surgery-related factors in decision making, besides the well-described importance of timing of PCI and a particular antiplatelet regimen. Although specific angiographic and procedural data may not be available, the presence of recognized clinical risk factors (e.g., diabetes, CHF, obesity, chronic kidney disease, ACS, prior ST) can be identified. Additional data such as stent type and number and coronary location of the stents, as well as the clinical indication for stent placement, can be obtained in many patients (Box 3.7). Although the individual risk associated with each factor is unknown, it is reasonable to believe that perioperative risk of ST and MACE is related

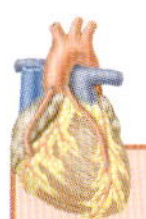

BOX 3.7   *Information Usually Available During Preoperative Evaluation*

Clinical

- Diabetes
- Heart failure
- Kidney dysfunction
- Prior myocardial infarction
- Prior stent thrombosis
- Cocaine use
- Cigarette smoking
- Type and duration of antiplatelet therapy

PCI Data

- Stent type
- Number of stents
- Date(s) and clinical indications for percutaneous coronary intervention
- Anatomic location of the stent(s)

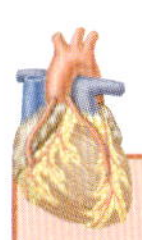

BOX 3.8   *Predictors of Perioperative Major Adverse Cardiac Events in Patients With Coronary Stents*

Clinical

- RCRI >2
- Urgent or emergent surgery
- Any stent <4–6 wk
- Elevated risk surgery
- Any stent <6 months post-ACS (particularly with positive biomarkers)
- DES <8–12 wk and SIHD
- Premature discontinuation of DAPT
- HTPR
- Major perioperative bleeding

Procedural

- Incomplete revascularization after PCI
- Persistent myocardial ischemia after PCI
- Ostial, calcified, long, or small lesions

ACS, Acute coronary syndrome; *DES,* drug-eluting stent; *DAPT,* dual antiplatelet therapy; *HTPR,* high on-treatment platelet reactivity; *PCI,* percutaneous coronary intervention; *RCRI,* revised cardiac risk index.

---

to the number of risk factors in each individual patient, with some (e.g., previous ACS or ST) having perhaps greater predictive value than others (Box 3.8). Similarly, although evidence for surgery-specific thrombotic risk is not widely available, it is reasonable to expect more complex surgeries to carry a higher risk of ST and perioperative MACE than more superficial procedures.

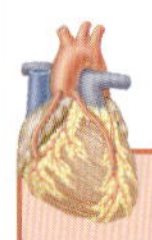

> **BOX 3.9** *Key Decision Points for Noncardiac Surgery*
>
> - Timing of surgery
> - Perioperative management of antiplatelet therapy
> - Impact on anesthetic techniques
> - Perioperative surveillance
> - Surgical venue with access to percutaneous coronary intervention capabilities

After an estimation of perioperative risk is made, the main decisions for elective NCS are timing of the surgery and perioperative management of APT. Additional considerations include the anesthetic technique, perioperative surveillance for myocardial ischemia, and whether to perform the procedure in a facility without onsite PCI capability (Box 3.9). For urgent or emergent procedures that cannot be delayed, attention should be focused primarily on the management of antihemostatic agents, minimizing the severity of bleeding, and close perioperative surveillance for ischemic or thrombotic events.

Timing of Surgery

This refers to the period between coronary stent placement and occurrence of the surgical procedure. For elective cases, the correct timing of surgery is strongly dependent on the clinical indication for APT. The main concern is primarily the risk for ST because of the presence of high platelet reactivity after PCI and the time course for endothelial stent coverage.

Cardiologists encountering candidates for elective PCI who are also scheduled for subsequent surgery have several alternatives. They first must consider whether to delay coronary stent placement and to manage the patient medically until after the surgical procedure takes place. In certain patients, this option might not be possible (patients with severe ischemia, ACS, high-risk lesions, or high-risk NCS). They traditionally follow a particular path if a future surgery date is known. For example, if surgery is required within 2 to 4 weeks, more often a balloon angioplasty will be recommended because it is relatively safe. In the past, if surgery was contemplated beyond 6 weeks, placement of a BMS was entertained, reserving a DES for those patients who will require surgery after 6 months. This approach, however, has been called into question because second- and third-generation DESs have a greater safety profile against LST than first-generation DESs or even BMSs, leading to a paradigm shift as evidenced in the most recent updates on DAPT for patients undergoing noncardiac surgical procedures (Table 3.8).

More commonly, patients present for previously unplanned surgery after PCI and stent placement. Evidence from multiple observational studies demonstrates that NCS during the first 6 weeks after coronary stenting constitutes the highest risk period for ST and MACEs, regardless of stent type and whether APT is continued. Thus unanimous agreement exists to withhold elective surgery during such period. Nonelective surgery must be performed at an institution with onsite PCI capability while maintaining DAPT or bridging therapy with IV platelet inhibitors and aggressive monitoring for thrombotic events.

It important to emphasize that NCS after such a waiting period is predominantly based on patients undergoing elective noncomplex PCI and does not necessarily

Table 3.8 ACC/AHA and ESC/EACTS Focus Update Recommendations for Elective Noncardiac Surgery in Patients With Preexisting Coronary Stents[a]

| | ACC/AHA (2016) | | | ESC/EACTS (2017) | |
Stent Type	PCI-NCS Interval (mo)	Action	Any Stent	PCI-NCS Interval (mo)	Action
BMS	<1	Delay	Any condition	<1	Delay
	≥1	Can proceed	Non-ACS/low risk	1–6	Should consider
				≥6	Can proceed
DES	≤3	Delay	ACS/high risk	1–6	May consider
	3–6	May consider		≥6	Can proceed
	≥6	Can proceed			

[a]ACC/AHA and ESC/EACTS recommendations on timing of elective surgery after percutaneous coronary intervention (PCI) stent placement in which the $P2Y_{12}$ inhibitor needs to be discontinued perioperatively. Aspirin (ASA) must be continued if possible. High risk = diffuse multivessel disease (especially in diabetes); three or more stents implanted; three or more lesions treated; stenting of last remaining patent coronary artery; bifurcation lesions; long, calcified, or ostial lesions; or left main disease.

NCS, Noncardiac surgery.

Modified from Levine GN, Bates ER, Buttk JA, et al; for the Focused Update Writing Group. ACC/AHA guideline focused update on duration of dual antiplatelet therapy in patients with coronary disease: a report of the American College of Cardiology/ American Heart Association Task Force on Clinical Practice Guidelines. *J Am Coll Cardiol.* 2016;68:1082–1115 and Valgimigli M, Bueno H, Byrne RA, et al. ESC focused update on dual antiplatelet therapy in coronary disease developed in collaboration with EACTS. *Eur Heart J.* 2018;39:213–260.

extend to patients with PCI for ACS. Indeed, retrospective data show the risk for perioperative MACEs for this population to be highest within 3 months after PCI. For such patients, as well as for those undergoing complex PCI or with increased ischemic burden (e.g., incomplete revascularization), it is reasonable to withhold elective surgery at least for 6 months and preferably for 12 months, if possible. Other patients who may require increased waiting time include individuals with poorly controlled clinical risk factors or those shown to exhibit HTPR.

BMSs have traditionally been touted as safer than DESs for patients requiring surgery within 1 year after PCI. Because endothelial stent coverage in most patients appears to be complete within weeks and the incidence of restenosis peaks between 4 and 12 months, some experts have advocated a safe window in which surgery should ideally be performed between 6 weeks after elective PCI and before restenosis becomes likely. Current guidelines recommend that NCS can be performed more than 4 to 6 weeks after BMS implantation. Recent studies, however, have shown that the risk of perioperative MACE with BMSs may be even greater than DESs, with clinical factors such as revised cardiac risk index of greater than 2, emergency surgery, and MI 6 months before NCS having a greater predictive value than stent type. These observations can be partially explained by selection bias, with sicker patients or those identified as having future NCS undergoing BMS placement in accordance with current practice and widespread use of safer newer generation DESs. Thus the higher rates of MACEs with BMSs are more likely explained by the patient's underlying disease rather than the influence of stent type on the surgical procedure.

In patients with DESs, the risk for perioperative MACEs, although lower after the first 6 to 8 weeks after PCI, remains elevated between 6 weeks and 6 months,

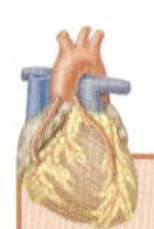

> **BOX 3.10** *Minimal Waiting Time and Duration of Dual Antiplatelet Therapy Before Elective Noncardiac Surgery*
>
> - BMS: SIHD and low risk: >6 wk
> - DES: SIHD and low risk: >8 wk <6 mo
> - BMS or /DES: ACS, complex PCI, or high thrombotic risk >6–12 mo
> - BRS: 12 mo
>
> *ACS,* Acute coronary syndrome; *BMS,* bare metal stent; *BRS,* bioresorbable stent; *DES,* drug-eluting stent; *PCI,* percutaneous coronary intervention; *SIHD,* stable ischemic heart disease.

particularly in high-risk patients undergoing complex procedures or in patients after ACS. Recent evidence based on stent registries strongly suggests that in selected low-risk patients with SIHD, elective surgery may be considered within such period of time, particularly in conditions in which outcomes may be strongly influenced by surgical delay or quality of life is significantly impaired. Additionally, published literature has consistently shown minimal incremental risk of NCS after 6 months; however, in patients with complex PCI and other risk factors for thrombotic complications, as well as those with BRSs, it may be prudent to wait more than 6 months and even 12 months (Box 3.10).

For time-sensitive NCS, an attempt should be made to defer the procedure for at least 8 to 12 weeks whenever possible. In such cases, every effort should be made to maintain DAPT, fully recognizing that the increase of bleeding may also lead to increased cardiac complications. Additionally, most studies address primarily major- or intermediate-risk surgery with very little information for patients undergoing low-risk procedures. Current available data suggest that performing ambulatory low-risk procedures after 4 to 6 weeks in patients with BMSs and longer than 3 months in low-risk patients with DESs may be relatively safe.

MANAGEMENT OF ANTIPLATELET THERAPY

Perioperative management of APT during NCS is one of the most important and controversial issues in coronary stent patients. For patients taking DAPT, a surgical or interventional procedure is considered the most common reason for temporary cessation of DAPT, thereby increasing the risk for perioperative MACEs. Alternatively, continuation of DAPT increases the perioperative risk and severity of bleeding, thus leading to additional complications, including increased risk for cardiac events.

Most controversies and guideline recommendations on perioperative APT have been centered primarily on the first 12 months after PCI, while being conspicuously austere beyond this time frame. As a result, many surgeons and interventional physicians indiscriminately withhold APT after 12 months even for low bleeding risk procedures. New evidence, however, shows additional benefits of 30 months of DAPT against ischemic or thrombotic syndromes in DES patients. This protection seems to extend to native coronaries as well and may require a reexamination of APT management in selected subjects undergoing NCS beyond 1 year.

Current guidelines provide a broad framework to guide clinicians in relation to the time of surgery. Thus a minimum of 4 to 6 weeks of DAPT is required for patients

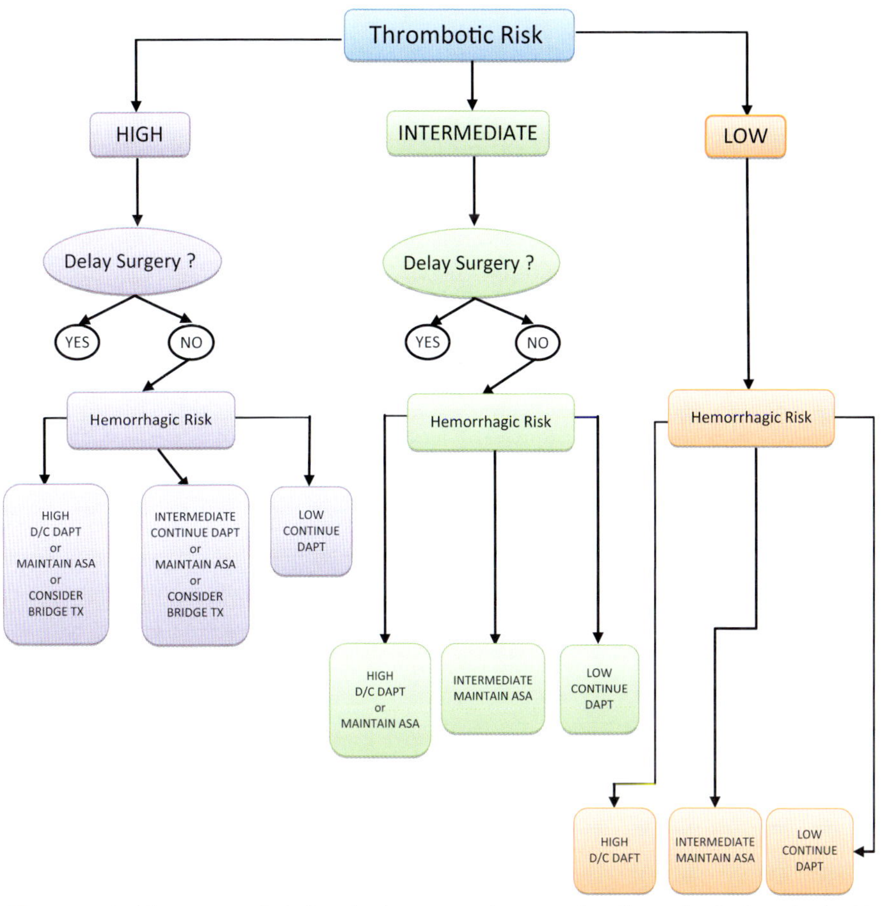

Fig. 3.6 Decision tree analysis for elective surgery, incorporating the patient's thrombotic risk (see Table 3.9) and surgical procedure's associated hemorrhagic risk (see Table 3.10). The therapeutic approach for each individual patient must also incorporate all known risk factors for perioperative major adverse cardiac events (see Boxes 3.7 and 3.8). *ASA,* Aspirin; *DAPT,* dual antiplatelet therapy.

with BMSs and 3 to 6 months for patients with DESs, with continuation of ASA monotherapy in most cases of SIHD unless contraindicated by the hemorrhagic risk. For patients following ACS or with a high ischemic or thrombotic risk, a minimum of 6 months and preferably 12 months of DAPT is indicated; those with BRSs require 1 year or perhaps longer as dictated by their thrombotic risk.

In the absence of well-designed randomized trials assessing the risk-to-benefit ratio of perioperative APT, most decisions should be based on the balance between thrombotic and hemorrhagic risks associated with each patient and surgical procedure (Fig. 3.6). Thrombotic risk is related to several procedural and clinical factors as well as the time from PCI to surgery, coronary lesions, and degree of surgical trauma (Table 3.9). Hemorrhagic risk is based on the type of surgical intervention (Table 3.10) plus the patient's inherent bleeding tendencies from additional comorbidities. It is important to recognize the lack of standard definition of surgery-specific degree of hemorrhage, with most classifications based largely on expert consensus. More recently, the Academic Research Consortium has proposed a standardized grading system for patients on APT and post-PCI bleeding (Table 3.11). Although not originally

Table 3.9 Perioperative Thrombotic Risk

High risk	BMS <6 wk after elective PCI or <6 mo after PCI for ACS DES <8 wk for SIHD, <6 mo after ACS, or complex PCI associated with high thrombotic risk[a] BRS first generation <12 mo <2 wk after balloon angioplasty Multiple clinical risk factors for ST Prior ST (particularly while on APT)
Intermediate risk	BMS >6 wk <6 mo for SIHD DES >8 wk <6 mo for SIHD DES or BMS >6 or <12 mo after ACS or complex PCI associated high thrombotic risk[a] BRS first generation 1–3 years Some clinical risk factors (except prior ST)
Low risk	BMS or DES >6 mo for SIHD DES or BMS for ACS or complex PCI >12 mo Few clinical risk factors

[a]For example, diffuse multivessel disease (specially in diabetes); three or more stents implanted; three or more lesions treated; stenting of last remaining patent coronary artery; bifurcation lesions; long, calcified, or ostial lesions; or left main disease.

ACS, Acute coronary syndrome; *BMS,* bare metal stent; *BRS,* bioresorbable stent; *DES,* drug-eluting stent; *PCI,* percutaneous coronary intervention; *SIHD,* stable ischemic heart disease; *ST,* stent thrombosis.

designed for NCS patients, this score may be useful in evaluating perioperative bleeding with platelet inhibitors.

Interruption of Antiplatelet Therapy

Interruption of DAPT (particularly both drugs) is associated with an increased risk of perioperative ST and other myocardial ischemic syndromes for several reasons. First, in many patients, stent struts might not be completely covered with endothelium. This property has been demonstrated to be much more frequent with first-generation DESs and those that incorporate a durable polymer, which can cause a localized chronic inflammatory vessel response. Second, an abrupt interruption of either ASA or a thienopyridine may be associated with a rebound phenomenon in which newer platelets generated by the bone marrow exhibit increased activation and aggregation to thrombotic stimuli. Multiple clinical studies have demonstrated unequivocally a peak in ischemic or thrombotic phenomena upon abrupt discontinuation of either ASA or clopidogrel. Whether this is due to platelet rebound or simply loss of the protective effect from APT is unclear. Third, some patients exhibit variable degrees of chronic HTPR, which may become fully expressed when DAPT is discontinued and in fact suffer from thrombotic events in stented areas or native atherosclerotic vessels.

Currently, because of the lack of good-quality evidence, the optimal period to perform NCS if surgical bleeding risk requires discontinuing DAPT is unknown. This is not surprising because each patient's thrombotic and hemorrhagic risk is different. Because wide variability to APT exists, future use of PFTs may prove advantageous by providing a tailored approach to DAPT before surgery, potentially minimizing bleeding and thrombotic risk.

Table 3.10 Hemorrhagic Risk

Surgery Related	Types of Procedures
Low risk: minimal morbidity or mortality risk from bleeding; transfusion from procedure is not likely	Minor plastic, orthopedic, general, gynecologic ENT procedures, EVAR, limb amputations Closed reductions of facial fractures Flexible cystoscopy or ureteroscopy Cataract surgery and intravitreal injections Tooth extractions, endodontic therapy GI endoscopy and biopsy, polypectomy (<1 cm) ERCP stent without sphincterotomy
Intermediate risk: moderate morbidity or mortality risk from bleeding; perioperative transfusion is likely	Intrathoracic (lobectomy, mediastinoscopy), intraabdominal, hemorrhoidectomy, obesity surgery, major orthopedic, urology, ENT, reconstructive surgery, GI polypectomy (>1 cm), esophageal dilation, PEG, variceal sclerotherapy, vitrectomy, trabeculectomy, ventriculoperitoneal shunt, multilevel spinal laminectomy
High risk: major risk of morbidity or mortality caused by substantial blood loss (acutely or protracted); high likelihood of major transfusion or surgical reintervention	Open thoracic or thoracoabdominal aortic surgery Esophagectomy, hepatic resection, transurethral resection of the prostate, TURBT, percutaneous lithotripsy, major femoral fractures, radical or debulking pelvic tumor surgery, multiple traumatic injuries, extensive burns, major spine surgery
High risk: bleeding into an enclosed space	Intracranial surgery, spinal canal surgery

ENT, Ear, nose, and throat; *ERCP,* endoscopic retrograde cholangiopancreatography; *EVAR,* endovascular aneurysm repair; *GI,* gastrointestinal; *PEG,* percutaneous endoscopic gastroscopy; *TURBT,* transurethral resection of bladder tumor.

Table 3.11 Bleeding Definition According to Academic Research Consortium

Type	Description
0	No bleeding
1	Nonactionable; patient does not seek studies, hospitalization, or treatment
2	Overt sign of hemorrhage requiring nonsurgical intervention, hospitalization, or increased level of care
3a	Overt bleeding with a 3 to 5 g/dL decrease in hemoglobin or requiring transfusion
3b	Overt bleeding with >5 g/dL decrease in hemoglobin or requiring surgical intervention or vasoactive drugs
3c	Intracranial hemorrhage, intraocular bleeding compromising vision
4	CABG-related bleeding
5	Fatal bleeding

CABG, Coronary artery bypass graft.
Modified from Mehran R, Rao SV, Bhatt DL, et al. Standardized bleeding definitions for cardiovascular clinical trials. A consensus report from the Bleeding Academic Research Consortium. *Circulation.* 2011;123:2736–2747.

Table 3.12	**Preoperative Interruption and Resumption of Antiplatelet Therapy**		
	Stop Before Surgery	**Resume[a]**	**Dose**
Oral Agent			
Aspirin	7 d	24 h postoperative	80–160 mg/d
Clopidogrel	5 d	24 h postoperative	Load with 300–600 mg followed by 75 mg/d
Prasugrel	7 d	24 h postoperative	Load with 60 mg; then 10 mg/d
Ticagrelor	3–5 d	24 h postoperative	Load with 180 mg followed by 90 mg twice daily
Intravenous Agent			
Tirofiban	4–8 h	4–6 h postoperative	0.1–0.15 µg/kg/min
Eptifibatide	4–6 h	4–6 h postoperative	2.0 µg/kg/min
Cangrelor	60–90 min	4–6 h postoperative	2–4 µg/kg/min

[a]Absent clinically significant bleeding. Intravenous agents can be discontinued upon reinstitution of oral dual antiplatelet therapy. Oral agents can be administered by nasogastric tube if the patient has not resumed oral intake.

For most patients, discontinuing DPAT means interruption of the adenosine antagonist while maintaining perioperative ASA because most elective and interventional procedures can safely be performed in patients receiving ASA. Certain operations may require withholding both agents (e.g., certain types of neurosurgery, urologic procedures, complex gastrointestinal endoscopy, or surgeries within an enclosed space) in which even minimal bleeding might cause significant complications. Discontinuation of DAPT (ADP antagonist) 1 week prior is necessary if a regional anesthetic or neuraxial technique is planned per current guidelines, and maintenance of ASA alone is generally considered safe. Selected patients probably can undergo peripheral nerve blocks while taking clopidogrel, but published experience is limited.

Currently, if one or both antiplatelet agents are discontinued, it is recommended that clopidogrel and ticagrelor be stopped 5 days before surgery; prasugrel and ASA should be stopped seven days before. With regard to ticagrelor, the recent ESC/EACT focused update recommends discontinuing ticagrelor only 3 days before surgery, but this is based on extrapolation from cardiac surgical patients because sufficient data on NCS are currently lacking. If an ischemic or thrombotic event occurs upon interruption of DAPT, limited evidence shows that it most commonly occurs 1 to 30 days after surgery because of persistence of a prothrombotic state. Thus it is imperative that DAPT be resumed as soon as possible, preferably within the first 24 hours. Reinstitution of the $P2Y_{12}$ inhibitor requires a loading dose, but ASA can be restarted with a normal maintenance dose (Table 3.12).

Continuation of Antiplatelet Therapy and Risk of Hemorrhage

In NCS, perioperative DAPT increases the likelihood of surgical blood loss requiring transfusion or reintervention by as much as 50%. Published reports, however, give conflicting results, suggesting that the risk for major bleeding may be surgery specific. For example, a large registry of vascular patients found no difference in bleeding complications based on the antiplatelet regimen, but in patients undergoing elective joint replacement or Mohs procedures, major bleeding complications were significantly higher. In general, there is agreement that DAPT should be continued in patients undergoing low-risk bleeding procedures. Nevertheless, it is important to recognize that most of the published evidence in NCS addresses patients on DAPT with clopidogrel, with very little information available regarding prasugrel or ticagrelor. In addition, only one study has addressed the effects of vorapaxar as part of perioperative DAPT.

The use of ASA monotherapy is also associated with increased surgical blood loss, but less than with DAPT. Previous studies including a meta-analysis of 50,000 patients showed more bleeding with ASA and no differences in outcome except in transurethral prostatectomy and intracranial surgery. A recent large randomized trial in NCS demonstrated a greater number of major bleeding events without reduction in thrombotic or ischemic events. In this study a minority (<5%) of patients had coronary stents, so the results may not be representative of this patient population. Current recommendations support continuing ASA, with decisions primarily centered on management of the $P2Y_{12}$ inhibitor unless the hemorrhagic risk by far exceeds the thrombotic risk.

Several management algorithms have been published, with the most comprehensive document put forth by combined Italian medical societies representing the Surgery After Stent Group. Although these are primarily based on expert consensus, subsequent validation studies correctly identified high risk groups for both thrombotic and hemorrhagic complications, as well as documented high degrees of compliance by practitioners.

It is important to emphasize that despite strong recommendations endorsed by different societies, a recent systematic review of all available evidence performed on behalf of the U.S. Department of Veterans Affairs failed to show any clear association between any given antiplatelet strategy and rates of perioperative MACE and bleeding. Ultimately, treatment recommendations should center on the careful individual evaluation of each patient's ischemic and thrombotic risk.

Bridging Therapy

This approach is reserved for selected patients who have a high thrombotic profile undergoing a procedure associated with high hemorrhagic risk, in whom DAPT must be suspended and surgery cannot be delayed. Antiplatelet agents are preferred because therapy is aimed at prevention of a platelet-rich thrombus. Although heparin has been advocated as a bridging agent, it is less than optimal because its beneficial effects on platelets are minimal or may even induce a prothrombotic effect.

Current agents available for bridging therapy are the short-acting GP IIb/IIIa inhibitors tirofiban and eptifibatide and the $P2Y_{12}$ antagonist cangrelor. This therapy calls for discontinuation of the $P2Y_{12}$ inhibitor 5 to 7 days before the surgical procedure. Patients are then admitted to the hospital and started on a continuous IV infusion (without a bolus) of either tirofiban or eptifibatide until 4 to 6 hours (tirofiban) or 4 to 8 hours (eptifibatide) before the planned procedure. The infusion is restarted postoperatively until oral DAPT can be reinstituted. Cangrelor represents an attractive alternative. Because of its very short half-life, an infusion of 0.75 µg/kg per minute can be continued until shortly before surgery. However, the use of cangrelor as a potential bridging agent has only been tested on patients undergoing cardiac surgery, with no published experience in NCS.

Although bridging therapy is relatively safe, ST can still occur, and there is an increased risk of bleeding. Furthermore, it is associated with increased hospitalization and costs.

Patients Undergoing Ambulatory Surgery

Patients with coronary stents undergoing ambulatory surgery raise the issue of safety in locations without an onsite cardiac catheterization laboratory. Although few data exist, current literature suggests that the incidence of MACEs is very low, although the risk of ST is still present.

Some authors have advocated that all surgical procedures be performed in facilities with immediate access to PCI capabilities. Such recommendations are impractical and economically burdensome because of the large number of patients undergoing ambulatory procedures. Currently, no official position has been promulgated by the various professional societies with most decisions driven by local and individual practice. A satellite center without PCI capabilities may be appropriate in patients who have undergone elective PCI, lack significant risk factors for ST, have exceeded the minimal duration of DAPT, and who undergo procedures that do not require interruption of any APT (e.g., high bleeding risk endoscopic intervention). More important, it is essential that practitioners establish protocols for treatment of STEMI and expeditious referral (<90 minutes) to a PCI center for immediate revascularization in the event of an ACS.

AN INTEGRATED APPROACH

When confronting NCS patients with coronary stents, clinicians face a potentially complex clinical conundrum that offers many challenges in efforts to find the optimal balance between thrombotic or ischemic risk and bleeding risk. This problem is compounded because interventional cardiology is undergoing rapid advances in stent technology and availability of newer antiplatelet drugs. This explosion of innovations frequently finds its way to clinical use wherein large numbers of patients receive new devices and drugs with which most perioperative physicians are relatively unfamiliar.

Inevitably, a significant percentage of individuals will require a surgical or interventional procedure, thus placing practitioners at a disadvantage because published evidence frequently lags behind clinical use. Current recommendations are an improvement from previous guidelines, but they are predominantly based on observational studies, which by their very nature are deficient because they are unable to control for the many variables that influence perioperative risk. Furthermore, the paucity of data regarding recent technologies such as BRSs or newer antiplatelet agents forces clinicians to extrapolate from the nonsurgical population. Last, techniques with significant potential for use in NCS (e.g., PFTs) still remain relatively unexplored. Such complexities highlight the importance of a multidisciplinary and regimented approach that is incorporated into an evidence-based comprehensive framework addressing surgery-specific risks, PCI and clinical risk factors, the pharmacologic profile of various antiplatelet agents, and the surgical venue. Only in this manner can it be said that the care of these patients is truly optimized.

SUGGESTED READING

Armstrong EJ, Graham LA, Waldo SW, et al. Incomplete revascularization is associated with an increased risk for major adverse cardiovascular events among patients undergoing noncardiac surgery. *J Am Coll Cardiol Intv*. 2017;10:329–338.

Armstrong EJ, Graham LA, Waldo SW, et al. Patient and lesion-specific characteristics predict risk of major adverse cardiovascular events among patients with previous percutaneous coronary intervention undergoing noncardiac surgery. *Catheter Cardiovasc Interv*. 2017;89:617–627.

Banerjee S, Angiolillo DJ, Boden WE, et al. Use of antiplatelet therapy/DAPT for post-PCI patients undergoing noncardiac surgery. *J Am Coll Cardiol.* 2017;69:1861–1870.

Bangalore S, Bezerra H, Rizik D, et al. The state of the Absorb bioresorbable scaffold. *JACC Cardiovasc Interv.* 2017;10:2349–2359.

Bønaa KH, Mannsver J, Wirsch R, NORSTENT Investigators, et al. Drug-eluting or bare-metal stents for coronary artery disease. *N Engl J Med.* 2016;375:1242–1252.

Childers CP, Maggard-Gibbons M, Shekelle PG. Antiplatelet therapy in patients with coronary stents undergoing elective noncardiac surgery: continue, stop, or something in between? *J Am Med Assoc.* 2017;318:120–121.

Columbo JA, Lambour AJ, Sundling RA, et al. A meta-analysis of the impact of aspirin, clopidogrel, and dual antiplatelet therapy on bleeding complications in noncardiac surgery. *Ann Surg.* 2017;May:[Epub ahead of print].

van Diepen S, Tricoci P, Podder M, et al. Efficacy and safety of vorapaxar in non-st-segment elevation acute coronary syndrome patients undergoing noncardiac surgery. *J Am Heart Assoc.* 2015;4:e002546.

Egholm G, Kristensen SD, Thim T, et al. Risk associated with surgery within 12 months after coronary stent implantation. *J Am Coll Cardiol.* 2016;68:2622–2632.

Essandoh M, Dalia AA, Albaghdadi M, et al. Perioperative management of dual-antiplatelet therapy in patients with newer-generation drug-eluting metallic stents and bioresorbable vascular scaffolds undergoing elective noncardiac surgery. *J Cardiothorac Vasc Anesth.* 2017;31:1857–1864.

Holcomb CN, Graham LA, Richman JS, et al. The incremental risk of of coronary stents on postoperative adverse events: a matched cohort study. *Ann Surg.* 2016;263:924–930.

Iqbal J, Onuma Y, Ormiston J, et al. Bioresorbable scaffolds: rationale, current status, challenges and future. *Eur Heart J.* 2014;35:765–776.

Lee S-Y, Hong M-K, Shin D-H, et al. Clinical outcomes of dual antiplatelet therapy after implantation of drug-eluting stents in patients with different cardiovascular risk factors. *Clin Res Cardiol.* 2017;106:165–173.

Levine GN, Bates ER, Buttk JA, et al; for the Focused Update Writing Group. ACC/AHA guideline focused update on duration of dual antiplatelet therapy in patients with coronary disease: a report of the American College of Cardiology/ American Heart Association Task Force on Clinical Practice Guidelines. *J Am Coll Cardiol.* 2016;68:1082–1115.

Maggard Gibbons M, Ulloa JG, Macqueen I, et al. Management of antiplatelet therapy among patients on antiplatelet therapy for coronary or cerebrovascular disease or with prior percutaneous cardiac interventions undergoing elective surgery: a systematic review; 2017. Us Dept of Veteran Affairs. https://www.hsrd.research.va.gov/publications/management_briefs/default.cfm?ManagementBriefsMenu=eBrief-no137&eBriefTitle=Systematic+Review%3A+Management+of+Antiplatelet+Therapy+among+Patients+Undergoing+Elective+Non-Cardiac+Surgery.

Mahmoud KD, Sanon S, Habermann EB, et al. Perioperative cardiovascular risk of prior coronary stent implantation among patients undergoing noncardiac surgery. *J Am Coll Cardiol.* 2016;67:1038–1049.

Palmerini T, Sangiorgi D, Valgimigli M, et al. Short versus long-term dual antiplatelet therapy after drug-eluting stent implantation : an individual patient data pairwise and network meta-analysis. *J Am Coll Cardiol.* 2015;65:1092–1102.

Palmerini T, Stone GW. Optimal duration of dual antiplatelet therapy after drug-eluting stent implantation: conceptual evolution based on emerging evidence. *Eur Heart J.* 2016;37:353–364.

Philip F, Stewart S, Southard JA. Very late stent thrombosis with second generation drug eluting stents compared to bare metal stents: network meta-analysis of primary percutaneous coronary intervention trials. *Circ Cardiovasc Interv.* 2016;88:38–48.

Rossini R, Angiolillo DJ, Musumeci G, et al. Antiplatelet therapy and outcome in patients undergoing surgery following coronary stenting: results of the Surgery After Stenting Registry *Catheter Cardiovasc Interv.* 2017;89:E13–E25.

Saia F, Belotti LMB, Guastaroba P, et al. Risk of adverse cardiac and bleeding events following cardiac and noncardiac surgery in patients with coronary stents. *Circ Cardiovasc Qual Outcomes.* 2016;9:39–47.

Sotomi Y, Onuma Y, Collet C, et al. Bioresorbable scaffold: the emerging reality and future directions. *Circ Res.* 2017;120:1341–1352.

Torrado J, Buckley L, Duran A, et al. Restenosis, stent thrombosis, and bleeding complications. *J Am Coll Cardiol.* 2018;71:1676–1695.

Valgimigli M, Bueno H, Byrne RA, et al; for the Task Force for dual antiplatelet therapy in coronary artery disease of the European Society of Cardiology (ESC) and of the European Association for Cardio-Thoracic Surgery (EACTS). 2017 ESC focused update on dual antiplatelet therapy in coronary disease developed in collaboration with EACTS. *Eur Heart J.* 2017;39(3):213–260.

Chapter 4

Cardiovascular Implantable Electronic Device Management in Noncardiac Surgery

Brett Cronin, MD • Timothy M. Maus, MD • Swapnil Khoche, MBBS, DNB • Marc A. Rozner, PhD, MD

Key Points

1. Active fixation leads can penetrate through structures (e.g., the thin-walled right atrium) during placement and present as pain, pneumomediastinum, or effusions.
2. Active rate modulation in cardiac implantable electrical devices (CIEDs) may result in heart rate changes intraoperatively related to changes in monitored parameters such as ventilation.
3. Mode switching allows for the identification of atrial tachyarrhythmias and the automatic conversion of pacemaker settings, which may have intraoperative hemodynamic consequences.
4. The currently approved leadless pacemaker system (e.g., Micra Transcatheter Pacemaker System; Medtronic) lacks a magnet sensor and therefore a magnet response.
5. Cardiac resynchronization therapy (CRT) with an automatic implantable cardioverter-defibrillator (AICD) (e.g., CRT-D) poses a unique problem for perioperative management because magnet application will only succeed in deactivating the AICD portion of the device.
6. Magnet application to an AICD is expected to disable tachyarrhythmia therapies; however, pacemaker-dependent patients with an AICD and an increased risk of EMI require perioperative programming.
7. Biotronik, Boston Scientific, and St. Jude Medical pacemakers have programmable magnet behavior.
8. The use of a magnet or programming to an asynchronous mode in a pacemaker with a ventricular lead could result in an R-on-T phenomenon and a malignant arrhythmia.
9. Currently, there is no recommendation for antibiotic prophylaxis before routine dental, gastrointestinal, or genitourinary procedures to prevent CIED infections.

In the future, anesthesiologists will likely be asked to take a more active role in the perioperative management of patients with cardiac implantable electronic devices (CIEDs). Therefore a basic knowledge of these devices (i.e., pacemakers and defibrillators) as well as the perioperative considerations is essential. This chapter provides the foundation required to effectively manage these devices during noncardiac surgery.

PACEMAKER BASICS

Pacemaker configurations include devices with leads in a single chamber, two chambers, or multiple chambers (e.g., biventricular pacing), which are denoted by the North American Society of Pacing and Electrophysiology, British Pacing and Electrophysiology Group, Generic (NBG) code (Table 4.1). Pacing and sensing can occur in the atrium, the ventricle, or both (Fig. 4.1) depending on the configuration and pacemaker programming. More complicated multichamber pacing and sensing schemes (e.g., dual-chamber pacing or cardiac resynchronization therapy [CRT]) may pose clinical challenges for anesthesiologists; however, they also provide for atrial-ventricular pacing or ventricular synchronicity and increased cardiac output.

Given the first position of the NBG code, which denotes the pacing chamber(s), the fifth position may seem redundant. However, it is used to denote multiple leads

Table 4.1	North American Society of Pacing and Electrophysiology/ British Pacing and Electrophysiology Group Revised (2002) Generic Pacemaker Code (NBG Code)				
Pacing Chamber	Sensing Chamber	Response	Rate Modulation		Multisite Pacing
O = None	O = None	O = None	O = None		O = None
A = Atrium	A = Atrium	I = Inhibited	R = Rate modulation		A = Atrium
V = Ventricle	V = Ventricle	T = Triggered			V = Ventricle
D = Dual	D = Dual	D = Dual			D = Dual

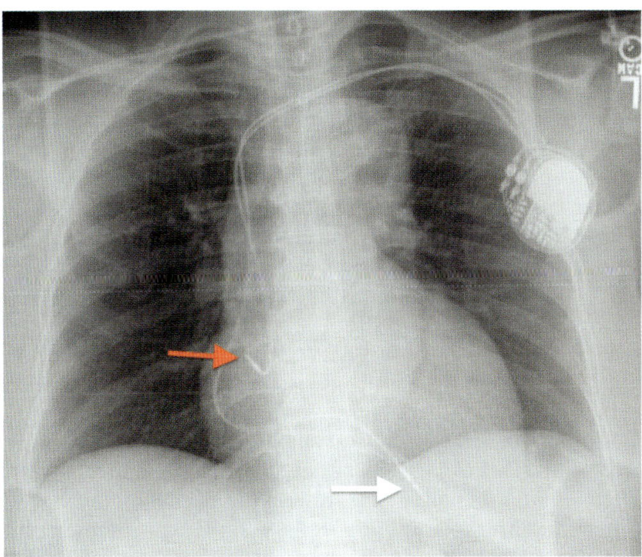

Fig. 4.1 Supine frontal chest radiograph showing a dual-chamber pacemaker with leads in the right atrium *(red arrow)* and right ventricle *(white arrow)* as well as the generator in the classic left pectoral location. (Note the difference between the pacing leads shown in this example and the shock coils of an implantable cardioverter-defibrillator located in the superior vena cava and right ventricle in Fig. 4.6.)

in a single chamber or leads in multiple chambers. Examples of multisite pacing would be multiple atrial leads to suppress atrial fibrillation or biventricular pacing for CRT. CRT-D (cardiac resynchronization therapy with defibrillation capability) in particular may pose a specific challenge for intraoperative management and is addressed later in the chapter. Rate modulation is also denoted by the NBG code, but additional information such as the indication for placement, magnet response, battery life, pacemaker dependence, rate enhancements, and mode switching, can only be determined by communicating with the device company or device interrogation.

Pacemaker Indications

Common indications for permanent pacing include symptomatic bradycardia from sinus node or atrioventricular (AV) node disease, long QT syndrome, hypertrophic obstructive cardiomyopathy (HOCM), and dilated cardiomyopathy.

Pacemaker Leads

Although knowledge regarding the exact type of leads implanted is not often necessary for the safe and appropriate perioperative management of CIEDs, a basic understanding of the lead types makes chest radiograph interpretation easier and helps determine the potential effects of electromagnetic interference (EMI). Furthermore, lead type can be very important during lead removal.

Pacemaker leads can be either bipolar or unipolar, with bipolar leads being more common in the United States. The chest radiograph in Fig. 4.1 is an example of a dual-chamber pacemaker with bipolar leads in the right atrium (RA) and right ventricle (RV). Bipolar leads contain both the anode and cathode within the lead itself, but in a unipolar system, the lead contains the cathode and the pulse generator itself functions as the anode. The shorter distance between the anode and cathode in a bipolar system reduces susceptibility to EMI specifically with regard to sensing. This shorter distance between anode and cathode can also result in smaller amplitude or even unrecognized pacer spikes on the intraoperative electrocardiogram (ECG). In contrast, the unipolar system results in electricity traveling a longer distance from the lead or cathode to the pulse generator or anode. This configuration requires the generator or "can" be positioned in the left pectoral region as well as an increased susceptibility to EMI.

Although bipolar leads are less susceptible to EMI, they have historically been larger in diameter and less durable than unipolar leads. However, durability in recent years has become closer to equivalent. Additional quoted advantages of bipolar leads include less pectoral muscle stimulation because they do not use an "active can" configuration and the ability to convert to unipolar pacing if indicated by the clinical situation.

Leads can also be broken down by their fixation mechanism. Fixation mechanism is important as active fixation leads are at risk of perforating thin-walled structures like the RA (Fig. 4.2) during placement. Perforation can result in significant pain, pneumomediastinum, or effusions. Occasionally, diaphragmatic pacing is associated with lead perforation. This can involve either diaphragm by direct stimulation of the diaphragm (left hemidiaphragm) or via stimulation of the phrenic nerve by the right atrial (right hemidiaphragm) or the coronary sinus (left hemidiaphragm) leads. Diaphragmatic pacing can be quite uncomfortable for the awake patient and may only require an alteration in voltage/pulse width or lead repositioning. However, it can be a sign of lead perforation and should elicit an investigation.

In preparation for lead removal, the length of time in situ and the fixation mechanism are vitally important. For example, tined leads are passive fixation leads (Fig. 4.3)

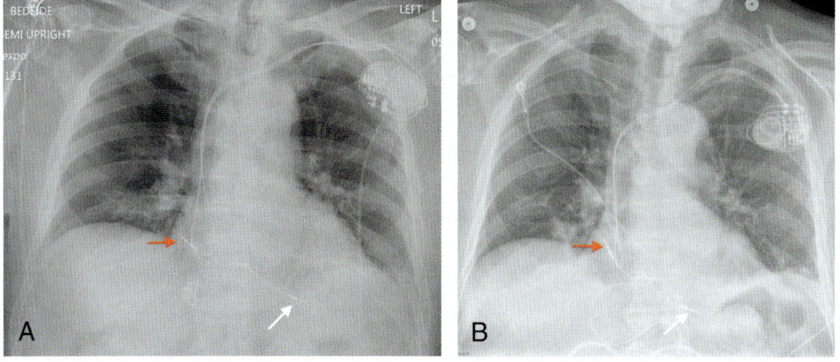

Fig. 4.2 (A) Upright frontal chest radiograph showing a dual-chamber pacemaker with a right atrial lead *(red arrow)* that has penetrated through the right atrial wall. This resulted in pneumomediastinum and significant pain. Right ventricular lead *(white arrow)*. (B) Upright frontal chest radiograph after the right atrial lead *(red arrow)* was appropriately repositioned.

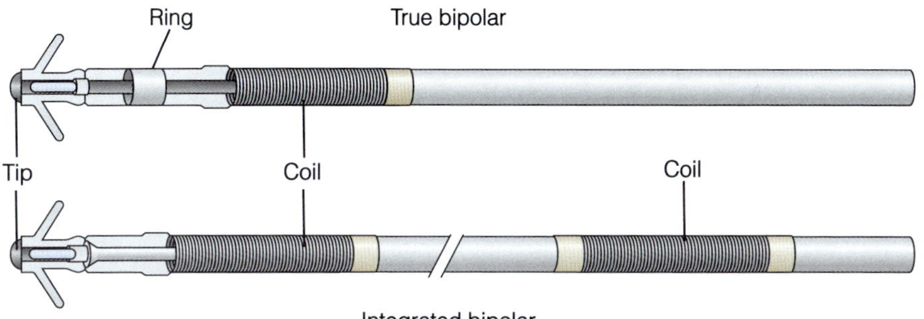

Fig. 4.3 True bipolar *(top)* and integrated bipolar *(bottom)* passive fixation leads. The true bipolar lead senses between the distal tip and the proximal ring, which are dedicated for pacing and sensing. True bipolar leads have a single coil. In contrast, integrated bipolar leads pace and sense between the tip and distal coil. The distal coil is used for sensing, pacing, and defibrillation. Integrated bipolar leads also contain a second, proximal coil, increasing the lead surface area for defibrillation. (From Bonow RO, Mann DL, Zipes DP, Libby P, eds. *Braunwald's Heart Disease.* 9th ed. Philadelphia: Elsevier; 2012.)

that are difficult to reposition or remove if ineffective because of their fixation mechanism and scar tissue formation. Luckily, they have fallen out of favor with most electrophysiologists. An additional type of passive fixation lead that is still in use today is covered in the discussion of CRT.

Rate Modulation

Rate modulation and rate adaptation, denoted by an R in the fourth position of the NBG code (see Table 4.1), are terms used to describe a pacemaker's ability to automatically change the heart rate in response to certain monitored parameters. Given that an estimated 85% of pacemakers implanted in the United States are rate responsive and 99% have this capability, anesthesiologists should be familiar with rate modulation in case an experienced programmer is not available preoperatively.

The monitored physiologic parameters that can induce rate changes include acceleration caused by motion; patient movement; QT interval; central venous temperature, oxygen saturation, or pH; right ventricular pressure; minute ventilation via thoracic impedance; physiologic impedance; heat; or a combination of acceleration and minute ventilation. When required, a pacemaker with rate modulation enabled can alter the heart rate and thus the cardiac output to meet metabolic demand.

Specifically, pacemakers that correlate an increase in respiratory rate and tidal volume with exercise and a need for increased cardiac output pose a challenge for anesthesiologists. The paced rate in these devices may inappropriately increase in response to mechanical hyperventilation, external respiratory rate monitoring, or even electrocautery. This results from monitoring respiratory rate and tidal volume via thoracic impedance between the lead and generator. On inspiration, the distance between the generator and the lead increases. In addition, the inspired gas in the thorax results in greater impedance to the small electrical signals emitted from the lead. The device then correlates the increase in thoracic impedance caused by distance as well as inspired gas with an increased respiratory rate or tidal volume and a need for greater cardiac output. Interestingly, patients with an exacerbation of congestive heart failure may present with a decrease in thoracic impedance as a result of associated pulmonary edema.

The American Society of Anesthesiologists (ASA) and Heart Rhythm Society (HRS), in the 2011 ASA Practice Advisory, provide a recommendation that rate-adaptive therapy should be disabled preoperatively if "advantageous." Intraoperative rate changes, which result from elective continuation of rate modulation or a lack of CIED programming resources, are usually benign. However, an increase in heart rate may be hemodynamically significant, unfavorable for certain comorbidities (e.g., coronary artery disease), or misinterpreted as patient discomfort. Therefore it is not surprising that device manufacturers have previously made more definitive recommendations that minute ventilation-driven rate-adaptive therapy should be programmed "off" during mechanical ventilation. Changes in rate because of active rate modulation can result from succinylcholine-induced muscle fasciculations, an oscillating saw, myoclonic jerks, postoperative shivering, electroconvulsive therapy (ECT), and QT alterations from medications, pH, or electrolytes. However, the most commonly encountered stimuli for rate changes in the operating room (OR) are electrocautery, external respiratory rate monitoring, and mechanical hyperventilation.

If active rate modulation results in an intolerable or undesirable increase in heart rate, a number of treatment options are available. The eliciting stimulus (e.g., hyperventilation or electrocautery) can be withdrawn, a magnet can place the pacemaker into an asynchronous mode (some caveats are discussed later), or CIED programming can disable rate modulation. Thankfully, minute ventilation rate modulation is only commonly found in the Boston Scientific and Sorin devices (Table 4.2). These Boston Scientific and Sorin devices may require perioperative programming given their rate modulation monitor in conjunction with their magnet mode rates of 100 beats/min and 96 beats/min, respectively. Magnet application as a means of addressing rate modulation in these devices may risk ischemia in patients with coronary artery disease.

Table 4.2 Pacemakers With Minute Ventilation Sensors

Boston Scientific/Guidant	Pulsar, Insignia, Altrua
Medtronic	Kappa
St. Jude (Telectronics)	Meta, Tempo
Sorin (ELA)	Brio, Chorus, Opus, Reply, Rhapsody, Symphony, Talent

From Kaplan JA, Reich DL, Savino JS. *Kaplan's Cardiac Anesthesia*. St. Louis: Elsevier; 2011:794.

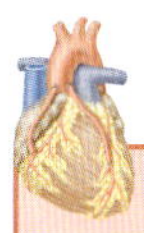

BOX 4.1   *Methods to Disable Rate Modulation*

- Cardiac implantable electrical device programming to disable rate modulation (preferred).
- Apply a magnet, which will place the pacemaker into an asynchronous mode.
- Remove the eliciting stimulus (e.g., hyperventilation or electrocautery).

Therefore disabling this function via programming may be more appropriate. Given that rate modulation via any monitored parameter offers no advantage to the patient in the OR, strong consideration should be given to disabling rate-adaptive therapy in the perioperative period (Box 4.1).

Multisite Pacing

At first glance, the fifth position of the NBG code (see Table 4.1) appears redundant given the possibility of "D" (dual) in the first position. Furthermore, the information conveyed by the fifth position is frequently omitted from notes regarding a device's mode (e.g., DDDR). However, the fifth position of the NBG code conveys unique and valuable information to the practitioner regarding either multiple leads in a single chamber or leads in multiple chambers. For example, in CRT, there are leads "in" both the RV and left ventricle (LV). This information would not be communicated by a "D" in the first position, which would simply denote leads in both the atrium and the ventricle (i.e., a dual-chamber pacemaker).

The goal of CRT is twofold: (1) to maintain sequential AV contraction and (2) to synchronize ventricular contraction of the RV and LV. A dual-chamber pacemaker successfully maintains sequential AV contraction between the RA and the RV; however, RV pacing often results in delayed depolarization of the LV inferior or inferolateral wall because of a conduction delay. CRT attempts to address this phenomenon in certain patient populations by placing a lead in the coronary sinus. The coronary sinus lead can then be used to pace the left ventricle from that inferolateral location with the goal being synchronized ventricular contraction and increased cardiac output. Interestingly, the coronary sinus or "CS lead" is another passive fixation lead that is frequently maintained in place by removing a guide, which allows the lead to take a bent shape in the vessel lumen. Given that this lead is placed in the coronary sinus, it results in epicardial pacing in contrast to the RA or RV leads, which are endocardial. The ultimate location of this coronary sinus lead has been generalized to the posterior or basal inferolateral location, but in fact optimization does vary (the process of optimization is beyond the scope of this text). However, despite optimal coronary sinus lead placement, approximately 30% of patients with severe LV systolic dysfunction do not respond to CRT. Determination of which patients will respond to CRT is an active field of investigation.

Indications for CRT, which is also frequently described as biventricular pacing, have expanded in recent years (Table 4.3). In 2012, an American College of Cardiology (ACC)/American Heart Association (AHA)/HRS update extended a class I indication to New York Heart Association (NYHA) class II patients with a left bundle branch block (LBBB) and QRS greater than 150 ms. A class IIa indication was also given to patients with an LBBB with QRS 120 to 149 ms or non-LBBB pattern with QRS greater than 150 ms. Therefore patients with CRT devices will likely become more

Table 4.3 Indications for Cardiac Resynchronization Therapy

	LVEF (%)	QRS Duration (ms)	NYHA Class	Bradycardia, Pacer Dependence
CRT-D	<35	>120	III, IV (I, II)	+/−
CRT-P	<35 (no ICD preferred)	>120	III, IV (I, II)	+/−

CRT, Cardiac resynchronization therapy; *CRT-D,* cardiac resynchronization therapy with automatic implantable cardioverter-defibrillator; *CRT-P,* biventricular pacing; ICD, implantable cardioverter-defibrillator; *LVEF,* left ventricular ejection fraction; *NYHA,* New York Heart Association.

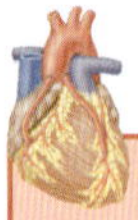

BOX 4.2 *Cardiac Resynchronization Therapy With Defibrillation Capability (CRT-D Devices) and Magnet Application*

- Because CRT-D devices contain an automatic implantable cardioverter-defibrillator, magnet application will only disable tachyarrhythmia therapies and NOT result in asynchronous pacing.
- Inhibition of biventricular pacing may result in a reduction in cardiac output and hypotension.

common in the OR. A small but sometimes confusing point is the documentation of either CRT-D or CRT-P. Although the indications are essentially the same (see Table 4.3), CRT-D implies pacing for CRT plus an automatic implantable cardioverter defibrillator (AICD), but CRT-P implies no AICD component. Because most patients who qualify for CRT also meet indications for AICD therapy, the majority of CRT patients will have CRT-D devices.

The CRT-D devices pose a unique problem for perioperative management because a magnet application will only succeed in deactivating the ICD portion of the device. Given that the goal of CRT is the synchronization of ventricular contraction and the associated increase in cardiac output, these patients might be considered "functionally" pacemaker dependent. This is a debatable position because CRT patients often have an "adequate" underlying rhythm. However, given the goal is to promote pacing, inhibition caused by EMI may result in a reduction in cardiac output. Therefore reprogramming CRT-D devices to an asynchronous mode would be required to guarantee continued pacing in the perioperative period when EMI is anticipated (Box 4.2).

Mode Switching

Although it is not present in the NBG code, mode switching can often be found in an interrogation note. Mode switching allows for device identification of atrial tachyarrhythmias and the automatic conversion of pacemaker settings. For example, atrial fibrillation can result in ventricular tachycardia in patients with a dual-chamber pacemaker. Without mode switching enabled, a DDDR pacemaker would track the atria (e.g., atrial fibrillation) and pace the ventricle resulting in ventricular tachycardia. This may be misdiagnosed as a run of ventricular tachycardia given the new wide complexes. With mode switching enabled, the pacemaker would automatically switch from DDDR to a VVIR mode and thus eliminate the atrial tracking function.

In certain situations, intraoperative mode switching can have significant hemodynamic consequences. For example, EMI (e.g., electrocautery) in the OR can be misinterpreted by the device as a supraventricular tachyarrhythmia. With mode switching enabled, the pacemaker may inappropriately switch to a VVIR setting. The subsequent loss of AV synchrony can result in a significant reduction in cardiac output and deterioration in hemodynamics. Although mode switching does not usually present significant challenges in the perioperative period, it can be used to a clinician's advantage. For example, the atrial tachyarrhythmia burden can be determined preoperatively from the number of mode switches listed in an interrogation note.

Pacemaker Failure

Pacemaker failure has three causes: (1) failure of capture, (2) lead failure, or (3) generator failure. Failure of capture secondary to a myocardial defect (i.e., no myocardial depolarizations despite generator output) is the most difficult problem to solve. Myocardial changes that can result in noncapture include myocardial ischemia or infarction, acid-base disturbances, electrolytes abnormalities, or abnormal antiarrhythmic drug levels. Sympathetic drugs, however, tend to lower pacing thresholds and therefore promote depolarization. Luckily, the other two causes of pacemaker failure—outright generator or lead failure—remain rare.

Leadless Transcatheter-Deployed Intracardiac Pacemakers

Given the potential complications related to transvenous pacing, which include problems with the leads as well as the pocket, a leadless pacing system offers certain potential advantages.

The Micra Transcatheter Pacemaker System (Medtronic) is a single-chamber ventricular pacemaker with accelerometer-based rate modulation capabilities. The device is positioned in the RV via a femoral percutaneous technique and subsequently secured with four tines at the distal end of the device (Fig. 4.4). Although estimated to be equivalent to other generators (e.g., >10 years), the longevity of the leadless device is unknown. In the event that the battery is exhausted or near exhaustion, the manufacturer contends that utilization of the "device off" mode and placement of a second neighboring device are options. Other options include percutaneous retrieval, which represents one of the highest risk procedures in interventional cardiology, or surgical explantation of the device. Although percutaneous retrieval has been documented, prior experience with the percutaneous extraction of chronic passive fixation transvenous leads would imply comparable difficulty with a long-term Micra device. This assumption is based on the characteristic fibrosis of chronically implanted devices and the similar fixation mechanism of the Micra device (i.e., four self-expanding electrically inactive nitinol tines).

Currently approved indications for the leadless device include tachycardia-bradycardia syndrome, symptomatic paroxysmal or permanent second- or third-degree AV block, bilateral bundle branch block, and paroxysmal or transient sinus node dysfunction with or without an AV conduction disorder. Contraindications to device implantation include the presence of another implanted cardiac device, mechanical tricuspid valve, or an inferior vena cava filter. Additional contraindications may include morbid obesity, unfavorable venous anatomy, or abnormal cardiac anatomy.

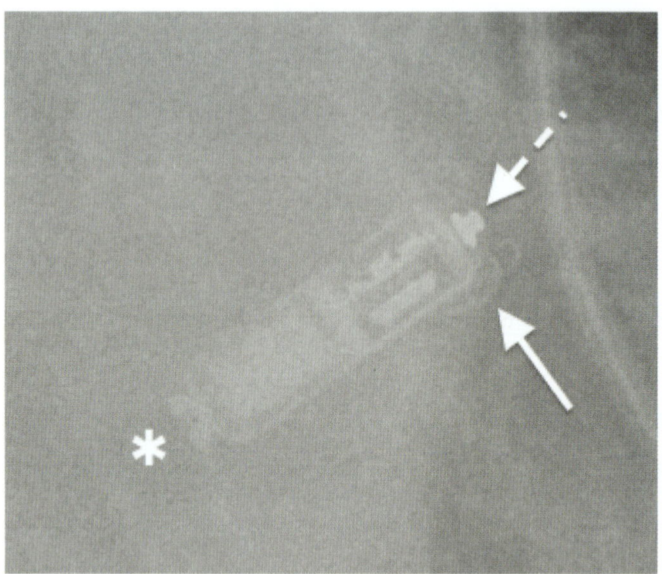

Fig. 4.4 Chest radiograph (magnified view) with a Medtronic Micra device in situ. One of the self-expanding nitinol tines is clearly visible *(solid arrow)* as well as the cathode *(dashed arrow)* and proximal retrieval feature *(asterisk)*.

Although the advent and use of the Micra system in the United States is exciting, it also poses new challenges for preoperative radiograph identification of leadless devices and perioperative management. Reports have indicated that appropriate interrogation software has not been readily available, which requires greater coordination with device representatives, and no magnet sensor. Medtronic has addressed the device interrogation issues; however, given the lack of a magnet response, early identification of these patients and proper interrogation are essential for perioperative management.

The Micra device has four functional modes (VVIR, VVI, VOO, OVO) and a "device off" mode. In the event of a device reset, the default is VVI at 65 beats/min. Similar to transvenous pacemakers, interactions between EMI and the leadless system can result in oversensing, tachyarrhythmias, tissue damage, and so on. However, unlike many traditional transvenous pacemakers, the Medtronic leadless device has received "magnetic resonance imaging (MRI) conditional" approval (see Special Situations for more information regarding MRI compatibility).

Alternatively, the St. Jude Nanostim (Fig. 4.5) leadless intracardiac pacemaker, which is currently approved for implant in countries outside of the United States, has a magnet sensor and response. Assuming appropriate battery life, a St. Jude Nanostim device will respond to a magnet applied over the apex of the heart by pacing at 100 beats/min for 8 beats followed by an asynchronous mode at 90 beats/min (65 beats/min elective replacement indicator) (Box 4.3).

AUTOMATIC IMPLANTABLE CARDIOVERTER-DEFIBRILLATOR BASICS

An AICD is a CIED that is able to detect and treat arrhythmias with antitachycardia pacing (ATP) or defibrillator shock via "shock coils" in the RV and occasionally the

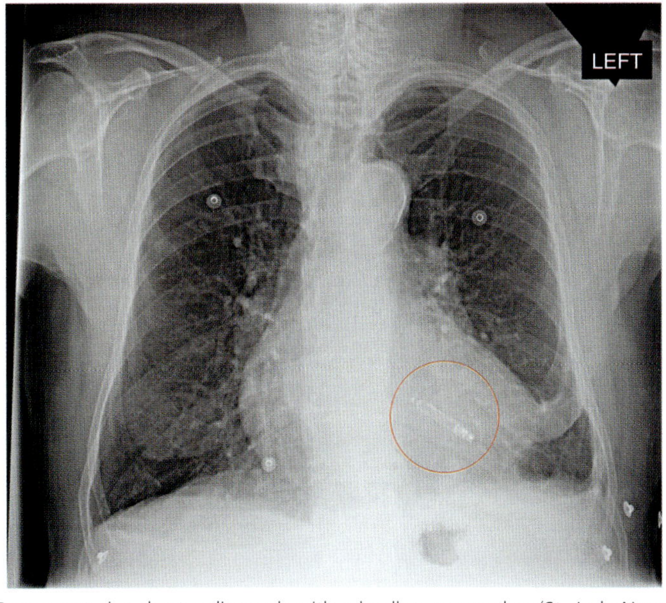

Fig. 4.5 Posteroanterior chest radiograph with a leadless pacemaker (St. Jude Nanostim) in the right ventricle *(circle)*, which is currently approved for implant outside of the United States. (Courtesy of Vivek Reddy, MD, Icahn School of Medicine at Mount Sinai, New York. From Rozner MA. Cardiac implantable cardiac devices. In Kaplan JA, ed. *Kaplan's Cardiac Anesthesia*. 7th ed. Philadelphia: Elsevier; 2017.)

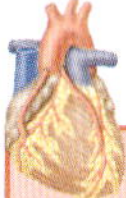

> **BOX 4.3**   *Leadless Transcatheter-Deployed Intracardiac Pacemakers and Magnets*
>
> - Medtronic Micra: no magnet response.
> - St. Jude Nanostim: a magnet applied over the apex of the heart induces asynchronous pacing at 90 beats/min (65 beats/min if at elective replacement interval).

superior vena cava. Treatment of identified ventricular tachyarrhythmias via overdrive pacing (i.e., ATP) or defibrillation depends on the diagnosis of either ventricular tachycardia or fibrillation. ATP or overdrive pacing, which typically occurs at lower rates (i.e., ventricular tachycardia), uses less energy—and thus less battery consumption—and is less painful so better tolerated by the awake patient. Given these advantages, most current AICDs can deliver some form of ATP while the capacitor charges for a shock. However, after a shock has been delivered, no further ATP will take place (Box 4.4).

The addition of a supraventricular coil (Fig. 4.6), which is denoted by the North American Society of Pacing and Electrophysiology/British Pacing and Electrophysiology Group Generic Defibrillator Code (NBD) code (Table 4.4), can be advantageous in differentiating supraventricular tachycardia from ventricular tachyarrhythmias. This differentiation is important because atrial fibrillation with rapid ventricular response and supraventricular tachycardia are the most common causes of inappropriate shock therapy, which occur in 20% to 40% of AICD patients. Whether inappropriate shocks injure patients remains a subject of considerable debate, but a significant number of

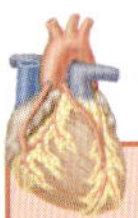

> ### BOX 4.4   *Automatic Implantable Cardioverter-Defibrillator Interrogation Reports*
>
> - Determine the indication for placement, date of placement, remaining battery life, and last interrogation.
> - Review the history of delivered therapies (i.e., how many times the patient has needed antitachycardia pacing, cardioversion, or defibrillation) and stored rhythms (i.e., ventricular tachycardia or ventricular fibrillation) since the last interrogation.
> - Determine the bradycardic pacing mode, rate, and dependence.

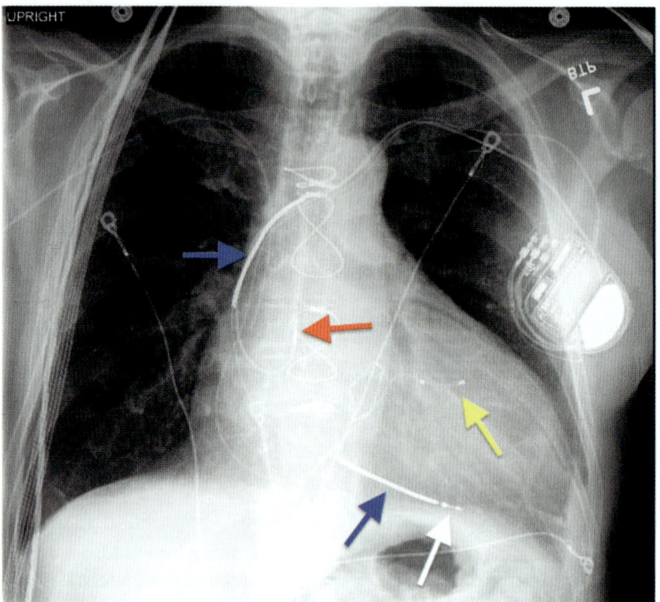

Fig. 4.6   Upright frontal chest radiograph showing a cardiac implantable electrical device with supraventricular/ventricular shock coils *(blue arrows)* and a bipolar pacing lead in the right ventricle *(white arrow)*, an atrial lead in the right atrium *(red arrow)*, and a coronary sinus lead *(yellow arrow)* for biventricular pacing. This is an example of a cardiac resynchronization therapy with defibrillation capability device.

Table 4.4	North American Society of Pacing and Electrophysiology/ British Pacing and Electrophysiology Group Generic Defibrillator Code (NBD Code)		
Shock Chamber	**Antitachycardia Pacing Chamber**	**Tachycardia Detection**	**Antibradycardia Pacing Chamber**
O = None	O = None	E = Electrogram	O = None
A = Atrium	A = Atrium	H = Hemodynamic	A = Atrium
V = Ventricle	V = Ventricle		V = Ventricle
D = Dual	D = Dual		D = Dual

patients who receive inappropriate shocks demonstrate elevated troponin levels in the absence of ischemia, and one death has been reported. Additionally, any AICD therapy (appropriate or inappropriate) has been associated with increased mortality.

Automatic Implantable Cardioverter-Defibrillator Indications

Initially, AICDs were implanted for hemodynamically significant ventricular tachycardia or fibrillation. New indications associated with sudden death include long QT syndrome, Brugada syndrome, arrhythmogenic RV dysplasia, and infiltrative cardiomyopathies. Recent studies also suggest that AICDs can be used for primary prevention of sudden death in patients with hypertrophic cardiomyopathy, postmyocardial infarction with an ejection fraction less than 30%, or cardiomyopathy with an ejection fraction of less than 35%. Finally, an AICD may be incorporated with CRT (e.g., CRT-D) in individuals with a dilated cardiomyopathy and a prolonged QRS interval. Although biventricular pacing (also known as CRT) has been shown to improve functional status and quality of life while reducing heart failure events, the addition of an AICD (i.e., CRT-D) has only been shown to reduce mortality rates in some studies.

In addition to tachyarrhythmia therapies, all AICDs are equipped with pacing capabilities; therefore the fourth position of the NBD code can be expanded to include all five pieces of information conveyed by the NBG code (Table 4.5). This expanded form is often referred to as the *label form*. Although pacing is advantageous when defibrillation results in a bradyarrhythmia, it also mandates perioperative programming in situations involving pacemaker-dependent patients and EMI.

Magnet Application

The application of a magnet to an AICD is expected to disable tachyarrhythmia therapies (Table 4.6). However, the typical magnet response may be disabled (e.g., some Boston Scientific and St. Jude Medical/Pacesetter devices) or ineffective. Reliable confirmation of appropriate magnet placement and suspension of antitachyarrhythmia therapies is only present in Boston Scientific AICDs (tone) and Sorin AICDs (pacing rate but not the mode; change to 90 beats/min if new or 80 beats/min if the battery is at elective replacement). Furthermore, the application of a magnet may not be a benign, immediately reversible process because there are case reports of magnet application permanently deactivating tachyarrhythmia therapy. Additional intraoperative concerns include the unrecognized displacement of the magnet and its lack of effect on the pacing function of the device. Although appropriate magnet application typically disables tachyarrhythmia therapies, it does not change the pacing function to an asynchronous mode. Therefore perioperative programming is mandatory for pacemaker-dependent patients with an AICD when EMI is likely (Box 4.5).

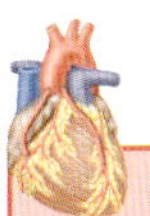

> **BOX 4.5**   *Automatic Implantable Cardioverter-Defibrillators and Magnet Application*
>
> - Magnet application for an automatic implantable cardioverter-defibrillator will have NO EFFECT on the underlying pacing functions.
> - Pacemaker-dependent patients require reprogramming to an asynchronous mode if electromagnetic interference is anticipated.

Table 4.5 Label Form: Expanded North American Society of Pacing and Electrophysiology/British Pacing and Electrophysiology Group Generic Defibrillator Code (NBD Code)

Shock Chamber	Antitachycardia Pacing Chamber	Tachycardia Detection	Pacing Chamber	Sensing Chamber	Response	Rate Modulation	Multisite Pacing
O = None A = Atrium V = Ventricle D = Dual	O = None A = Atrium V = Ventricle D = Dual	E = Electrogram H = Hemodynamic	O = None A = Atrium V = Ventricle D = Dual	O = None A = Atrium V = Ventricle D = Dual	O = None I = Inhibited T = Triggered D = Dual	O = None R = Rate Modulation	O = None A = Atrium V = Ventricle D = Dual

Table 4.6 Automatic Implantable Cardioverter-Defibrillator Response to Magnet Placement[a]

ICD Manufacturer	Magnet Modes	Magnet Mode Designation	Effect on Tachy Therapy	Effect on Brady Therapy (Regular Pacing)	Magnet Mode Confirmation
Biotronik			Disables	No effect	None
Boston Scientific (Guidant Medical, CPI)	Transvenous BSC: all BOS (except 119, 203) x-ray labels	ON (default)	Disables	No effect	Short beep every second or constant tone[b]
		OFF	No effect	No effect	None
	Transvenous GDT, CPI	ON (default)	Disables	No effect	Short beep with each R wave, or constant tone[b]
	BOS 119, BOS 203 x-ray labels	OFF	No effect	No effect	None
	Subcutaneous		Disables	No effect. S-ICD has no regular pacing. However, postshock pacing (VVI, 50 beats/min, 30 seconds, nonprogrammable) is terminated.	Short beep with each R wave, whether ICD therapy is on or off, for the first 60 seconds of magnet application. Thereafter, no confirmation.
Medtronic	AT-500[c]		Disables	No effect	None
	All others[d]		Disables	No effect	

Continued

Table 4.6 Automatic Implantable Cardioverter-Defibrillator Response to Magnet Placement[a]—cont'd

ICD Manufacturer	Magnet Modes	Magnet Mode Designation	Effect on Tachy Therapy	Effect on Brady Therapy (Regular Pacing)	Magnet Mode Confirmation
Pacesetter and St. Jude Medical		Normal (default)	Disables	No effect	
Sorin (was ELA Medical)		Ignore	No effect Disables	No effect The pacing rate, but not mode, changes to 96 beats/min (new device) declining to 80 beats/min, indicating elective replacement time.	None Pacing rate changes as noted.

[a]Effect(s) of appropriately placing a magnet over an ICD are shown. Some manufacturers have multiple responses that can be determined by the x-ray identifier. If the magnet response is programmable, the second column shows the various magnet modes available. The first mode shown is the default mode. A device reset from electromagnetic interference might produce some other mode (e.g., magnet mode disabled). Column 3 shows the effect on antitachycardia therapy (defibrillation, cardioversion, and antitachycardia pacing) for the magnet mode shown in Column 2. Only ICDs from Sorin Medical alter their antibradycardia pacing rate upon magnet placement, and this pacing rate can be used to predict remaining battery life provided that the patient's native heart rate is less than the magnet rate. Only ICDs from Boston Scientific/Guidant/CPI produce reliable audio feedback for confirmation of magnet placement. For devices from Pacesetter/St. Jude Medical, a device interrogation is required to determine the magnet mode.

[b]Any Boston Scientific/Guidant/CPI ICD that does not emit sound when a magnet is applied should undergo an immediate device interrogation. A stethoscope might be needed; for electronic stethoscopes, only the "Diaphragm" mode should be used because filtering in the "Bell" mode might not permit the sound to be transmitted to the earpiece.

For Boston Scientific/Guidant/CPI ICDs, if magnet mode is programmed to ON, appropriate magnet placement disables tachy detection and therapy, and tachy therapies remain disabled for as long as the magnet remains appropriately applied. When magnet mode is enabled in these devices, the ICD will emit either a constant tone or a beep to identify appropriate magnet placement. If the device emits a constant tone, then tachy therapy is disabled whether or not a magnet is present, and tachy therapy will not be present even after the magnet is removed. If any of these ICDs emit a beep (ICDs with GDT or CPI x-ray codes emit each beep with any paced or sensed R wave; ICDs with BOS or BSC x-ray code emits a beep every second), then a properly working ICD will be enabled for tachy therapy upon magnet removal.

Note that the "Change Tachy Mode with Magnet" feature is present only in very few remaining GDT and CPI x-ray labeled devices. When programmed ON, after 30 seconds of continuous magnet application, the tachy mode will toggle (i.e., it will switch from enabled when the magnet is removed [beeping with magnet correctly applied] to permanently disabled [constant tone when magnet is correctly applied] or vice versa). This mode has been phased out for most BOS/GDT/CPI ICD families, and software in programmers since October of 2009 is designed to disable and eliminate this feature.

[c]The Medtronic AT-500 series atrial defibrillators provide antitachycardia pacing in the atrium ONLY and usually after a delay often exceeding 1 minute from onset of atrial tachyarrhythmia. They do not have any shock coils on any lead and are very difficult to distinguish from a conventional two-chamber pacemaker. They have NO apparent magnet response. The x-ray identifier on these devices includes the Medtronic "M," but the first character is "I." All other Medtronic cardiac generators have the Medtronic "M" with the first letter identifier "P."

[d]Some Medtronic ICDs will emit a tone for 15 to 30 seconds when a magnet is placed on the device. However, this tone is not continuous with magnet placement, and it will not be interrupted with immediate magnet removal. As a result, the tone cannot be used for confirmation of appropriate magnet placement.

ICD, Implantable cardioverter-defibrillator; *S-ICD*, subcutaneous implantable cardioverter-defibrillator.

Subcutaneous Implantable Cardioverter-Defibrillators

The development of the subcutaneous implantable cardioverter-defibrillator (S-ICD) (Fig. 4.7) has further complicated AICD management because no specific recommendations have been published regarding the perioperative management of these devices. Furthermore, S-ICDs possess several fundamental differences from traditional transvenous AICDs. S-ICDs are larger than their transvenous counterparts, cannot

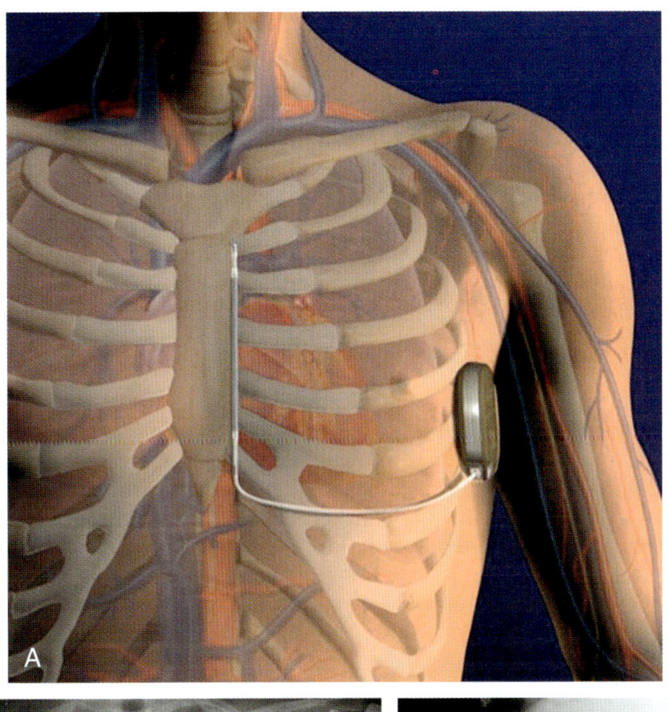

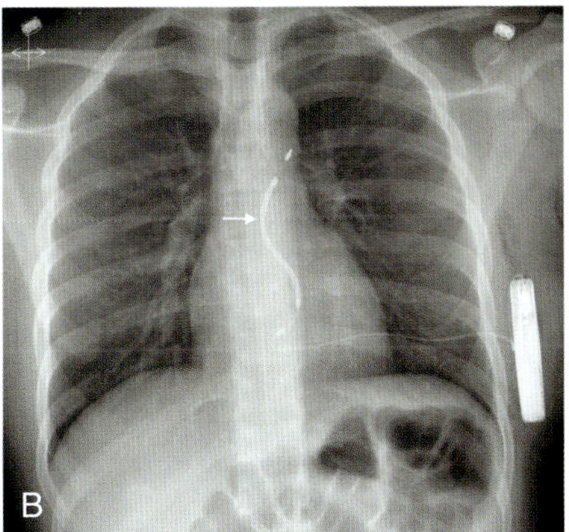

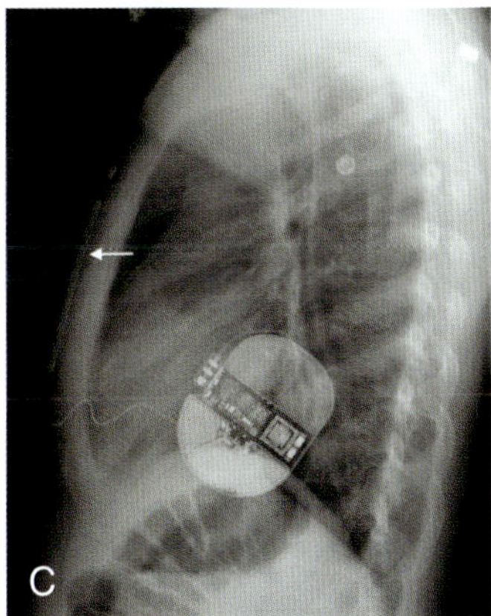

Fig. 4.7 (A) The Boston Scientific subcutaneous implantable cardioverter-defibrillator (S-ICD). The generator is implanted along the lateral chest wall with a subcutaneous lead tunneled into position over the heart. (B) Supine chest radiograph demonstrating an S-ICD generator along the lateral chest wall and tunneled lead *(arrow)*. (C) Lateral chest radiograph again demonstrating an S-ICD generator and tunneled lead *(arrow)*. (A, From Rozner MA. Cardiac implantable cardiac devices. In Kaplan JA, ed. *Kaplan's Cardiac Anesthesia*. 7th ed. Philadelphia: Elsevier; 2017.)

provide antitachycardia or sustained antibradycardia pacing (antibradycardia pacing only after shock therapy), and generally have higher defibrillations thresholds. However, the S-ICD response to magnet application is similar to traditional transvenous AICDs. Magnet application in the Boston Scientific devices is expected to disable tachyarrhythmia therapy. Given that these devices have no regular pacing function, magnet application has no effect on pacing. Rather, magnet application only disables postshock pacing (VVI, 50 beats/min for 30 seconds, nonprogrammable).

PREOPERATIVE PREPARATION FOR A PATIENT WITH A CARDIAC IMPLANTABLE ELECTRICAL DEVICE

In addition to a thorough past medical and surgical history, essential preoperative information includes the indication for the device, the current settings, the date of the last interrogation, the battery life and lead thresholds at the time of interrogation, and the magnet response. The practitioner must also determine pacemaker dependency. Determination of pacing dependence is difficult because there is no strict definition. However, patients who have undergone AV node ablation, have an underlying significant ventricular bradyarrhythmia, or have a high percentage paced on interrogation are often labeled *pacemaker dependent*. Reprogramming a pacemaker to VVI at 30 beats/min in the preoperative area can also be used to investigate underlying activity.

Although a wealth of information can be gained from a wallet card provided by the patient, medical records, or the company, individuals often present for surgery with little to no information regarding their devices. Therefore alternative investigative techniques must be used to attain the required information. Some approaches (e.g., attempting programmers from all five device companies to determine the manufacturer, which assumes the device is functional, or calling all five companies) are time consuming and may not instill a sense of confidence in the practitioner (Table 4.7). An alternative involves magnet application to narrow the field of the potential manufacturers by the magnet mode rate (Table 4.8). This technique requires assumptions regarding the programmed magnet response (i.e., Biotronik, Boston Scientific, and St. Jude devices) and battery life of the device. However, it can be used to quickly identify a newly implanted Medtronic or Sorin pacemaker given the consistent, unique magnet response.

Alternatively, a chest radiograph can be used to determine the device type (pacemaker vs. CRT-P vs. AICD vs. CRT-D), number of leads implanted, and device company as well. The prevalence of preoperative chest radiographs as well as the ability to magnify sections of radiographs (e.g., the generator) make identifying the device type, number of leads, and device company possible. It should begin by differentiating between a pacemaker (see Fig. 4.1) and an AICD (Fig. 4.8). The number of leads present can then help the practitioner identify the pacing scheme, differentiating among single-chamber (Fig. 4.9), dual-chamber (see Fig. 4.1), or biventricular (Fig. 4.10). The

Table 4.7	Device Manufacturer Contact Numbers
Manufacturer	**Phone Number**
Medtronic	800-633-8766
St. Jude Medical/Abbott (Telectronics)	800-722-3423
Boston Scientific (Guidant, Intermedics)	800-227-3422
Sorin	800-352-6466
Biotronik	800-547-0394

Table 4.8	**Pacemaker Magnet Mode Rates by Company**[a]					
	St. Jude	Medtronic	Biotronik	Boston Scientific	Sorin	Intermedics
Rate	100[b]	85	70–90	100	96	65 asynchronous beats and then the magnet is ignored
ERI	86	65	80	85	80	

[a]Biotronik, Boston Scientific, and St. Jude Medical generators have programmable magnet behavior.

[b]Older St. Jude models have an asynchronous rate of 98.6 beats/min, the St. Jude Pacesetter rate is model specific, VARIO mode is a repeating sequence, and the Nanostim rate is 100 beats/min for 8 cycles followed by 90 beats/min (elective replacement interval [ERI], 65 beats/min).

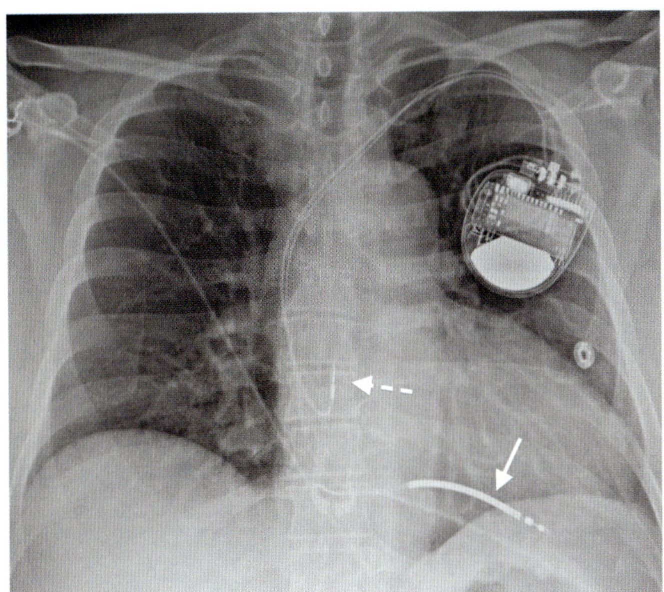

Fig. 4.8 Chest radiograph of an automatic implantable cardioverter-defibrillator (AICD). This is a dual-chamber device with one lead in the right atrium *(dashed arrow)* and another in the right ventricle *(solid arrow)*. A defibrillation coil is present, which differentiates it as an AICD.

practitioner can also determine if an AICD has a single defibrillation coil (see Fig. 4.8), has two coils, or possesses CRT capability (see Fig. 4.6). Finally, radiographic markings (e.g., alphanumeric codes), the shape of the battery, the shape of the generator, or the header orientation can be used to identify the device company (Fig. 4.11). After the device company has been identified, the patient and device can be confirmed over the phone, and an industry representative or management team can be requested for assistance or interrogation as needed. (See Suggested Reading at the end of the chapter for a chest radiograph algorithm.)

After the device manufacturer has been determined, contacting the company (technical support or local representative) can provide a wealth of information. Support personnel can confirm the patient and device, the potential magnet responses, and the expected effect of magnet removal (Box 4.6). Depending on the specific device, situation, and surgical procedure, this may be enough information to proceed.

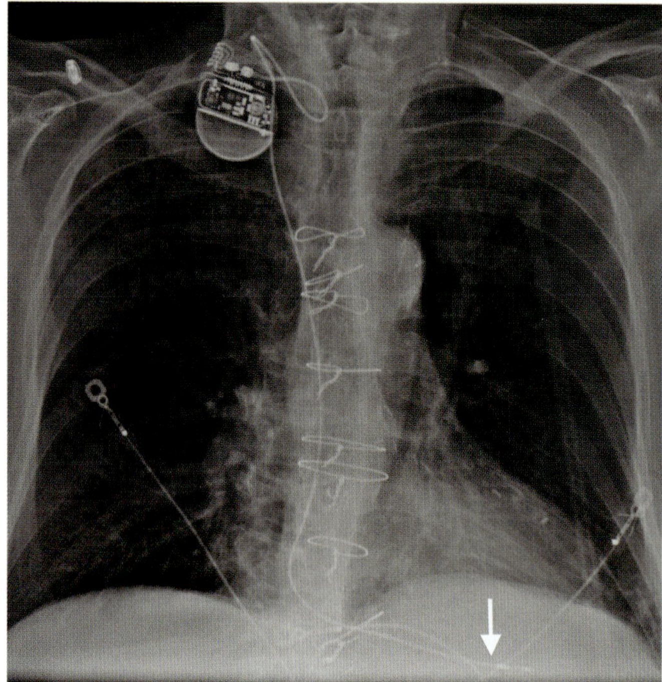

Fig. 4.9 Chest radiograph of a pacemaker with a single lead in the right ventricle (*arrow*). This is likely a temporary transvenous pacemaker given the position of the generator and venous access (i.e., right internal jugular).

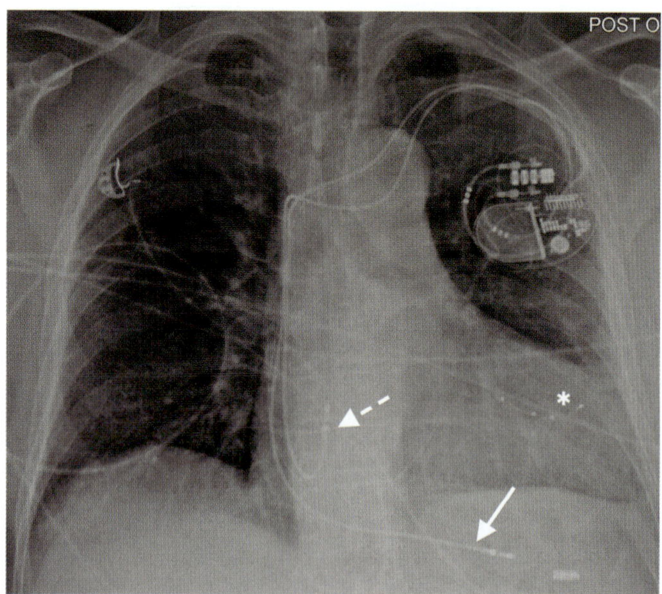

Fig. 4.10 Chest radiograph of a cardiac resynchronization therapy pacing device with a lead in the right atrium (*dashed arrow*), right ventricle (*solid arrow*), and coronary sinus (*asterisk*).

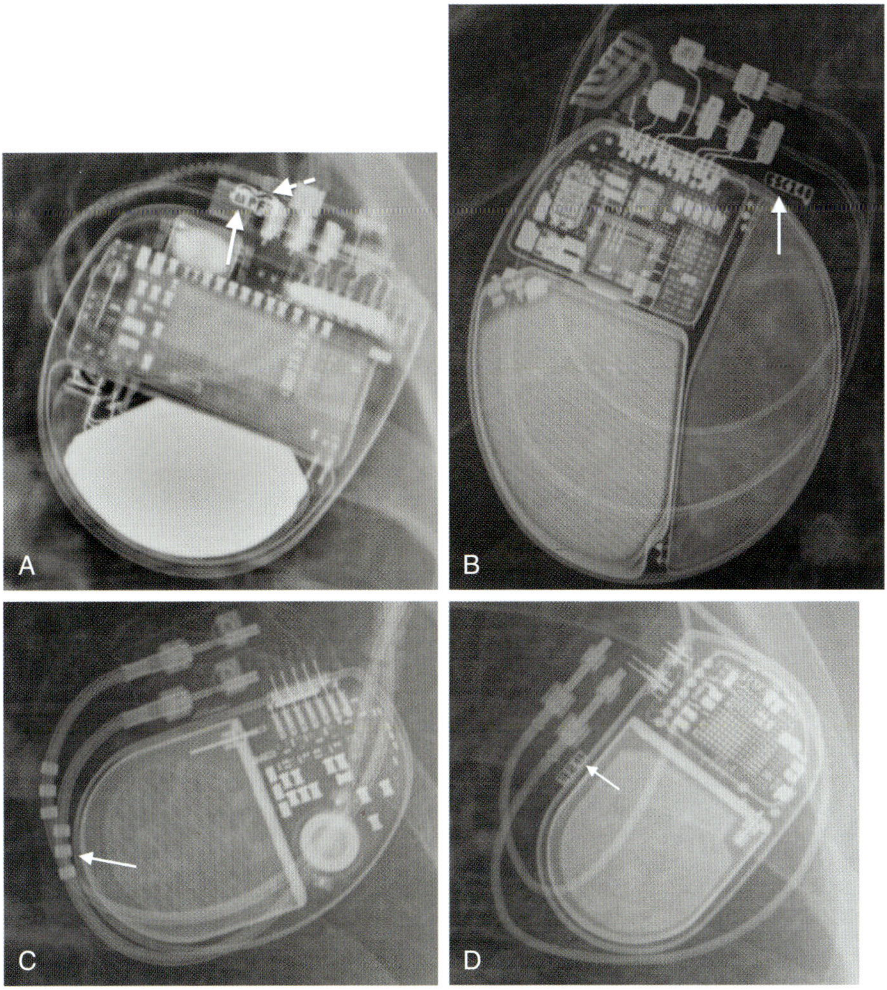

Fig. 4.11 Chest radiographs with magnification of the generator and characteristic radiographic markings. (A) Medtronic device with the Medtronic symbol *(solid arrow)* and magnetic resonance conditional marking *(dashed arrow)*. (B) Boston Scientific device with characteristic radiographic marking *(arrow)*. (C) St. Jude dual-chamber device with MR conditional leads denoted by the three radiographic rings *(arrow)*. (D) Biotronik device and symbol *(arrow)*.

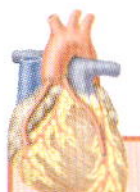

> **BOX 4.6**   *Programmable Magnet Response*
>
> - Biotronik, Boston Scientific, and St. Jude Devices have programmable responses to magnet application.
> - A recent interrogation or confirmation on an interrogation report is required to guarantee an asynchronous response.

A common misconception is that the device companies have a centralized record system to store and access previous interrogations. Although remote interrogation records may be made available, the patient and technical representative ultimately can only provide so much information, and an interrogation or recent interrogation note is required to determine pacemaker dependence, current mode, status of the battery and leads, programmed magnet mode, and so on. The American Society of Anesthesiologists recommends that "CIED function [is] ideally assessed by a comprehensive evaluation of the device" within 3 months of the procedure. The HRS recommends that a pacemaker be interrogated within 12 months, ICD within 6 months, and CRT device within 3 to 6 months of surgery. Although electronic medical records have made locating a recent interrogation report easier, locating this vital information in medical records is often still difficult.

Finally, to formulate a perioperative CIED management plan, the likelihood of EMI must be determined. The location and nature of the surgery are generally predictive of EMI.

Electromagnetic Interference

Although the myriad number of current CIED options presents a challenge for anesthesiologists, the technological advancements have also made these devices more resistant to EMI. Newer CIEDs use noise protection algorithms, filters (bandpass), and circuit shields to help minimize EMI. An additional explanation for the reduction in EMI is the trend to implant pacemakers with bipolar rather than unipolar leads. As previously mentioned, bipolar leads are more resistant to EMI because the anode and cathode are both contained within the lead itself. In contrast, unipolar leads are more susceptible to EMI because the distance between the anode (pulse generator) and cathode (tip of the lead) is much greater.

Despite these improvements, EMI can still occur and is the crux of any perioperative management plan (Fig. 4.12) is determining the likelihood of encountering interference. EMI can result from any device that emits radiofrequency (RF) waves between 0 and 10^9 Hz. The expansive list of potential EMI sources includes, but is not limited to, electrocautery, external defibrillation, ECT, and RF waves used in ablation procedures. In addition, the RF scanning systems used to identify retained surgical material can interfere with pacing, and some manufacturers recommend reprogramming to an asynchronous pacing mode.

Although a potential source of EMI may be present, EMI may still be unlikely. For example, the potential for interaction is considered to be markedly reduced if the distance from the electrocautery current to the CIED generator and leads is greater than 6 inches. One protocol further defines a critical zone of increased risk of EMI to include the area from the mandible to the xiphoid. Furthermore, it is the current belief that for operative procedures below the umbilicus, electrocautery does not interfere with a generator and leads that are located in the upper chest.

There are additional techniques other than absolute distance that can reduce the possibility or effect of EMI such as the use of bipolar as opposed to monopolar electrocautery, short bursts of electrocautery (<4 seconds, separated by at least 2 seconds), lower electrocautery power settings, nonblended cutting electrocautery, use of an ultrasonic cutting device (i.e., harmonic scalpel), and proper positioning of the electrocautery return pad to minimize return current interaction with the device. Proper electrocautery return pad placement may be the shoulder contralateral to the device for head and neck surgery or placement on the ipsilateral arm with the wire prepped into the field for breast or axillary cases. Although proper use of electrocautery and bipolar leads have significantly decreased EMI, it is difficult to predict what effects

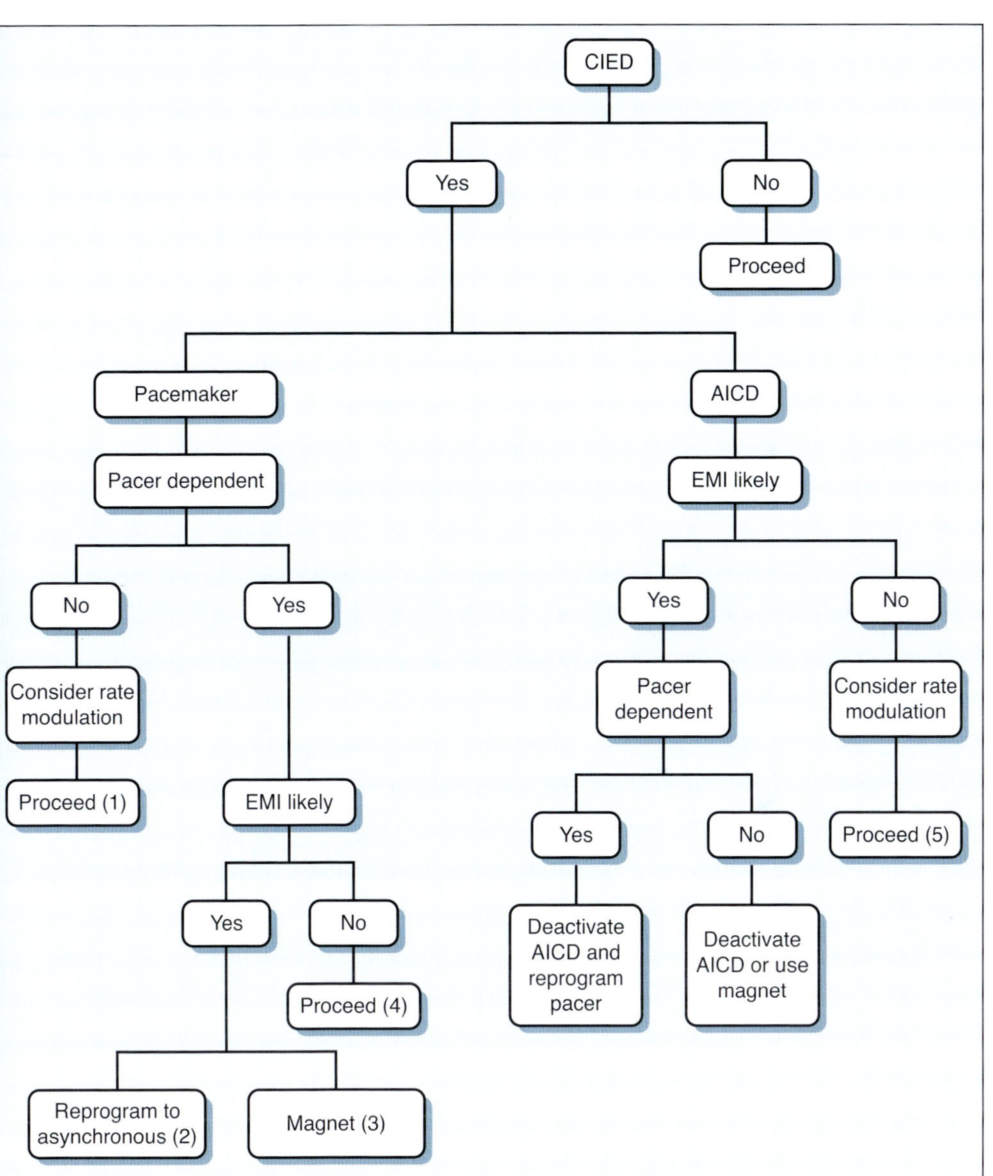

Fig. 4.12 General approach to perioperative cardiovascular implantable electronic device (CIED) management. Additional considerations: (1) have magnet available; (2) be aware of potential R-on-T phenomenon if applicable; (3) consider magnet mode settings, patient comorbidities, and potential R-on-T phenomenon; (4) complete preoperative CIED assessment, have magnet available, and consider rate modulation; and (5) have a magnet available. *AICD,* Automatic implantable cardioverter-defibrillator; *EMI,* electromagnetic interference.

if any will occur in the OR because no testing of EMI and CIEDs is currently required before a device is brought to market.

Preoperative Evaluation: Summary

The current recommendations from the ASA/HRS are very clear that an appropriate preoperative evaluation involves communication between the operative team and the primary CIED management team as well as direction from the primary CIED management team. In addition to consultation with the management team and a current interrogation (i.e., within 12 months for pacemakers and 6 months for ICDs), the ASA/HRS recommends that certain key pieces of information regarding the device and operation be determined (Box 4.7).

Current Recommendations

It is challenging to develop a perioperative CIED management algorithm that is universally applicable. Therefore it should not surprise practitioners that recommendations regarding the perioperative management of CIEDs vary according to the organization. Similarly, it is not surprising that the current recommendations from the ASA and HRS focus on an individualized, multidisciplinary approach with less reliance on direction from industry employed allied health professionals and increased involvement of the primary CIED management team. Given that the ASA/HRS recommendations are the standard by which anesthesiologists will be judged, it seems prudent to adhere to those guidelines. Although these recommendations excel at optimizing patient safety, it should be noted that strict adherence to the recommendations may not always be feasible because of the clinical situation or resources available. Alternative protocols for device management, such as the Pacing And Cardioversion Electronic Devices Perioperative Protocol (PACED-OP), advocate for more selective criteria for CIED reprogramming in an effort to operate within the confines of restricted resources and avoid reprogramming errors.

In response to high rates of reprogramming and interrogation, which require resources and personnel and create the potential for pre- and postprocedure programming errors, the PACED-OP protocol attempted to develop a simplified perioperative management algorithm. The PACED-OP protocol only required device reprogramming when EMI was expected within a critical zone (i.e., the area between the mandible and the xiphoid) and the patient was pacemaker dependent or had an AICD. Pacemaker dependency was also simplified to encompass individuals who had a preoperative ECG displaying a paced rhythm (Fig. 4.13). AICDs were managed with a magnet if

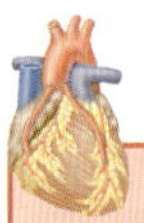

> **BOX 4.7** **Essential Elements of Cardiac Implantable Electrical Device Preoperative Evaluation**
>
> - Procedure: type, anatomical location, patient position, potential sources of electromagnetic interference, anticipated cardioversion or defibrillation, surgical venue, and postoperative disposition
> - Device: type, manufacture, model, indication for the device, battery longevity, date of lead placement, mode and programming, pacemaker dependency and underlying rhythm, recent therapies, response to magnet application, recent device alerts, and pacing thresholds

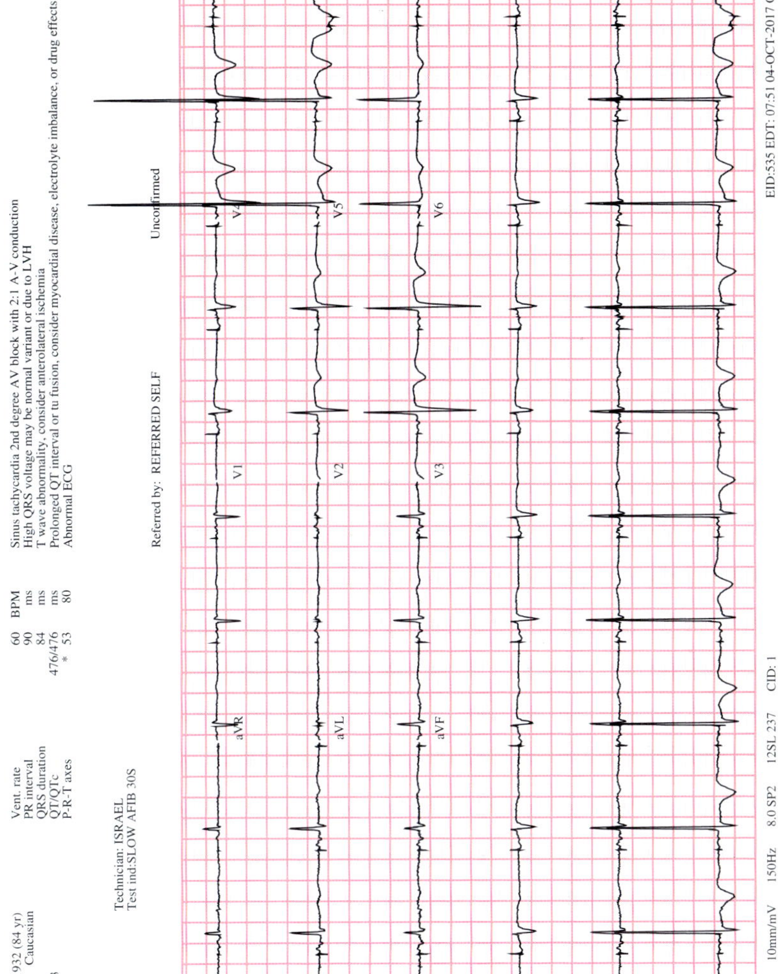

Fig. 4.13 Preoperative electrocardiogram displaying an atrial paced rhythm at the lower rate limit (60 beats/min) in a patient with a dual-chamber pacemaker.

Table 4.9 PACED-OP Protocol Summary

Clinical Situation	Management
1. Pacemaker dependent or AICD + EMI in critical zone	1. Reprogram preoperatively and interrogate postoperatively
2. AICD + EMI outside the critical zone	2. Apply magnet (exception: devices with a reed switch)
3. Pacemaker-dependent patient + EMI outside the critical zone + bradycardia postoperatively	3. Interrogate postoperatively

AICD, Automatic implantable cardioverter-defibrillator; *EMI,* electromagnetic interference; *PACED-OP,* Pacing And Cardioversion Electronic Devices Perioperative Protocol.

EMI was anticipated outside the critical zone. Exceptions were AICDs that contained a reed switch, which were reprogrammed. Postoperatively, additional CIED interrogation was only recommended if an ECG identified bradycardia in a pacemaker-dependent patient after electrocautery was used outside the critical zone (Table 4.9).

Even though multiple organizations have recently released recommendations that call for increased involvement of the primary CIED management team and perioperative interrogation or reprogramming, anecdotes imply these devices are frequently managed by magnet application or EMI avoidance. However, it must be stated that the recommendations clearly favor interrogation and reprogramming over magnet application. Although comprehensive perioperative CIED services are staffed by anesthesiologists at some large academic centers, the majority of management teams that complete the perioperative interrogation and programming described are a division of cardiology.

INTRAOPERATIVE MANAGEMENT OF A PATIENT WITH A CARDIAC IMPLANTABLE ELECTRICAL DEVICE

Although not applicable to every situation, a general approach to perioperative CIED management is presented in Fig. 4.12. As shown, perioperative management largely relies on determining the patient's CIED dependence and EMI potential. Based on the risk assessment, CIED management may require a magnet to be available, the use of a magnet, or interrogation and reprogramming. As previously mentioned, rate responsiveness and other rate enhancements (e.g., hysteresis, sleep rate, AV search) should be considered when reprogramming because these options may be misinterpreted as pacing system malfunction instead of mechanisms to reduce or prevent RV pacing.

A historic staple of CIED perioperative management has been the application of a magnet. Although reliance on a magnet is not preferred by the societal guidelines and may not be the most elegant of techniques, it is applicable in some situations. However, knowing the magnet mode rate for pacemakers (see Table 4.8) and the device responses for AICDs (see Table 4.6) before making this decision is vital. Please note that Table 4.8 is drastically oversimplified. For example, some pacemaker magnet modes are programmable (e.g., Biotronik, Boston Scientific, and St. Jude Medical). These devices can be programmed to respond to magnet application with asynchronous pacing, a brief period of asynchronous pacing followed by a return to the original settings (Biotronik), synchronous pacing without rate responsiveness (Biotronik), no response (e.g., magnet response off in Boston Scientific and St. Jude Medical devices), data collection only and no change in pacing (Boston Scientific and St. Jude Medical), asynchronous pacing at a model-specific rate (e.g., Pacesetter, St. Jude Medical), or a repeating sequence (e.g., Vario Mode, St. Jude Medical). Intermedics (now Boston Scientific) devices respond to magnet application with asynchronous pacing for only 65 beats. Therefore the use of a magnet may not result in sustained asynchronous pacing (e.g., 10 cycles of 90 beats/min in an asynchronous mode followed by a return to programmed mode and rate in Biotronik devices) or only result in data collection, or the pacemaker may not respond to magnet placement on account of programming (e.g., safety mode after an electrical reset or magnet mode programmed off). If sustained asynchronous pacing is desired and not obtained with magnet application in St. Jude, Biotronik, or Boston Scientific devices, consultation and programming may be required. Alternatively, confirmation of magnet response may be possible if the data from a recent remote interrogation are made available by a device representative. For a detailed, specific list, see Chapter 5 in *Kaplan's Cardiac Anesthesia,* 7th edition, or contact the manufacturer for additional information.

A few other considerations regarding magnet application merit special attention. Placing a pacemaker in an asynchronous mode may not be benign and therefore should not be taken lightly or without careful consideration. The use of a magnet or programming to an asynchronous mode in a pacemaker with a ventricular lead could result in an R-on-T phenomenon and significant arrhythmia. Furthermore, the use of a magnet may result in AV dyssynchrony, a reduction in stroke volume, or a set rate that is disadvantageous in the setting of certain comorbidities (e.g., coronary artery disease).

Although no special monitoring or anesthetic technique is required for the patient with a pacemaker, monitoring of the patient should include the ability to detect mechanical systoles since EMI, as well as devices such as a nerve stimulator, can interfere with QRS complexes and pacemaker spikes on the ECG. Mechanical systoles are best evaluated by pulse oximetry, plethysmography, or an arterial waveform. With regard to anesthetic technique, no studies have proven one technique superior. However, reports have documented QT prolongation with isoflurane or sevoflurane, and medications such as dexmedetomidine or high-dose opiates may suppress underlying electrical activity rendering the patient pacemaker dependent. Similarly, no anesthetic techniques have proven superior in patients with AICDs. Many of these patients have severely depressed systolic function, dilated ventricular cavities, and significant valvular pathology. Therefore the anesthetic technique is mainly dictated by the underlying physiologic derangements.

It is also important to note that when tachyarrhythmia therapies are programmed off, an external defibrillator should be readily available—and practitioners should be familiar with its application—until therapies are reenabled. Placement of external pads before disabling the device is recommended. In addition, medications to manipulate hemodynamics (e.g., inotropes, vasopressors), heart rate (e.g., anticholinergics, β-blockers, calcium channel blockers), and rhythm (e.g., antiarrhythmics) should be readily available.

Alternatively, if magnet application is used instead of programming, it can be removed to deliver an internal shock if indicated. Reliance on a magnet for the intraoperative management of an AICD poses a particular challenge because (1) the magnet response can be programmed off (see Table 4.6), (2) magnet application has previously permanently disabled tachyarrhythmia therapies (e.g., Guidant AICDs before a software update in 2009), (3) a limited number of AICDs lack a magnet response, and (4) the magnet has to be reliably secured over the device and out of

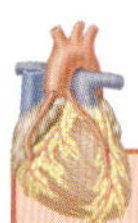

> **BOX 4.8** *Disabling Tachyarrhythmia Therapies in the Perioperative Period*
>
> - Changes to cardiac implantable electrical device programming should be documented in the medical record (i.e., interrogation report).
> - Alternative means of cardioversion or defibrillation and emergency medications must be readily available (e.g., external pads, defibrillator, code medications).
> - Tachyarrhythmia therapies should be reenabled at the conclusion of the procedure and again documented in the medical record (i.e., interrogation report).

the surgical field. These challenges are not to be taken lightly as inappropriate ATP or defibrillation can result in significant battery depletion or myocardial injury. Navigating these situations is best accomplished through proper preoperative preparation and reliance on the device company technical support (Box 4.8).

SPECIAL SITUATIONS

Imaging Patients With Cardiac Implantable Electrical Devices

Frequently, patients with CIEDs require a computed tomography (CT) scan or MRI. CT scans directly over the generator can rarely cause oversensing and pacing inhibition. MRI represents another imaging modality that requires special attention in patients with CIEDs. More recently, a large number of patients with CIEDs have undergone MRIs when the benefit outweighed the theoretical risk to the patient. In fact, more than 3000 patients with CIEDs have undergone MRIs without significant incident, other than an occasional device electrical reset. In the United States, pacemakers manufactured by Biotronik and Medtronic carry "MR conditional" labeling. Although the Food and Drug Administration believes that unconditional or MR "safe" labeling of CIEDs for MRI is unlikely, these select devices (Fig. 4.14) can undergo MRI with certain additional conditions. However, pacing-dependent patients remain at increased risk, and most centers will not perform an MRI on a pacing-dependent patient with an ICD.

Lithotripsy

Consideration should be given to programming the pacing function out of an atrial-paced mode for lithotripsy procedures. Some lithotriptors are designed to fire on the R wave, and the atrial pacing stimulus could be misinterpreted as the contraction of the ventricle.

ANTIBIOTIC PROPHYLAXIS

Antimicrobial prophylaxis at the time of CIED placement is recommended and typically achieved by the administration of an antibiotic with activity against staphylococci (e.g., cefazolin or vancomycin) before incision. However, there is currently no

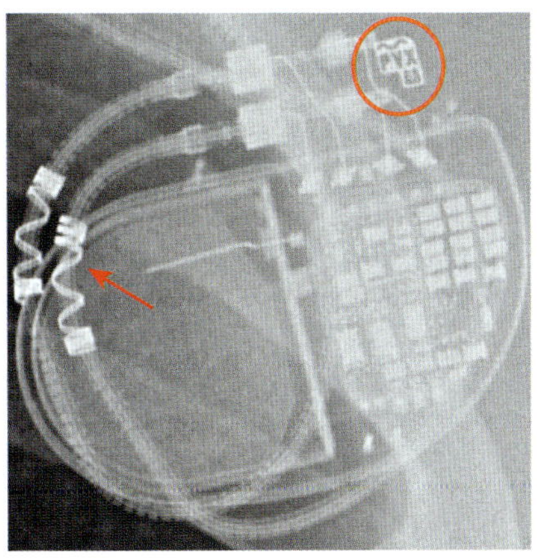

Fig. 4.14 Medtronic Advisa MR conditional pacemaker. Note the additional marking on the logo above "PVX" that is used by Medtronic to identify their magnetic resonance (MR) conditional devices. This particular generator also has MR conditional leads, which also have special x-ray identifiers *(arrow)*. (From Rozner MA. Cardiac implantable cardiac devices. In Kaplan JA, ed. *Kaplan's Cardiac Anesthesia*. 7th ed. Philadelphia: Elsevier; 2017.)

recommendation for antibiotic prophylaxis before routine dental, gastrointestinal, or genitourinary procedures to prevent CIED infections. This recommendation against routine antibiotic prophylaxis for dental or other invasive procedures not directly related to device manipulation solely for the purpose of CIED infection prevention is based on the premise that the risk of prophylaxis (e.g., development of antibiotic-resistant pathogens, allergic reactions, cost) outweighs the unproven benefit.

POTENTIAL ADVERSE OUTCOMES

Aside from preoperative preparation (i.e., knowledge regarding the model type, dependency, magnet mode, EMI potential) and a well-thought-out perioperative management plan, a thorough understanding of the potential complications or adverse outcomes is paramount to the successful perioperative management of a patient with a CIED. For example, central venous catheter placement can result in coronary sinus lead displacement and loss of biventricular pacing. Early recognition and action by the anesthesiologist can be facilitated by the published experience of others and known EMI interactions.

The list of potential complications and case reports surrounding CIEDs is extensive. EMI from monopolar electrocautery or RF ablation can result in oversensing and inhibition of pacemakers, inappropriate tachyarrhythmia therapy from AICDs, device reset, pulse generator damage, lead damage, inappropriate rate-adaptive heart rate changes, inappropriate mode switching, impedance changes, and tissue damage via conduction through device leads. A recent study has identified a trend toward alterations in threshold and sensing in devices that required reprogramming postoperatively. One proposed explanation is changes in lead tissue interaction from intraoperative EMI. However, other studies present contrary evidence and suggest that these interactions are uncommon.

External cardioversion or defibrillation can also potentially result in tissue damage via conduction through leads or device reset. Therefore it is recommended that tachyarrhythmia therapies be reenabled either by removing a magnet or reprogramming to allow for device-delivered therapy. If this is not feasible or effective, then emergency guidelines must be followed. In an effort to minimize current through the device or leads, the pads should be placed as far away from the generator as possible and perpendicular to the axis of the CIED (e.g., anterior-posterior).

Finally, although therapeutic radiation in patients with CIEDs is not contraindicated, it should be recognized that ionizing radiation could result in damage to the pulse generator or lead insulation. Recent evidence suggests that modern AICDs may be more susceptible to radiation damage than pacemakers. The damage incurred can result in electrical resets or AICDs unable to deliver a high-voltage shock. Therefore it is recommended that the device be shielded or relocated and interrogation be completed during as well as at the completion of radiation treatment.

POSTOPERATIVE MANAGEMENT OF A PATIENT WITH A CARDIAC IMPLANTABLE ELECTRICAL DEVICE

Postoperatively, practitioners are faced with the dilemma of postoperative interrogation. Programming to asynchronous modes or disabling tachyarrhythmia therapies preoperatively mandates postoperative interrogation. However, for devices that were not reprogrammed and functioned normally in the perioperative period, the recommendation is more nebulous. For nonreprogrammed pacemakers, most manufacturers recommend interrogation to ensure proper functioning and remaining battery life if monopolar electrocautery was used in the perioperative period. The ASA recommends that a postoperative check may not be needed if the device was evaluated appropriately preoperatively, no perioperative programming was required, no EMI was encountered, no blood transfused, and no problems were encountered. The HRS/ASA suggests that for hemodynamically challenging cases or when EMI was likely (e.g., external cardioversions, RF ablation, cardiothoracic surgery), an evaluation should be completed before discharge. Conversely, for low-risk procedures (e.g., inferior to the umbilicus) when the device functioned as expected in the perioperative period, then an evaluation can be completed as an outpatient within 30 days. Overall, the preferred and safest practice is to ensure that a CIED is functioning properly in the postoperative period with a thorough interrogation by a qualified practitioner. As previously stated, any perioperative programming or CIED dysfunction mandates a postoperative interrogation to restore the original settings or troubleshoot the device. Finally, whenever an interrogation is completed, proper documentation (i.e., a report) should be included in the patient's medical record.

SUGGESTED READING

American Society of Anesthesiologists. Practice advisory for the perioperative management of patients with cardiac implantable electronic devices: pacemakers and implantable cardioverter-defibrillators: an updated report by the American Society of Anesthesiologists task force on perioperative management of patients with cardiac implantable electronic devices. *Anesthesiology*. 2011;114(2):247–261.

Anand NK, Maguire DP. Anesthetic implications for patient with rate-responsive pacemakers. *Semin Cardiothorac Vasc Anesth*. 2005;9(3):251–259.

Baddour LM, Epstein AE, Erickson CC, et al. Update on cardiovascular implantable electronic device infections and their management: a scientific statement from the American Heart Association. *Circulation*. 2010;121(3):458–477.

Cheng A, Nazarian S, Spragg DD, et al. Effects of surgical and endoscopic electrocautery on modern-day permanent pacemaker and implantable cardioverter-defibrillator systems. *PACE*. 2008;31:344–350.

Costelloe CM, Murphy WA Jr, Gladish GW, et al. Radiography of pacemakers and implantable cardioverter defibrillators. *AJR Am J Roentgenol*. 2012;199:1252–1258.

Cronin B, Essandoh MK. Perioperative interrogation of St. Jude cardiovascular internal electrical devices for anesthesiologists. *J Cardiothorac Vasc Anesth*. 2018;32:982–1000.

Crossley GH, Poole JE, Rozner MA, et al. The Heart Rhythm Society/American Society of Anesthesiologists Expert Consensus Statement on the perioperative management of patients with implantable defibrillators, pacemakers and arrhythmia monitors: facilities and patient management: executive summary. *Heart Rhythm*. 2011;8:e1–e18.

Healey JS, Merchant R, Simpson S, et al. Canadian Cardiovascular Society/Canadian Anesthesiologists' Society/Canadian Heart Rhythm Society joint position statement on the perioperative management of patients with implanted pacemakers, defibrillators, and neurostimulating devices. *Can J Cardiol*. 2012;28(2):141–151.

Jacob S, Shahzad MA, Maheshwari R, et al. Cardiac rhythm device identification algorithm using x-rays: CaRDIA-X. *Heart Rhythm*. 2011;8(6):915–922.

Madhavan M, Mulpuru S, McLeod C, et al. Advances and future directions in cardiac pacemakers. *J Am Coll Cardiol*. 2017;69:212–235.

Mahlow WJ, Craft RM, Misulia NL, et al. A perioperative management algorithm for cardiac rhythm management devices: the PACED-OP protocol. *PACE*. 2013;36:238–248.

Mickus GJ, Soliman GI, Reed RR, et al. Perioperative management of a leadless pacemaker: the paucity of evidence-based guidelines. *J Cardiothorac Vasc Anesth*. 2016;30:1594–1698.

Moss AJ, Hall WJ, Cannom DS, et al. Cardiac-resynchronization therapy for the prevention of heart-failure events. *N Engl J Med*. 2009;361:1329–1338.

Mulpuru S, Madhavan M, McLeod C, et al. Cardiac pacemakers: function, troubleshooting, and management. *J Am Coll Cardiol*. 2017;69:189–210.

Nazarian S, Hansford R, Roguin A, et al. A prospective evaluation of a protocol for magnetic resonance imaging of patients with implanted cardiac devices. *Ann Intern Med*. 2011;155:415–424.

Rasmussen MJ, Friedman PA, Hammill SC, et al. Unintentional deactivation of implantable cardioverter-defibrillators in health care settings. *Mayo Clin Proc*. 2002;77:855–859.

Reynolds D, Duray GZ, Omar R, et al. A leadless intracardiac transcatheter pacing system. *N Engl J of Med*. 2016;374:533–541.

Rooke GA, Bowdle TA. Perioperative management of pacemakers and implantable cardioverter defibrillators: it's not just about the magnet. *Anesth Analg*. 2013;117:292–294.

Schulman PM, Rozner MA. Use caution when applying magnets to pacemakers or defibrillators for surgery. *Anesth Analg*. 2013;117:422–427.

Squara F, Chik WW, Benhayon D, et al. Development and validation of a novel algorithm based on the ECG magnet response for rapid identification of an unknown pacemaker. *Heart Rhythm*. 2014;11:1367–1376.

Stone ME, Salter B, Fischer A. Perioperative management of patients with cardiac implantable electronic devices. *Br J Anaesth*. 2011;107(suppl 1):i16–i26.

Stone ME, Apinis A. Current perioperative management of the patient with a cardiac rhythm management device. *Semin Cardiothorac Vasc Anesth*. 2009;13(1):31–43.

Thompson A, Mahajan A. Perioperative management of cardiovascular implantable electronic devices: what every anesthesiologist needs to know. *Anesth Analg*. 2013;116(2):276–277.

Weiss R, Knight BP, Gold MR, et al. Safety and efficacy of a totally subcutaneous implantable-cardioverter-defibrillator. *Circulation*. 2013;128:944–953.

Chapter 5

Left Ventricular Assist Device–Supported Patient Presenting for Noncardiac Surgery

Marc E. Stone, MD

Key Points

1. Regardless of the level of complexity or invasiveness of the planned procedure, the perioperative considerations and the anesthetic approach to left ventricular assist device (LVAD)–supported patients are the same because the removal of sympathetic tone by sedation or induction of general anesthesia should be expected to initially exert the same effect on the physiology of ventricular assist device (VAD)-supported patients regardless of the planned procedure.
2. A team-based approach and preoperative planning regarding intraoperative management and postoperative recovery location are key to the successful perioperative management of VAD-supported patients presenting for noncardiac surgery.
3. An understanding of the physiology of the VAD-supported state is the key to safe intraoperative management.
4. No specific sedatives or anesthetic agents are contraindicated because of the presence of a VAD, but the required anticoagulation often precludes major regional techniques.
5. Most patients with a modern nonpulsatile left VAD (LVAD) do exhibit pulsatility of their circulation; however, they can lose this pulsatility after induction because of the relative hypovolemia and vasodilation that accompany an anesthetic, bringing considerations of appropriate monitoring.
6. Optimization of volume status will help maintain pulsatility of the circulation in a VAD-supported patient.
7. Intraoperative changes to baseline VAD settings are rarely (if ever) needed in a VAD-supported patient who was optimized on these settings when not anesthetized.

ROLE OF VENTRICULAR ASSIST DEVICES IN THE MANAGEMENT OF HEART FAILURE

The prevalence of heart failure (HF) worldwide is estimated to be about 26 million people. In the United States alone, there are approximately 5.7 million adults with HF, and this number is projected to increase to approximately 8 million by the year 2030. Mechanical circulatory support (MCS) with a left ventricular assist device (LVAD) is now the standard management for patients with chronic refractory HF. The goals of LVAD support are twofold: (1) to decompress the failing left ventricle, thus dramatically reducing left ventricular (LV) myocardial oxygen demand (which, in certain circumstances, may promote recovery of the failing myocardium), and (2) to maintain adequate systemic perfusion to avert cardiogenic shock. The pump itself is attached to the heart and great vessels by cannulae that allow continuous collection of blood returning to the left side of the heart and ejection of that blood into the aorta.

According to the latest data from the Interagency Registry for Mechanically Assisted Circulatory Support (INTERMACS), there are currently 2000 to 3000 LVAD implantations annually at approximately 160 centers in the United States alone. Table 5.1 outlines the current indications for long-term LVAD support, as well as the current frequency and current success of each indication in the United States.

Until 2009, bridge to transplantation (BTT) was the most common indication for implantation of a durable LVAD, but the approval of the HeartMate II for destination therapy (DT) in 2010 heralded a new era of MCS because before that, a durable device that could provide years of support did not exist. Continuous-flow (CF) devices (e.g., the HeartMate II) have now been used to provide support for 100% of patients implanted for DT since 2010, as well as for more than 95% of all other LVAD indications. The first generation of pulsatile, implantable devices is essentially no longer in use.

The most common indication for LVAD implantation is now DT (see Table 5.1), with BTC the second most common indication and BTT (the traditional indication before 2010) now third most common. Overall, all-comer survival with a durable

Table 5.1 Indications, Explanations, Current Frequency, and Current Success Rates for Implantations of Durable LVADs in the United States

Indication	Explanation	Current U.S. Frequency (%)	Current U.S. Success
Bridge to transplantation	The LVAD is used to bridge the patient with chronic, progressive heart failure to transplantation. This includes patients with an acute exacerbation of chronic heart failure.	26	86% alive at 1 year 31% transplanted 55% still supported
Bridge to candidacy	The LVAD is used to restore systemic perfusion to an adequate level and thus improve multisystem organ failure such that the patient might be an acceptable transplant candidate.	37	84% alive at 1 year 20% transplanted 64% still supported
Destination therapy	The LVAD is used as a final, permanent management strategy for end-stage, refractory heart failure in a transplant-ineligible patient.	46	>75% alive at 1 year >50% alive at 3 years

LVAD, Left ventricular assist device.

LVAD now approaches 80% at 1 year, and the 4-year survival rate now approaches 50%. As the survival rate has increased, the number of patients supported by LVADs requiring interventional and diagnostic procedures and noncardiac surgery (NCS) procedures has increased. The volume of NCS in LVAD-supported patients varies from institution to institution and practice to practice, but current trends indicate that the vast majority of NCS procedures performed in this population are now diagnostic and therapeutic endoscopies. Although supported patients still tend to receive their care in the academic VAD centers, there has been some expansion into the private practice settings and even some endoscopy centers.

INTERMACS

INTERMACS is a North American registry database sponsored by the National Heart, Lung and Blood Institute; the Food and Drug Administration (FDA); and the Centers for Medicare and Medicaid Services (CMS). Centered at the University of Alabama at Birmingham, INTERMACS was established in 2005 for patients receiving long-term MCS therapy with implantable, durable devices to treat advanced HF. Essentially, INTERMACS collects clinical data about VAD patients as it happens. Postimplant follow-up data are collected at 1 week, 1 month, 3 months, and 6 months and every 6 months thereafter. Major outcomes after implant (e.g., death, transplant, explant, rehospitalization, and adverse events) are entered by implanting centers as such events occur and at defined follow-up time points, along with more "complex" endpoints (e.g., the patient's level of function and quality of life), which are critical to the evaluation of current MCS therapy, for which improvements in both survival and function have been compelling. These indices are becoming increasingly important as survival improves, and new devices will be compared for outcomes beyond simple survival. A similar European-based database called EuroMACS exists in Europe, and there is also a database of pediatric MCS called PEDIMACS. A new international database maintained by the International Society for Heart and Lung Transplantation (ISHLT) called IMACS now exists, and reports of the international experience will soon provide data regarding international outcomes.

Regarding LVAD implantation by indication, the most recent INTERMACS data available at the time of this writing report that DT continues to be the most prevalent indication for LVAD implantation, having increased to 45.7% of all implants in 2014 (compared with 14.7% in 2006 and 2007, and 28.6% between 2008 and 2011). In the sixth annual report (released in 2014), BTC was the second most common modern indication for VADs, with BTT in third place, but in the seventh annual report (released in 2015), 30% of patients were already listed for transplantation at the time of implantation, with an additional 23% implanted as a BTC. "Bridge to recovery" with short-term VADs continues to constitute only a very small percentage of the usage of this technology in the most current report (0.2% in 2014). Additional data available from INTERMACS regard survival by both timing of implantation and by type of device.

The INTERMACS profile (also called the INTERMACS level) describes the clinical condition of the patient on a scale from 1 to 7, with a numerically lower profile indicating more severe illness. A level 7 patient is simply in the advanced stages of HF (e.g., New York Heart Association class III), and the clinical condition of the patient gets worse as the INTERMACS profile number gets lower. For example, a level 4 patient has symptoms at rest, a level 3 patient is essentially hemodynamically stable but inotrope dependent, a level 2 patient is deteriorating despite inotropes, and a level 1 patient is essentially in cardiogenic shock despite maximal therapy.

The experience has been that if a durable LVAD is implanted too early (at numerically higher INTERMACS levels), the risks of adverse events outweigh the benefits. Conversely, if the VAD is not implanted until the patient is already likely developing multisystem organ failure (e.g., level 1), the likelihood of ultimate rescue is low, and the survival rate is poor. Survival data suggest that implantation of durable LVADs when the patient is level 3 or 4 would be ideal to balance the risks and benefits. Large multicenter head-to-head trials conducted in the modern era with modern devices (e.g., Momentum 3, Endurance) have reported the profile of risks and benefits associated with each of the modern devices (see Suggested Reading).

SPECIFIC DEVICES IN CURRENT USE

The two most commonly implanted FDA-approved durable devices in the United States are the HeartMate II (Abbott) and the HeartWare HVAD (Medtronic). The Heartmate 3 is a relatively recently introduced implantable, durable device that has received FDA approval for certain indications, although approval of other indications is still pending at the time of this writing.

HeartMate II

The HeartMate II (HM II; Fig. 5.1) is currently the most commonly implanted durable LVAD in the United States and in many countries around the world. The HM II is a miniaturized "second-generation" continuous axial flow pump that was FDA approved as a BTT in 2008 and as DT in 2010. According to the manufacturer, more than 16,000

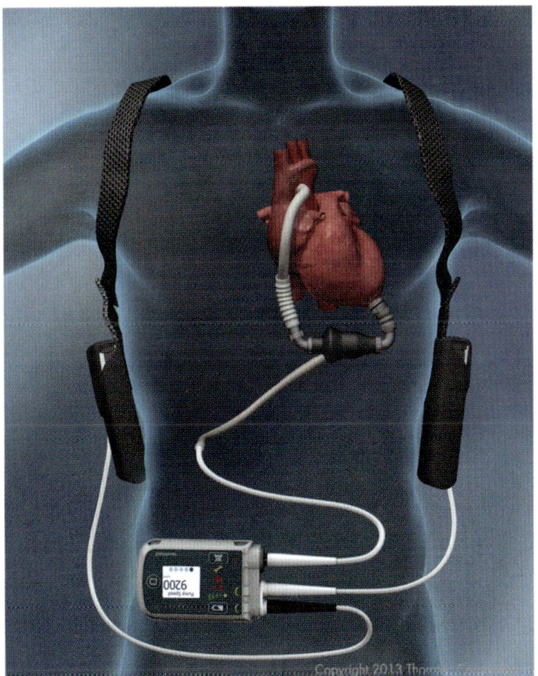

Fig. 5.1 HeartMate II. (Courtesy Abbott/Thoratec, Inc., Pleasanton, CA.)

patients worldwide have received the HM II, with the longest duration of support more than 8 years. Although the impeller is the only moving part, it is stabilized at both ends by bearings. Current postimplantation protocols call for warfarin anticoagulation to an international normalized ratio (INR) of 2.5 to 3.5 plus aspirin. The currently reported rate of successful BTT with the HM II is approximately 86%. Fig. 5.2 shows and discusses details regarding parameters displayed on the HM II clinical control screen.

HeartWare HVAD

The HeartWare HVAD (Fig. 5.3) is a miniaturized CF centrifugal pump with a magnetically driven, hydrodynamically suspended impeller (the impeller floats in the blood without any bearings). This device is implanted within the pericardium without any significant intervening "inflow cannula"; it directly abuts the LV apex. This design provides for potential use in patients with smaller body surface areas and ostensibly results in shorter surgical implantation times. The HVAD was approved as a BTT in 2012. According to the manufacturer, more than 10,000 patients worldwide have received the HVAD, with the longest duration of support more than 7 years. Current postimplantation protocols call for warfarin anticoagulation to an INR of 2.0 to 3.0 plus aspirin. The manufacturer also recommends testing for aspirin resistance and, if detected, the adjunctive use of clopidogrel, dipyridamole, or both. The currently reported rate of successful BTT with the HVAD is 88% to 90%. The HVAD was recently approved as a DT device in the United States as a result of the ENDURANCE trial and the ENDURANCE supplemental trial. Experience with the HVAD as an implantable right ventricular assist device (RVAD) is accruing. Fig. 5.4 shows and discusses details regarding parameters displayed on the HeartWare clinical control screen.

HeartMate 3

The HeartMate 3 (HM 3, Thoratec, Pleasanton, CA; see Fig. 5.5) is a miniaturized CF centrifugal pump with a magnetically driven, magnetically suspended impeller. It is implanted within the pericardium and thus shares some of the potential advantages of the HVAD. Design features ostensibly improve hemocompatibility and reduce the risk of thrombus formation. Similar to the HM II and the HVAD, the HM 3 can reportedly produce 10 L/min of flow. The HM 3 was demonstrated to be noninferior to the HM II in the MOMENTUM 3 trial regarding survival free from either disabling stroke or reoperation for device malfunction at 6 months after implantation. This third-generation device was FDA approved for "short-term indications" in 2017, and its evaluation for "long-term indications" (e.g., DT) is ongoing.

PERIOPERATIVE MANAGEMENT

The perioperative management of an LVAD-supported patient can be divided into preoperative assessment and planning for the case, intraoperative management, and postoperative considerations.

Overview of the Preoperative Assessment

Regardless of the venue or level of complexity or invasiveness of the planned procedure, the perioperative considerations and the anesthetic approach to the LVAD-supported

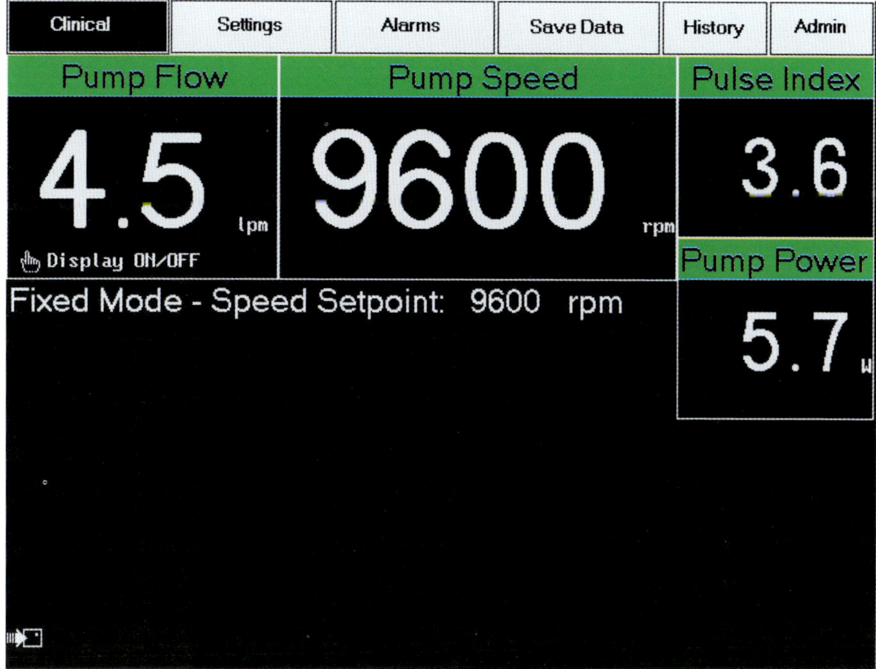

Fig. 5.2 Clinical control screen of the HeartMate II (HM II). **Pump flow** is continuous estimate of the output from the device (derived from the speed of the impeller and the power it takes to achieve that speed). Flows encountered clinically usually range from 4 to 6 L/min, but the device is capable of flowing up to 10 L/min. If the outflow is less than the lower limit set as the alarm condition, three dashes (—) will be displayed in this box instead of a number. This does not necessarily mean there is no outflow. It only means there is less flow than the lower limit set for the alarm. There is a very loud screeching alarm annunciated from the controller if there is no outflow. This is an exceedingly rare thing to encounter. The **pump speed** is the number of revolutions per minute (rpm) at which the impeller is rotating. In most situations, this is a set and fixed value. Speeds encountered clinically are usually in the range of 9000 to 10,000 rpm, but some centers run the ventricular assist device (VAD) at lower rotational speeds to allow the left ventricle (LV) to do more work. Increases in speed will facilitate ventricular unloading by increasing flow through the pump. If the amount of flow exceeds the available volume in the ventricle, a "suckdown" will occur. Decreasing the speed can potentially increase the volume in the LV, although initial steps to increase LV volume would ideally involve infusing volume or supporting right ventricle (RV) function as needed. The **pulsatility index (PI)** is a unitless index of how much pulsatility the device senses as a result of ventricular contractions. Initially, the failed ventricle contributes very little (which is why a VAD was needed) but as the excessive wall tension is decreased in the failing ventricle as a result of VAD action, the ventricle begins to recover, and as long as volume in the LV is optimized, the ventricle will again begin to contract, forcing little pulses through the VAD, as well as through the aortic valve. The PI can be used as a trend to assist with optimization of volume status. PI values around 2 to 3 are typical when there is little pulsatility and the VAD is doing most or all of the work. PI values of 4 to 6 are typical when the partially decompressed ventricle recovers. The PI will decrease with hypovolemia and will increase with myocardial recovery. Thus a low (or falling) PI likely indicates the need to increase the volume status or possibly to increase contractility. RV dysfunction can lead to a decreased filling of the LV. **Pump power** is the energy required to spin the impeller at the set speed and is partially determined by flow. Increases in speed or flow or resistance to flow will require increased power. Power is generally in the range of 5 to 7 W. A sudden increase in the power requirement may suggest significantly increased afterload, but it can also suggest thrombus or other obstruction to rotor rotation. These will be exceedingly rare events. Abrupt increases in power not explainable by an increase in pump speed should always be investigated. A gradual increase in power to high levels over time suggests developing thrombus in the pump.

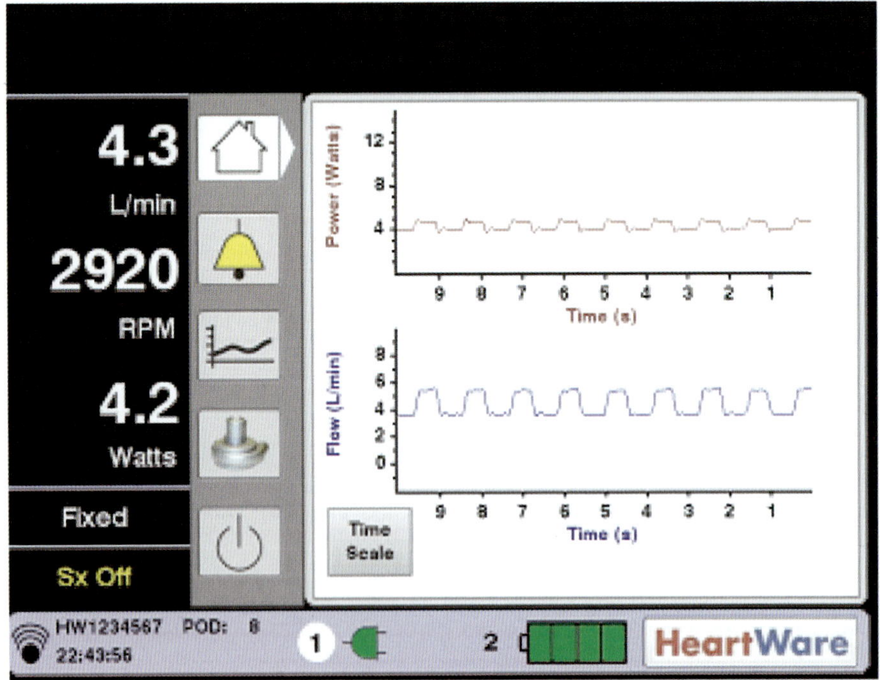

Fig. 5.3 HeartWare HVAD. (Courtesy HeartWare Inc., Framingham, MA.)

Fig. 5.4

Fig. 5.4, cont'd Clinical control screen of the HVAD. The left side of the HVAD control screen shows a continuous estimate of the output from the device in liters per minute *(top left)*, the speed at which the impeller is rotating in revolutions per minute (rpm) (below the output), a readout of the power consumption in watts (below the pump speed), the mode of operation (in this case, a "fixed" speed) and the status of "the suction alarm." In the panel to the right are the power and flow waveforms. At the bottom of the screen are indicators of A/C mains power and a battery status meter. According to the manufacturer, the **flow estimation** *(top left)* should be used as a trending tool only. The readout of device flow is derived from the speed of the impeller, the power it takes to achieve that speed, and the blood viscosity. The viscosity is calculated from the patient's hematocrit, so to obtain the most accurate estimate of flows with this device, the patient's hematocrit must be input into the monitor and the hematocrit updated whenever it changes by 5% or more in either direction. Flows encountered clinically usually range from 4 to 6 L/min, but the device is capable of flowing up to 10 L/min. The amount of flow a centrifugal pump can generate is dependent on a number of factors to do with the diameter and geometry of the impeller, the capacity of the motor, and so on. However, of great importance is the pressure differential across the pump, visualized on the flow rpm at which the impeller is rotating. In most situations, this is a set and fixed value. Speeds encountered clinically are usually in the range of 2400 to 3200 rpm, but the device range is from 1800 to 4000 rpm. Increases in speed will facilitate ventricular unloading by increasing flow through the pump. If the amount of flow exceeds the available volume in the ventricle, a "suckdown" will occur. Infusing volume or decreasing the speed will increase the volume in the left ventricle. **Power** is the power required to spin the impeller at the set speed and is partially determined by flow. Increases in speed or flow or resistance to flow will require increased power. Power is generally in the range of 5 to 7 W. A sudden increase in the power requirement may suggest significantly increased afterload, but it can also suggest thrombus or other obstruction to rotor rotation. These will be exceedingly rare events. Abrupt increases in power not explainable by an increase in pump speed should always be investigated. A gradual increase in power to high levels over time suggests developing thrombus in the pump. The HVAD provides no numeric readout of the pulsatility, but one can physically see the pulse pressure on the **flow waveform**. The peaks are the flow during systole and the troughs during diastole, so the difference, in effect, reflects the "pulse pressure" or "pulsatility" of the patient during support. Of course, the difference in velocity is coming from LV contraction, forcing blood through the pump at a higher velocity during systole. This waveform can help greatly with fluid management in real time because just as in a patient without a VAD, one can increase the pulse pressure by administering fluid to optimize volume status. Maintenance of a pulse pressure is also important to prevent retrograde flow through the pump, as well as to prevent suction events. In general, the diastolic flows should be kept greater than 2 L/min, and there should be at least 2 L/min difference between systolic and diastolic flows. Even though suckdown events are rare, one nice feature of the HVAD in this regard is the "suckdown" detection and alarm. The HVAD controller establishes a diastolic flow baseline. If the diastolic flow falls to less than 40% of the established baseline for more than 10 seconds, the suckdown detection alarm will be annunciated. It would be optimal, however, to observe that the diastolic flow is decreasing and proactively prevent suckdown events from occurring in the first place. For example, volume status might be augmented if hypovolemia or vasodilation is believed to be the problem. If right ventricular (RV) dysfunction results in underfilling of the left ventricle, then RV function would be supported with inotropes, decrease the PVR, or both.

---

patient are the same because the removal of sympathetic tone by sedation or induction of general anesthesia should be expected to exert the same initial effect on the physiology of the VAD-supported patient regardless of the planned procedure. Thus a thorough, thoughtful assessment of the VAD-supported patient is mandatory, even for what appear to be the most minor of cases, because (1) even an ambulatory and seemingly uncompromised VAD-supported patient may have some level of underlying renal, hepatic, pulmonary, or central nervous system insufficiency, and (2) the physiology of the VAD-supported state can be adversely affected by inadequate optimization before and during the anesthetic. It should also be appreciated that deterioration in the perioperative period may preclude full recovery or may disqualify a patient from later heart transplantation.

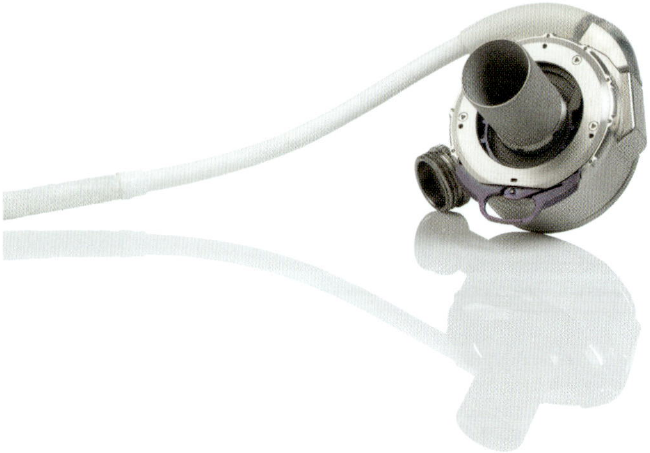

Fig. 5.5 HeartMate 3. (Courtesy Abbott/Thoratec, Inc., Pleasanton, CA.)

If the clinician has questions or concerns, the importance of communicating in advance whenever possible about key issues with a knowledgeable colleague, the physician managing the VAD, the surgeon, and dedicated VAD staff cannot be over-emphasized. Fortunately, experience has shown that the anesthetic management of a VAD-supported patient is not so different from that for a nonsupported patient, but an additional level of advanced planning is required. In addition to the usual areas of anesthetic inquiry at the preanesthetic assessment (e.g., airway, dentition, functional status, allergies), Table 5.2 outlines specific areas of focus and consideration during the preanesthetic assessment of a VAD-supported patient, and key areas are discussed in more detail later.

Planning Appropriate Perioperative Anticoagulation

Preoperative planning by the anesthesiologist, surgeon, and cardiologist managing the VAD must determine how anticoagulation will be managed for the perioperative period. An INR of approximately two to three times normal is required for both the HM II and the HVAD to prevent thrombus formation and potential thromboembolism. Maintenance is usually with warfarin and aspirin (and antiplatelet agents in some patients). In elective cases in which bleeding risk is substantial, warfarin can be discontinued or the patient bridged to surgery with heparin, but it would be imprudent to automatically "discontinue heparin on call to the operating room (OR)" or advise a patient to stop warfarin without preoperative discussion with the physician managing the VAD. In general, the amount of anticoagulation can be safely reduced for the immediate perioperative period to the lower limits of manufacturers' recommendations (which may allow for brief periods without any), but most semi-invasive procedures (e.g., endoscopies) and many general surgical procedures can be safely performed with mild levels of anticoagulation (exceptions include ophthalmologic procedures, neurosurgery, and spine surgery). When needed, infusions of fresh-frozen plasma (FFP), cryoprecipitate, or platelets may be guided by point-of-care (POC) tests (e.g., partial thromboplastin time, INR, thromboelastography, rotational thromboelastometry)

Table 5.2	Specific Areas of Preanesthetic Inquiry and Consideration for Ventricular Assist Device–Supported Patients
Area of Focus	**Rationale**
End-organ insufficiency	Even seemingly uncompromised VAD-supported patients may exist with varying degrees of renal, hepatic, pulmonary, or CNS insufficiency. The pathophysiology of the current surgical disease and any coexisting disease states must be taken into account when planning the optimization of the VAD-supported patient for surgery.
Presence of a CIED	It is common for LVAD-supported patients to have an ICD or a pacemaker. Perioperative management of pacemakers and ICDs is the same as for any other patient undergoing the same procedure (discussed further in the text).
Anticoagulation	Preoperative discussions about the appropriate level of anticoagulation for the case must take place in advance with the physician managing the VAD-supported patient and the surgeon (discussed further in the text).
Type of LVAD present	The name of the LVAD present must be known, especially if seeking advice from knowledgeable colleagues about planned management.
Baseline LVAD settings and parameters of function	Perioperative changes to VAD settings are rarely needed in a VAD-supported patient who was optimized on these settings when not anesthetized, so it is helpful to make note of the stable baseline settings and parameters of VAD function before altering the sympathetic tone and volume status with the delivery of an anesthetic because some of the baseline parameters potentially serve as targets during optimization. The clinical control screens of the HM II and the HVAD are depicted in Figs. 5.2 and 5.4.
Staffing	Appropriate anesthesia staffing for these procedures (e.g., cardiac vs. noncardiac trained personnel) is based on the status of the patient, the nature of the procedure, and the culture and resources of the institution and surgical venue (discussed further in the text).

CIED, Cardiac implantable electronic device; *CNS,* central nervous system; *HM,* HeartMate; *ICD,* implantable cardioverter-defibrillator; *LVAD,* left ventricular assist device; *VAD,* ventricular assist device.

to achieve goals. The administration of vitamin K or factor concentrates to reverse anticoagulation is not recommended.

Management of a Cardiac Implantable Electronic Device

Pacemakers and implantable cardioverter-defibrillators (ICDs) should be managed in the same fashion as for any other patient undergoing the same procedure. It is critical to understand that a cardiac implantable electrical device (CIED) is *either* a pacemaker *or* an ICD. Whereas pacemakers provide pacing, ICDs provide antitachycardia therapies (e.g., shocks and antitachycardia pacing). However, ICDs (with the exception of the recently introduced subcutaneous ICD) have potential backup pacing settings in case defibrillation results in bradycardia or asystole. ICDs can also be programmed to provide full-time pacing as needed (e.g., for pacemaker-dependent patients who also have an indication for an ICD; see Chapter 4).

Preoperatively, for the highest level of patient safety, it must be ascertained what device is present, programmed settings, level of device dependency, and confirmed that the device is functioning as intended. A review of the chest radiograph can easily establish lead locations (e.g., right atrium, right ventricle, coronary sinus) and if a device is a pacemaker or an ICD. A 12-lead electrocardiogram can help to establish pacemaker dependency because the presence of pacemaker spikes before every P-wave or QRS complex suggests dependency. However, the actual percentage paced can only be established by formal device interrogation. The risk of electromagnetic interference (EMI) during the procedure should be assessed, bearing in mind that EMI (e.g., from the surgical electrocautery unit) will most likely inhibit or otherwise interfere with the intended function of a pacemaker or trigger the delivery of antitachycardia therapies from an ICD. Electrocautery grounding pads should always be positioned distal to the site of surgery with respect to the CIED so that current does not cross the device.

Although there is some controversy surrounding cases in which the potential source of EMI is sufficiently far away from the CIED (e.g., >15 cm), current recommendations still hold that ICD therapies should be disabled and pacing settings reprogrammed to an asynchronous (nonsensing) mode for pacemaker-dependent patients. There is no reason to empirically reprogram *nondependent* patients to an asynchronous mode, and in fact, this could cause harm if pacing impulses compete with a spontaneous rhythm (e.g., R-on-T phenomenon resulting in ventricular fibrillation).

Temporary reprogramming of a CIED for the perioperative period can be accomplished with a manufacturer-specific programmer and/or a magnet. Magnet application effectively disables the primary sensing function(s) of a CIED; however, what exactly will be disabled depends on what device is present. Magnet application to the vast majority of pacemakers should cause the pacemaker to pace asynchronously, which will protect the patient from EMI. Pacemakers with adequate battery longevity will pace asynchronously at higher rates than pacemakers with little remaining battery life (e.g., 85–100 beats/min vs. 65 beats/min, respectively). Magnet application to an ICD should disable the antitachycardia therapies but will have no effect on any pacing settings. Therefore magnet application to an ICD in a pacemaker-dependent patient will *not* protect the pacing settings from interference, and the patient will require formal reprogramming of at least the pacing settings preoperatively. (A magnet could be used intraoperatively to disable the ICD therapies.)

When feasible, it is likely safer and more convenient to use a magnet to control the behavior of a CIED intraoperatively because magnet removal will restore the behavior of the device to the preoperative baseline settings. An ICD that was temporarily disabled by magnet application will again be "live" when the magnet is removed and thus enable rapid defibrillation if needed intraoperatively. Reliance on a magnet also permits discharge from the monitored recovery setting without the need for formal interrogation and reprogramming. Removal of a magnet from a pacemaker will restore the baseline "sensing" mode (e.g., DDD, VVI). Although not routinely warranted, there are some clinical situations in which a formal device interrogation is recommended postoperatively, including:

1. Patients who had formal reprogramming of their device preoperatively
2. Patients who underwent "hemodynamically challenging" procedures involving large fluid shifts or transfusions that may have resulted in altered lead impedances
3. Patients who experienced a cardiac arrest intraoperatively requiring resuscitation, defibrillation, and so on

4. Patients who underwent cardiac or thoracic surgery, during which the leads may have been dislodged or damaged, or the device affected by high levels of EMI in close proximity to the device

Perioperative decision-making algorithms exist in the peer-reviewed published literature and practice advisories, but key to the use of such an algorithm is an understanding of what device is present, how it is programmed (including the magnet response; usually it is programmed "on"), the level of CIED dependency, and that it is functioning as intended.

Baseline Parameters of Ventricular Assist Device Function

Figs. 5.2 and 5.4 depict the clinical control screens of the HM II and the HVAD, and the figure legends discuss various aspects of those parameters.

Appropriate Staffing of the Case

Even though cardiac-trained personnel still staff all noncardiac cases and procedures on VAD-supported patients in some institutions, it has been demonstrated in experienced, high-volume centers that noncardiac trained anesthesiologists can safely and confidently provide anesthetic care to VAD-supported patients after a period of education and experience. Certainly, minor cases or procedures (e.g., endoscopies, computed tomography scans, cystoscopies) on baseline stable VAD patients who are not on any pharmacologic support and lack other major comorbidities can be safely performed by most board-certified noncardiac anesthesiologists. One factor that has facilitated this culture change in certified VAD centers is the requirement by the CMS for the involvement of a VAD team not only for transport to and from the procedure, but that a "VAD-certified person" must be in the room for the duration of the procedure. Ideally, these cases would be scheduled during daylight hours and can safely take place in their usual locations (e.g., procedural suites). From the standpoint of the anesthesia provider, if questions or concerns exist after appropriate preanesthetic assessment, consultation with cardiac colleagues and discussions with the physician managing the VAD should precede OR entry. However, if the patient at baseline requires pharmacologic support, has major comorbidities, or if the case involves predicted large fluid shifts or potential periods of hemodynamic upheaval or is urgent or emergent, the case should ideally be done by a cardiac-trained anesthesiologist. Even so, the perioperative involvement of the VAD team must be assured as for any other case regardless of the anesthesia team being "VAD knowledgeable" as mandated by CMS.

INTRAOPERATIVE ANESTHETIC MANAGEMENT

The vast majority of the time, clinicians must simply ensure continued optimization of the usual determinants of hemodynamics (preload, afterload, heart rate, and contractility) during the anesthetic, just as they would for any patient. In general, maintaining adequate volume status is likely the key to maintaining hemodynamic stability, although assuring adequate right ventricular contractility and avoidance of increased pulmonary vascular resistance (PVR) are important as well. That said, the basis of the safe and effective perioperative anesthetic management of the VAD-supported patient is a working understanding of the physiology of the VAD-supported state and how all the various aspects come together.

Key Points of Physiology

There are three essential points of physiology and three intrinsic myocardial mechanisms that must be understood (or can be manipulated) to maintain optimal hemodynamics perioperatively:

- Ventricular interdependence
- Series circulatory effects
- Ventriculoarterial coupling
- The Frank-Starling mechanism
- The Anrep effect
- The Bowditch effect

Ventricular Interdependence

Both ventricles are bounded by, and exist within, the pericardium. Thus geometric changes of one ventricle (e.g., caused by volume or pressure overload) necessarily affect the geometry of the other, and geometrical changes of a ventricle decrease the effectiveness of its contractility. The continuous nature of the muscle fibers between the free wall of the right ventricle (RV) and the left ventricle (LV), as well as the sharing of a common interventricular septum (IVS), results in mechanical interactions between the ventricles and an anatomic coupling of their respective contractility. It is known that leftward septal shift (e.g., caused by excessive decompression of the LV by LVAD action or overfilling of the RV) has a deleterious effect on RV contractility; however, when clinically significant decreases in RV output occur, it is on account of an alteration of muscle fiber orientation and not simply the change in position of the IVS (i.e., leftward shift). In fact, it has long been demonstrated that as long as septal function is unimpaired, the RV free wall is dispensable where overall RV pressure development and volume outflow are concerned because it is really the contraction of the IVS that "wrings" blood out from the RV.

Series Circulatory Effects

The output of the RV fills the LVAD, and the LVAD output subsequently becomes the preload of the RV. Thus optimal LVAD function requires at least adequate RV "function" (which conceptually includes adequate RV preload, adequate RV contractility, or a pulmonary vascular resistance that permits blood to move from the right side to the left).

Ventriculoarterial Coupling

No matter how depressed the intrinsic systolic function of a ventricle, the ability of a ventricle to function as a pump can be improved by decreasing the afterload against which it must pump. This is ventriculoarterial coupling. Thus, afterload reduction (as tolerated) is a key principle in the modern management of both left- and right-sided ventricular failure and has applications during both acute and chronic situations. Acute RV dysfunction, for example, responds particularly well to selective pulmonary vasodilatation, and chronic LV dysfunction is routinely managed with inodilators. Acute LV dysfunction, on the other hand, is often accompanied by significant hypotension, limiting the use of systemic afterload reduction.

Frank-Starling Mechanism

The Frank-Starling law holds that increased stretch on the myocytes (to a point) increases the force of their contraction. As the ventricle fills, the potential force of the myocardial contraction increases because stretching of the muscle fibers increases the affinity of troponin C for calcium, causing a greater number of actin–myosin cross-bridges to form within the muscle fibers. The force that any single cardiac muscle fiber generates is proportional to the initial sarcomere length (also known as preload), and the stretch on the individual fibers is related to the end-diastolic volume of the left and right ventricles.

In the human heart, maximal force is generated with an initial sarcomere length of 2.2 μm, a length that is rarely exceeded in the normal heart. Initial lengths longer or shorter than this optimal value will decrease the force the muscle can achieve. At longer sarcomere lengths, there is less overlap of the thin and thick filaments, and at shorter sarcomere lengths, the myofilaments exhibit a decreased sensitivity for calcium.

Anrep Effect

The Anrep effect is an intrinsic myocardial reflex, or an autoregulation mechanism, maintained even in the denervated heart, in which myocardial contractility increases with increasing afterload. Initially, acutely increased aortic resistance to ejection results in a decreased stroke volume (and therefore an increased end-diastolic volume) that increases the force of contraction through the Frank-Starling mechanism. However, it has been demonstrated that contractility continues to increase starting around 10 to 15 minutes after the initial sudden stretch through the Anrep effect. Without the Anrep effect, an increase in aortic pressure would result in a sustained decrease in stroke volume, which might compromise cardiac output. This effect was originally described in 1912 by the Russian physiologist Gleb von Anrep, details of the mechanism were further elucidated from 1950 to 1980, and sophisticated investigations into this mechanism continue to the present time. Modern investigations have revealed the Anrep effect to be a very complex mechanism involving angiotensin II, endothelin, the mineralocorticoid receptor, the epidermal growth factor receptor, mitochondrial reactive oxygen species, redox-sensitive kinases upstream myocardial Na^+/H^+ exchanger (NHE1), NHE1 activation, increase in intracellular Na^+ concentration, and increase in Ca^{2+} transient amplitude through the Na^+/Ca^{2+} exchanger.

Bowditch Effect

The prime manner by which the heart achieves an increased contractility in response to increased metabolic demand is via an increase in heart rate. This is the Bowditch effect. Effectively, increases in heart rate result in an increase in contractility and an increase in cardiac output. The putative mechanism underlying the Bowditch effect is similar to the mechanism by which digoxin acts. Increased heart rates challenge the efficiency of the Na^+/K^+-ATPase, and calcium builds up (which is inotropic in myocardial tissue). The Bowditch effect also reportedly exerts a lusitropic effect, whereby increases in heart rate increase relaxation, improving diastolic function.

Specific Intraoperative Actions

Table 5.3 outlines specific intraoperative actions, the anesthetic management, and monitoring of a VAD-supported patient. Key areas are discussed in more detail in the next sections.

Table 5.3   **Specific Intraoperative Actions and Considerations for Ventricular Assist Device–Supported Patients**

Intraoperative Intervention	Rationale
Plug it in!	A low battery situation will not occur if the device is kept plugged in. Furthermore, the full control console can only be used (and the displayed parameters of device function to aid optimization) when the device is plugged in.
Prophylactic antibiotics	Appropriate antibiotics must be used because VADs are large foreign bodies that cannot be adequately sterilized if infected.
Anticoagulation	The anticoagulation strategy that was determined in advance should be adhered to, but further manipulations may be required if significant surgical bleeding is encountered.
Anesthetic agents and techniques	No specific sedatives or anesthetic agents are contraindicated because of the presence of a VAD (but the unsupported, potentially dysfunctional RV should be taken into account), and the required anticoagulation often precludes major regional techniques.
Monitoring	Standard ASA monitors should always be used. Because baseline pulsatility may decrease with anesthetic induction, a noninvasive blood pressure cuff and pulse oximetry may become unreliable, suggesting the need for an invasive arterial monitoring catheter and cerebral oximetry for cases involving large fluid shifts or if pulsatility is low at baseline or cannot be maintained. The need for central venous access should be considered on a case-by-case basis.
Displayed parameters of LVAD function	Perioperative changes to VAD settings are rarely needed in a VAD-supported patient who was optimized on these settings when not anesthetized. As discussed in the text, the preoperative baseline parameters (noted at the preanesthetic assessment) can help to serve as targets during intraoperative optimization. Optimization will more often require compensation with volume infusion and manipulations of afterload during an anesthetic than changes to previously stable VAD settings.

ASA, American Society of Anesthesiologist; *LVAD,* left ventricular assist device; *RV,* right ventricle; *VAD,* ventricular assist device.

Plug It In!

Transport to the OR will be on battery power. A pair of wearable, rechargeable modern LVAD batteries last for 4 to 8 hours (depending on the charge status, the number of previous charging cycles, and the hemodynamic condition of the patient). Similar to all other critical, life-support, and lifesaving equipment in the OR, whenever feasible, the device should be kept plugged in and the backup batteries charged. Additionally, the full control console and the reported parameters of VAD function used to guide optimization can only be used when the device is plugged in.

Appropriate Antibiotic Coverage

Preoperative antibiotic coverage for most procedures often includes broad-spectrum coverage, taking local flora into account. Coverage for gram-negative organisms and anaerobes is prudent for intraabdominal procedures. Antifungals should be considered in patients who may be at higher risk, which may include recent treatment with an antibiotic course or multiple indwelling catheters. Most infections associated with VADs tend to occur in the percutaneous tract through which the driveline exits, but it must be appreciated that VADs are large foreign bodies that when infected may not be adequately treated. The VAD driveline itself should not be prepped with povidone iodine–containing solutions because these can result in breakdown of the plastic. When necessary, drivelines can be draped out of the field or covered temporarily with a sterile drape.

Anticoagulation

As already discussed, when needed, POC and standard laboratory testing of the parameters of coagulation and hemostasis can be used to achieve the preoperatively determined goals for intraoperative anticoagulation or further refinements as warranted during the case. Infusions of FFP, cryoprecipitate, or platelets may sometimes be needed if significant surgical bleeding is encountered, but the administration of vitamin K or factor concentrates to acutely and completely reverse anticoagulation is not recommended. As needed, consultation with the physician managing the VAD is encouraged.

Anesthetic Agents and Techniques

No specific anesthetic agents are contraindicated because of the presence of a VAD, and the choice of agents and dosages used should be appropriate for the procedure, but should take into account the potentially dysfunctional unsupported right ventricle, as well as any other existing comorbidities. Most VAD-supported patients receive a general anesthetic because of the requisite anticoagulation, but in selected cases, superficial regional blocks under ultrasound guidance or a regional intravenous technique (e.g., a Bier block) may be appropriate. Major conduction anesthetics (e.g., spinals and epidurals) are generally contraindicated. Intubation and extubation criteria are the same as for any patient. In fact, early (if not immediate postoperative) extubation is desirable because prolonged intubation predisposes to pulmonary infection and requires prolonged sedation. There is no reason for patients to remain intubated just because they are supported by a VAD. As well, the miniaturized nature of the modern devices currently in use (and the fact that they are no longer implanted in a preperitoneal location) no longer relegates the LVAD-supported patient to "full stomach" status, as was the case with the large, pulsatile first-generation devices.

Monitoring

Standard ASA monitors should always be used, but the potential loss of pulsatility portends the unreliability of a noninvasive blood pressure (NIBP) cuff and pulse oximetry. Pulsatility of the circulation in a VAD-supported patient refers to contractility of the LV forcing an increased systolic velocity of blood either through the LVAD, out the aortic valve, or both. Although most patients with a modern nonpulsatile LVAD do exhibit pulsatility of their circulation when the LV partially recovers after VAD implantation, they can lose this pulsatility after induction because of the relative hypovolemia and vasodilation that accompany an anesthetic induction. Furthermore, VAD patients always lose pulsatility if they get significantly hypovolemic from blood loss or major fluid shifts. An NIBP cuff and pulse oximeter will work as long as sufficient pulsatility is maintained through optimization of the volume status presented to the LV (or optimization of RV function and pulmonary vascular resistance). Figs. 5.2 and 5.4 show and discuss the clinical control screens of the HM II and the HVAD from which information is obtained to assist with optimization and maintenance of pulsatility. An arterial line catheter often needed for cases with anticipated major

5

fluid shifts and can also be used to assess oxygenation when needed. Cerebral oximetry is increasingly being used when the pulse oximeter becomes unreliable. Transthoracic echocardiography (TTE) or transesophageal echocardiography (TEE) is not generally necessary unless clinical management questions arise. The VAD console already describes the cardiac output and LV volume status (see Figs. 5.2 and 5.4), so the actual utility of a central venous access or a pulmonary artery (PA) catheter should be carefully assessed for a given patient, particularly for minor procedures and procedures not expected to result in large volume shifts. The risks of line sepsis, arrhythmias, and pneumothorax from central catheter placement must be weighed against the potential utility, which include following the trends of cardiac output and derived hemodynamic indices to help guide fluid management and inotropic support, the ability to measure SVO_2, the ability to assess the efficacy of interventions to lower PA pressures, and the ability to provide pacing. Echocardiography, especially TEE, is likely to be the most helpful monitor if a management dilemma arises.

PUTTING IT ALL TOGETHER: OPTIMIZATION DURING THE INTRAOPERATIVE PERIOD

A consideration of the physiology of the VAD-supported state, the principles outlined in the earlier sections, and the parameters of VAD function displayed on the clinical control screen provide a clear management strategy for VAD-supported patients who present for NCS.

Volume status must be maintained and optimized for the LVAD patient for the same reasons as any other patient receiving an anesthetic and is often the key to maintaining pulsatility of the circulation (through optimization of Starling's forces and the Anrep effect to optimize contractility). As discussed earlier, the pulsatility index of the HM II, and the information presented on the HVAD clinical screen (e.g., the diastolic baseline and the pulse pressure displayed) can be of assistance in optimizing and maintaining volume status. The goal for perioperative fluid management is to maintain a euvolemic, if not slightly hypervolemic state (assuming the unsupported and potentially dysfunctional RV is able to handle the volume load). The effect of surgical positioning or retractors must be considered as they may influence preload to the RV and high intrathoracic pressure (e.g., from excessively large tidal volumes) should be avoided because it impedes venous return to the heart. An "empty" LV also shifts the interventricular septum (IVS) to the left, which will decrease RV function through the principle of ventricular interdependence and the septal architectural disadvantage that comes from the change of IVS position, which reduces IVS contractility. A relative state of hypovolemia may occur in the LV if the RV fails to get blood across the pulmonary circulation for any reason, and sometimes there is a need to decrease pulmonary vascular resistance (the principle of ventriculoarterial coupling) or support RV contractility. Apart from usual small boluses of vasoconstrictors at the time of induction, significant compensation for anesthetic effects on vasomotor tone is infrequently needed as long as volume status is kept optimized. Judiciously raising the heart rate can also assist contractility (the Bowditch effect).

When all this is taken into account, changes to previously stable VAD settings are the least likely initial maneuver undertaken to correct hemodynamic instability resulting from vasodilation and loss of sympathetic tone after anesthetic induction or blood loss. Instead, systemic vasodilatation should be corrected with judicious manipulations of vascular resistance and the correction of hypovolemia. If the amount of blood removed from the LV by continuous VAD action exceeds the amount of blood present, a "suckdown" can occur. A decreasing pulsatility index of the HM II or a decreasing diastolic flow baseline of the HVAD (as well as the suction alarm of the HVAD) can herald an impending suction event. Assuming the volume status is adequate, a suction event will be a rare occurrence, but the usual initial management of such an event would entail volume infusion. If RV dysfunction is suspected, then inotropic support, selective pulmonary vasodilatation, or both would be used. Again, TEE or TTE could assist with a determination of the etiology of the problem. Theoretically, a temporary decrease in VAD speed could help to break the suction event, but caution is advised in this regard unless performed by an experienced VAD operator.

POSTOPERATIVE CONSIDERATIONS

Table 5.4 outlines the postanesthetic considerations for VAD-supported patients presenting for NCS.

Table 5.4	Specific Postanesthetic Considerations for Ventricular Assist Device–Supported Patient
Area of Focus	**Rationale**
Appropriate recovery setting	The location of patient recovery (e.g., PACU vs. ICU vs. VAD floor, if available) may bear discussion in advance to ensure the receiving staff on duty are able to care for an LVAD patient. Excessive anxiety on the part of the nursing or other receiving staff is not in the best interest of the patient but is generally amenable to education and experience over time.
Plug it in!	The patient will be transported on battery power from the OR to the recovery location, and it is prudent to reconnect the VAD to A/C power and the system base unit on arrival. Backup batteries should be maintained in their chargers.
Continued optimization	Optimization of all parameters of hemodynamics must continue into the postoperative period. Volume status must be maintained and all factors avoided that could contribute to elevated PVR (e.g., hypercarbia, hypoxia, hypothermia, acidemia, pain). Effective pain management is essential not only for patient comfort but also to avoid increases in the PVR that may strain the potentially dysfunctional, unsupported RV.
CIEDs	Baseline pacemaker or ICD settings should be restored before discharge from a monitored setting. If a magnet was used to keep an ICD inactive intraoperatively, removal of the magnet will reactivate the ICD. Similarly, magnet removal from a pacemaker will restore baseline programming. Any CIED settings that were formally reprogrammed with a manufacturer-specific programming device will need to be similarly restored. Device interrogation will not routinely be necessary except as discussed in the text.
Baseline LVAD settings and parameters of function	Perioperative changes to VAD settings are rarely needed in a VAD-supported patient who was optimized on these settings when not anesthetized, so it is helpful to make note of the stable baseline settings and parameters of VAD function before altering the sympathetic nervous system tone and volume status with the delivery of an anesthetic because some of the baseline parameters potentially serve as targets during optimization. The clinical control screens of the HM II and the HVAD are depicted in Figs. 5.2 and 5.4.

Continued

Table 5.4	Specific Postanesthetic Considerations for Ventricular Assist Device–Supported Patient—cont'd	
Area of Focus	**Rationale**	
Coordination with knowledgeable VAD personnel	The transportation of the VAD-supported patient from one location to another should be coordinated with and assisted by knowledgeable personnel who can ensure the batteries are correctly connected and that the system is functioning as intended before and after transport.	

CIED, Cardiac implantable electronic device; *HM*, HeartMate; *ICD*, implantable cardioverter-defibrillator; *ICU*, intensive care unit; *LVAD*, left ventricular assist device; *OR*, operating room; *PACU*, postanesthesia care unit; *PVR*, pulmonary vascular resistance; *RV*, right ventricle; *VAD*, ventricular assist device.

SUGGESTED READING

Heart Failure and VAD Statistics

Heidenreich PA, Albert NM, Allen LA, et al; on behalf of the American Heart Association Advocacy Coordinating Committee; Council on Arteriosclerosis, Thrombosis and Vascular Biology; Council on Cardiovascular Radiology and Intervention; Council on Clinical Cardiology; Council on Epidemiology and Prevention; Stroke Council. Forecasting the impact of heart failure in the United States: a policy statement from the American Heart Association. *Circ Heart Fail*. 2013;6:606–619.
Kirklin JK, Naftel DC, Pagani FD, et al. Seventh INTERMACS annual report: 15,000 patients and counting. *J Heart Lung Transplant*. 2015;34:1495–1504.
Mozzafarian D, Benjamin EJ, Go AS, et al; on behalf of the American Heart Association Statistics Committee and Stroke Statistics Subcommittee. Heart disease and stroke statistics—2016 update: a report from the American Heart Association. *Circulation*. 2016;133:e38–e360.

Devices

Mathis M, Sathishkumar S, Kheterpal S, et al. Complications, risk factors, and staffing patterns for noncardiac surger in patients with left ventricular assist devices. *Anesthesiology*. 2017;126:450–460.
Mehra MR, Naka Y, Uriel N, et al; for the MOMENTUM 3 investigators. A fully magnetically levitated circulatory pump for advanced heart failure. *N Engl J Med*. 2017;376(5):440–450.
Rogers JG, Pagani FD, Tatooles AJ, et al; for the ENDURANCE Trial investigators. Intrapericardial left ventricular assist device for advanced heart failure. *N Engl J Med*. 2017;376(5):451–460.
Rose EA, Gelijns AC, Moskowitz AJ, et al. Long-term use of a left ventricular assist device for end-stage heart failure. *N Engl J Med*. 2001;345(20):1435–1443.
Schmitto JD, Hanke JS, Rojas SV, Avsar M, Haverich A. First implantation in man of a new magnetically levitated left ventricular assist device (HeartMate III). *J Heart Lung Transplant*. 2015;34:858–860.
Stoicea N, Cardozo F, Joseph N, et al. Pro: Cardiothoracic anesthesiologists should provide anesthetic care for patients with VADs undergoing noncardiac surgery. *J Cardiothorac Vasc Anesth*. 2017;31:378–381. (For "Con," see pp 382–387.)
Stone ME, Hinchey J, Sattler C, Evans A. Trends in the management of patients with left ventricular assist devices presenting for non-cardiac surgery—a ten year institutional experience. *Semin Cardiothorac Vasc Anesth*. 2016;20(3):197–204.
Stulak JM, Davis ME, Haglund N, et al. Adverse events in contemporary continuous-flow left ventricular assist devices: A multi-institutional comparison shows significant differences. *J Thorac Cardiovasc Surg*. 2016;151:177–189.

VAD Physiology

Cingolani HE, Pérez NG, Cingolani OH, et al. The Anrep effect: 100 years later. *Am J Physiol Heart Circ Physiol.* 2013;304:H175–H182.
Saleh S, Liakopoulos OJ, Buckberg GD. The septal motor of biventricular function. *Eur J CT Surg.* 2006;29s: S126–S138.
Santamore WP, Gray L Jr. Left ventricular contributions to right ventricular systolic function during LVAD support. *Ann Thorac Surg.* 1996;61:350–356.

Chapter 6

Anesthesia for Noncardiac Surgery After Heart Transplant

Swapnil Khoche, MBBS, DNB • Brett Cronin, MD

> **Key Points**
>
> 1. Cardiac transplant is the definitive treatment of advanced heart failure and has demonstrated improving outcomes and long-term survival.
> 2. The transplanted heart receives no neural modulatory signal in the posttransplant period and is dependent on filling and humoral catecholamines.
> 3. Mild restrictive physiology is the norm even with well-functioning grafts, and peak exercise capacity is reduced under even optimal circumstances.
> 4. The risk of rejection decreases with time after transplant and is associated with a reduction in immunosuppression and surveillance. The diagnosis of rejection is via biopsy with management centered around increased immunosuppression.
> 5. Cardiac allograft vasculopathy is a late form of diffuse coronary occlusion that causes graft dysfunction, which is difficult to treat by conventional means.
> 6. Anemia, infection, renal dysfunction, and hypertension are common side effects of immunosuppression. Multiple interactions exist between anesthetic drugs and immunosuppressants.
> 7. There is no contraindication to any anesthesia technique provided it maintains preload, sinus rhythm, and afterload.
> 8. There is a higher risk of infection and bleeding complications with regional anesthetic techniques in this patient population.

Heart transplantation (HT) means a new lease on life for people with end-stage heart disease who have failed maximal medical therapy. Since its introduction by Dr. Christiaan Barnard more than 50 years ago, HT has rapidly become a viable and reliable treatment option for advanced heart failure (HF). More than 100,000 transplants have been performed to date, and more than 4000 procedures are being performed yearly. A 5-year survival rate of more than 70% and a median survival of more than 10 years serve as a testament to the vast strides forward in patient selection, surgical technique, and immunosuppression (Fig. 6.1). Noncardiac surgery is required in 15% to 47% of these patients, with a higher mortality risk for emergent procedures. Thus with an increasing number of patients surviving and remaining functional long after HT, it is no longer practical to have specialized teams and centers perform noncardiac procedures on transplant recipients exclusively. Furthermore, a large proportion of these procedures are of an urgent nature, and prolonged evaluation, optimization, or transfer to a major academic center is often not possible.

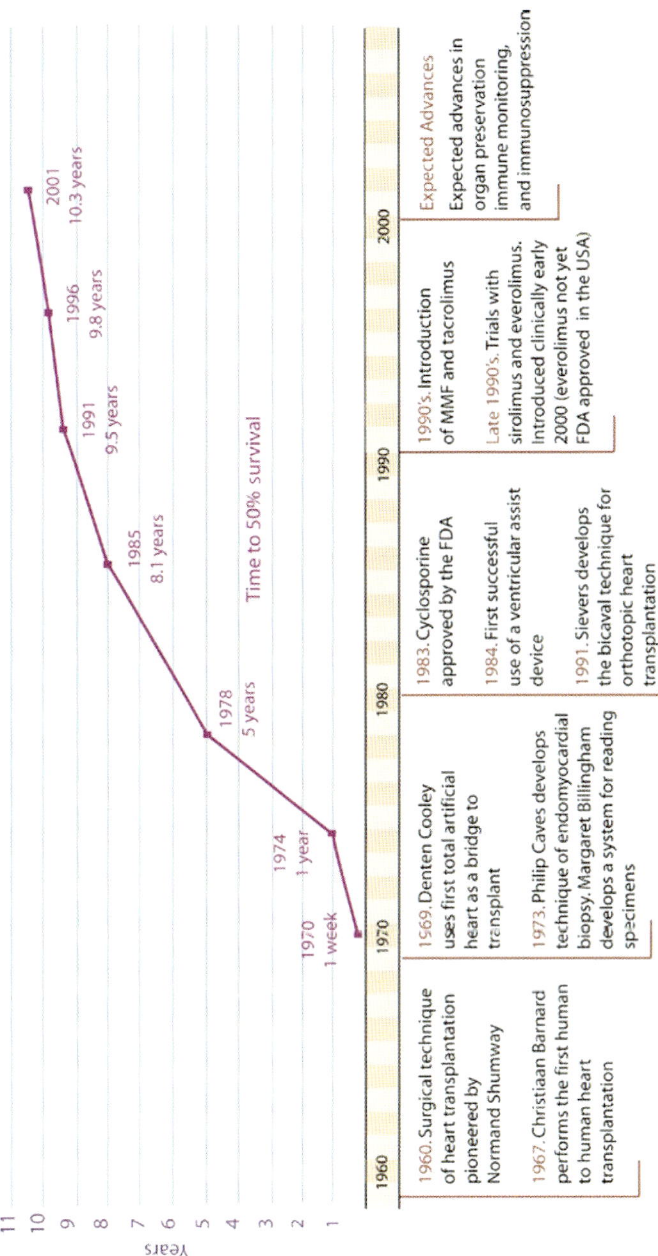

Fig. 6.1 Heart transplantation milestones and expected survival. *FDA*, Federal Drug Administration; *MMF*, mycophenolate mofetil. (From Hunt SA, Haddad F. The changing face of heart transplantation. *J Am Coll Cardiol.* 2008;52:587-598.)

6

Given this scenario, it is imperative for anesthesiologists to have a comprehensive knowledge of the physiology of the transplanted heart, the pharmacologic implications of immunosuppressive therapy, the complications of immunosuppressive therapy, and the anesthetic options for this subpopulation. The HT population presents a number of challenges because management of HT recipients is evolving. For example, the standard evaluation tools for risk assessment such as the Revised Cardiac Risk Index or guidelines from American Heart Association do not address risk stratification for this particular subgroup, and there are no clear guidelines for preoperative testing. Therefore the goal of this chapter is to provide a brief overview of the following:

1. Physiologic attributes of the transplanted heart
2. Immunosuppressive medications and their perioperative management
3. Preoperative assessment and optimization
4. Perioperative monitoring and management

PHYSIOLOGIC ATTRIBUTES OF THE TRANSPLANTED HEART

The Transplanted Heart and the Cardiovascular System

Before transplantation, patients with advanced HF display varying degrees of systolic or diastolic dysfunction (or both). Whereas the former leads to a decrease in ejection fraction and cardiac output, the latter results in higher filling pressures. The reduction in cardiac output results in a reduction of blood, oxygen, and nutrient supply to end organs, which is only compounded by partial venous congestion. After HT cardiac output improves, and end-organ perfusion is largely restored. However, transplantation does not completely restore the patient to a nonpathologic state.

Anatomic Correlates

Despite the advances made in the management of HF, immunosuppression, and postoperative care, the surgical technique remains largely unchanged from the one described in the 1960s. The donor heart is anastomosed to the native circulation primarily in one of two ways. Biatrial anastomosis, which involves suturing of the native atria to the donor atria, was the standard approach originally and is technically simpler because it preserves the connections to the recipient atrium. The risk of sinus node injury is higher with the biatrial technique, as is the chance of hemodynamic problems associated with altered atrial geometry, size, and flow. Of note, with the biatrial technique, dual p-waves may be seen on the electrocardiogram (ECG) because of activation of native atrial tissue and can sometimes mimic atrial flutter. In addition, the sewing cuff can be seen as a ridge in the atria and can be confused for thrombi or endocarditis. Therefore knowledge of the surgical technique can often be beneficial to avoid misdiagnoses. The biatrial technique has been largely replaced by the bicaval technique. The bicaval technique involves anastomoses at the level of the great vessels—the superior and inferior vena cava—and a line of left atrial tissue encircling the pulmonary vessels. This technique has been associated with a reduction in sinus node dysfunction, tricuspid regurgitation, atrial fibrillation, and atrial dilation after transplant. The bicaval technique has also been shown to confer a small but significant survival advantage compared to the biatrial approach (Box 6.1).

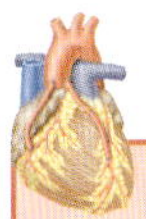

<table>
<tr><td colspan="2" style="background:#f5c9a8;">BOX 6.1   Heart Transplant Bicaval Technique</td></tr>
<tr><td>

- Advantages: reduction in sinus node dysfunction, tricuspid regurgitation, atrial fibrillation, and atrial dilation after transplant; also, small significant survival advantage
- Disadvantage: more complex technique

</td></tr>
</table>

Reinnervation

The normal heart is innervated by sympathetic and parasympathetic fibers of the autonomic nervous system. Whereas sympathetic innervation to the heart is from the cervical ganglia and upper thoracic (T1–T4) sympathetic chain, branches of the vagus nerves contribute the parasympathetic input. The cardiac plexus, which contains the postganglionic sympathetic and preganglionic parasympathetic fibers, is located at the base of the heart. The autonomic nervous system is also the conduit by which a supply of visceral sensory fibers is supplied to the pericardium. During transplantation, postganglionic neural axons innervating the heart are transected. Within days, cardiac stores of norepinephrine are exhausted, and autonomic influence over the heart ceases. After a variable period of 6 to 12 months, partial reinnervation of the transplanted heart has been shown to occur (see later). However, it remains incomplete and variable for many years after transplant. Thus in the early postoperative period, the transplanted heart is only subject to manipulation via humoral catecholamines.

As a consequence of efferent denervation, sympathetic stimulation and chronotropic responses to exercise, stress, and hypovolemia are not seen. This also includes blunting of baroreceptor responses (e.g., responses to laryngoscopy and intubation). Afferent denervation, on the other hand, impedes vasoregulatory responses by means of the renin-angiotensin axis, and the perception of pain secondary to ischemia (angina) is lost. Transplanted hearts demonstrate a high resting heart rate (90–100 beats/min) without much variability (Table 6.1). Eventually, nerve sprouting occurs, and reinnervation proceeds along the left ventricle into the sinoatrial node and then to the coronaries, in that chronological order. Parasympathetic reinnervation tends to lag behind sympathetic reinnervation; in theory, there could be a state where the transplanted heart could have "unbalanced" autonomic input with sympathetic predominance. With the passage of time, the resting heart rate slows down, and rate variability reappears (see Table 6.1). The clinical implications of this pattern of cessation and gradual restoration of neural input to the transplanted heart are many and are discussed later in the text (Box 6.2).

Filling Patterns

The filling pressures of an immediate posttransplant heart are significantly elevated. The elevated filling pressures are likely related to ischemic myocardial injury, rejection, volume overload, or a preexisting pulmonary vascular abnormality. Over time, this transitions to a mild rightward shift on the Frank-Starling curve during rest. However, circulating brain natriuretic peptide (BNP) levels are elevated even with normal hemodynamic parameters, suggesting some atrial stretch. The filling pressures, which are significantly elevated immediately after transplant, typically never fully return to normal, suggesting a mild restrictive physiology. Donor recipient size mismatch, increased afterload in the form of hypertension, and rejection are all proposed mechanisms.

Table 6.1　Normal Physiologic Parameters After Heart Transplantation

	Normal	Early Posttransplant	Late Posttransplant
Heart rate: rest (beats/min)	60–80	100–120	80–100
Heart rate: exercise	Early rise	Slow rise	Intermediate
Heart rate: peak	+++	+	++
Heart rate variability	++	Decreased	Variable
Systolic BP (mm Hg)	100–120	No change	Increased
Stroke volume (mL)	Normal	Slightly decreased	Decreased
Cardiac output (L/min)	4–5	No change	No change
Ejection fraction: rest (%)	60–70	No change	No change
Ejection fraction: exercise	+++	+	++
SVR (dynes/sec/cm^5)	700–1600	+	++

BP, Blood pressure; *SVR,* systemic vascular resistance.

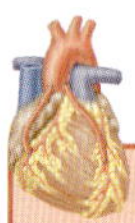

BOX 6.2　*The Transplanted Heart and the Autonomic Nervous System*

- Postganglionic neural axons innervating the heart are transected during transplant.
- The newly transplanted heart is only subject to manipulation via humoral catecholamines.
- Reinnervation can occur within 6–12 months posttransplant.

Often the end result is an abrupt rise in left ventricular filling pressures in response to fluid challenges, which makes these patients prone to pulmonary and systemic venous congestion. Mild rejection does not affect function significantly, although both systolic and diastolic function are adversely affected when rejection reaches severe proportions. Overall, this calls for caution with fluid challenges in the face of hypotension and vigilance toward volume status under anesthesia.

Exercise Response

Compared with their own pretransplant status, the exercise capacity of HT recipients shows improvement, but it is still reduced compared with that of healthy control participants. In healthy persons, withdrawal of vagal tone at the onset of exercise results in an initial increase in heart rate, which then results in an increased cardiac output. In HT recipients, the heart rate increase is slower, and the maximal heart rate achieved is lower (see Table 6.1). During exercise, an initial increase in cardiac output results from an increase in stroke volume and preload, but later during exercise, improved contractility and heart rate augmentation from circulating catecholamines take over. This neurohumoral response is exaggerated in HT recipients and may represent compensation for denervation. In addition, elevated pulmonary resistance and impairment in skeletal muscle function contribute to the reduction in maximal exercise capacity in HT recipients. HF in the pretransplant period, chronic oxygen debt, and steroid use generally lead to muscle fiber atrophy in this patient population. However, exercise training can result in a restoration of muscle mass, strength, and endurance after transplant. In a variety of clinical situations, exercise tolerance has been successfully used as a predictor of a patient's ability to undergo the stress of anesthesia and surgery. It is no different for a transplant recipient presenting for noncardiac surgery.

Receptors and Drug Response

An increase in the number and the sensitivity of β-adrenergic receptors is present posttransplant. As a consequence, the transplanted heart demonstrates augmented responses to directly acting β-adrenergic antagonists. Resting coronary blood flow increases because of an absence of sympathetic tone. However, scrotonin hypersensitivity (likely related to endothelial damage) causes decreased flow reserve in the transplanted heart. Abnormalities of response to endothelium-derived vasodilators such as substance P and acetylcholine have been noted, although the response to non–endothelium-derived vasodilators such as adenosine and dipyridamole is preserved. As previously noted, coronary demand-supply mismatch does not result in ischemic pain or angina in transplanted patients, so surveillance is required to identify coronary vasculopathy, which results in ischemia, even in the absence of symptoms.

Complications After Transplantation

Although rejection, infection, and cancer all come to mind as common complications posttransplant, the total list of complications is fairly long. In fact, surviving recipients have hypertension (97%), severe renal insufficiency (14%), hyperlipidemia (93%), diabetes (39%), and angiographic coronary allograph vasculopathy (CAV) (52%) by 10 years postcardiac transplantation. Many of these have a profound impact on outcomes in the perioperative period and the delivery of an anesthetic.

Rejection

Early success of HT was limited by organ rejection, and the evolution of the procedure has centered around methods to counteract and manage rejection. The risk of allograft rejection is the highest within 3 to 6 months of transplantation and decreases significantly after 1 year. Symptoms from rejection can be insidious and nonspecific, and surveillance biopsies at established intervals posttransplant are often necessary to make the diagnosis. The histologic hallmark of rejection is an inflammatory response directed against the grafted organ. The most feared type of rejection is the hyperacute variety, which manifests soon after restoration of circulation to the transplanted heart and is related to preformed antibodies to human leukocyte antigens (HLAs). This phenomenon has nearly been eliminated thanks to the development of prospective cytotoxic crossmatches. The newer variant of this technique is the "virtual crossmatch," in which a profile of recipient cytotoxic antibodies against antigens is created. This virtual crossmatch avoids the need for the recipient's blood to be matched against donor antigens when an organ becomes available.

Cell-mediated immunity has been recognized as the primary offender in rejection, although increasingly, antibody-mediated rejection is being recognized to play an equally important role. Frequently, cell-mediated rejection occurs 3 to 6 months after transplant and generally results in myocyte necrosis. The diagnosis is made by endomyocardial biopsy, and the severity is then graded between 1 and 3, the latter being most severe. Antibody-mediated rejection (AMR) usually results from preformed circulating antibodies. It was previously believed that AMR did not have a significant contribution to rejection that occurred multiple months after transplant. It is now known that humoral responses can occur and do contribute to rejection in the later phases as well. AMR is usually accompanied by early graft dysfunction, allograft vasculopathy, and hemodynamic compromise.

Treatment for AMR is initiated in patients with the clinical features of HF or ventricular dysfunction, irrespective of histologic evidence of cellular infiltrates. Symptoms of AMR can be nonspecific and include fatigue, unexplained weight gain, edema, or atrial fibrillation. This requires a high index of suspicion on the part of the treating physician. Endomyocardial biopsy via the internal jugular or femoral vein remains the gold standard for diagnosis. It is performed with decreasing frequency after the transplant (i.e., weekly for the first month, twice in the second month, and monthly for the next 4 months) per guidelines from the International Society of Heart and Lung Transplantation. Biopsy results can help differentiate between cell- and antibody-mediated rejection. However, it has the disadvantage of being invasive and sometimes requires general anesthesia. In addition, patchy inflammatory infiltrates may be missed on random biopsy sampling, and a histologic diagnosis may signal that significant myocardial damage has already occurred. Diastolic dysfunction and tissue Doppler imaging, using echocardiography, has shown some promise with a high negative predictive value when no abnormalities are detected. However, these echocardiographic modalities are nonspecific and have limited utility in the early detection of rejection. Cardiac magnetic resonance imaging has also shown some promise as a noninvasive test to detect rejection relatively early by using myocardial contrast enhancement. Serum markers such as troponins and BNP are nonspecific in the low-positive range and are not elevated until late in the disease process. The only Food and Drug Administration–approved noninvasive test used in routine clinical practice involves the creation of a genetic profile and identification of genetic markers that are suggestive of susceptibility to rejection. In a recent trial, this technique was shown to be comparable with endomyocardial biopsy in monitoring for rejection.

Treatment of rejection is guided by the severity and the nature of rejection as seen on biopsy. For asymptomatic patients with cellular rejection, it may suffice to increase the therapeutic levels of therapy. For coexisting cardiac dysfunction, pulse steroid therapy is used, and patients taking cyclosporine are switched to tacrolimus. It is important to remember that patients with asymptomatic humoral rejection are at a higher risk for allograft vasculopathy. Patients with AMR who are symptomatic are more aggressively managed with pulse steroids and occasionally intravenous (IV) γ-globulin. A detailed description of the therapy is beyond the scope of this text, but the principles are summarized in Table 6.2. Support with inotropes, intraaortic balloon pump counterpulsation, or extracorporeal membrane oxygenation may be required in patients with cardiogenic shock.

When transplant recipients present for noncardiac surgery, it is important to review their transplant and follow-up records to note the incidence, timing, and nature of rejection as well its management. Graft dysfunction is an ominous feature and should be discussed with the primary treatment team. As noted, patients with humoral rejection are at a higher risk of allograft vasculopathy (discussed later). The chronic administration or multiple courses of steroids can result in adrenal suppression and should be considered if this patient population is hemodynamically unstable in the perioperative period. Finally, the management of any circulatory support devices (e.g., ECMO) and associated anticoagulation must be considered.

Cardiac Allograft Vasculopathy

Coronary allograft vasculopathy (CAV) has been a major impediment to the long-term survival of HT recipients, with one-third of the HT patients developing CAV after

Table 6.2 Treatment of Cardiac Transplant Rejection

Immune Response	No Symptoms	Reduced Ejection Fraction	Failure or Shock
Cellular	Increase CNI; oral steroid bolus with taper	Oral steroid bolus with taper or IV pulse steroid	IV pulse steroid; cytolytic therapy; plasmapheresis; IVIG; inotropic support; IABP or ECMO; retransplantation
Humoral	No treatment (?)	Oral steroid bolus with taper or IV pulse steroid ± IVIG	

CNI, Calcineurin inhibitor; *ECMO*, extracorporeal membrane oxygenation; *IABP*, intraaortic balloon pump; *IV*, intravenous; *IVIG*, intravenous γ-globulin.
From Patel JK, Kittleson M, Kobashigawa JA. Cardiac allograft rejection. *Surgeon*. 2011;9:160-167.

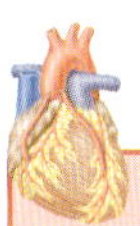

BOX 6.3 *Cardiac Allograft Vasculopathy*

- Affects one-third of heart transplant recipients at 5 years
- Presents as diffuse, concentric, hyperplastic lesions that affect the entire coronary tree
- Risk factors include general cardiac risk factors (e.g., obesity, hypertension, smoking, diabetes) as well as reperfusion injury, organ preservation, human leukocyte antigen compatibility, rejection, and cytomegalovirus infection

5 years. Little advancement has been made in prevention, and the incidence of CAV has not decreased dramatically in the past 20 years. It remains one of the major long-term (i.e., >1 year posttransplant) causes of mortality. CAV begins with a complex interaction between immune and nonimmune factors that eventually results in endothelial injury and subsequently an excessive fibroproliferative response. CAV is characterized by diffuse, concentric, hyperplastic lesions that affect the entire coronary tree. This is in contrast to native coronary atherosclerosis, in which the lesions are eccentric and distributed in a patchy, focal manner in the proximal epicardial vessels.

Endothelial injury is the final common pathway for this complex process, and it results in an excessive tissue repair response characterized by cell proliferation, fibrosis, and luminal narrowing. The previously mentioned nonimmune factors include not only general cardiac risk factors such as obesity, hypertension, smoking, and diabetes but also some modifiers unique to HT such as reperfusion injury and organ preservation. Growing evidence points to HLA compatibility, rejection, and CMV infection having roles in the pathogenesis as well. Calcification on imaging, which is common with native disease, is uncommon with CAV. Because angina is uncommon due to denervation at transplant, CAV manifests in much more sinister forms such as congestive HF, arrhythmias, or sudden cardiac death. This makes routine surveillance essential for diagnosis, which is difficult even when CAV is suspected. Myocardial perfusion imaging and stress echocardiography have limited diagnostic accuracy, though their prognostic utility is better. Coronary angiography combined with intravascular ultrasound is currently the standard for diagnosis, with an increase of 0.5 mm or more in intimal thickness within the first year after transplantation a powerful predictor of all-cause mortality, myocardial infarction, and angiographic abnormalities (Box 6.3).

The management of CAV hinges on primary prevention and early treatment. Blood pressure control, specifically using vasodilators such as calcium channel blockers and angiotensin-converting enzyme inhibitors, has been shown to delay CAV. The role of appropriate immunosuppression and treatment of rejection in the management of CAV cannot be overemphasized. The inhibition of vascular smooth muscle and fibroblast proliferation by sirolimus and everolimus can be helpful but their indiscriminate use is associated with intolerance, infections, and impaired wound healing. Because of the diffuse and hyperplastic nature of the disease, angiographic relief of stenosis is neither easy nor very successful. Retransplantation remains the definitive treatment for this complicated and grave condition; however, it possesses significant technical and ethical challenges. In general, it should be suspected that some degree of CAV is present in HT recipients who are 1 year out from transplantation and presenting for noncardiac surgery. Asymptomatic does not mean disease free in this special population, and all diagnostic studies need to be carefully reviewed. If these studies cannot be accessed before the procedure, then management decisions should be made assuming some coronary stenosis is present.

Infection

Unfortunately, immunosuppression is a double-edged sword, bringing with it the risks of malignancy and infection. The risk of infection decreases over time, likely reflecting alterations in immune suppression. In the immediate postoperative period, nosocomial or iatrogenic infections predominate. Between 1 and 6 months, opportunistic infections and activation of latent infection occurs. After 6 months, community-acquired infections are more common. Improved bacterial and viral prophylaxis has resulted in a decrease in infections with pneumocystis, cytomegalovirus (CMV), *Listeria* spp., *Nocardia* spp., and *Toxoplasma* spp. Prophylactic therapy generally includes sulfamethoxazole and trimethoprim for *Pneumocystis carinii*, ganciclovir for CMV, acyclovir for herpes simplex virus, pyrimethamine for toxoplasmosis, and nystatin for *Candida* spp. Antifungal prophylaxis and treatments have improved as well, resulting in improved survival despite emergence of resistant candida and *Aspergillus* strains. These treatments should be continued in the perioperative period, which mandates that clinicians should be aware of the possible drug interactions. In addition, strict aseptic technique in the perioperative care of these patients is paramount, particularly for invasive hemodynamic monitoring placement, urinary catheterization, and other invasive procedures. Additional antibiotic prophylaxis should be individualized with attention toward the specific patient, the procedure, and the bacterial spectrum. It is important to note that fever and leukocytosis do not usually accompany infection in transplant recipients, so vigilance is required to avoid progression to catastrophic sepsis.

IMMUNOSUPPRESSIVE MEDICATIONS AND THEIR PERIOPERATIVE MANAGEMENT

Immunosuppression

Advances in immunosuppression have been the driving force behind the success of HT as a procedure. Technically, it involves induction (high-intensity initiation of therapy), maintenance, and reversal of rejection, if applicable. The function of immunosuppressive drugs is to prevent or ameliorate rejection while minimally impacting normal physiology. Immunosuppressant medications have three main effects: therapy (i.e., suppression of rejection), unwanted results of immunosuppression (e.g., infection and cancer), and nonimmune cytotoxicity. Most of these drugs act by depleting lymphocytes, diverting the traffic for the ones that exist, or blocking response pathways if lymphocytes become activated. Generally, suppression of humoral immunity is better tolerated than suppression of cell-mediated immunity because of the absence of cytokine release and thus fewer side effects.

Native and memory T lymphocytes are involved in the process of alloimmunity, especially those that are sensitized to HLA. This is thought to stem from previous infection with viral agents that cross-react with the HLA domains. After activation and transformation in the lymphoid tissue surrounding the graft, effector T cells emerge and orchestrate an inflammatory response. This is carried out in conjunction with B lymphocytes, which mediate a humoral antibody response. This process has a characteristic histopathologic appearance with deposition of complement C4a. As previously stated, antibody-mediated rejection is associated with more severe hemodynamic compromise and worse outcome, with the primary site for damage being the capillary endothelium. The process of rejection can take days to reach its peak, which may be after the patient has been discharged from the initial procedure.

Induction Therapy

The efficacy of induction therapy is debated, and it is currently recommended only for select patients. The benefits of induction therapy include a reduction in steroid use and a delay in the initiation of calcineurin inhibitors. There is, however, a relative paucity of data on its long-term adverse effects with regard to infection and malignancy.

Induction is usually carried out using the following two types of drugs (Table 6.3):

1. Depleting protein-type drugs (e.g., OKT3 or muromonab-CD3, antithymocyte globulin): These act by destroying T cells and B cells. Their administration results in cytokine release, which can have systemic effects. These medications are also associated with an increased incidence of lymphoproliferative disorders.

Table 6.3 Induction Agents for Immunosuppression and Common Side Effects

Drug	Target	Effect	Major Side Effect
Depleting Protein-Type Drugs			
ATG: rabbit, horse	Binding of antigens, including CD45	Rapid depletion of T and B cells	Leucopenia, low platelets, cytokine release syndrome, serum sickness
Anti-CD3 antibodies (muromonab CD3)	Binding of CD3	Rapid depletion of T cells	Cytokine release syndrome, serum sickness
Nondepleting Protein Drugs			
IL-2 receptor antagonist (basiliximab)	Inhibition of IL-2 receptor	Prevention of proliferation and differentiation of T cells	No major side effect
Anti-CD52 antibodies (alemtuzumab)	Binding of CD52	Rapid depletion of T and B cells	Persistent leucopenia

ATG, Antithymocyte globulin; *CD,* cluster of differentiation; *IL,* interleukin.

6

2. Nondepleting protein drugs (e.g., monoclonal antibodies and fusion proteins): These medications suppress the immune system without the destruction of lymphocytes. In general, they have limited efficacy but a much better side effect profile.

Maintenance Therapy

Maintenance therapy attempts to achieve graft–host adaptation while minimizing the aforementioned complications. To this end, maintenance therapy typically consists of a corticosteroid, a calcineurin inhibitor (e.g., cyclosporine or tacrolimus), and an antiproliferative agent (e.g., mycophenolate). Steroids are used for a limited period of time, with an effort to keep its duration between 1 and 5 years. Tacrolimus continues to be the preferred calcineurin inhibitor and is preferred in cases with higher chances of rejection, hypertension, and hyperlipidemia; cyclosporine is used more commonly with diabetes mellitus. Sirolimus, an inhibitor of mammalian target of rapamycin (mTOR) receptor, has shown promise in reduction of nephrotoxicity, CAV, and cardiac morbidity.

Rejection

Acute rejection, when it is cellular and associated with significant hemodynamic compromise, is treated with either high-dose steroids or antithymocyte globulin. Severe humoral rejection that causes hemodynamic compromise is usually managed with high-dose corticosteroids and plasmapheresis followed by IV immunoglobulin or rituximab (a B cell–depleting monoclonal anti-CD20 antibody).

Interactions of Immunosuppressant Medications and Anesthetic Drugs

The world of immunosuppressant medications is evolving rapidly, and the interactions they share with anesthesia drugs are numerous and complicated. However, general concepts such as serum concentrations remain constant and should not be overlooked. It is important to remember that massive fluid shifts can result in alterations in serum levels. This is particularly important when it comes to drugs such as cyclosporine and tacrolimus because a reduction in their efficacy can either precipitate or worsen organ rejection. Also, because of reductions in gastric emptying, levels of medications may be subtherapeutic if orally administered just before induction. Alternatively, common medications such as calcium channel blockers can increase levels of immunosuppressant medications. Thus monitoring of drug levels is essential because dose adjustments may be needed to maintain therapeutic levels in the perioperative period.

Cyclosporine is perhaps the most studied agent in terms of its interaction with anesthetic drugs. Patients receiving cyclosporine may require a lower initial dose of nondepolarizing muscle relaxant, and the therapeutic effect may be prolonged. Cyclosporine may also reduce the seizure threshold; therefore avoidance of hyperventilation while under anesthesia when possible is prudent. This is also true of tacrolimus. Cyclosporine and tacrolimus are also known to cause decreases in renal blood flow and glomerular filtration rate. These effects can be compounded by other nephrotoxic medications commonly administered in the perioperative period such as nonsteroidal antiinflammatory drugs (NSAIDs), ranitidine, cotrimoxazole, and gentamycin. Therefore when possible, the use of additional nephrotoxic agents should be avoided in the perioperative period.

Many drugs, including the commonly used immunosuppressants and antifungal agents, are metabolized through the cytochrome P450 (CYP450) enzyme system and extruded from cells by the multiple drug resistance transporter protein, P-glycoprotein. Drugs such as midazolam, verapamil, and erythromycin are inhibitors of the P-glycoprotein system and can enhance the effects as well as the toxicity of the immunosuppressants that are substrates for it. Furthermore, both CYP450 and P-glycoprotein exhibit genetic polymorphisms, which can result in significant differences in drug metabolism. Intraoperative factors such as hypothermia may also have a direct effect on important drug concentrations via an effect on metabolism pathways. For example, hypothermia during or after surgery can result in the reduced clearance of and higher levels of drugs metabolized by the P450 system (e.g., immunosuppressants). Another example of reduced metabolism and elimination involves the shared extrahepatic glucuronidation pathways of propofol and mycophenolate, which could potentially result in decreased elimination if coadministered. Finally, anesthetic drugs have been shown to influence cell-mediated immunity, assist tumor growth, and affect neurodegenerative protein accumulation. The clinical impact of these properties over a short anesthetic is probably not significant but may accumulate if repeated procedures are carried out in a short period of time (Box 6.4).

For additional information regarding drugs that affect immunosuppressant levels, immunosuppressants that may impact perioperative management, and drugs that may result in renal dysfunction if coadministered with immunosuppressants, see Tables 6.4 and 6.5 and Box 6.5.

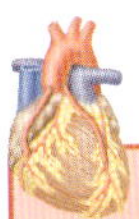

BOX 6.4   *Anesthesia and Immunosuppressant Medications*

- Fluid shifts can alter serum levels.
- Calcium channel blockers can increase serum levels.
- Cyclosporine and tacrolimus can prolong the therapeutic effect of nondepolarizing muscle relaxants.
- Hypothermia can result in the reduced clearance of and higher levels of drugs metabolized by the P450 system (e.g., immunosuppressants).

Table 6.4   **Drugs That Affect Immunosuppressive Drug Levels**

Drugs That Increase Levels	Drugs That Decrease Levels
Bromocriptine	Carbamazepine
Chloroquine	Octreotide
Cimetidine	Phenobarbital
Clarithromycin	Phenytoin
Cotrimoxazole	Rifampicin
Danazol	Ticlopidine
Diltiazem	
Erythromycin	
Fluconazole, itraconazole	
Metoclopramide	
Nicardipine	
Verapamil	

Modified from Kostopanagiotou G, Smyrniotis V, Arkadopoulos N, et al. Anesthetic and perioperative management of adult transplant recipients in nontransplant surgery. *Anesth Analg.* 1999;89:613-622.

Table 6.5 **Side Effects of Immunosuppressives That Affect Anesthesia Management**

Side Effect	CyA	Tacrolimus	Aza	Steroids	MMF	ATG	OKT3
Anemia	−	−	+	−	+	−	−
Leukopenia	−	−	+	−	+	+	+
Thrombocytopenia	−	−	+	−	+	−	−
Hypertension	++	+	−	+	−	−	−
Diabetes	+	++	−	++	−	−	−
Neurotoxicity	+	+	−	+	−	−	−
Renal insufficiency	+	++	−	−	−	−	−
Anaphylaxis	−	−	−	−	−	+	+
Fever	−	−	−	−	−	+	+

ATG, Antithymocyte globulin; *Aza*, azathioprine; *CyA*, cyclosporine; *MMF*, mycophenolate mofetil; *OKT3*, monoclonal antibodies against CD3 antigen; −, no effect; +, mild effect; ++, significant effect.

Modified from Kostopanagiotou G, Smyrniotis V, et al. Anesthetic and perioperative management of adult transplant recipients in nontransplant surgery. *Anesth Analg.* 1999;89:613-622.

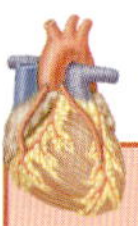

BOX 6.5   *Drugs That Impair Renal Dysfunction When Given With Cyclosporine or Tacrolimus*

Amphotericin
Cimetidine
Ranitidine
Melphalan
Nonsteroidal antiinflammatory drugs
Cotrimoxazole
Vancomycin
Tobramycin
Gentamycin

Modified from Kostopanagiotou G, Smyrniotis V, Arkadopoulos N, et al. Anesthetic and perioperative management of adult transplant recipients in nontransplant surgery. *Anesth Analg.* 1999;89:613-622.

PREOPERATIVE ASSESSMENT AND OPTIMIZATION

Preoperative Evaluation and Testing

The perioperative management of a transplant recipient begins with elucidating the details of the transplant procedure, such as the indication, date, success, and postoperative course. Contact with the primary transplant team may provide this information and may also yield the latest diagnostic information and laboratory studies, which are ultimately relevant to perioperative management. The focus of the preoperative assessment is to assess graft function (echocardiography), rejection status (endomyocardial biopsy), coronary artery disease (intravascular ultrasound or angiography), functional status, and end-organ involvement. For these purposes, evaluation based on symptoms and clinical pictures has to be augmented by a review of previous studies or if not recent then the completion of new ones. The previously detailed potential complications and interactions should be carefully investigated and ruled out. It is important to communicate the patient's CMV status with the blood bank because CMV-seronegative recipients require products from CMV-negative donors. If blood products are required, use of leukodepleted, irradiated cells reduces the likelihood of graft-versus-host disease. Perioperative consultation with a transplant microbiologist can be helpful to both screen for infection and devise an individual antimicrobial prophylaxis plan according to the patient's infection profile, the proposed procedure, and the duration since transplant. In the absence of significant shunt or intracardiac prosthetic material, infectious endocarditis prophylaxis is usually not necessary for noncardiac surgery. Finally, healthcare providers must also be sensitive to the fact that these patients can, despite improved physical status and indices, have subtle mental and psychiatric ailments such as depression.

The preoperative evaluation must take into account duration since the transplant because the patient's physiology, complications and risks undergo a transition approximately 1 year after the procedure. The risk of rejection is higher during the first phase, and thus immunosuppression is more intense as well. This produces a higher incidence of complications, such as anemia or leukopenia from mycophenolate, diabetes or hypertension from steroids, and renal dysfunction from calcineurin inhibitors. Graft dysfunction, volume status changes, and deconditioning are common before 1 year as well. For these reasons, elective surgery should be deferred until the end of the first year, and patients presenting for urgent procedures are ideally managed in consultation with an expert (e.g., cardiothoracic anesthesiologist). After the first year, the risk of rejection falls, and immunosuppression intensity can be reduced. However, the risk of CAV increases, and depending on monitoring protocols at individual institutions, patients are required to undergo angiography with intravascular ultrasonography every 1 to 2 years. Therefore most procedures can be conducted without subspecialist help, but the practitioner should have a high degree of suspicion for CAV as the time from transplantation increases (Box 6.6).

In terms of cardiac tests, the preoperative ECG may show dual P-waves or pacing spikes from a cardiovascular implantable electronic device (CIED). First-degree atrioventricular (AV) block, right bundle branch block, and atrial flutter can be seen as well. To obtain information regarding CIED dependence and recent arrhythmia episodes, all CIEDs should be interrogated before surgery. Depending on the type and proximity of any anticipated electrical interference, conversion to asynchronous mode in pacemaker-dependent patients and discontinuation of antitachycardia and defibrillator therapies may be required. If tachyarrhythmia therapies are disabled, continuous monitoring with easy access to external pacing and defibrillation is required, as are interrogation and programming at the conclusion of the procedure. New arrhythmias identified in the course of CIED interrogation or preoperative evaluation may indicate

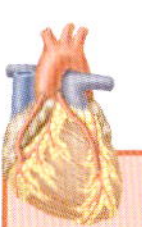

> **BOX 6.6** *Time Since Transplantation and Complications*
>
> - <1 year: rejection, graft dysfunction, fluid overload, anemia or leukopenia, diabetes, renal dysfunction, and deconditioning
> - >1 year: coronary artery disease (e.g., cardiac allograft vasculopathy)

6

graft dysfunction or CAV and should be investigated thoroughly. Imaging studies such as echocardiography can provide valuable information about systolic function, diastolic function, and valvular competence. The presence of diastolic dysfunction may signal rejection, and systolic dysfunction could be a sign of CAV. Finally, pertinent preoperative fluid laboratory tests include hematology, chemistry, coagulation, and liver enzyme studies, which may identify end-organ dysfunction from either hypoperfusion or immunosuppressant-induced toxicity.

Perioperative Immunosuppressant Management

Immunosuppressants, in consultation with the transplant service, should be continued perioperatively. Disruption of oral intake may necessitate substitution with IV formulations. Given the required conversion of oral to IV formulations, as well as potential differences among formulations (e.g., the IV preparation of calcineurin inhibitors is more nephrotoxicity than oral preparations at equipotent doses), it is prudent to involve a knowledgeable pharmacist. It is also important to note that mTOR inhibitors can also affect wound healing, and dose reductions or interruption may be advisable. Perioperative steroid administration in patients administered steroids preoperatively, on the other hand, is a more controversial issue. It has been suggested that patients receiving immunosuppressive doses of steroids do not need additional doses of steroids for surgery and that hypotension under anesthesia is more often related to hypovolemia rather than adrenal insufficiency. Furthermore, excessive steroid administration is associated with gastric erosions, hyperglycemia, infection risk, and psychological disturbances. The authors do not routinely administer steroids in patients who are on steroid therapy if they receive their daily dose of steroids on the day of surgery. If faced with refractory hypotension (i.e., not responsive to fluids and vasopressor administration), then 25 mg of hydrocortisone may be administered intravenously. A lower threshold for steroid administration should exist in cases in which steroid therapy was recently discontinued, when there is coexisting infection, or when the surgery is major and invasive.

PERIOPERATIVE MONITORING AND MANAGEMENT

Monitoring

Patients are aware of the increased risk they face as transplant recipients, so judicious premedication can help alleviate anxiety and improve their experience. ECG monitoring for myocardial ischemia detection is critical, as it is for changes in heart rate and AV nodal conduction caused by the anesthetic drugs used perioperatively. The absence of usual cardiovascular responses to light anesthesia requires increased vigilance to ensure anesthetic depth and a depth-of-anesthesia monitor (i.e., processed electroencephalogram) should be used when appropriate. Specialized monitoring should be based on the patient's condition, the proposed procedure, the nature of the procedure (e.g., emergent), blood loss, and anticipated fluid shifts. The pulmonary artery catheter can be useful if large fluid shifts are expected, especially if there is preexisting cardiac dysfunction. Transesophageal echocardiography is a useful, minimally invasive monitor to guide fluid therapy, monitor global cardiac function, and titrate vasoactive and inotropic medications. As previously mentioned, strict aseptic precaution and infection prevention during placement of invasive monitors cannot be overemphasized in this particularly vulnerable population.

Anesthetic Technique

The choice of anesthetic technique requires individualization. There is no clear contraindication to any anesthetic technique; sedation, regional, and general techniques have all been used successfully. The anesthetic goals should include maintenance of preload, preservation of sinus rhythm, avoidance of sudden changes in afterload, and careful monitoring for intraoperative complications. Laparoscopic procedures can be carried out safely provided sudden fluctuations in preload and afterload (as can occur with insufflation and desufflation) are detected and managed expeditiously.

Although the use of a laryngeal mask airway is an acceptable alternative to endotracheal intubation in the face of favorable anatomy and no contraindications, oral intubation of the trachea is preferable to the nasal route to reduce infection risk. Gingival hyperplasia related to cyclosporine is possible, and airway anatomy can be altered by lymphoproliferative disorders. It can complicate airway management and make ventilation difficult if airway compression is present. Vocal cord dysfunction from prolonged intubation previously or tracheal stenosis secondary to a prior tracheostomy can contribute to difficulty in airway management as well. HT patients generally manifest reduced time to desaturation during apnea. This can be related to atelectasis, pleural effusions, or an increase in extravascular lung water. All these factors make it necessary to have both expertise and equipment available to secure the airway expeditiously.

Regional anesthesia administration may be contraindicated by thrombocytopenia and the susceptibility to infection means that blocks should be carried out under strict asepsis and catheter removal should occur as soon as possible. The more gradual, controlled onset of blockade with an epidural may be advantageous compared with a spinal anesthetic in these patients because their chronotropic response to an acute reduction in afterload may be impaired. Vigilance during block onset is mandatory because hemodynamic responses can be unpredictable and severe.

Pregnancy is feasible and indeed reported in HT recipients. Pregnancy is accompanied by an increase in blood volume and cardiac output, which a well-functioning transplanted heart can handle without problem. Immunosuppressives are not necessarily teratogenic and do not need to be discontinued during pregnancy. However, the risks of infection, chronic hypertension, pregnancy-induced hypertension, preterm labor, and rejection are increased. These patients have a higher likelihood of requiring a cesarean section for delivery as well. Neuraxial anesthesia is an acceptable choice for both labor analgesia and cesarean delivery provided coagulopathy does not exist and care is taken to maintain preload in the face of vasodilation.

Intraoperative Management

Hemodynamic management principles should take into account the altered physiology of a transplanted heart. Drugs using the sympathetic nervous system are poorly efficacious, and drugs with direct and indirect effects (e.g., ephedrine) will manifest only the direct effects (Table 6.6). Normal responses should be expected from epinephrine, norepinephrine, glucagon, isoproterenol, and metaraminol. Levosimendan, a calcium sensitizer, has been shown to improve cardiac function in the graft and can reduce inotrope requirements. Drugs that alter vascular tone such as phenylephrine, nitroglycerin, and vasopressin will work normally; however, the compensatory responses of heart rate adjustment will not be present early in the posttransplant period. If anything, this results in a slight augmentation of their clinical effects. The response to adenosine can be exaggerated as well, and the drug is best avoided in this population. Because of denervation, it would be plausible that cholinergic drugs such as reversal

Table 6.6 Cardiovascular Effects of Drugs on Normal and Transplanted Hearts

		Heart Rate		Blood Pressure	
Drug	Type of Action	Normal	Transplanted	Normal	Transplanted
Atropine	Indirect	Increase	None	None	None
Ephedrine	Direct and indirect	Increase	Small increase	Increase	Small increase
Epinephrine	Direct	Increase	Increase	Increase	Increase
Phenylephrine	Direct	Decrease	None	Increase	Increase

Modified from Ashary N, Kaye AD, Hegazi AR, Frost EAM. Anesthetic considerations in the patient with a heart transplant. *Heart Dis*. 2002;4:191-198.

agents will have little effect on heart rate. However, neostigmine is well known to cause bradycardia and even cardiac arrest when used for neuromuscular blockade reversal, although the exact mechanism has been unclear. Preadministration of glycopyrrolate and the ready availability of direct chronotropic agents are essential when administering neostigmine to these patients. Sugammadex presents a good alternative to neostigmine because it is devoid of significant cardiac effects.

Patients on immunosuppression are at increased risk for renal injury, and the use of nephrotoxic drugs such as NSAIDs, or aminoglycoside antibiotics should be avoided. In fact, any maneuver or procedure (e.g., laparoscopy) that negatively impacts renal perfusion can cause or aggravate renal dysfunction. In the absence of end-organ dysfunction, the choice of opiates or muscle relaxants is based on the surgery and anticipated recovery. Special attention needs to be given to patient positioning and padding given the ecchymosis and osteoporosis that often accompany steroid therapy.

Postoperative Management

Postoperative care is similar to other patients with attention to adequate analgesia, normothermia, and hydration. However, HT recipients possess an increased risk of arrhythmias, and a lower threshold should exist for monitoring via telemetry in the postoperative period. If immunosuppression was interrupted, then resumption of immunosuppression should occur as soon as oral intake is permitted or IV formulations allow. A heightened awareness needs to exist regarding postoperative infection and wound healing. For these reasons, intravascular catheters and drains need to be removed as soon as possible. Finally, because this patient population is at higher than normal risk for deep vein thrombosis, thromboprophylaxis should be instituted as soon as possible.

CONCLUSION

Heart transplantation continues to improve the length and quality of life for patients with end-stage HF. The advances in immunosuppression protocols and organ preservation and the use of more specific immune monitoring tools are likely to move cardiac transplantation closer to its original goal of near-normal physiology for recipients.

With knowledge of the current physiologic differences, practitioners can safely care for heart transplant recipients undergoing noncardiac surgery. Organ transplantation is often described as the exchange of one disease state for another, although with modern medicine, this exchange is fast becoming a more propitious one.

SUGGESTED READING

Anaizi N. Drug interactions involving immunosuppressive agents. *Graft*. 2001;4(4):232.

Awad M, Czer LSC, Hou M, et al. Early denervation and later reinnervation of the heart following cardiac transplantation: a review. *J Am Heart Assoc*. 2016;5:e004070.

Chih S, Chong AY, Mielniczuk LM, Bhatt DL, Beanlands RSB. Allograft vasculopathy. *J Am Coll Cardiol*. 2016;68:80.

Colvin-Adams M, Smith JM, Hcubner BM, et al. OPTN/SRTR 2013 annual data report: heart. *Am J Transplant*. 2015;15:1–28.

Everly MJ, Bloom RD, Tsai DE, Trofe J. Posttransplant lymphoproliferative disorder. *Ann Pharmacother*. 2007;41:1850–1858.

Fishman JA. Infection in solid-organ transplant recipients. *N Engl J Med*. 2007;357:2601–2614.

Fontes ML, Rosenbaum SH. Noncardiac surgery after heart transplantation. *Anesthesiol Clin N Am*. 1997;15:207–220.

Hamon D, Taleski J, Vaseghi M, Shivkumar K, Boyle NG. Arrhythmias in the heart transplant patient. *Arrhythm Electrophysiol Rev*. 2014;3:149–155.

Hunt SA, Haddad F. The changing face of heart transplantation. *J Am Coll Cardiol*. 2008;52:587–598.

Jurgens PT, Aquilante CL, Page RL, Ambardekar AV. Perioperative management of cardiac transplant recipients undergoing noncardiac surgery: unique challenges created by advancements in care. *Semin Cardiothorac Vasc Anesth*. 2017;21:235–244.

Kittleson M, Kobashigawa J. Cardiac transplantation: curreent outcomes and contemporary controversies. *JACC Heart Fail*. 2017;5:858–868.

Kobashigawa J, Olymbios M. Physiology of the transplanted heart. In: Kobashigawa J, eds. *Clinical Guide to Heart Transplantation*. Cham: Springer International Publishing; 2017:81–93.

Kostopanagiotou G, Smyrniotis V, Arkadopoulos N, et al. Anesthetic and perioperative management of adult transplant recipients in nontransplant surgery. *Anesth Analg*. 1999;89:613.

Lindenfeld J, Miller GG, Shakar SF, et al. Drug therapy in the heart transplant recipient. *Circulation*. 2004;110:3858.

Lund LH, Edwards LB, Kucheryavaya AY, et al. The registry of the international society for heart and lung transplantation: thirty-first official adult heart transplant report—2014; focus theme: retransplantation. *J Heart Lung Transplant*. 2014;33(10):996–1008.

McKellar S. Clinical firsts: Christiaan Barnard's heart transplantation. *N Engl J Med*. 2017;377:2211–2213.

Page RL, Miller GG, Lindenfeld J. Drug therapy in the heart transplant recipient: part iv: drug–drug interactions. *Circulation*. 2005;111:230–239.

Patel JK, Kittleson M, Kobashigawa JA. Cardiac allograft rejection. *Surgeon*. 2011;9:160–167.

Ramsingh D, Harvey R, Runyon A, Benggon M. Anesthesia for heart transplantation. *Anesthesiol Clin*. 2017;35:453 471.

Söderlund C, Rådegran G. Immunosuppressive therapies after heart transplantation—the balance between under- and over-immunosuppression. *Transplant Rev*. 2015;29:181–189.

Spann JC, Van Meter C. Cardiac transplantation. *Surg Clin North Am*. 1998;78(5):679–690.

Swanevelder J, Gordon P, Brink J, et al. Fifty years: reflections since the first successful heart transplant. *J Cardiothorac Vasc Anesth*. 2018;32:14–18.

Valantine H. Cardiac allograft vasculopathy after heart transplantation: risk factors and management. *J Heart Lung Transplant*. 2004;23(5, suppl):S187–S193.

Chapter 7

Pulmonary Hypertension in Noncardiac Surgical Patients

Dean Bowker, MD • Dalia Banks, MD, FASE

Key Points

1. Pulmonary hypertension (PH) is a rare disease with a high degree of morbidity and mortality for patients undergoing noncardiac surgery.
2. PH, although having several classification schemes, can be largely divided into high pulmonary venous pressure (typically from left-sided heart disease) and normal pulmonary venous pressure (typically from lung, embolic, or intrinsic disease).
3. The morbidity and mortality from PH rest on the impact of significant afterload to the right ventricle, which normally works against a low-resistance circuit. The right ventricular (RV) dysfunction leads to the symptomatology of low cardiac output (CO) and venous congestion.
4. The initial presenting symptom for a patient with PH is dyspnea on exertion caused by the inability of the right ventricle to provide an adequate CO in the presence of increasing afterload. Signs and symptoms of frank RV failure such as jugular venous distention, hepatomegaly, ascites, and peripheral edema are often late findings and portend a poor prognosis.
5. The pillars of hemodynamic management of a patient with PH include maintaining coronary perfusion pressure via systemic vasopressors, reduction of pulmonary pressures via selective pulmonary vasodilation and maintenance of RV contractility via inodilators.
6. During anesthesia, preventing increases in pulmonary vascular resistance (PVR) is imperative through avoidance of hypoxia, hypercarbia, and acidosis.
7. Regional anesthetics such as neuraxial and peripheral techniques are useful as primary anesthetics or as adjuncts to general anesthesia. Care must be exercised in sedation during regional block placement or during monitored anesthesia care. Postoperative regional anesthesia may help to prevent postoperative pain with attendant increases in PVR as well as to reduce narcotic-induced hypoventilation.
8. Several novel therapies aimed at reducing pulmonary pressures are used in patients preoperatively such as phosphodiesterase inhibitors and prostaglandins. These medications should be continued perioperatively because abrupt cessation may lead to lethal rebound PH.
9. Echocardiography and right heart catheterization are key components in the preoperative workup. Both modalities provide insight into the right heart's response to increased afterload as well as the potential use of pulmonary vasodilators perioperatively.
10. Factors suggestive of perioperative decompensation include right atrial pressure greater than 12 mm Hg, RV end-diastolic pressure greater than 15 mm Hg, mean pulmonary artery pressure greater than 55 mm Hg, PVR greater than 1000 dynes $\cdot$ s $\cdot$ cm^{-5}, cardiac index less than 2 L/min per m^2, and a lack of a vasodilator response.

> 11. Patients with factors suggestive of decompensation should have elective cases delayed until the patient is hemodynamically optimized.
> 12. Postoperatively, patients with severe PH require adequate monitoring in an intensive care unit to continue appropriate hemodynamic management as well as avoidance of hypoxia, hypercarbia, acidosis, and pain.

Pulmonary arterial hypertension (PAH) is a disorder in which flow to the pulmonary arterial circulation is constrained because of vascular remodeling and proliferation, resulting in increased pulmonary vascular resistance (PVR) and ending with right heart failure and death. PAH is a rare disease, with an estimated prevalence of 1% of the global population and an incidence of 1 to 2 cases per million people in the United States.

Pulmonary hypertension (PH), whether from PAH or another cause, is a known risk factor for perioperative complications, with an increased perioperative morbidity and mortality.

The choice of anesthetic technique together with patient and surgical characteristics are crucial factors in perioperative management. The main principles of perioperative management are to avoid systemic hypotension, as well as acute elevations in pulmonary arterial pressure, as both can lead to right ventricular (RV) ischemia and failure. This chapter focuses on perioperative management of pulmonary hypertension patients undergoing noncardiac surgery.

CLASSIFICATION OF PULMONARY HYPERTENSION

By definition, PH constitutes a mean pulmonary artery pressure (mPAP) greater than 25 mm Hg and a PVR greater than 300 dynes $\cdot$ s $\cdot$ cm^{-5}. Severe PH is defined as an mPAP greater than 50 mm Hg and a PVR greater than 600 dynes $\cdot$ s $\cdot$ cm^{-5}.

Pulmonary hypertension classification began in 1973 at the World Health Organization (WHO) conference and has since undergone multiple changes as the appreciation of the disease and treatment of PH has evolved. The Fourth World Symposium on PH held in 2008 in Dana Point, California, was the first international meeting to focus not only on PAH but also on other forms of PH caused by left heart disease, chronic lung disease, chronic venous thromboembolism, and other related diseases. Consensus during the recent Fifth World Symposium on PH was to maintain the same classification of PH into five distinct subgroups of patients sharing specific features (Box 7.1).

Another classification of PH assessed by right heart catheterization (RHC) divides PH into precapillary and postcapillary groups. Precapillary PH (groups I, III, IV, and V of the Fifth World Symposium classification) is characterized by mPAP greater than 25 mm Hg with normal pulmonary capillary wedge pressure (PCWP; i.e., <15 mm Hg, with a PVR >300 dynes $\cdot$ s $\cdot$ cm^{-5}). Postcapillary PH (group II), the most common form of PH, is caused by left heart disease and is characterized by mPAP greater than 25 mm Hg and PCWP greater than 15 mm Hg with normal PVR. Differentiating PAH from pulmonary venous hypertension (PVH) in group II is important given the high prevalence of left heart disease (Table 7.1).

IDIOPATHIC PULMONARY ARTERIAL HYPERTENSION

Idiopathic pulmonary arterial hypertension (IPAH) is a rare, debilitating disorder that affects the pulmonary vasculature, leading to PH and, consequently, right heart

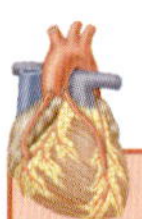

> **BOX 7.1** *Revised World Health Organization Classification of Pulmonary Hypertension*
>
> - Group I: IPAH, heritable PAH, HIV infection, and other subtypes of PAH
> - Group II: left heart disease, cardiomyopathies and LV failure, aortic and mitral valvular pathologies
> - Group III: respiratory disease and hypoxemia, COPD, sleep disorders, and ILD
> - Group IV: CTEPH
> - Group V: miscellaneous causes
>
> *COPD*, Chronic obstructive pulmonary disease; *CTEPH*, chronic thromboembolic pulmonary hypertension; *HIV*, human immunodeficiency virus; *ILD*, interstitial lung disease; *IPAH*, idiopathic pulmonary arterial hypertension; *LV*, left ventricular; *PAH*, pulmonary arterial hypertension.

Table 7.1 Comparison of Pulmonary Arterial Hypertension and Pulmonary Venous Hypertension

	Pulmonary Arterial Hypertension	Pulmonary Venous Hypertension
RA size	Enlarged	May be enlarged
LA size	Small	Large
Interatrial septum	Bows from right to left	Bows from left to right
RVOT notching	Common	Rare
Aortic pressure	Normal or low	Normal or high
PCWP (mm Hg)	<15	>15
PADP-PCWP (mm Hg)	>7	<5

LA, Left atrial; *PADP*, pulmonary artery diastolic pressure; *PCWP*, pulmonary capillary wedge pressure; *RA*, right atrial; *RVOT*, right ventricular outflow tract.

failure and death. IPAH, associated with a prothrombotic diathesis, excessive endothelial proliferation, and antiapoptotic cells within the vascular lumen, is identified when no other cause for the PH is identified. The endothelium displays an imbalance between vasoconstrictors relative to vasodilators.

"Plexogenic pulmonary arteriopathy" is the pathologic hallmark of primary PH, and it reflects a dysregulation of phenotypically altered endothelial growth.

Idiopathic pulmonary arterial hypertension is a panvasculopathy mostly affecting small and medium-size arterial vessels with a wide range of abnormalities, including intimal hyperplasia, medial hypertrophy, adventitial proliferation, and plexiform arteriopathy.

PATHOGENESIS

The pulmonary vasculature is a low-pressure, high-flow circuit balancing vasodilation and constriction, with a tendency toward vasodilation. The endothelium modulates vascular smooth muscle cell activity through the production of various vasodilators (prostacyclin and nitric oxide [NO]) and vasoconstrictors (thromboxane A_2 and

140

endothelin). The endothelium of the lung is markedly different from endothelium of the systemic vasculature. Although the stimuli that trigger primary PAH may differ, an undefined injury to the endothelium occurs that causes increased coagulation, proliferation, and vasoconstriction that are instrumental to the development of PAH. Mediator imbalance results in pulmonary vasoconstriction that leads to the disordered endothelial cell proliferation in combination with proliferation of intimal cells that form the characteristic plexiform lesions.

There is, however, no specific histopathologic lesion that defines primary PAH. Evidence of proliferative and obliterative intimal lesions composed of myofibroblasts is found in the pulmonary arteries and arterioles from increased production of endothelial mediators. Additionally, thickened arterial smooth muscle (isolated medial hypertrophy), destruction and fibrosis of vessel walls, and in situ thrombosis lead to stiffening of the arteries and greater vasoconstriction. Eventually, the endothelial mediators that maintain the low-pressure, high-flow pulmonary circulation (NO, endothelium-derived hyperpolarizing factor, natriuretic peptides, adrenomedullin, and α_2-agonists) are lost, and PA pressure increases at rest and with exercise. Regardless of the primary pathophysiologic pathways to PAH, a similar endpoint is reached.

Hypercoagulability is enhanced by increased platelet activity and elevated levels of serotonin, plasminogen activator inhibitor, and fibrinopeptide A together with a decrease in thrombomodulin levels. Endothelin (ET)-1, a potent vasoconstrictor, was found in high levels in arterial plasma compared with venous plasma in IPAH, suggesting that ET-1 may contribute to elevated PVR in these patients.

Idiopathic pulmonary arterial hypertension has been associated with increased local expression of ET-1 in pulmonary vascular endothelial cells, contributing to the pathogenesis of PAH. Additionally, the inhibition of voltage-gated (Kv) channels raises the membrane potential activating the voltage gated L-type calcium channel, which increases the calcium levels, leading to vasoconstriction and possibly initiating cell proliferation.

CLINICAL MANIFESTATIONS

The diagnosis of PH is often significantly delayed because of the nonspecific symptoms that may mimic known underlying pulmonary or cardiac disorders. Gradual onset of shortness of breath is the earliest and most common symptom of PH reflecting an inability to increase cardiac output (CO) in proportion to activity. Right-sided chest pain is prevalent in PH despite normal coronary arteries. Additional symptoms include syncope, fatigue, and worsening peripheral edema. Hemoptysis may occur as a result of rupture of dilated and distended pulmonary vessels. Enlarged pulmonary arteries may compress the recurrent laryngeal nerve, leading to hoarseness in these patients.

Physical examination focuses on signs of PH, right ventricular hypertrophy (RVH), and right-heart failure (Table 7.2). Accentuation of the pulmonic component of the second heart sound might be the only finding on physical examination and is easily overlooked. Hepatomegaly and peripheral edema, although less subtle on physical examination, typically signify advanced PH with concomitant right heart failure.

The first step in diagnosing PH is having a high index of suspicion in patients with these described signs and symptoms or those at risk such as coexisting left heart disease or pulmonary disease. Chest radiography and electrocardiogram (ECG) may display markers indicative of PH such as enlarged pulmonary arteries or right-axis deviation, respectively, but with very low specificity. Provided there is a high index of suspicion from the history and physical examination, echocardiography is the most

Table 7.2 Features of the Physical Examination Pertinent to the Evaluation of Pulmonary Hypertension

Sign	Implication
Physical Signs That Reflect the Severity of PH	
Accentuated pulmonary component of S_2 (audible at apex in >90%)	High pulmonary pressure increases force of pulmonic valve closure
Early systolic click	Sudden interruption of opening of pulmonary valve into high-pressure artery
Midsystolic ejection murmur	Turbulent transvalvular pulmonary outflow
Left parasternal lift	High RV pressure and hypertrophy present
RV S_4 (in 38%)	High RV pressure and hypertrophy present
Increased jugular a-wave	Poor RV compliance
Physical Signs That Suggest Moderate to Severe PH	
Holosystolic murmur that increases with inspiration	Tricuspid regurgitation
Increased jugular v-waves	
Pulsatile liver	
Diastolic murmur	Pulmonary regurgitation
Hepatojugular reflux	High central venous pressure
Advanced PH with RV failure	
RV S_3 (in 23%)	RV dysfunction
Distention of jugular veins	RV dysfunction, tricuspid regurgitation, or both
Hepatomegaly	RV dysfunction, tricuspid regurgitation, or both
Peripheral edema (in 32%)	
Ascites	
Low blood pressure, diminished pulse pressure, cool extremities	Reduced CO, peripheral vasoconstriction
Physical Signs That Suggest Possible Underlying Cause or Associations of PH	
Central cyanosis	Abnormal V/Q, intrapulmonary shunt, hypoxemia, pulmonary-to-systemic shunt
Clubbing	Congenital heart disease, pulmonary venopathy
Cardiac auscultatory findings, including systolic murmurs, diastolic murmurs, opening snap, and gallop	Congenital or acquired heart or valvular disease
Rales, dullness, or decreased breath sounds	Pulmonary congestion or effusion or both
Fine rales, accessory muscle use, wheezing, protracted expiration, productive cough	Pulmonary parenchymal disease
Obesity, kyphoscoliosis, enlarged tonsils	Possible substrate for disordered ventilation
Sclerodactyly, arthritis, telangiectasia, Raynaud phenomenon, rash	Connective tissue disorder
Peripheral venous insufficiency or obstruction	Possible venous thrombosis
Venous stasis ulcers	Possible sickle cell disease
Pulmonary vascular bruits	Chronic thromboembolic PH
Splenomegaly, spider angiomata, palmary erythema, icterus, caput medusa, ascites	Portal hypertension

CO, Cardiac output; *PH,* pulmonary hypertension; *RV,* right ventricular; *V/Q,* ventilation/perfusion.

appropriate next step. Echocardiography is sensitive to the effects of PH on the right heart and estimation of pulmonary artery (PA) pressures is possible in the presence of tricuspid regurgitation. Additional details of the echocardiographic examination of patients with PH is included below. Computed tomography (CT) and magnetic resonance (MR) imaging are new techniques available to further explore the diagnosis. RHC with assessment of PVR and right atrial (RA) and ventricular pressures together with left-sided pressure estimation are required to confirm the diagnosis and to define the hemodynamic profile with greater precision. Fig. 7.1 outlines an algorithm for the evaluation of PAH.

The number of patients with PH related to pulmonary venous hypertension, chronic lung disease with hypoxemia, and thromboembolic disease pulmonary disease is far greater than the number of patients with IPAH. The term "secondary" PAH is being used less because of the many therapies for PAH regardless of etiology and often the underlying disease overshadows the clinical manifestations of PAH. After the etiology of PAH is identified, treatment should begin immediately with the goal of preventing the onset of right heart failure. Unfortunately, at presentation, PAH has often progressed to the point that the value of any treatment is limited to palliation of incapacitating symptoms. Decisions about whether institution of therapy and the specific therapy chosen are made on a case-by-case basis and are best performed at centers with experience in managing PH. One factor in the evaluation of patients includes an assessment of RV function, typically by echocardiography and RHC, because the presence of RV dysfunction plays a major role in prognosis.

RIGHT VENTRICULAR PATHOPHYSIOLOGY: EFFECT OF PULMONARY HYPERTENSION ON THE RIGHT VENTRICLE

The right ventricle is a unique, asymmetric, crescent-shape structure that is designed to accommodate the entire venous return while maintaining a low RA pressure and providing sustained low-pressure perfusion through the lungs. Normally, the RV receives coronary blood supply throughout the cardiac cycle (i.e., during systole and diastole) because of the continuous coronary perfusion pressure gradient between the aorta and the right ventricle. Caution must be applied when treating systemic hypertension in a patient with severe PH as this can compromise RV perfusion pressure, leading to ischemia in an already compromised ventricle.

Unlike the left ventricle, which generates high pressure to optimize organ perfusion, the right ventricle ejects blood from the right atrium to the lungs via the low-pressure, low-resistance, high-compliance circuit of the pulmonary vascular bed. Functionally and anatomically, the right ventricle is adapted for the generation of sustained low-pressure perfusion. The right ventricle is divided by a circular muscular band that separates the inflow portion; the sinus, which generates pressure during systole; and the outflow portion, the conus, which regulates this pressure. RV contraction occurs in three phases; first, contraction of the papillary muscles; then a bellows-like peristaltic movement of the RV free wall toward the interventricular septum (IVS); and, finally, contraction of the left ventricle causes a "wringing" type of motion of the IVS that further empties the RV. The net effect is the generation of pressure starting from the apex moving toward the compliant conus, which is able to decrease the peak RV and PA pressures, thereby prolonging ejection.

The RV tolerates small changes in venous return well without changing end-diastolic pressure or volume; however, this is not true with larger amounts of venous return. The RV pressure-volume loop has a triangular shape in contrast to the rectangular shape of the LV pressure-volume loop, meaning that the right ventricle has longer

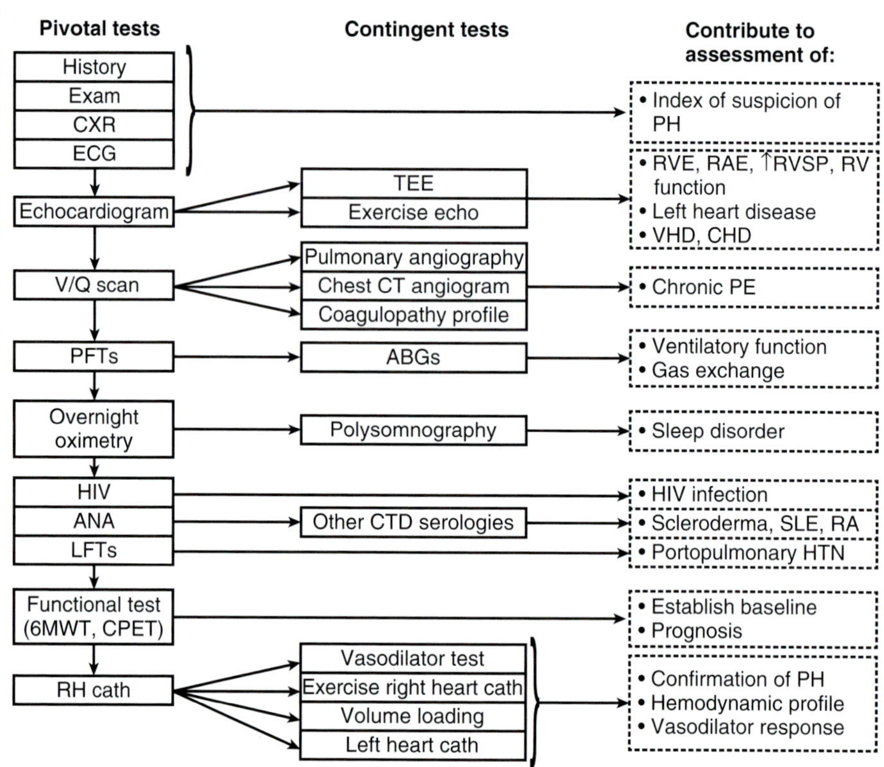

Fig. 7.1 Diagnostic approach to pulmonary arterial hypertension (PAH). The diagnosis of idiopathic pulmonary arterial hypertension (IPAH) is one of excluding all other reasonable possibilities. Pivotal tests are those that are essential to establishing a diagnosis of any type of PAH either by identification of criteria of associated disease or exclusion of diagnoses other than IPAH. All pivotal tests are required for a definitive diagnosis and baseline characterization. An abnormality of one assessment (e.g., obstructive pulmonary disease on pulmonary function tests) does not preclude that another abnormality (e.g., chronic thromboembolic disease on ventilation/perfusion scan and pulmonary angiogram) is contributing or predominant. Contingent tests are recommended to elucidate or confirm results of the pivotal tests and need only be performed in the appropriate clinical context. The combination of pivotal and appropriate contingent tests contributes to assessment of the differential diagnoses in the right-hand column. It should be recognized that definitive diagnosis may require additional specific evaluations not necessarily included in this general guideline. *ABG,* Arterial blood gas; *ANA,* antinuclear antibody serology; *CHD,* congenital heart disease; *CPET,* cardiopulmonary exercise test; *CT,* computed tomography; *CTD,* connective tissue disease; *CXR,* chest radiography; *ECG,* electrocardiogram; *HIV,* human immunodeficiency virus screening; *HTN,* hypertension; *LFT,* liver function test; *PE,* pulmonary embolism; *PFT,* pulmonary function test; *PH,* pulmonary hypertension; *RA,* rheumatoid arthritis; *RAE,* right atrial enlargement; *RH cath,* right heart catheterization; *RVE,* right ventricular enlargement; *RVSP,* right ventricular systolic pressure; *6MWT,* 6-minute walk test; *SLE,* systemic lupus erythematosus; *TEE,* transesophageal echocardiography; *VHD,* valvular heart disease. (From McLaughlin VV, Archer SL, Badesch DB, et al. ACCF/AHA 2009 expert consensus document on pulmonary hypertension: a report of the American College of Cardiology Foundation Task Force on Expert Consensus Documents. *J Am Coll Cardiol.* 2009;53:1573.)

periods of ejection and shorter periods of isovolumetric contraction and relaxation. The prolonged low-pressure ejection of the right ventricle is very sensitive to changes in PA pressures as is seen with PH. Consequently, the RV pressure–volume loop adapts to the same rectangular shape as the left ventricular (LV) pressure-volume loop, with prolonged isovolumetric contraction and a shortened ejection time causing an increase in myocardial oxygen consumption. When acute or chronic RV dysfunction ensues, the thin-walled, crescent shape allows the RV to accommodate a large increase in preload with minimal change in RV end-diastolic pressure (RVEDP). Consequently, the initial primary compensatory mechanism of RV dysfunction is dilation that is usually well tolerated. Compared with the left ventricle, the normal right ventricle has half the wall thickness (~5 mm) and performs one quarter the stroke work. The IVS is responsible for approximately half the RV CO; in fact, during RV infarction with loss of the RV free wall, the septum continues to generate RV systolic pressure.

It is important to note that the afterload effect on RV systolic function is typically more significant than the afterload effect on LV performance. Increased RV afterload not only decreases the RV ejection fraction in a linear fashion; it also leads to increased RV wall tension and RV oxygen demand, thereby increasing susceptibility to ischemia. After RV afterload increases and ventricular dilation ensues, decreased RV oxygen supply compromises RV contractility. Normally, the IVS is shifted toward the RV free wall, contributing to RV ejection. However, when the RV pressure increases, the IVS paradoxically shifts toward the left ventricle, impairing its contribution to RV ejection. The decreased RV output and septal shift toward the LV result in decreased LV filling, decreased LV output, and systemic hypotension, further reducing RV perfusion and oxygen supply. Increasing the systemic vascular resistance (SVR) can help increase LV pressure, counter the septal shift, and thereby restore the contribution of the IVS to RV ejection. Systemic vasoconstrictors can therefore be used to increase RV ejection in addition to increasing coronary perfusion pressure.

DIAGNOSTIC EVALUATION

The development of acute or chronic right heart failure is a devastating end-stage complication of PH that is associated with significant morbidity and mortality. Evidence of significant RV dysfunction should prompt a reevaluation of the need for elective surgery and will significantly impact the anesthetic management if the decision is made to proceed. Therefore a key component of the evaluation of PH is the assessment of the ability of the RV to compensate for the elevated afterload. There are several ways to diagnose right ventricular failure (RVF). In addition to the clinical signs and symptoms detailed earlier, which are very nonspecific, there are diagnostic modalities such as cardiac biomarkers, cardiac MRI, echocardiography, and RHC, which are more definitive and may reveal contributing causes (Box 7.2). Cardiac MRI accurately assesses RV size and function, low RV stroke volume, and RV dilation; impaired LV filling independently predicts mortality.

Predictors of survival after the first year of therapy with epoprostenol include functional class and improvement in exercise tolerance, cardiac index (CI), and mean PA pressure. A 6-minute walk test (6MW) was found to be an independent predictor of survival in several studies, leading to use of this test as the primary endpoint for many prospective trials. N-terminal pro–brain natriuretic peptide (NT-proBNP) levels are independent predictors of survival and correlate well with RV enlargement and dysfunction. The presence of cardiac troponin T potentially suggests RV ischemia and therefore confers poor prognosis (Box 7.3).

Echocardiography is an easy, accessible bedside technique for diagnosing and following patients suspected of having PH. Echocardiography easily assesses RA and RV enlargement, reduced RV function, displacement of the IVS, and tricuspid regurgitation. Furthermore, the echocardiography finding of a pericardial effusion has proven a consistent predictor of death.

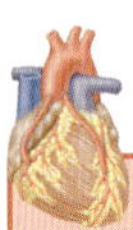

BOX 7.2   *Causes of Right Ventricular Failure*

RV Pressure Overload

- Pulmonary embolism
- Pulmonary hypertension
- Pulmonary stenosis
- Pericardial disease
- Left-sided valvular disease
- Left-sided cardiomyopathy
- RV outflow obstruction
- After cardiac and lung transplantation

RV Volume Overload

- Tricuspid regurgitation
- Pulmonary regurgitation
- Intracardiac shunt

RV, Right ventricular.

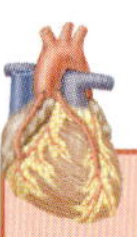

BOX 7.3   *Assessment of Right Ventricular Dysfunction*

ECG

- T inversion in leads V_1 to V_4 or lead III and aVF
- Sinus tachycardia
- New RBBB
- S1Q3T3 pattern

ECHO (+TEE)

- RV dilation (without mitral valve lesion and LV disease)
- RV free wall motion hypokinesia with sparing of apex (McConnell sign)
- Increased RV afterload
- Change to a more concentric RV morphology
- PH as TR with jet velocity >2.8 m/s
- Paradoxical septal motion
- 60/60 sign
- Lack of inspiratory collapse of the IVC
- Pulmonary artery dilation and RA enlargement

Right Heart Catheterization

- Evidence of pulmonary arterial obstruction (precapillary pressure >20 mm Hg with PCWP <19 mm Hg)
- Impaired LV diastolic filling

Increased Levels of Biomarkers

- cTnT >0.07 µg/L
- proBNP ≥600 ng/L

cTnT, Cardiac troponin T; *ECG*, electrocardiogram; *ECHO*, echocardiogram; *IVC*, inferior vena cava; *LV*, left ventricular; *PCWP*, pulmonary capillary wedge pressure; *PH*, pulmonary hypertension; *proBNP*, pro–brain natriuretic peptide; *RA*, right atrial; *RBBB*, right bundle branch block; *RV*, right ventricular; *TEE*, transesophageal echocardiography; *TR*, tricuspid regurgitation.

There are two simple visual methods to assess RV chamber size: (1) RV chamber area relative to LV chamber area in the midesophageal four-chamber view and (2) RV extension relative to the apex of the heart. RV dilation is severe when the RV area is more than the LV area, and the RV apex extends beyond the LV apex. Echocardiographic evaluation of RV wall thickness may also serve to evaluate global RV performance in conditions of RV pressure overload causing compensatory RVH. RVH may be diagnosed when the RV free wall thickness is greater than 5 mm at end-diastole. Common etiologies of RV pressure overload causing secondary RVH include pulmonary stenosis (PS) and PH from mitral stenosis, pulmonary embolism, chronic thromboembolic pulmonary hypertension (CTEPH), or other causes. When RV dysfunction ensues, the compensatory RV dilation causes the normal complex RV geometry to change from a triangular, crescent shape to a more ellipsoid, circular, D shape. Although such changes point to RV dysfunction, they do not distinguish whether the RV dysfunction is related to RV volume overload, RV pressure overload, or both. Echocardiographic evaluation of the shape and motion of the IVS may be useful to differentiate between RV volume overload versus RV pressure overload pathology.

Right Ventricular Volume Overload

Normally, the IVS is curved in a convex fashion toward the RV during the entire cardiac cycle as a result of its motion being controlled by the more abundant and centrally located LV muscle mass. As the RV progressively dilates and hypertrophies such that the RV mass increases to equal that of the LV, the convex shape of the IVS begins to flatten. Moreover, when RV volume and mass exceed that of the LV, paradoxical septal motion appears such that the IVS abnormally bows toward the LV. In cases of RV volume overload, this abnormal bowing is seen most prominently at end-diastole because this is the time that corresponds with maximal RV volume (Fig. 7.2).

Additional signs of RV volume overload include RA enlargement, dilation of the tricuspid annulus or hepatic or great veins, and leftward deviation of the atrial septum.

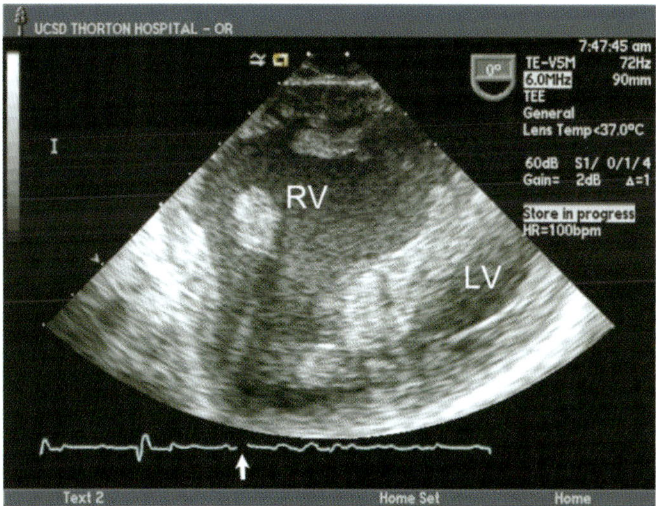

Fig. 7.2 Transgastric mid-papillary short-axis view demonstrating right ventricular volume overload. Note the interventricular septal flattening during end-diastole. The arrow points to the associated electrocardiogram denoting end-diastole. *LV,* Left ventricle; *RV,* right ventricle.

Such findings of RV volume overload suggest severe tricuspid regurgitation (TR), intracardiac shunts, or PH (caused by left-sided heart disease or intrinsic lung disease).

Right Ventricular Pressure Overload

Although RV pressure overload alone may occur because of PS or PH, pure RV pressure overload is uncommon in adult hearts because RV hypertension is usually associated with TR and RV dilation. Initially, RV pressure overload reduces the normal motion and curvature of the IVS toward the RV and causes the appearance of abnormal IVS flattening throughout the cardiac cycle. As RV pressure overload progresses to more severe RVH, the center of mass of the heart shifts toward the RV. This causes a characteristic paradoxical septal motion of the IVS bowing toward the LV that is most pronounced at end-systole when RV systolic afterload is at its peak (i.e., the time when RV pressure is the highest; Fig. 7.3). When comparing the paradoxical septal motions of RV pressure overload versus RV volume overload, the key point to remember is that the most pronounced IVS bowing toward the LV occurs at end-systole with RV pressure overload and at end-diastole with RV volume overload.

Tricuspid annular plane systolic excursion (TAPSE) is another method to assess global RV systolic function. TAPSE refers to the long-axis, apex-to-base lateral tricuspid annulus systolic excursion. Because of the relatively fixed septal attachment of the tricuspid annulus, its displacement is asymmetric, and TAPSE appears more as a hinge-like motion. Normal TAPSE is 17 mm or greater toward the cardiac apex, and reductions in TAPSE values are suggestive of RV systolic dysfunction.

Right heart catheterization remains the gold standard in assessment of hemodynamics in patients with PH as well as a confirmatory method for diagnosis. RHC is performed in patients who have suspected PH after the initial screening. This procedure focuses on measuring PA pressure, PVR, and the effects of vasodilator therapy on the pulmonary circulation. The underlying principle for vasodilator testing

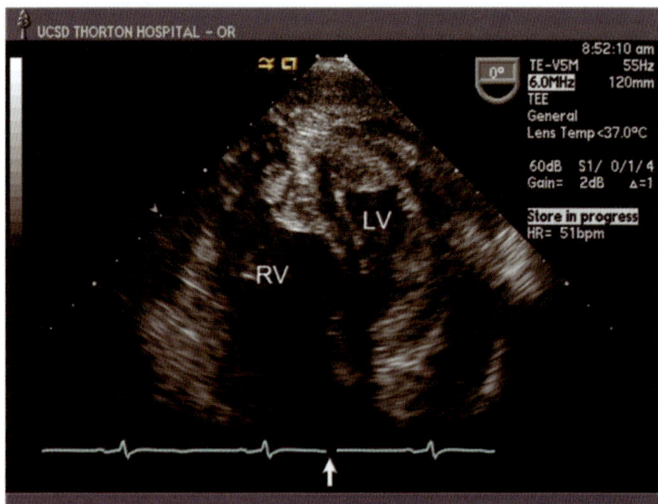

Fig. 7.3 Transgastric mid-papillary short-axis view demonstrating right ventricular pressure overload. Note the interventricular septal flattening yielding a D-shaped left ventricle in systole. *Arrow* points to the associated electrocardiogram denoting end-systole. *LV,* Left ventricle; *RV,* right ventricle.

as a diagnostic step is identifying patients who are responders to vasodilator therapy because these patients are more likely to benefit from treatments with medications such as oral calcium channel blockers. Inhaled NO is most commonly used in acute vasodilator testing, but intravenous (IV) epoprostenol and IV adenosine are acceptable alternatives. A positive result of vasodilator testing is defined as a decrease in mPAP of at least 10 mm Hg to an absolute mPAP of less than 40 mm Hg without decreasing the CO.

TREATMENT OPTIONS FOR PULMONARY HYPERTENSION

Patients with PH may present for surgery on a wide variety of pulmonary vasodilators or other medications (Table 7.3). Improper perioperative management can have profound and perhaps lethal consequences, so familiarity with these medications and their management is imperative. Treatments in patients with PAH are geared toward improving symptoms and quality of life. Another important objective is to lower PAP and normalize CO as early in the disease process as possible before RVF ensues.

Diuretics are indicated in patients with RVF as evidenced by elevated jugular venous pressure, lower extremity edema, and ascites. It is not unusual for these patients to require oxygen to maintain saturation above 90% to prevent further hypoxia-induced vasoconstriction.

Patients whose vasodilator test result was positive may be treated with calcium channel blockers such as nifedipine. Alternative or additional therapy should be instituted if patients do not improve to functional class I or II on their current treatment.

The prostacyclin pathway agonists are an important class of vasodilators used for the treatment of PH. In addition to direct vasodilatory effects, they inhibit platelet aggregation via adenylate cyclase activation and resultant increases in cyclic adenosine monophosphate (cAMP) within platelets. Prostacyclin therapy also contains valuable antiinflammatory properties that are directed at the various pathologic mechanisms considered responsible for PAH. Continuous epoprostenol (prostaglandin I_2 [PGI_2]) infusion therapy (Flolan) was found to improve hemodynamics and exercise tolerance and to prolong survival. Several open-label randomized trials demonstrated significant improvements of the primary endpoint, a 6MW test. IV epoprostenol is titrated based on relief of symptoms or side effects, but most experts would not exceed a dose between 25 and 40 ng/kg per minute for most adult patients when used as monotherapy. Common side effects include headache, jaw pain, flushing, nausea, diarrhea, skin rash, and musculoskeletal pain. Infusion interruptions can lead to rebound PH, severe systemic hypotension, and cardiovascular collapse, so it is critically important that these infusions be continued throughout the perioperative period. Epoprostenol use should be limited to centers experienced with its administration and with systematic follow-up of patients.

Because epoprostenol therapy requires continuous IV administration to be efficacious, alternate forms have been created: oral (beraprost), subcutaneous (treprostinil), and inhaled (iloprost). Treprostinil, a stable prostanoid with an elimination half-life of about 4.5 hours, has been shown to produce modest improvements in a 6MW test and is approved for use in patients with functional class II, III, and IV. Iloprost is another prostanoid that is delivered by the inhalation method. Iloprost has shown improvements in function in patients with functional class III and IV with IPAH or PAH caused by connective tissue disease or inoperable patients with CTEPH disease. Common side effects include cough, headache, flushing, and jaw pain. Iloprost is approved for functional class III and IV PAH.

Table 7.3   Pharmaceutical Agents Utilized to Lower Pulmonary Arterial Pressures

Drug: Generic Name (Brand Name)	Mechanism of Action	Route of Administration	Typical Dose	Notes
Calcium Channel Blockers				
Nifedipine (Adalat, Procardia)	Calcium channel blocker	PO	30–240 mg	Used as outpatient therapy when vasoactivity responsiveness is demonstrated
Prostacyclin Pathway Agonists				
Epoprostenol (Flolan, Veletri)	Prostacyclin analogue (PGI_2)	Continuous IV	2–25 ng/kg/min	Inhibits platelet aggregation Abrupt cessation may lead to rebound pulmonary hypertension
Beraprost	Prostacyclin analogue	PO	60–180 µg/day	
Treprostinil (Tyvaso, Remodulin, Orenitram)	Prostacyclin analogue	SC	1.25 ng/kg/min; increase by 1.25–2.5 ng/kg/ min per week	May also be delivered by inhalation
Iloprost (Ventavis)	Prostacyclin analogue	Intermittently Inhaled	2.5–5 µg/dose 6 to 9 times/day	Hemodynamic effect lasts ~90 min
Thromboxane Inhibition				
Terbogrel	Thromboxane A_2 receptor antagonist	PO		Remains investigatory
Endothelin Receptor Antagonists				
Bosentan (Tracleer)	Endothelin-1 receptor antagonist	PO	62.5–125 mg BID	Potentially hepatotoxic; requires LFTs
Sitaxsentan (Thelin)	Endothelin receptor antagonist	PO		Removed from market because of hepatotoxicity
Ambrisentan (Letairis)	Type A endothelin receptor antagonist	PO	5–10 mg every day	Not indicated in existing hepatic impairment; requires LFTs

Cyclic GMP mediators				
Nitric oxide (INOmax)	cGMP-mediated smooth muscle relaxation	Continuous Inhaled	10–40 ppm	Can be delivered by face mask, nasal cannula, or endotracheal tube Uses commercially available delivery system to monitor NO and NO_2 Abrupt cessation may lead to rebound pulmonary hypertension
Sildenafil (Revatio)	PDE-5 inhibitor	PO	5–20 mg TID	May also be provided IV
Tadalafil (Adcirca)	PDE-5 inhibitor	PO	40 every day	
Riociguat (Adempas)	Stimulates soluble guanylate cyclase yielding increased cGMP	PO	1–2.5 mg PO TID	Indicated for persistent or recurrent CTEPH after surgery or inoperable CTEPH
Inodilators				
Dobutamine (Dobutrex)	β-Adrenergic stimulation	IV infusion	5–20 µg/kg/min	Be cautious with systemic vasodilation; consider coadministering vasopressor
Milrinone (Primacor)	PDE-3 inhibitor	IV Infusion	0.25–0.75 µg/kg/min	Be cautious with systemic vasodilation; consider coadministering vasopressor

BID, Twice a day; *cGMP,* cyclic guanosine monophosphate; *CTEPH,* chronic thromboembolic pulmonary hypertension; *IV,* intravenous; *LFT,* liver function text; *NO,* nitric oxide; NO_2, nitrogen dioxide; *PDE,* phosphodiesterase; *PGI₂,* prostaglandin I₂; *PO,* oral; *SC,* subcutaneous; *TID,* three times a day.

151

Newer agents targeting thromboxane inhibition (terbogrel) and endothelin-receptor antagonism (bosentan, sitaxsentan, and ambrisentan) have also been developed. Bosentan, a promising endothelin (ET) receptor antagonist, works by blocking ET-1 vasoconstriction effect on the pulmonary circulation. Patients with PAH have been found to have high levels of circulating ET-1, which correlate with the severity and prognosis of IPAH. Bosentan has been found to increase functional status and CI while decreasing PVR. The Food and Drug Administration requires that liver function tests be checked monthly and hematocrit every 3 months to ensure safety in these patients.

Phosphodiesterase (PDE) inhibitors also play an important role in the treatment of PH. NO exerts its vasodilatory effect by its ability to augment and sustain cyclic guanosine monophosphate (cGMP) content in vascular smooth muscle, and the brief vasodilatory effect of cGMP is due to its rapid breakdown by PDEs. Thus decreased endothelial NO levels and increased PDE-5 expression and activity in lung tissue and RV myocardium contribute to PAH. PDE-5 inhibitors, such as sildenafil and tadalafil, act by blocking the PDE enzymes that inactivate the second messenger (cGMP) for the vasodilating signals in lung tissues (see Table 7.3). Sildenafil monotherapy has been found to significantly improve mPAP, exercise capacity, and WHO functional class.

Tadalafil, a longer-acting PDE inhibitor, is well tolerated and associated with improved quality of life and time to clinical deterioration. Sildenafil and tadalafil are both indicated for use in patients with mild to moderately severe symptoms (WHO class II or III), but for patients with severe (class IV) symptoms, IV epoprostenol or treprostinil is preferred.

Combination therapy is an attractive option considering the availability of medications with different mechanisms of action. The goal of combination therapy should be to maximize efficacy while reducing side effects.

Despite all the advances in the medical treatment for PAH, invasive therapies are still a valid option for patients who are refractory to medical treatments, with worsening right heart failure leading to poor quality of life. It is in these patients that interventional and surgical therapeutic options should be considered, including atrial septostomy and lung or combined heart and lung transplantation. For CTEPH patients, pulmonary thromboendarterectomy is the treatment of choice. With the latest advances in cardiac surgery, ventricular assist devices have proven effective and may be another viable option for patients with severe refractory right heart failure (Fig. 7.4).

Primary PH is associated with a prothrombotic state, with increased levels of tissue plasminogen activator inhibitor-1, and decreased tissue factor pathway inhibitor. Consequently, anticoagulation is recommended, and prospective and retrospective studies have proven increased survival with warfarin therapy in PAH patients.

The medical management of patients with PH is complex and evolving. As detailed earlier, medications may include oxygen, diuretics, several classes of vasodilators, and anticoagulants in addition to any medications for the management of comorbid conditions. Diuretic management should be targeted toward maintaining a euvolemic state because the RV may only tolerate a narrow range of loading conditions. Typically, patients are maintained on their preoperative vasodilators throughout the perioperative period as abrupt cessation of medications can lead to rebound PH with associated circulatory collapse. For this reason, hypotensive episodes in patients with continuous infusions should be treated with vasopressors and inotropes rather than reductions in their vasodilator dose. Anticoagulants are typically held preoperatively to minimize intraoperative bleeding risk.

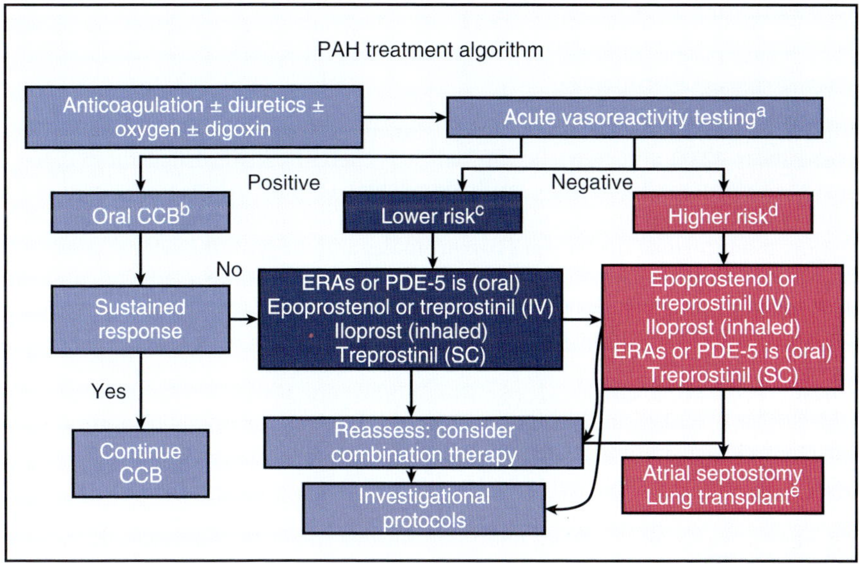

Fig. 7.4 Treatment algorithm for pulmonary arterial hypertension (PAH). Background therapies include warfarin anticoagulation, which is recommended in all patients with idiotapthic pulmonary arterial hypertension (IPAH) without contraindication. Diuretics are used for management of right heart failure. Oxygen is recommended to maintain oxygen saturation greater than 90%. [a]Acute vasodilator testing should be performed in all IPAH patients who may be potential candidates for long-term therapy with calcium channel blockers (CCBs). [b]Patients with PAH caused by conditions other than IPAH have a very low rate of long-term responsiveness to oral CCBs, and the value of acute vasodilator testing in such patients needs to be individualized. Patients with IPAH in whom CCB therapy would not be considered, such as those with right heart failure or hemodynamic instability, should not undergo acute vasodilator testing. CCBs are indicated only for patients who have a positive acute vasodilator response, and such patients need to be followed closely both for safety and efficacy. [c]For patients who did not have a positive acute vasodilator testing and are considered lower risk based on clinical assessment, oral therapy with an endothelin receptor antagonist or a phosphodiesterase (PDE5) inhibitor would be the first line of therapy recommended. If an oral regimen is not appropriate, the other treatments would need to be considered based on the patient's profile and side effects and risk of each therapy. [d]For patients who are considered high risk based on clinical assessment, continuous treatment with intravenous (IV) prostacyclin (epoprostenol or treprostinil) would be the first line of therapy recommended. If a patient is not a candidate for continuous IV treatment, the other therapies would have to be considered based on patient's profile and side effects and risk of each treatment. Epoprostenol improves exercise capacity, hemodynamics, and survival in IPAH and is the preferred treatment option for the most critically ill patients. Although expensive and difficult to administer, epoprostenol is the only therapy for PAH that has been shown to prolong survival. Treprostinil may be delivered via either continuous IV or subcutaneous (SC) infusion. Iloprost is a prostacyclin analogue delivered by an adaptive aerosolized device six times daily. The endothelin receptor antagonists are oral therapies that improve exercise capacity in PAH. Liver function tests must be monitored indefinitely on a monthly basis. PDE inhibitors also improve exercise capacity. Combination therapy should be considered when patients are not responding adequately to initial monotherapy. [e]Timing for lung transplantation and/or atrial septostomy is challenging and is reserved for patients who progress despite optimal medical treatment. (From McLaughlin VV, Archer SL, Badesch DB, et al. ACCF/AHA 2009 expert consensus document on pulmonary hypertension: a report of the American College of Cardiology Foundation Task Force on Expert Consensus Documents. *J Am Coll Cardiol.* 2009;53:1573.)

ANESTHETIC MANAGEMENT

Preoperative Evaluation

Patients with PH undergoing noncardiac surgery have significantly increased risk of morbidity (~42%) and mortality (~7%). It is therefore critical that these patients have had thorough preoperative evaluation, which should include assessment of the patient's functional status and severity of disease as detailed earlier. Other important considerations include the patient's comorbidities and the type of surgery. Collectively, this will dictate exactly what testing is necessary, but typical initial preoperative studies often include complete blood count (CBC), complete metabolic panel, coagulation studies, ECG, echocardiography, chest radiography, and RHC. Blood gases and pulmonary function tests may also be helpful in patients with lung disease. These tests are useful for ensuring preoperative optimization.

A CBC can be helpful in identifying multiple areas for potential optimization. Leukocytosis may point to a latent infectious process. These are important to identify because the low SVR and high CO of a sepsis state are very poorly tolerated in these patients. Furthermore, patients on chronic vasodilator or inotropic infusions may be at increased risk for bloodstream infections. Anemia reduces oxygen-carrying capacity and delivery to an already overworked right ventricle, with significantly increased oxygen demand. Thrombocytopenia secondary to hepatic congestion may lead to increased surgical blood loss; the hypovolemia associated with the blood loss may be poorly tolerated because the right ventricle depends on adequate preload to overcome the high PVR.

The complete metabolic panel can identify electrolyte abnormalities, which may predispose to arrhythmias that can cause severe instability in patients with PH, and a metabolic acidosis increases PVR and may indicate inadequate tissue perfusion. Chronic kidney disease (CKD) is a predictor of increased perioperative morbidity and mortality. The results of liver function tests and coagulation studies may be abnormal in patients with right heart failure and resultant congestive hepatopathy, and these patients may be at increased risk for bleeding.

The echocardiographic evaluation of patients with PH is essential and has already been described in detail, but concerning findings include increased RA size, severe TR, a severely dilated right ventricle, RVH, reduced TAPSE or other indicators of RV performance, paradoxical motion of the IVS consistent with volume or pressure overload, and presence of a pericardial effusion. An ECG should also be performed to assess for right-axis deviation, baseline rhythm or conduction disturbances, or evidence of coexisting coronary artery disease.

Preoperative RHC is indicated for quantification of PH severity, assessment of RV function, and determination of responsiveness to vasodilators. Collectively, this information is valuable for risk stratification and intraoperative management. Findings of RHC that indicate significant RV dysfunction and high risk of perioperative morbidity and mortality include RA pressure greater than 12 mm Hg, RVEDP greater than 15 mm Hg, mPAP greater than 55 mm Hg, PVR greater than 1000 dynes $\cdot$ s $\cdot$ cm^{-5}, CI less than 2 L/min per m^2, and a lack of a vasodilator response.

In patients with coexisting lung disease or left-sided congestive heart failure, arterial blood gas testing may be helpful to screen for signs of hypoxia or baseline respiratory acidosis. Chest radiography and pulmonary function tests can also be helpful in identifying and optimizing coexisting lung pathology.

Other predictors of morbidity and mortality among patients with PH include a history of PE, CKD, poor functional status, intermediate or high-risk surgical procedure, emergency surgery, RV systolic pressure greater than 66% of systemic systolic pressure, and the use of intraoperative vasopressors. Given the complexity of the condition and its management, it may be helpful to have the assistance of pulmonologists and cardiologists to ensure that the patient is medically optimized before any elective procedure. Cancellation or postponement should be considered in any patient presenting with an exacerbation of heart failure symptoms, severe hypoxia, or metabolic acidosis.

Choice of Anesthetic Technique

The most appropriate anesthetic technique will largely be dictated by the surgical procedure. However, given the known morbidity and mortality associated with general anesthesia in patients with PH, it is reasonable to favor regional or neuraxial anesthesia when possible. These approaches may potentially avoid the deleterious effects of positive-pressure ventilation on PVR and RV function as well as the possibility of difficult postoperative weaning from the ventilator. Furthermore, regional or neuraxial techniques can block pain-induced increases in PVR both during the procedure and postoperatively while minimizing the use of opioids. Therefore catheter techniques that can provide days of analgesia may be preferable, especially if significant postoperative pain is anticipated.

If a neuraxial anesthetic is chosen, the anesthesiologist must proceed with caution because the associated sympathectomy may be poorly tolerated in patients with PH. Although a single-shot subarachnoid injection can result in sudden-onset severe hypotension, an epidural catheter allows gradual titration of medication to effect, which may help avoid dramatic decreases in SVR. Placement of an epidural catheter is therefore recommended over the use of a single-shot subarachnoid block.

Although regional anesthetic techniques may allow for avoidance of endotracheal intubation and positive-pressure ventilation, the accompanying sedation that is frequently administered in the operating room (OR) can be problematic for patients with PH. Great care must be taken to avoid respiratory depression or airway compromise in this population. This generally means that patients who are prone to airway obstruction, who are unable to lie flat, or who may require more than very light sedation may not be good candidates for total regional techniques.

Intraoperative Monitoring

Special consideration should be given to the monitoring strategy for these patients. In addition to standard American Society of Anesthesiologists monitors, these patients usually require invasive monitoring to facilitate optimal control of their hemodynamics.

Insertion of an arterial catheter before induction of anesthesia is standard for patients with moderate to severe PH because it allows for real-time monitoring of blood pressure during one of the riskiest stages of the anesthetic. Furthermore, waveform analysis or pulse pressure variation can be assessed for clues regarding the patient's current CO and volume responsiveness. Finally, arterial access facilitates frequent arterial blood gases, which are helpful to ensure that hypoxia and hypercapnia are avoided.

Placement of a central venous catheter is useful for prompt delivery and titration of vasoactive medications. Furthermore, monitoring of central venous pressure (CVP) can provide helpful information regarding right heart loading conditions and optimal fluid management, although the value of CVP as a monitor of volume responsiveness has been questioned. Trending of central venous blood gases can also provide insight into the adequacy of the CO.

The insertion of pulmonary arterial (PA) catheters has come under question because several studies have failed to show benefit, and others have shown an increased risk of adverse events. However, the real-time monitoring of PA pressures and their responses to various interventions may be helpful. Furthermore, the use of the thermodilution technique allows for easy, rapid assessment of CO, and the mixed venous oxygen saturation can provide information about the adequacy of end-organ perfusion. Therefore PA catheter placement is generally recommended for patients with PH that is severe or in patients who are undergoing moderate- to high-risk surgical procedures.

Intraoperative transesophageal echocardiography (TEE) can be useful for continuous, real-time monitoring of RV function, tricuspid regurgitation, and volume status. Furthermore, TEE can be used to estimate and follow PA pressures and CO. Although no current guidelines exist for the use of TEE in the intraoperative management of patients with PH, in experienced hands, this can be a valuable tool for rapidly diagnosing causes of hemodynamic instability and assessing responsiveness to therapeutic interventions.

Hemodynamic Goals

A thorough understanding of the pathophysiology of PH and RVF as already detailed informs the hemodynamic management strategy for the perioperative period. Because the right ventricles of patients with PH may have marginal cardiac reserve, the central aim is to protect the right ventricle by minimizing myocardial oxygen demand and maximizing oxygen supply while maintaining adequate CO. This is a complex interaction that is guided by several interrelated factors. One approach is to individually consider the following determinants of myocardial performance: preload, afterload, contractility, heart rate, and rhythm.

The preload or wall stress at end-diastole that the right ventricle encounters is one of the major determinants of its stroke volume and CO. Although not strictly accurate, in clinical contexts, the term *preload* is often used to indicate end-diastolic volume. In patients with PH, the right ventricle may only adequately function within a narrow range of preload conditions (i.e., euvolemia). On the one hand, if the preload is too low because of hypovolemia or decreased venous return (e.g., with initiation of positive-pressure ventilation), the right ventricle will not be able to generate sufficient pressures to overcome the high afterload of the pulmonary vasculature. On the other hand, the right ventricle may already be maximally dilated and unable to compensate for further increases in preload, leading to decreased pump efficiency, increased wall stress, increased myocardial oxygen demand, decreased coronary perfusion, ischemia, and decreased CO.

This balance can be especially difficult to maintain given the absence of a great clinical monitor for preload assessment. The CVP is often used as a surrogate for assessing or at least trending RV loading conditions, but its failure to accurately predict volume status or volume responsiveness is well established. Although there are devices designed to assess volume responsiveness based on pulse contour analysis, these have not yet been validated in patients with PH. TEE can easily show RV volume and provide some information regarding RV compliance, but it is important to note that these patients often have extensive ventricular remodeling that may result in dramatic dilation of the right ventricle even in the compensated state. Thus a single snapshot is probably inadequate. It is therefore important to continually assess the relationship between volume status and CO in an ongoing process of integration of all available information.

Another important contributor to stroke volume and CO is afterload, which is defined as the wall stress of the ventricle during ejection. This is particularly important in patients with PH. Although the development of hypertrophy allows the RV to overcome a much higher afterload than would otherwise be tolerated, these patients

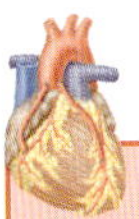

> **BOX 7.4** **_Factors to Avoid During Anesthesia for Patients With Pulmonary Hypertension_**
>
> - Hypoxia
> - Hypercarbia
> - Metabolic acidosis
> - Pain and light anesthesia
> - Nitrous oxide
> - Systemic vasodilation
> - Excessive volume administration
> - Hypovolemia
> - Excessively high tidal volumes
> - Excessively low tidal volumes

may be at the limit of their ability to compensate. Any further increases in RV afterload may not be tolerated, leading to a cycle of decreased RV output, decreased LV output, decreased coronary perfusion, RV ischemia, and a further decline in RV output.

The PVR is the primary determinant of RV afterload in patients without pulmonic valve stenosis or RV outflow tract obstruction. Several factors may increase PVR in the perioperative period, including pain, hypothermia, hypoxia, hypercapnia, metabolic acidosis, vasopressors, nitrous oxide, and mechanical ventilation with excessively high or low tidal volumes. It is therefore important to keep these in mind throughout the perioperative management of patients with PH (Box 7.4).

Although premedication may be necessary in extremely anxious patients, anxiolytics should be administered judiciously because of the potential for oversedation, respiratory depression, and resultant hypoxic or hypercapnic increases in PVR. Ideally, the patient should be given supplemental oxygen and monitored closely before any sedatives are administered. After thorough preoxygenation, the induction of anesthesia should be conducted in such a manner that the provider can quickly take over ventilation for the patient to minimize periods of apnea, and the sympathetic response to laryngoscopy and surgical stimulation must be blunted to avoid associated rises in PVR. Administering a higher inspired oxygen concentration on the ventilator can provide a margin of safety against hypoxia. Later, a robust respiratory drive should be confirmed before removal of the breathing tube, so excessive opioid use should be avoided if extubation is planned for the end of the procedure. Depending on the severity of disease and the type of surgery, it may be appropriate to leave the endotracheal tube in place so that careful weaning from the ventilator may be accomplished in the intensive care unit (ICU). Additionally, adequate postoperative analgesia will help avoid pain-associated rises in PVR. The use of multimodal analgesics and nerve block techniques may be helpful to this end.

There are many ways in which mechanical ventilation may lead to increases in afterload for the RV. Clearly, hypoventilation should be avoided, so the respiratory rate should be set to maintain a low to normal $PaCO_2$ (arterial partial pressure of carbon dioxide) while avoiding air-trapping and associated overdistention of the lungs. Hyperexpansion of the lungs stretches the alveolar vessels, increasing their resistance, while lower volumes and atelectasis increase resistance within the extraalveolar vessels through decreased radial traction. Because total PVR is dependent on both alveolar and extra-alveolar vessels, the PVR tends to be lowest at functional residual capacity. Excessive positive end-expiratory pressure (PEEP) can also increase PVR by direct compression of the pulmonary vasculature. Therefore it is recommended that patients with PH be ventilated with low to moderate tidal volumes and low levels of PEEP to avoid atelectasis. Recruitment maneuvers are helpful for treating atelectasis and improving ventilation-perfusion matching.

The use of IV and inhaled vasodilators is a key component of the management of patients with PVR and RV afterload in the perioperative period. A review of pulmonary vasodilators used in the outpatient treatment of patients with PH has already been provided, but in general, patients should be continued on their baseline regimens. The use of vasodilators during the perioperative period is detailed later in this chapter.

One important distinction is that in patients with PH caused by elevated pulmonary venous pressures (i.e., secondary to left heart failure), afterload reduction for the left ventricle using systemic vasodilators may result in reduced PA pressures and improved RV function. This must be balanced against the need to maintain an adequate coronary perfusion pressure.

Contractility is the next main determinant of CO, and it is defined as the intrinsic ability of the myocardium to shorten or squeeze. This is commonly thought of in terms of the stroke volume generated for a given preload and afterload. Several factors can negatively impact the contractility of the right ventricle in PH patients undergoing noncardiac surgical procedures.

Anesthetic agents can impair RV contractility either through their direct negative inotropic properties or by decreasing coronary perfusion through their reductions in SVR. As detailed earlier, the elevated RV pressures often seen in patients with PH are both an impediment to coronary perfusion and a cause of increased myocardial oxygen demand. Therefore it is imperative that systemic blood pressure be maintained to ensure an adequate coronary perfusion gradient is preserved. This should be accomplished first with the administration of vasopressors while potential sources of hypotension are investigated and treated. In addition to anesthetic side effects, these may include hypovolemia, sepsis, or a failing right ventricle.

Another important principle to understand when thinking about RV contractility is that of ventricular interdependence. It has been reported that the shared ventricular septum contributes up to 40% of the RV stroke volume, but in patients with a dilated, failing right ventricle, the septum is displaced toward the left ventricle, which results in impaired RV contractility as well as LV systolic and diastolic dysfunction. This explains why a right ventricle at the limit of compensation can rapidly progress into a spiral of reduced RV contractility, reduced LV function, systemic hypotension, and RV ischemia with further declines in contractility. The use of vasopressors can help interrupt this process by increasing coronary perfusion and increasing LV systolic pressure, which may help push the septum back toward the RV. Inotropes are also important in the treatment and prevention of RV failure by augmenting RV stroke volume, reducing RV dilation and ventricular septal deviation, and augmenting coronary perfusion. The use of vasopressors and inotropes in the perioperative period will be discussed below.

Heart rate can have dramatic effects on CO, myocardial oxygen consumption, and coronary perfusion. An understanding of these relationships is important to the proper intraoperative management of patients with PH. Because CO is equal to stroke volume multiplied by heart rate, it is clear that large increases or decreases in heart rate can have profound impacts on overall CO. Furthermore, bradycardia can lead to overdistention of the RV, increased wall tension, increased oxygen consumption, and reduced myocardial efficiency. However, this must be balanced against the fact that at excessively high heart rates, diastolic filling time is reduced, leading to inadequate stroke volume and CO. As the RV pressures rise, the right ventricle, which is normally perfused throughout the cardiac cycle, may only receive blood flow during diastole. In this case, tachycardia not only increases myocardial oxygen demand but also reduces coronary perfusion by reducing the time spent in diastole. Given the compromised myocardial perfusion and CO that occur at excessively high and low heart rates, it is recommended that these patients' heart rates be kept between 60 and 90 beats/min.

One other determinant of myocardial performance that needs to be considered is the rhythm. Although sinus rhythm is almost always hemodynamically preferable, it is especially important in patients with PH and borderline RV function. The atrioventricular synchrony afforded by sinus rhythm is critical to optimizing RV diastolic filling, and without it, some patients may experience rapid hemodynamic deterioration. Furthermore, because many patients with PH have dilated atria, they may be at increased risk for developing atrial arrhythmias such as atrial fibrillation. During the perioperative management of these patients, the anesthesiologist should be prepared to rapidly administer synchronized cardioversion to restore sinus rhythm in the event that such an arrhythmia is poorly tolerated. Pharmacologic rate or rhythm control (or both) may be attempted first depending on the stability of the patient, but care should be taken to avoid agents with negative inotropic effects.

Intraoperative Pharmacologic Management

The main classes of pharmacologic agents available to the anesthesiologist for the intraoperative hemodynamic management of patients with PH include vasodilators, inodilators, inotropes, and vasopressors (see Table 7.3).

Vasodilating medications are administered to the patients with PH with the goal of reducing PVR and thus RV afterload. However, most of these medications can also result in systemic hypotension and reduced coronary artery perfusion, so they should be used with caution. As reviewed in detail earlier, several classes of pulmonary vasodilators are used in the outpatient treatment of patients with PH. In general, these medications should be continued through the day of surgery.

In the OR, the use of inhaled pulmonary vasodilators such as NO has proven to be useful for both reduction of PVR and improvement in ventilation/perfusion (V/Q) matching. These medications are rapidly metabolized, so they tend to have minimal systemic vasodilatory effects while producing significant reductions in PA pressure. Because they are delivered via inhalation, they result in selective vasodilation of the PA vasculature in regions of the lungs that are well ventilated, thus improving V/Q matching. This results in more efficient gas exchange within the lungs, with the potential for significantly enhanced oxygenation and ventilation.

Inhaled NO rapidly diffuses from alveoli to the pulmonary vascular smooth muscle, where it mediates its vasodilatory properties by stimulating production of cGMP, which results in decreased intracellular calcium and reductions in smooth muscle tone. When NO reaches the bloodstream, it is metabolized within seconds, and its duration of effect is only a few minutes. This facilitates relatively selective vasodilation within the pulmonary vasculature without associated systemic hypotension. The typical dose used is 20 parts per million (ppm); higher doses run the risk of inducing methemoglobinemia or pulmonary injury from the toxic metabolite nitrogen dioxide. Doses greater than 40 ppm offer minimal additional clinical benefit. Other potential downsides of this medication include significant cost, potential inhibition of platelet aggregation, and the significant rebound PH that can occur with abrupt discontinuation. Therefore inhaled NO started in the OR should be continued postoperatively and weaned according to protocol (Box 7.5).

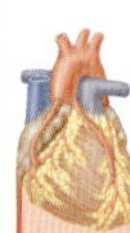

> **BOX 7.5**   *Setting Up Inhaled Nitric Oxide in the Operating Room*
>
> - Bring the iNO delivery device to the OR (contact responsible department, respiratory technician, pharmacy to deliver).
> - Install the iNO delivery adaptor inline to the inspiratory limb of the ventilator circle.
> - Ensure the iNO delivery line is attached to adaptor.
> - Place the sampling line adaptor proximally (closer to the patient).
> - Resume and ensure adequate ventilation and flows.
> - Open the NO cylinder on the iNO delivery device to allow NO flow to the adaptor.
> - Set the delivery device to the desired parts per million (ppm).
> - Observe the monitor for appropriate NO and NO_2 levels.
>
> *iNO,* Inhaled nitric oxide; *NO,* nitric; *NO_2,* nitrogen dioxide; *OR,* operating room.

The prostacyclin epoprostenol can also be delivered via inhalation. The prostacyclins have been reviewed in detail earlier in this chapter, but it is worth noting that the inhaled formulation is thought to be associated with less systemic hypotension. However, concerns about impaired platelet aggregation remain. Inhaled epoprostenol is delivered via jet nebulizer attached to the inspiratory limb of the breathing circuit. A concentration of 20,000 ng/mL nebulized with oxygen flows of 2 to 3 L/min delivers about 8 mL/h or 38 ng/kg per minute for a 70-kg patient. Doses above 50 ng/kg per minute do not provide additional clinical benefit, may contribute to systemic hypotension, and are not recommended. Similar to inhaled NO, abrupt discontinuation of this medication can cause life-threatening rebound increases in PVR. Therefore it is typically weaned in the postoperative period by reducing the concentration by 50% every 2 to 4 hours as tolerated.

The inodilators compose another class of medications that can be very useful in the perioperative treatment of patients with PH who are not able to generate an adequate CO in the face of excessive PVR. These medications, named for their inotropic and vasodilatory properties, are able to augment CO by increasing contractility and reducing afterload. Although reductions in PVR are clearly desirable, simultaneous dilation of the systemic vasculature can cause hypotension with impaired coronary perfusion.

Dobutamine is an inodilator with primarily β_1-adrenergic receptor activation, somewhat less β_2 activity, and minimal α_1 stimulation. β_1 stimulation results in cAMP-mediated positive inotropic and chronotropic effects. Whereas doses up to 5 µg/kg per minute primarily result in increased myocardial contractility, doses greater than 10 µg/kg per minute may result in tachycardia with increased myocardial oxygen demand. Because the vasodilatory β_2 effects overcome the minimal α_1 activity, this medication is associated with reductions in SVR and PVR, making it well suited for supporting the RV of patients with PH as long as systemic hypotension is avoided.

Milrinone, another inodilator, works by inhibiting PDE-3 with resultant increases in cAMP. This leads to increased myocardial contractility and decreased PVR and SVR via reductions in vascular smooth muscle tone. Doses range between 0.1 and 0.75 µg/kg per minute and should be titrated as necessary. Although milrinone results in less tachycardia than high-dose dobutamine, significant hypotension may occur. Avoidance of a loading dose and starting with lower doses may reduce this risk. Hypotension may be long-lasting in patients with impaired renal function; in these patients, milrinone should be given at reduced doses or avoided altogether. Because milrinone and dobutamine increase cAMP by separate mechanisms, their concurrent use may be synergistic, and for both medications, it may be necessary to administer them with a vasopressor to maintain systemic blood pressure and coronary perfusion.

The calcium sensitizer levosimendan is an additional medication with positive inotropic and vasodilatory properties. Whereas the inotropic effects are mediated through an enhanced myocardial contractile response to calcium, the vasodilation is enacted by opening potassium channels in the vascular smooth muscle. Although in theory this should result in improved CO without increasing myocardial oxygen consumption, studies have failed to show significant mortality benefit over dobutamine in patients with acute heart failure requiring inotropic support. This medication remains investigational in the United States, but it has been approved for use in Europe and South America.

Although the combined vasodilatory and inotropic effects of medications such as dobutamine make them a great choice for supporting the failing right ventricle in many patients with PH, it should be noted that the subset of patients with CTEPH are an exception. These patients do not typically respond well to vasodilators as the lesions responsible for their elevated PVR are relatively fixed. Because the goals of pharmacologic ventricular support are more focused on increasing contractility and maintaining coronary perfusion, the use of inotropes such as dopamine or epinephrine is preferable in this patient population.

Dopamine is an inotropic medication with dopaminergic and adrenergic receptor activity with different hemodynamic effects occurring within different ranges of doses. Doses less than 5 µg/kg per minute are thought to primarily cause dopamine receptor stimulation with associated increases in renal and mesenteric blood flow. However, low-dose dopamine has not been shown to help prevent or treat acute kidney injury. Between 5 and 10 µg/kg per minute, dopamine and β_1 activity results in increased heart rate, myocardial contractility, and CO. At these doses, dopamine has been shown to increase CO without increasing PVR; however, at doses greater than 10 µg/kg per minute, α_1 effects begin to predominate, with increased vasoconstriction and resultant elevations in systemic and pulmonary blood pressures. It should be noted that there is significant overlap between ranges, and there may be great variability in hemodynamic responses between patients.

Epinephrine is another medication with inotropic and vasoconstricting properties. It works by stimulating α-, β_1-, and β_2-adrenergic receptors to produce increases in heart rate, myocardial contractility, and vascular smooth muscle tone. Although at low doses β_2 receptor activation may produce vasodilation within certain vascular beds, α_1 activity typically results in increases in both SVR and PVR to a similar degree. In the event of a rapidly deteriorating RV, boluses of dilute epinephrine may be required to restore RV function and avoid cardiac arrest.

One final class of medications that is indispensable to the intraoperative management of patients with PH is the vasopressors. As discussed in detail earlier, it is important to avoid increases in PVR that may further stress a right ventricle that is already on the brink of failure, but it is also critical to maintain coronary perfusion by avoiding precipitous drops in systemic blood pressure. Given that most IV or volatile anesthetics will decrease SVR to some degree, the judicious administration of vasopressors may be necessary to counter this effect. Although phenylephrine, an α_1 agonist, is commonly used for this purpose, it results in equal increases in both SVR and PVR. Norepinephrine, a mixed α_1/β_1 agonist, also increases SVR, but it may increase PVR to a lesser degree than phenylephrine. There is evidence that vasopressin results in selective increases in SVR without affecting PVR and may potentially cause modest pulmonary vasodilation. Vasopressin infusions of 0.01 to 0.04 U/min may therefore be the best choice for the treatment of reduced SVR in patients with PH.

Postoperative Considerations

Because of the multitude of risks that patients with PH face in the postoperative period, they remain at increased risk for morbidity and mortality for several days. It is therefore important to have a well-developed plan for the postoperative management of these patients. Such a plan should address monitoring, pain control, ventilator weaning, and management of volume status and hemodynamics. The hemodynamic goals of the intraoperative period still remain a priority, and care should be taken to avoid hypothermia, hypoxia, hypercarbia, acidosis, pain, and volume overload.

Given the relatively narrow range of physiologic conditions tolerated by some patients with PH, it is important that they are monitored appropriately throughout their postoperative course. The degree of postoperative monitoring needed dictates where the patient is cared for immediately after any procedure. Some patients may require admission to the ICU, and others may recover in the postanesthesia care unit. This will depend on the severity of disease, invasiveness of the surgery, type of anesthesia administered, stability of the patient, and the need for ongoing ventilator or vasoactive medication management.

Pain control can be challenging in these patients, so a plan for pain management should be carefully developed preoperatively. Although opioids are central to many postoperative pain management regimens, the associated sedative and respiratory depressant effects can lead to hypoxia or hypercarbia, with increased PVR that may be poorly tolerated in patients with PH. Therefore attempts should be made to minimize opioid administration through the use of multimodal and regional analgesic strategies when appropriate. This may include perioperative use of acetaminophen, gabapentin, ketorolac, and regional or neuraxial nerve blocks (single injection or continuous infusion via catheter).

Although excessive sedation and respiratory depression must be avoided, it is equally important to adequately control pain because pain-induced catecholamine surges may lead to increased PVR and tachycardia, which stress the RV. It may be advisable to consult with an acute pain management service preoperatively if postoperative pain control is predicted to be difficult with minimal opioid use. Such cases include very painful procedures, patients with opioid tolerance, and those for whom regional or neuraxial analgesic techniques are not appropriate. In some cases, it may be necessary for the patient to remain mechanically ventilated until the surgical pain subsides enough to allow for reduced narcotic administration.

Although many patients can be successfully extubated at the end of the surgery, the clinician should have a lower threshold for continuing mechanical ventilation into the postoperative period in patients with PH. Before removal of the endotracheal tube, the patient must be alert with an intact respiratory drive, neuromuscular blockade fully reversed, surgical pain adequately controlled, and the risk of postoperative respiratory compromise should be minimal. In patients with sleep apnea or who have undergone long procedures, the risk of oversedation or airway compromise leading to hypoxia or hypercarbia may necessitate postoperative mechanical ventilation. This may also be necessary in patients with poorly controlled pain, intrinsic lung disease, difficulty with oxygenation or ventilation during the procedure, ongoing metabolic acidosis, or the potential for large fluid shifts postoperatively.

In any patient undergoing surgery, dramatic fluid shifts are possible in the first few days of the postoperative period, and this may account for significant perioperative morbidity and mortality. As discussed in a previous section, the right ventricles of patients with PH may only be able to maintain adequate CO over a narrow range of loading conditions. Therefore PH patients may need close monitoring of volume status, and to maintain euvolemia, a diuretic or judicious IV fluid administration may be necessary.

Finally, for patients who require intraoperative administration of vasodilators or inotropes, care must be taken to taper these medications safely. This typically requires ICU admission, with careful monitoring for signs of rebound increases in PVR or RV failure, while the patient is weaned off these medications or transitioned to her or his outpatient regimen.

CONCLUSION

Although PH is a relatively uncommon condition among patients undergoing noncardiac surgery, it is strongly associated with increased perioperative morbidity and mortality. Therefore it is essential that the clinician tasked with caring for these patients possess a thorough understanding of the pathophysiology and medical management of PH and RV failure. The central principle guiding the perioperative management of these patients is to avoid increases in PVR and decreases in systemic blood pressure because both can lead to RV ischemia and failure. To properly care for these patients, a carefully crafted, comprehensive perioperative management plan should be developed with input from surgical, anesthetic, and medical specialists.

SUGGESTED READING

Barnett CF, Alvarez P, Park MH. Pulmonary arterial hypertension: diagnosis and treatment. *Cardiol Clin.* 2016;34(3):375–389.

Elmi-Sarabi M, Deschamps A, Delisle S, et al. Aerosolized vasodilators for the treatment of pulmonary hypertension in cardiac surgical patients: a systematic review and meta-analysis. *Anesth Analg.* 2017;125(2):393–402.

Fischer LG, Van Aken H, Bürkle H. Management of pulmonary hypertension: physiological and pharmacological considerations for anesthesiologists. *Anesth Analg.* 2003;96(6):1603–1616.

Galiè N, Humbert M, Vachiery JL, et al. 2015 ESC/ERS guidelines for the diagnosis and treatment of pulmonary hypertension: the Joint Task Force for the diagnosis and treatment of pulmonary hypertension of the European Society of Cardiology (ESC) and the European Respiratory Society (ERS): endorsed by: Association for European Paediatric and Congenital Cardiology (AEPC), International Society for Heart and Lung Transplantation (ISHLT). *Eur Respir J.* 2015;46:903–975.

Galiè N, Saia F, Palazzini M, et al. Left main coronary artery compression in patients with pulmonary arterial hypertension and angina. *J Am Coll Cardiol.* 2017;69:2808–2817.

Gille J, Seyfarth HJ, Gerlach S, et al. Perioperative anesthesiological management of patients with pulmonary hypertension. *Anesthesiology Research and Practice.* 2012;16. Article ID 356982.

Hosseinian L. Pulmonary hypertension and noncardiac surgery: implications for the anesthesiologist. *J Cardiothorac Vasc Anesth.* 2014;28(4):1064–1074.

Kamenskaya O, Klinkova A, Loginova I, et al. Factors affecting the quality of life before and after surgery in patients with chronic thromboembolic pulmonary hypertension. *Qual Life Res.* 2017.

Kaw R, Pasupuleti V, Deshpande A. Pulmonary hypertension: an important predictor of outcomes in patients undergoing non-cardiac surgery. *Respir Med.* 2011;105(4):619–624.

McGlothlin D, Ivascu N, Heerdt P. Anesthesia and pulmonary hypertension. *Prog Cardiovasc Dis.* 2012;55(2):199–217.

Memon HA, Park MH. Pulmonary arterial hypertension in women. *Methodist Debakey Cardiovasc J.* 2017;13(4):224–237.

Meyer S, McLaughlin VV, Seyfarth HJ, et al. Outcomes of noncardiac, nonobstetric surgery in patients with PAH: an international prospective survey. *Eur Respir J.* 2013;41(6):1302–1307.

Minai OA, Yared JP, Kaw R, et al. Perioperative risk and management in patients with pulmonary hypertension. *Chest.* 2013;144(1):329–340.

Pilkington SA, Taboada D, Martinez G. Pulmonary hypertension and its management in patients undergoing non-cardiac surgery. *Anaesthesia.* 2015;70(1):56–70.

Price LC, Dimopoulos K, Marino P, et al. The CRASH report: emergency management dilemmas facing acute physicians in patients with pulmonary arterial hypertension. *Thorax.* 2017;pii: thoraxjnl-2016-209725.

Price LC, Wort SJ, Finney SJ, Marino PS, Brett SJ. Pulmonary vascular and right ventricular dysfunction in adult critical care: current and emerging options for management: a systematic literature review. *Crit Care*. 2010;14(5):R169.

Ramakrishna G, Sprung J, Ravi BS, et al. Impact of pulmonary hypertension on the outcomes of noncardiac surgery: predictors of perioperative morbidity and mortality. *J Am Coll Cardiol*. 2005;45(10):1691–1699.

Rush B, Biagioni BJ, Berger L, et al. Mechanical ventilation outcomes in patients with pulmonary hypertension in the United States: A national retrospective cohort analysis. *J Intensive Care Med*. 2016.

Strumpher J, Jacobsohn E. Pulmonary hypertension and right ventricular dysfunction: physiology and perioperative management. *J Cardiothorac Vasc Anesth*. 2011;25(4):687–704.

Chapter 8

Adult Congenital Heart Disease in Noncardiac Surgery

Victor C. Baum, MD • Duncan G. De Souza, MD, FRCPC •
Brett Cronin, MD • Timothy M. Maus, MD

Key Points

1. Because of successes in treating congenital cardiac lesions, there are currently as many as or more adults than children with congenital heart disease (CHD).
2. Noncardiac anesthesiologists see these patients for a vast array of ailments and injuries requiring surgery.
3. If at all possible, noncardiac surgery on adult patients with moderate to complex CHD should be performed at an adult congenital heart center with the consultation of an anesthesiologist experienced with adult CHD.
4. Delegation of one anesthesiologist as the liaison with the cardiology service for preoperative evaluation and triage of adult CHD patients is helpful.
5. All relevant cardiac tests and evaluations should be reviewed in advance.
6. Sketching out the anatomy and path(s) of blood flow is often an easy and enlightening aid in simplifying apparently very complex lesions.

Advances in perioperative care for children with congenital heart disease (CHD) over the past several decades have resulted in an ever-increasing number of these children reaching adulthood with their cardiac lesions palliated or repaired. The first paper on adult CHD, published in 1973, is of increasing interest to the medical community. The field has grown such that several texts are now devoted to it, and a dedicated specialty society, the International Society for Adult Congenital Heart Disease (http://www.isachd.org), was formed in the 1990s. Each year an estimated 32,000 new cases of CHD occur in the United States and 1.5 million worldwide. More than 85% of infants born with CHD are expected to grow to adulthood. It is estimated that there are more than 1 million adults with CHD in the United States and 1.2 million in Europe, and this population is growing at approximately 5% per year; 55% of these adults remain at moderate to high risk, and more than 115,000 in the United States have complex disease. The increasing survival of children with complex disease has shifted the spectrum of adults with CHD. Once it was thought that adults represent milder degrees of disease, but this is now changing. Annual admissions for adults with CHD have increased significantly faster than those for children, and adults now account for 37% of admissions for those with CHD. As many adults as children have congenital cardiac defects considered severe. As an example to support the increased life expectancy of this patient group, the leading cause of death in adults with acyanotic CHD in the

United States is currently coronary artery disease. (Arrhythmia remains the leading cause of death for cyanotic patients, as it was for acyanotic patients before 1990.) Not surprisingly, the mortality rate in adults with CHD is increased with increased disease severity, with 77% of deaths from cardiovascular causes. Adults with CHD are seen for common ailments of aging and trauma that require surgical intervention. Additionally, women of childbearing age with CHD may become pregnant. They must cope with the added physiologic demands of pregnancy and require analgesia for labor and anesthesia for cesarean delivery.

Even though CHD carries implications for lifelong medical problems, a significant number of patients, even those with lesions deemed severe, do not have continuing cardiology follow-up despite ongoing general medical care. These patients bring with them anatomic and physiologic complexities of which physicians accustomed to caring for adults may be unaware, as well as medical problems associated with aging or pregnancy that might not be familiar to physicians used to caring for children. This is even more complicated because a significant number of these patients are unaware of their cardiac diagnosis, and having lived with their disease for many years, these patients self-limit exercise or think of themselves as asymptomatic when in fact they are not. This problem has led to the establishment of the growing subspecialty of adult CHD (ACHD). The mortality rate for adult CHD patients decreased after the introduction of specialized ACHD centers, with less than half dying of cardiovascular diseases. Adult patients with moderate or complex CHD are therefore recommended to be cared for in specialized ACHD centers. An informed anesthesiologist is a critical member of the team required to care optimally for these patients. Despite this recommendation, the majority of adult patients with CHD having ambulatory surgery appear not to be having their surgery at ACHD centers.

NONCARDIAC SURGERY IN ADULTS WITH CONGENITAL HEART DISEASE

As expected, young adults (aged 18 to 39 years) with a history of cardiac surgery have an increased risk of a series of serious morbidities and mortality after noncardiac surgery. High-risk patients include, but are not limited to, those with Fontan physiology; cyanotic disease; severe pulmonary arterial hypertension; and complex disease with residua such as heart failure, valve disease or the need for anticoagulation, or the potential for malignant arrhythmias.

Adults with CHD represent approximately 0.1% of admissions, and this has increased from about 0.07% to 0.18% from 2002 to 2009. The fraction of adult CHD admissions associated with noncardiac surgery also increased over this time period. Most were cared for in nonteaching hospitals. CHD confers an incremental mortality risk with both children and adults with CHD having noncardiac inpatient surgery. The mortality rate appears highest for those with the most complex lesions. Risk factors for noncardiac surgery include heart failure, pulmonary hypertension, and cyanosis.

GENERAL NONCARDIAC ISSUES WITH LONG-STANDING CONGENITAL HEART DISEASE

A variety of organ systems can be affected by long-standing CHD; these are summarized in Boxes 8.1 and 8.2. Because CHD can be one manifestation of a multiorgan genetic or dysmorphic syndrome, all patients require a full review of systems and examination.

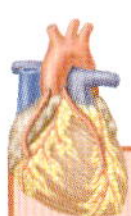

> **BOX 8.1**   *Potential Noncardiac Organ Involvement in Patients With Congenital Heart Disease*

Potential Respiratory Implications

- Decreased compliance (with increased pulmonary blood flow or impediment to pulmonary venous drainage)
- Compression of airways by large, hypertensive pulmonary arteries
- Compression of bronchioles
- Scoliosis
- Hemoptysis (with end-stage Eisenmenger syndrome)
- Phrenic nerve injury (prior thoracic surgery)
- Recurrent laryngeal nerve injury (prior thoracic surgery; very rarely from encroachment of cardiac structures)
- Blunted ventilatory response to hypoxemia (with cyanosis)
- Underestimation of $PaCO_2$ by capnometry in cyanotic patients

Potential Hematologic Implications

- Symptomatic hyperviscosity
- Bleeding diathesis
- Abnormal von Willebrand factor
- Artifactually elevated prothrombin or partial thromboplastin times with erythrocytic blood
- Artifactual thrombocytopenia with erythrocytic blood
- Gallstones

Potential Renal Implication

- Hyperuricemia and arthralgias (with cyanosis)

Potential Neurologic Implications

- Paradoxical emboli
- Brain abscess (with right-to-left shunts)
- Seizure (from old brain abscess focus)
- Intrathoracic nerve injury (iatrogenic phrenic, recurrent laryngeal, or sympathetic trunk injury)

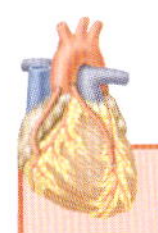

> **BOX 8.2**   *Noncardiac Organ Systems With Potential Involvement by Long-Standing Congenital Heart Disease*

- Pulmonary
- Hematologic
- Renal
- Neurologic
- Vasculature
- Genitourinary (pregnancy)
- Psychosocial

Pulmonary

Any lesion that results in either increased pulmonary blood flow or pulmonary venous obstruction can cause increased pulmonary interstitial fluid with decreased pulmonary compliance and increased work of breathing. Patients with cyanotic heart disease have increased minute ventilation and maintain normocarbia. These patients have a normal ventilatory response to hypercapnia but a blunted response to hypoxemia that normalizes after corrective surgery and the establishment of normoxia. End-tidal CO_2 underestimates arterial $PaCO_2$ in cyanotic patients with decreased, normal, or even increased pulmonary blood flow.

Although enlarged hypertensive pulmonary arteries or an enlarged left atrium can impinge on bronchi in children, this is rare in adults. Late-stage Eisenmenger syndrome can result in hemoptysis, and patients with Eisenmenger physiology and erythrocytosis can develop thrombosis of upper lobe pulmonary arteries. Prior thoracic surgery could have injured the phrenic nerve with resultant diaphragmatic paresis or paralysis.

In an attempt to increase pulmonary blood flow, large collateral vessels originating from the aorta may have developed. These are sometimes embolized in the catheterization laboratory before thoracic surgery to prevent excessive intraoperative blood loss.

Hematologic

Hematologic manifestations of chronic CHD are primarily a consequence of long-standing cyanosis and incorporate abnormalities of both hemostasis and red blood cell (RBC) regulation. Long-standing hypoxemia causes increased erythropoietin production in the kidney and resultant increased RBC mass. Because solely RBC production is affected, these patients are correctly referred to as erythrocytotic rather than polycythemic. There is, however, a fairly poor relationship among oxygen saturation, RBC mass, and 2,3-diphosphoglycerate. The oxygen-hemoglobin dissociation curve is normal or minimally shifted to the right. Most patients have established an equilibrium state at which they have a stable hematocrit and are iron replete. Some patients, however, develop excessive hematocrits and are iron deficient, causing a hyperviscous state. Iron-deficient RBCs are less deformable and cause increased viscosity for the same hematocrit. This is a strong independent predictor of thrombosis in the setting of Eisenmenger syndrome. Symptoms of hyperviscosity are uncommon and typically develop only at hematocrits exceeding 65%, provided the patient is iron replete. Iron deficiency also shifts the oxygen-hemoglobin dissociation curve to the right, decreasing oxygen affinity in the lungs. Iron deficiency can be the result of misguided attempts to lower the hematocrit by means of repeated phlebotomies.

Symptomatic hyperviscosity is the indication for treatment to temporarily relieve symptoms. It is not indicated to treat otherwise asymptomatic elevated hematocrits (generally hemoglobin >20 g/dL and hematocrit >65%). Treatment is by means of a partial isovolumic exchange transfusion, and it is assumed that the increased hematocrit is not related to dehydration. Partial isovolumic exchange transfusion usually results in regression of symptoms within 24 hours. It is rare to require exchange of more than 1 unit of blood. Preoperatively, phlebotomized blood can be banked for autologous perioperative retransfusion if required. Elective preoperative isovolumic exchange transfusion has decreased the incidence of hemorrhagic complications of surgery. Hyperviscosity and erythrocytosis can cause cerebral venous thrombosis in younger children, but it is not a problem in adults, regardless of the hematocrit. Protracted preoperative fasts need to be avoided in erythrocytotic patients because they can be accompanied by rapid elevations in the hematocrit.

Bleeding dyscrasias have been described in up to 20% of patients. A variety of clotting abnormalities have been described in association with cyanotic CHD but none uniformly. Bleeding dyscrasias are uncommon until the hematocrit exceeds 65%, although excessive surgical bleeding can occur at lower hematocrits. Generally, higher hematocrits are associated with a greater bleeding diathesis. Abnormalities of a variety of factors in both the intrinsic and extrinsic coagulation pathways have been described. Fibrinolytic pathways are normal.

The decreased plasma volume in erythrocytotic blood can result in spuriously elevated measures of the prothrombin and partial thromboplastin times, and the fixed amount of anticoagulant in the collection tube will be excessive because it presumes a normal plasma volume in the blood sample. Erythrocytotic blood has more RBCs and less plasma in the same volume. If informed in advance of a patient's hematocrit, the clinical laboratory can provide an appropriate sample tube.

Platelet counts are typically normal or occasionally low, but bleeding is not due to thrombocytopenia. Platelets are reported per milliliter of blood, not per milliliter of plasma. When corrected for the decreased plasma fraction in erythrocytotic blood, the total plasma platelet count is closer to normal. That said, abnormalities in platelet function and life span have on occasion been reported. Patients with low-pressure conduits (Fontan pathway) or synthetic vascular anastomoses are often maintained on antiplatelet drugs.

Cyanotic erythrocytotic patients have excessive hemoglobin turnover, and adults have an increased incidence of calcium bilirubinate gallstones. Biliary colic can develop years after cyanosis has been resolved by cardiac surgery.

A variety of mechanical factors can also affect excessive surgical bleeding in patients with cyanotic CHD. These factors include increased tissue capillary density, elevated systemic venous pressure, aortopulmonary and transpleural collaterals that have developed to increase pulmonary blood flow, and prior thoracic surgery. Aprotinin and ε-aminocaproic acid improve postoperative hemostasis in patients with cyanotic CHD. The results with tranexamic acid have been mixed.

Renal

Some degree of renal insufficiency is common in adults with CHD, and the severity is a predictor of death. Moderate or severe renal dysfunction (estimated glomerular filtration rate [GFR] of <60 mL/min per m^2) carries a fivefold increased risk of death at 6-year follow-up compared with patients with normal GFR and a threefold increase over those with mild elevations in GFR. Renal dysfunction is particularly prevalent in cyanotic patients and those with poor cardiac function. Adult patients with cyanotic CHD can develop abnormal renal histology with hypercellular glomeruli and basement membrane thickening, focal interstitial fibrosis, tubular atrophy, and hyalinized afferent and efferent arterioles. Cyanotic CHD is often accompanied by elevations in plasma uric acid levels that are caused by inappropriately low fractional uric acid excretion. Decreased urate reabsorption is thought to result from renal hypoperfusion with a high filtration fraction. Despite the elevated uric acid levels, urate stones and urate nephropathy are rare. Although arthralgias are common, true gouty arthritis is less frequent than would be expected from the degree of hyperuricemia.

Neurologic

Adults with persistent or potential intracardiac shunts remain at risk for paradoxical embolism. Paradoxical emboli can occur even through shunts that are predominantly left-to-right because during the cardiac cycle, there can be small transient reversals of the shunt direction. It has been said that, unlike in children, adults with cyanotic CHD are not at risk for the development of cerebral thrombosis despite the hematocrit. However, this assertion has been challenged with the suggestion that an association of stroke occurs, not with RBC mass but with iron deficiency and repeated phlebotomy. Adults do, however, remain at risk for the development of brain abscess. A healed childhood brain abscess can provide the nidus for the development of seizures throughout life.

Prior thoracic surgery can result in permanent peripheral nerve damage. Surgery at the apices of the lungs is particularly associated with the risk of nerve damage. These operations would include Blalock-Taussig shunts, ligation of patent ductus arteriosus (PDA), banding of the pulmonary artery, and repair of aortic coarctation. Nerves that are susceptible to injury include the recurrent laryngeal nerve, the phrenic nerve, and the sympathetic chain. The incidence of migraine headaches is higher in adults with CHD compared with a control group with acquired heart disease (45% vs. 11%) and is increased in left-to-right, right-to-left, and no-shunt groups.

Vasculature

Vessel abnormalities can be congenital or iatrogenic. They can affect the suitability of vessels for cannulation by the anesthesiologist or measurement of correct pressures. These abnormalities are described in Table 8.1.

Pregnancy

The physiologic changes of pregnancy, labor, and delivery can significantly alter the physiologic status of women with CHD, and mortality and morbidity are increased in mothers with CHD. Several texts are available that specifically discuss issues of pregnant women with CHD in more detail than is possible here. Management and clinical outcomes during pregnancy and delivery for several cardiac lesions are included under the later discussions of these lesions.

Table 8.1 **Potential Vascular Access Issues**	
Vessel	**Possible Problem**
Femoral vein(s)	May have been ligated if cardiac catheterization was done by cutdown. Large therapeutic catheters in infants often thrombose femoral veins.
Inferior vena cava	Some lesions, particularly when associated with heterotaxy (polysplenia) have discontinuity of the inferior vena cava; will not be able to pass a catheter from the groin to the right atrium.
Left subclavian and pedal arteries	Distal blood pressure will be low in the presence of coarctation of the aorta or following subclavian flap repair (subclavian artery only) and variably so if postoperative recoarctation; pulses can be absent or palpable with abnormal blood pressure.
Subclavian artery	Blood pressure low with classic Blalock-Taussig shunt on that side and variably so with modified Blalock-Taussig shunt.
Right subclavian artery	Blood pressure artifactually high with supravalvular aortic stenosis (Coanda effect).
Superior vena cava	Risk of catheter-related thrombosis with Glenn operation.

Although cardiac complications, spontaneous abortions, premature delivery, thrombotic complications, peripartum endocarditis, and poor fetal outcomes can occur, successful pregnancy to term with vaginal delivery is possible for most patients with congenital defects. High-risk factors for mothers and fetuses include pulmonary hypertension, depressed ventricular function, Marfan syndrome with dilated aortic root, cyanosis, severe left heart obstructive lesions, and pressure (vs. volume) lesions. Eisenmenger physiology is a particular risk factor. Up to 47% of cyanotic women have worsening of functional capacity during pregnancy. Hematocrits greater than 44% are associated with birth weights less than 50th percentile, and fetal death is about 90% or more with hemoglobin levels greater than 18 g/dL or oxygen saturation less than 85%, with most losses in the first trimester. The increases in stroke volume and cardiac output during pregnancy can stress an already pressure-overloaded ventricle. The decrease in systemic vascular resistance that accompanies pregnancy is better tolerated by women with regurgitant lesions and typically offsets the added insult of pregnancy-related hypervolemia. The decrease in systemic vascular resistance can, however, increase right-to-left shunting. Hypervolemia can be problematic in patients with poor ventricular function. Maternal cyanosis is associated with increased incidences of prematurity and intrauterine growth retardation. Profound cyanosis is associated with a high rate of spontaneous abortion. Endocarditis prophylaxis is not currently recommended for vaginal deliveries. The recurrence risk of any congenital cardiac defect in a newborn is 2.3% with one affected older sibling (any defect), 7.3% with two affected older siblings, and 6.7% if the mother has a congenital cardiac defect but only 2.1% if the father is affected. However, it has become apparent that recurrence risk can be specific to the type of maternal defect and the underlying genetic basis. If possible, pregnancies in mothers with CHD should be managed in a high-risk obstetric center with cardiologists experienced with the care of ACHD and with early consultation with the obstetric anesthesia service. Women on long-term anticoagulation likely need peripartum modifications, and postpartum thromboembolism is a potential significant problem. Anesthesiologists generally encounter pregnant patients well into the last trimester. Most of the major physiologic changes associated with pregnancy occur before the third trimester, and if patients have maintained good functional status to this point, they will have demonstrated themselves to be in a relatively low-risk group. Pregnancy is a stress test, and if they have successfully arrived at the mid to late third trimester, it is more likely that they will successfully tolerate delivery. Also, many high-risk women will have been counseled to avoid pregnancy. There is no a priori reason to favor an instrumented or cesarean delivery over a vaginal one. This is an obstetric, not cardiologic, decision. That said, there is a common belief that women with ACHD will not tolerate the "stress" of labor, particularly bearing down in the second stage. However, a well-functioning epidural makes uterine contractions easy to tolerate. Furthermore, avoidance of second-stage pushing is an option as long as progress is being made and can be combined with a maneuver such as low-outlet vacuum or forceps to facilitate delivery. The third stage can be accompanied by an autotransfusion of placental blood or potentially with hypovolemia with uterine atony and hemorrhage. If oxytocic drugs are required, the hemodynamic effects must be kept in mind. Oxytocin will decrease systemic vascular resistance and increase heart rate and pulmonary vascular resistance (PVR). Methylergonovine will increase systemic vascular resistance. These rapid changes in loading conditions can be poorly tolerated in mothers with fixed cardiac output, and pulmonary edema or heart failure can develop.

Some mothers take medications for their cardiac condition, including antiar-rhythmics. In general, these are safe for the infant. Exceptions include β-blockers, which can interfere with fetal growth and the response of the fetus to the stress of labor, and amiodarone, which can affect fetal thyroid function. Maternal cardioversion appears to be safe for fetuses at all stages because of the low intensity of the electrical field at the uterus. However, fetuses should be monitored throughout the procedure. Women with implanted internal defibrillators have carried successfully to term. If cardiopulmonary bypass (CPB) is required during pregnancy, it carries with it increased fetal risk, particularly if hypothermia is used.

Psychosocial

Teenagers with CHD are certainly no different from other teenagers in that issues of denial, a sense of immortality, and risk-taking behavior can affect optimal care for these youngsters. Bodies that carry scars from prior surgery and physical limitations can complicate the body-conscious teenage years. Although most adolescents and adults with CHD function well, adults with CHD are less likely to be married or cohabitating and are more likely to be living with their parents. There are several reports of the psychosocial outcomes of adolescent and adult patients, but there are no well-done controlled studies. It has been suggested that depression is common and can exacerbate the clinical consequences of the cardiac defect.

Adolescent CHD patients have higher medical care expenses than the general population, and they can have difficulty in obtaining life and health insurance after they can no longer be covered under their parents' policies. Life insurance is somewhat more available to adult CHD patients than in the past; however, policies vary widely among insurers.

The issue of denial or lack of awareness of their cardiac condition is very relevant in teenagers and young adults. While they are children, these patients rely on their parents to ensure regular cardiac appointments are kept and surveillance echocardiograms are done.

Unfortunately, young adults with ACHD often do not appreciate their physiologic limitations because they have lived with them their entire lives. Many often lack basic knowledge of their cardiac condition. Sadly, this can result in ACHD patients being lost to follow-up until they arrive in their local emergency department with an urgent condition requiring surgery.

CARDIAC ISSUES

The basic hemodynamic effects of an anatomic cardiac lesion can be modified by time and by the superimposed effects of chronic cyanosis, pulmonary disease, or the effects of aging. Although surgical cure is the goal, true universal cure, without residua, sequelae, or complications, is uncommon on a population-wide basis. Exceptions include closure of a nonpulmonary hypertensive PDA or atrial septal defect (ASD), probably in childhood. Although there have been reports of series of surgeries on adults with CHD, the wide variety of defects and sequelae from prior surgery make generalizations difficult, if not impossible. Poor myocardial function can be inherent in the CHD, but it can also be affected by long-standing cyanosis or superimposed surgical injury, including inadequate intraoperative myocardial protection. This is particularly true of adults who had their cardiac repair several decades ago when myocardial protection may not have been as good and when repair was undertaken at an older age. Postoperative arrhythmias are common, particularly when surgery entails long atrial suture lines, and the incidence of atrial arrhythmias increases with time, either as a primary sequela or as an indicator of diminished cardiac function. Thrombi can be found in these atria precluding immediate cardioversion. Bradyarrhythmias can be secondary to surgical injury to the sinus node or conducting tissue or can be a component of the cardiac defect.

The number of cardiac lesions and subtypes, together with the large number of contemporary and obsolescent palliative and corrective surgical procedures, make a complete discussion of all CHD impossible. Readers are referred to one of the current texts on pediatric cardiac anesthesia for more detailed descriptions of these lesions, the available surgical repairs, and the anesthetic implications during primary repair. Some general perioperative guidelines to caring for these patients are offered in Box 8.3. This chapter provides a discussion of the more common and physiologically important defects that will be encountered in an adult CHD population.

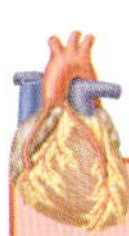

BOX 8.3   *General Approach to Anesthesia for Patients With Congenital Heart Disease*

General

- The best care for both cardiac and noncardiac surgery in adult patients with congenital heart disease (CHD) is afforded in a center with a multidisciplinary team experienced in the care of adults with CHD and knowledgeable about both the anatomy and physiology of CHD and the manifestations and considerations specific to adults with CHD.

Preoperative

- Review most recent laboratory data, catheterization, and echocardiogram and other imaging data. The most recent office letter from the cardiologist is often most helpful. Obtain and review them in advance.
- Drawing a diagram of the heart with saturations, pressures, and direction of blood flow often clarifies complex and superficially unfamiliar anatomy and physiology.
- Avoid prolonged fast if patient is erythrocytotic to avoid hemoconcentration.
- There is no generalized contraindication to preoperative sedation.

Intraoperative

- Large-bore IV access for redo sternotomy and cyanotic patients
- Avoid air bubbles in all IV catheters. There can be transient right-to-left shunting even in lesions with predominant left-to-right shunting. (Filters are available but will severely restrict ability to give volume and blood.)
- Apply external defibrillator pads for patients with poor cardiac function.
- Use appropriate endocarditis prophylaxis (orally or intravenously before skin incision).
- Consider antifibrinolytic therapy, especially for patients with prior sternotomy.
- Use transesophageal echocardiography for major surgery.
- Modulate pulmonary and systemic vascular resistances as appropriate pharmacologically and by modifications in ventilation.

Postoperative

- Provide appropriate pain control (cyanotic patients have normal ventilatory response to hypercarbia and narcotics). Maintain hematocrit appropriate for arterial saturation.
- Maintain venous pressures appropriate for altered ventricular diastolic compliance or presence of beneficial atrial level shunting.
- PaO_2 may not increase significantly with the application of supplemental oxygen in the face of right-to-left shunting. Similarly, neither will it decrease much with the withdrawal of oxygen (in the absence of lung pathology).

8

Aortic Stenosis

Valvar aortic stenosis is the most common congenital heart defect, but it is often not seen in that light because it typically does not cause problems until adulthood. Most aortic stenosis in adults is caused by a congenitally bicuspid valve that does not become problematic until late middle age or beyond, although endocarditis risk is lifelong. Congenital aortic stenosis can on some occasions, however, become severe enough to warrant surgical correction in adolescence or young adulthood, in addition to those severely affected valves that present in infancy. When symptoms (angina, syncope, near-syncope, heart failure) develop, survival is markedly shortened. The median survival periods are 5 years after the development of angina, 3 years after syncope, and 2 years after heart failure. Anesthetic management of aortic stenosis does not vary whether the stenosis is congenital or acquired.

Most mothers with aortic stenosis can successfully carry pregnancies to term and have vaginal deliveries. Severe stenosis (valve area <1.0 cm^2) can result in clinical deterioration and maternal and fetal death. Hemodynamic monitoring during delivery with maintenance of adequate preload and avoidance of hypotension is critical.

Aortopulmonary Shunts

Depending on their age, adult patients may have had one or more of several aortopulmonary shunts to palliate cyanosis during childhood. These are shown in Fig. 8.1. Although lifesaving, these shunts had considerable shortcomings in the long term.

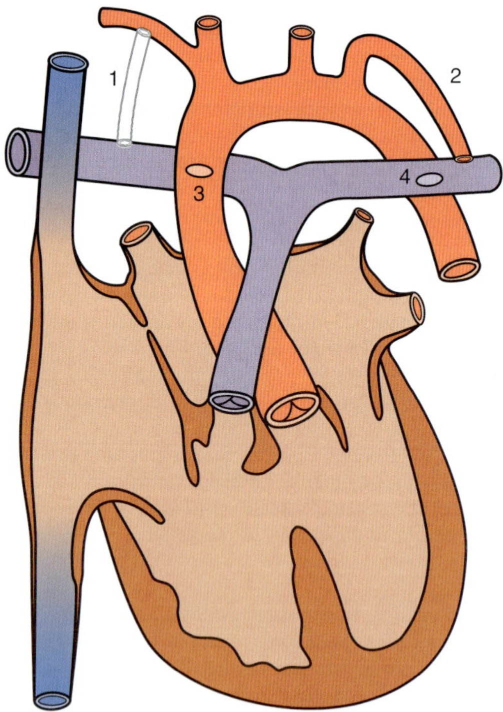

Fig. 8.1 The various aortopulmonary anastomoses. The illustrated heart is one with tetralogy of Fallot. The anastomoses are the modified Blalock-Taussig *(1)*, classic Blalock-Taussig *(2)*, Waterston (Waterston-Cooley) *(3)*, and Potts *(4)*. (From Baum VC. The adult with congenital heart disease. *J Cardiothorac Vasc Anesth*. 1996;10:261.)

All were inherently inefficient because some of the oxygenated blood returning through the pulmonary veins to the left atrium and ventricle would then return to the lungs through the shunt, thus volume loading the ventricle. It was difficult to quantify the size of the earlier shunts, such as the Waterston (side-to-side ascending aorta to right pulmonary artery) and Potts (side-to-side descending aorta to left pulmonary artery). If too small, the patient was left excessively cyanotic; if too large, there was pulmonary overcirculation and the risk of developing pulmonary vascular disease. Waterston shunts, in fact, could on occasion distribute blood flow unequally, resulting in a hyperperfused, hypertensive ipsilateral (right) pulmonary artery and a hypoperfused contralateral (left) pulmonary artery. There were also surgical issues when complete repair became possible. Takedown of Waterston shunts often required a pulmonary arterioplasty to correct a deformity of the pulmonary artery at the site of the anastomosis, and the posteriorly located Potts anastomoses could not be taken down from a median sternotomy. Patients with a classic Blalock-Taussig shunt almost always lack palpable pulses on the side of the shunt and arm length as well as strength can be mildly affected. Even if there is a palpable pulse (from collateral flow around the shoulder), blood pressure obtained from that arm will be artifactually low. After a modified Blalock-Taussig shunt (using a piece of Gore-Tex tubing instead of an end-to-side anastomosis of the subclavian and pulmonary arteries), there can be a blood pressure disparity between the arms. To ensure a valid measurement, preoperative blood pressure should be measured in both arms.

Atrial Septal Defect and Partial Anomalous Pulmonary Venous Return

There are several anatomic types of ASD (Fig. 8.2). The most common type—and, if otherwise undefined, the presumptive type—is the secundum type located in the

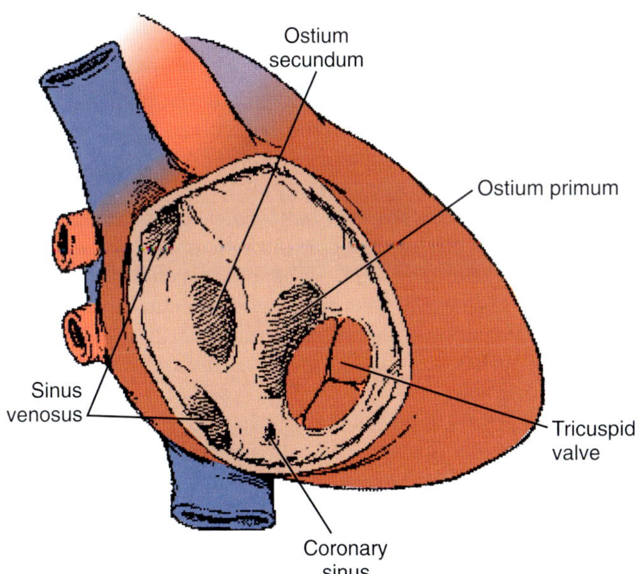

Fig. 8.2 Types of atrial septal defects. (From Nichols DG, Cameron DE, Greeley WG, et al, eds. *Critical Heart Disease in Infants and Children*. St. Louis: Mosby; 1995.)

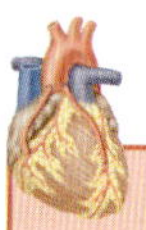

> **BOX 8.4** *Complications of Atrial Septal Defect in Adulthood*
>
> - Paradoxical emboli
> - Effort dyspnea
> - Atrial tachyarrhythmias
> - Right-sided failure with pregnancy
> - Pulmonary hypertension
> - Increase in right-sided failure with decrease in left ventricular compliance with aging
> - Mitral insufficiency

midseptum. The primum type at the lower end of the atrial septum is a component of endocardial cushion defects, the most primitive of which is the common atrioventricular (AV) canal (see later). The sinus venosus type, high in the septum near the entry of the superior vena cava, is almost always associated with partial anomalous pulmonary venous return, most frequently drainage of the right upper pulmonary vein to the low superior vena cava. An uncommon atrial septal–type defect occurs when blood passes from the left atrium to the right via an unroofed coronary sinus. For purposes of this section, only secundum defects are considered, although the natural histories of all of the defects are similar (Box 8.4).

Both the natural history and the postoperative outcome of ASDs and the physiologically related partial anomalous venous return are similar. Because the symptoms and clinical findings of an ASD can be quite subtle and patients often remain asymptomatic until adulthood, ASDs represent approximately one-third of all CHD discovered in adults. Although asymptomatic survival to adulthood is common, significant shunts ($\dot{Q}p/\dot{Q}s$ >1.5:1) will probably cause symptoms over time, and paradoxical emboli can occur through defects with smaller shunts. Surgical repair of restrictive lesions 5 mm or less in size does not impact the natural history. Thus surgical closure of small lesions is not indicated in the absence of paradoxical emboli. Effort dyspnea occurs in 30% by the third decade of life and atrial flutter or fibrillation in about 10% by age 40 years. The avoidance of complications developing in adulthood provides the rationale for surgical repair of asymptomatic children. The mortality rate for a patient with an uncorrected ASD is 6% per year after 40 years of age, and essentially all patients older than 60 years of age are symptomatic. Large unrepaired defects can cause death from atrial tachyarrhythmias or right ventricular failure in 30- to 40-year-old patients. With the decreased left ventricular diastolic compliance accompanying the systemic hypertension or coronary artery disease that is common with aging, left-to-right shunting increases with age. Unlike ventricular or ductal level shunts, pulmonary vascular disease typically does not develop until after the age of 40 years. Mitral insufficiency can be found in adult patients and is significant in about 15%. Paradoxical emboli remain a lifelong risk.

Late closure of the defect, after 5 years of age, has been associated with incomplete resolution of right ventricular dilation. Left ventricular dysfunction has been reported in some patients having defect closure in adulthood, and closure, particularly in middle age, may not prevent the development of atrial tachyarrhythmias or stroke. Survival of patients without pulmonary vascular disease has been reported to be best if operated on before 24 years of age, intermediate if operated on between 25 and 41 years of age, and worst if operated on thereafter. However, more recent series have shown that even at ages after 40 years, surgical repair provides an overall survival and complication-free benefit compared with medical management, although pulmonary artery hypertension can progress even after surgical closure if done late. Surgical morbidity in these patients is primarily atrial fibrillation, atrial flutter, or junctional rhythm. Current practice is to close these defects in adults in the catheterization laboratory via transvascular devices if anatomically practical. For example, there needs to be an adequate rim of septum around the defect to which the device can attach. Device closure is inappropriate if the defect is associated with anomalous pulmonary venous drainage. The indications for closure with a transvascular device are the same as for surgical closure. Surgical closure of ASD also lends itself to a thoracoscopic approach.

An otherwise uncomplicated secundum ASD, unlike most congenital cardiac defects, is not associated with an increased endocarditis risk. Presumably, this is because the shunt, although potentially large, is low pressure and not associated with jet lesions of the endocardium from turbulent flow. Although some discussion is given to onset times with intravenous or inhalation induction agents, clinical differences are hard to notice with the modern low-solubility volatile agents. Thermodilution cardiac output reflects pulmonary blood flow, which will be in excess of systemic blood flow. Pulmonary arterial catheters are not routinely indicated. Patients generally tolerate any appropriate anesthetic; however, particular care should be taken in patients with pulmonary arterial hypertension or right-sided failure.

The vast majority of women with an ASD tolerate pregnancy well. However, the normal hypervolemia associated with pregnancy can result in heart failure in women with large defects. Hypovolemia accompanying delivery can result in right-to-left shunting through the defect, and there is a risk of pulmonary thromboembolism or paradoxical embolism.

Coarctation of the Aorta

Unrepaired coarctation of the aorta in an adult brings with it significant morbidity and mortality. Mortality rates are 25% by age 20 years, 50% by age 30 years, 75% by age 50 years, and 90% by age 60 years. Left ventricular aneurysms, rupture of cerebral aneurysms, and dissection of a postcoarctation aneurysm all contribute to the excessive mortality rates. Left ventricular failure can occur in patients older than 40 years of age with unrepaired lesions. If repair is not undertaken early, there is incremental risk for the development of premature coronary atherosclerosis. Even with surgery, coronary artery disease remains the leading cause of death 11 to 25 years after surgery. Coarctation is accompanied by a bicuspid aortic valve in the majority of patients. Although endocarditis of this abnormal valve is a lifelong risk, these valves often do not become stenotic until middle age or later. Coarctation can also be associated with mitral valve abnormalities (Box 8.5).

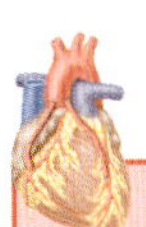

BOX 8.5 *Complications of Aortic Coarctation in Adulthood*

- Left ventricular failure
- Premature coronary atherosclerosis
- Rupture of cerebral aneurysm
- Aneurysm at site of coarctation repair
- Complications of associated bicuspid aortic valve
- Exacerbation of hypertension during pregnancy

Aneurysms at the site of coarctation repair can develop years later, and restenosis can develop in adolescence or adulthood as well. Persistent systemic hypertension is common after coarctation repair. The risk of hypertension parallels the duration of unrepaired coarctation. Adult patients require continued periodic follow-up for hypertension. A pressure gradient of 20 mm Hg or more (less in the presence of extensive collaterals) is an indication for treatment. Recoarctation can be treated surgically or by balloon angioplasty with stenting.

Pregnancy can exacerbate preexisting hypertension in women with unrepaired lesions, increasing the risk of aortic dissection or rupture, heart failure, angina, and rupture of a circle of Willis aneurysm. Adequate blood pressure control during pregnancy is paramount in these women. Most aortic ruptures during pregnancy occur during labor and delivery. Presumably, epidural analgesia would moderate hypertension during delivery.

Congenitally Corrected Transposition of the Great Vessels (L-Transposition, Ventricular Inversion)

"Transposition" in this context refers solely to the fact that the aorta arises anterior to the pulmonary artery. It bears no reference to the origin of blood in the aorta or pulmonary artery or to the ventricle of origin of those vessels. In levo-transposition of the great vessels (L-TGV), as a consequence of the embryonic heart tube rotating to the left (levo) rather than to the right, the flow of blood is through normal vena cava to the right atrium, through a mitral valve to a right-sided morphologic left ventricle, to the pulmonary artery, through the pulmonary circulation, to the left atrium, through a tricuspid valve to a left-sided morphologic right ventricle, and then to the aorta (Fig. 8.3). The L refers to the fact that the aorta originates anterior and to the left (levo) of the pulmonary artery. Although anatomically altered, the physiologic flow of blood is appropriate, and there are no associated shunts. L-TGV is frequently associated with other cardiac lesions, most commonly a ventricular

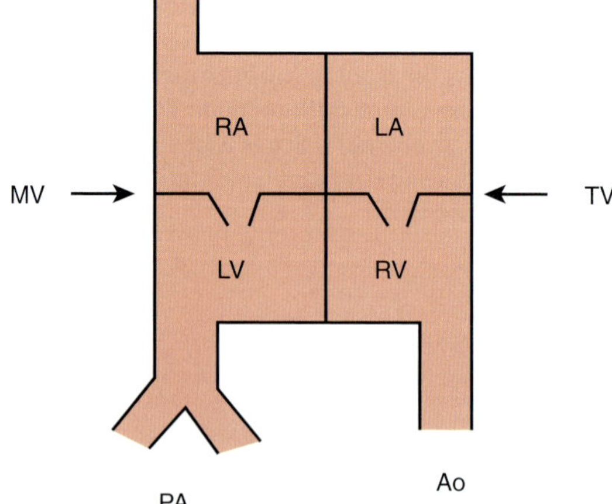

Fig. 8.3 Diagram of the anatomy of left transposition of the great arteries. Note that the atrioventricular valves are associated with the "usual" ventricle. *Ao,* Aorta; *LA,* left atrium; *LV,* morphologic left ventricle; *MV,* mitral valve; *PA,* pulmonary artery; *RA,* right atrium; *RV,* morphologic right ventricle; *TV,* tricuspid valve.

septal defect (VSD), subpulmonic stenosis, heart block, or systemic AV (tricuspid) valve regurgitation. In the absence of any of these associated cardiac defects, L-TGV is usually asymptomatic through infancy and childhood. When L-transposition is an isolated lesion, most patients maintain normal biventricular function through early adulthood and can attain a normal lifespan. However, the relatively thin-walled morphologic right ventricle is not well suited to eject blood against systemic pressure. Over a lifetime, the right ventricle can fail, and the patient will develop heart failure.

Systemic AV (tricuspid) valve insufficiency may not develop until later in life, resulting in approximately 60% of patients being diagnosed as adults. Dysfunction of the right (the systemic) ventricle can develop with aging, and asymptomatic aging is relatively uncommon. By age 45 years, heart failure will be present in 67% of patients with associated lesions and 25% of those without. Resynchronization therapy for severe ventricular dysfunction can be problematic because of significant abnormal cardiac venous drainage with variations in coronary sinus anatomy. These patients can be born with congenital heart block, which can progress in degree. Second- or third-degree heart block occurs at a rate of about 2% per year. More than 75% of patients develop some degree of heart block, although the intrinsic pacemaker remains above the His bundle with a narrow QRS complex. Chronic subpulmonary (left) ventricular pacing can be associated with a deterioration in systemic (right) ventricular function. L-TGV can be associated with an Ebstein-like deformity of the systemic AV (tricuspid) valve, and there can be a bundle of Kent, causing the Wolff-Parkinson-White (WPW) syndrome associated with the abnormal valve. There is a significant incidence of tricuspid valve insufficiency in the systemic ventricle, and this is higher still in patients with an Ebstein deformity of the valve. Anesthetic management depends on the presence of any associated lesions and the adequacy of right (systemic) ventricular function.

Although women generally do well with pregnancy, the physiologic stresses of pregnancy and delivery can result in ventricular or valvular dysfunction, particularly with baseline dysfunction or an insufficient systemic AV valve. However, even if these develop, pregnancy can be successfully managed. The decrease in systemic vascular resistance associated with both pregnancy and neuraxial analgesia might be advantageous to women with tricuspid (systemic) valve insufficiency. The acute autotransfusion associated with delivery could potentially cause problems for women with existing diminished systemic ventricular function. Pregnancy may result in a sustained deterioration in right (systemic) ventricular function.

Ebstein Anomaly of the Tricuspid Valve

This defect, one of arrested or incomplete delamination of the embryonic tricuspid valve from the right ventricular myocardium resulting in apically displaced valve tissue, is the most common cause of congenital tricuspid insufficiency. The septal leaflet tends to be the most dysplastic. The anterior leaflet tends to be large and redundant. The defect is associated with a patent foramen ovale or a secundum ASD and "atrialization" of part of the right ventricle. The displacement of the tricuspid valve toward the right ventricular apex results in a portion of the right ventricle being above the tricuspid valve and becoming functionally part of the right atrium. Apicalization of the tricuspid valve results in a portion of the heart above the valve having a ventricular intracardiac electrogram (it is ventricular myocardium) but atrial pressures (it lies above the tricuspid valve). The right atrium can be massively enlarged, and the right ventricle, lacking the inflow portion that is now part of the right atrium, is smaller than usual with varying degrees of pulmonic stenosis. Patients with L-TGV can have an Ebstein or Ebstein-like anomaly of a left-sided tricuspid valve. This anomaly is also on occasion associated with left ventricular noncompaction.

Symptoms vary based on the amount of displacement of the valve and the size of the smaller-than-normal right ventricle. Cyanosis from atrial-level right-to-left shunting can be a neonatal phenomenon that resolves with the normal postnatal decrease in PVR, only to recur in adolescence or adulthood. Very mild disease is quite compatible with asymptomatic survival into adulthood. About half develop arrhythmias, typically supraventricular tachyarrhythmias. When symptoms develop, disability rapidly progresses.

Ebstein valves are often associated with a right-sided bypass tract, causing WPW syndrome. This is of concern because 25% to 30% of patients develop supraventricular tachyarrhythmias. The dilated right atrium is also ready substrate for the development of atrial fibrillation. In addition to a decrease in cardiac performance, atrial fibrillation is also potentially very dangerous in patients with underlying WPW because very high atrial rates can be conducted to the ventricle through the bypass tract. The major concerns when anesthetizing patients who have Ebstein anomaly include decreased cardiac output, right-to-left atrial-level shunting with cyanosis, and the propensity for atrial tachyarrhythmias. The right atria of these patients are very sensitive, and arrhythmias are easily induced by catheters or guidewires passed into the right atrium or during surgical manipulation. Arrhythmias remain a concern into the postoperative period. Supraventricular arrhythmias should be treated aggressively. If associated with significant hypotension, the arrhythmia needs to be electrically cardioverted. In the absence of marked cyanosis, pregnancy and delivery are generally well tolerated. There is, however, an increased incidence of prematurity and fetal loss. Birth weights are lower in infants of cyanotic mothers, and the incidence of CHD is increased in offspring.

Eisenmenger Syndrome

Eisenmenger syndrome has come to describe the clinical setting in which a large left-to-right cardiac shunt results in the development of pulmonary hypertension. Although early on the pulmonary vasculature remains reactive, with continued insult, pulmonary hypertension becomes fixed and does not respond to pulmonary vasodilators. Ultimately, the level of PVR is so high that the shunt reverses and becomes right-to-left. Clinically, patients who are cyanotic from intracardiac right-to-left shunting are deemed to have Eisenmenger physiology even though their PVR may not yet truly be fixed. This is the intermediate phase of the disease before progression to a truly fixed PVR. That is, at baseline, they shunt right-to-left but may still retain some pulmonary vascular reactivity in the presence of vasodilating agents such as oxygen or nitric oxide. The degree of reactivity can be determined in the catheterization laboratory by measuring the pulmonary blood flow on room air, pure oxygen, and pure oxygen with nitric oxide added. The development of pulmonary vascular disease is dependent on shear rate. Lesions with high shear rates, such as a large VSD or a large PDA, can result in pulmonary hypertension in early childhood. Lesions such as an ASD with high pulmonary blood flow, but low pressure may not result in pulmonary vascular disease until late middle age. Pulmonary vascular disease progression is also accelerated in patients living at high altitudes.

The most common presenting symptom is dyspnea on exertion. Additional symptoms include palpitations, edema, hemoptysis, syncope, hyperpnea, and, of course, increasing cyanosis. Hepatic synthetic function can be altered from the elevated central venous pressure. There can be central nervous system symptoms from increased blood viscosity from the erythrocytosis associated with cyanosis. Right ventricular ischemia is a possibility. Patients may be on chronic therapy with drugs such as intravenous prostacyclin, an oral phosphodiesterase 5 inhibitor such as sildenafil (e.g., Revatio), an oral endothelin receptor antagonist such as bosentan (e.g., Tracleer), a prostanoid, or a soluble guanylate cyclase stimulator such as riociguat (Adempas). Because of the risk of pulmonary thromboses, patients may be on chronic anticoagulants.

Eisenmenger physiology is compatible with survival into adulthood. However, reported rates of survival after diagnosis vary, probably based on the relatively long life expectancy and variability in the time of diagnosis. The median survival period is reported as 53 years but with wide variation; survival rates of 80% at 10 years after diagnosis and 42% at 25 years have been reported. Recent data suggest worse long-term survival. Syncope, increased central venous pressure, and arterial desaturation to less than 85% are all associated with poor short-term outcomes. Other factors associated with death include syncope, age at presentation, functional status, supraventricular arrhythmias, elevated right atrial pressure, renal insufficiency, severe right ventricular dysfunction, and trisomy 21. Most deaths are sudden cardiac deaths. Other causes of death include heart failure, hemoptysis, brain abscess, thromboembolism, and complications of pregnancy and noncardiac surgery. These patients face potentially significant perioperative risks. Findings of Eisenmenger syndrome are summarized in Box 8.6.

Surgical closure of cardiac defects with fixed pulmonary vascular hypertension is associated with very high mortality rates. Lung or heart-lung transplantation is a surgical alternative. Although several surgical series report survival after heart-lung or single- or double-lung transplantation performed for primary pulmonary hypertension, it is unclear if this cohort of patients is similar to patients with Eisenmenger physiology.

When noncardiac surgery is deemed essential and time permits, a preoperative cardiac catheterization may be helpful to determine the presence of pulmonary reactivity to oxygen or nitric oxide. Fixed PVR precludes rapid adaptation to perioperative hemodynamic changes. Changes in systemic vascular resistance are mirrored by changes in intracardiac shunting. A decrease in systemic vascular resistance is accompanied by increased right-to-left shunting and a decrease in systemic oxygen saturation. In addition, an acute fall in systemic resistance can impair left ventricular filling with the right ventricular encroachment. Systemic vasodilators, including regional

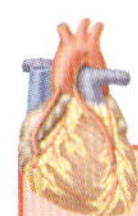

BOX 8.6 *Findings in Eisenmenger Syndrome*

- Physical examination: loud pulmonic component of the second heart sound, single or narrowly split second heart sound, Graham-Steell murmur of pulmonary insufficiency, pulmonic ejection sound ("click")
- Chest radiography: decreased peripheral pulmonary arterial markings with prominent central pulmonary vessels ("pruning")
- Electrocardiogram: right ventricular hypertrophy
- Impaired exercise tolerance
- Exertional dyspnea
- Palpitations (often caused by atrial fibrillation or flutter)
- Complications from erythrocytosis or hyperviscosity
- Hemoptysis from pulmonary infarction, rupture of pulmonary vessels, or aortopulmonary collateral vessels
- Complications from paradoxical embolization
- Syncope from inadequate cardiac output or arrhythmias
- Heart failure (usually end stage)

anesthesia, should be used with caution, and close assessment of intravascular volume is important. Epidural analgesia has been used successfully in patients with Eisenmenger physiology, but the local anesthetic must be delivered slowly and incrementally with close observation of blood pressure and oxygen saturation. Postoperative postural hypotension can also increase the degree of right-to-left shunting, and these patients should change position slowly. All intravenous catheters must be maintained free of air bubbles.

Placement of pulmonary artery catheters in these patients is problematic for a variety of reasons, and they are of less utility than might be expected. Pulmonary arterial hypertension is a risk factor for pulmonary artery rupture from a pulmonary artery catheter. Rupture is particularly worrisome in these cyanotic patients, who can also have hemostatic deficits associated with erythrocytosis. Abnormal intracardiac anatomy and right-to-left shunting can make successful passage into the pulmonary artery difficult without fluoroscopy. Relative resistances of the pulmonary and systemic beds are reflected in the systemic oxygen saturation, readily measured by pulse oximetry, so measures of pulmonary artery pressure are not required. In addition, in the presence of right-to-left shunting, thermodilution cardiac outputs do not accurately reflect systemic output. Thus, the value of pulmonary artery catheters in these patients is minimal at best, and they essentially are never indicated. The one potential exception is the patient with an ASD who is at risk of developing right ventricular failure if suprasystemic right ventricular pressure develops.

Fixed PVR is by definition unresponsive to pharmacologic or physiologic manipulation, but as previously mentioned, only patients at the true end stage of disease have fixed PVR. Thus, the clinician must still avoid factors known to increase PVR, including hypothermia, hypercarbia, acidosis, hypoxia, and α-adrenergic agonists. Although the last of these is commonly listed to be avoided, in the face of pulmonary vascular disease caused by intracardiac shunting, the systemic vasoconstrictive effects predominate, and systemic oxygen saturation increases.

Nerve blocks offer an attractive alternative to general anesthesia if otherwise appropriate. Although the mortality rate in nerve block cases was found to be less than that for general anesthesia cases (5% vs 15%), a difference in the relative risk between the type of anesthetic and type (complexity) of surgery could not be identified.

If patients have general anesthesia, consideration should be given to postoperative observation in an intensive or intermediate care unit. Because of the increased perioperative risk, patients should be observed overnight, particularly if they have not had recent surgery or anesthesia, because their responses will be unknown. Ambulatory surgery is possible for patients having uncomplicated minor surgery under sedation or nerve block.

Although the perioperative mortality risk in the past has been estimated to be as high as 30%, estimates of mortality rates after noncardiac surgery in adulthood from more current series suggest that the mortality risk from noncardiac surgery or anesthetics is less than previously quoted. Mortality rates have ranged from 7% down to 3.8% from small single-center studies. In one series, 26% of patients developed significant systemic hypotension, and 17% developed oxygen desaturation intraoperatively. Not surprisingly, hypoxemia was preceded by systemic hypotension. The incidence of hypotension was worse with propofol and inhalation inductions, and the authors found that use of a vasopressor during induction was helpful. The authors reported that the only two deaths in their series occurred after monitored anesthesia care: the first patient developed hypoxic respiratory failure 2 hours after transesophageal echocardiography (TEE) and cardioversion, and the second patient died on postoperative day 6 after TEE, cardioversion, and upper and lower endoscopy.

Pregnancy carries very high risks of death and premature delivery. About 20% to 30% of pregnancies result in spontaneous abortions, and premature delivery occurs in about half. At least half of newborns have intrauterine growth retardation. About 30% to 45% of all pregnancies end in maternal death intrapartum or during the first postpartum week, and a successful first pregnancy does not preclude maternal death during a subsequent pregnancy. The hemodynamic changes of both pregnancy and delivery increase maternal risk. Pulmonary microembolism and macroembolism have caused peripartum maternal deaths, even days after delivery. Factors influencing mortality include thromboembolism (44%), hypovolemia (26%), and preeclampsia (18%). The mortality rate is similar with cesarean section or vaginal delivery, and both carry significantly higher mortality rates than that for spontaneous abortion. The mortality rate for laboring women who received regional anesthesia was found to be 24%. Most of these women died several hours after delivery. Pregnancy should be discouraged in these women. Women who do become pregnant should be closely monitored with arterial catheters during delivery. Epidural analgesia, delivered slowly and incrementally, can moderate many of the deleterious hemodynamic changes of active labor. Pulmonary arterial catheters are of little to no use during delivery. Prompt treatment of blood loss and hypotension during delivery is vital. Postpartum observation should be in an intensive care setting.

Endocardial Cushion Defects (Atrioventricular Canal Defects)

The endocardial cushions are the embryonic cardiac tissues that form the crux of the heart—the primum (lower) atrial septum, the posterior basal part of the ventricular septum, the septal leaflet of the tricuspid valve, and the anterior leaflet of the mitral valve. The endocardial cushion defects then consist of one or more of a primum ASD, inlet VSD, cleft septal leaflet of the tricuspid valve, or cleft anterior leaflet of the mitral valve. The most primitive form is the complete AV canal. In this defect, there is a single large AV valve with mitral and tricuspid components with large ASDs and VSDs. This valve is usually "balanced." In the more complex, unbalanced defects, one component of the valve can be predominant, and this large valve is not centered over the ventricular septum, leading to underfilling of one of the ventricles. Three-dimensional echocardiography can be particularly useful in delineating the specific anatomy with these lesions. These defects can occur alone or can be part of more complex cardiac defects such as tetralogy of Fallot or single ventricle. Half of all children with Down syndrome have CHD; half of these children have an endocardial cushion defect. These lesions are marked by a typical electrocardiogram (ECG) with first-degree block and a superior QRS axis with a counterclockwise QRS loop. Although adults with unrepaired complete AV canal will likely have developed inoperable pulmonary arterial hypertension, partial canal defects can sometimes be first diagnosed in adults and can be appropriate candidates for surgical repair.

Fontan Physiology

In 1968, performing the operation that now bears his name, Fontan and colleagues proved that it was possible to deliver the entire systemic venous return to the lungs without the benefit of a ventricular pump. The Fontan operation was a landmark development in CHD because it established a "normal" series circulation in patients with a single ventricle. The price to be paid for a series circulation is the unique physiologic demand of passive pulmonary blood flow. Complications never envisioned at the time of the original operation have occurred, necessitating significant changes in operative technique. Fontan's original operation (Fig. 8.4) was soon modified to an atriopulmonary connection (Fig. 8.5). The original strict eligibility criteria have been liberalized, but patients meeting as many of the criteria as possible still have the best prognosis for good long-term survival. By the mid-1980s, it became clear that success of Fontan circulation was based on an unobstructed pathway from systemic veins to pulmonary artery, a pulmonary vasculature that was free from anatomic distortion (e.g., from previous Blalock-Taussig shunt), low PVR, and good ventricular function without significant AV valve regurgitation. The incorporation of the atrium in the Fontan pathway proved disappointing. The atrium lost its contractile function,

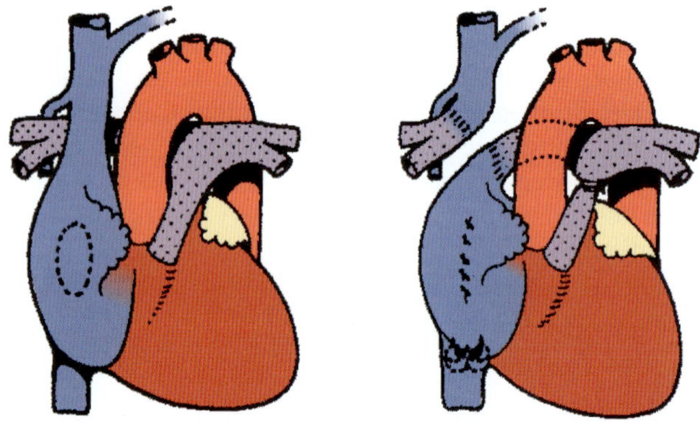

Fig. 8.4 Original Fontan operation. Note the classic Glenn shunt connecting the superior vena cava to the right pulmonary artery and the homografts at the inferior vena cava–right atrial junction and connecting the right atrium to the left pulmonary artery. (From Fontan F, Baudet E. Surgical repair of tricuspid atresia. *Thorax.* 1971;26:240.)

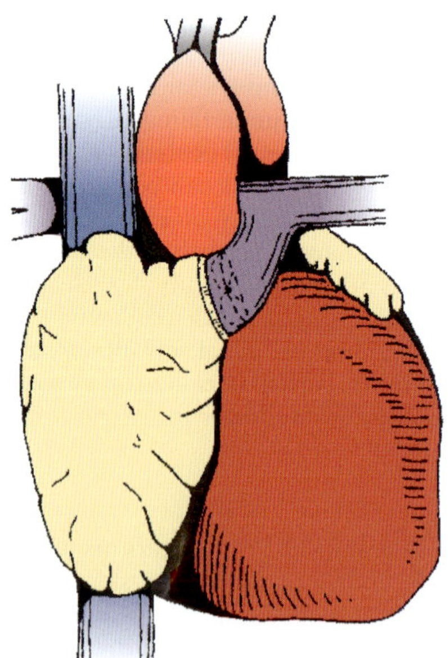

Fig. 8.5 Atriopulmonary modification of the Fontan operation. (From Kreutzer G, Galindez E, Bono H, et al. An operation for the correction of tricuspid atresia. *J Thorac Cardiovasc Surg.* 1973;66:613.)

184

providing no assistance to pulmonary blood flow and causing serious complications. Understanding these complications and how the Fontan operation has evolved is the key to managing these challenging patients whose complex CHD has been palliated, not cured.

Complications *(Box 8.7)*

The dilated, noncontractile atrium serves as a reservoir of blood and a ready source of thrombus. Pulmonary embolization will impair the passive blood flow necessary for successful Fontan circulation. Atrial thrombus could embolize paradoxically through residual right-to-left shunts. Patients are also at risk for arterial thrombosis, secondary to a mild hypercoagulable state. Given the morbidity associated with thromboembolism, it seems reasonable to put all Fontan patients on aspirin. Those who display further potential for thrombosis such as low cardiac output state, atrial arrhythmia with significant atrial dilation, or marked venous hypertension may benefit from warfarin (Coumadin).

Fontan patients show a steady increase in atrial tachyarrhythmias with an incidence of more than 50% at 20 years. Changes in surgical technique evolved in part to decrease the rate of atrial arrhythmias. Although initial results were promising, unfortunately, much of this benefit is lost with longer-term follow-up. Fontan patients tolerate tachycardia very poorly, and acute episodes usually require urgent treatment using medical therapy to control ventricular rate or cardioversion. Late-onset atrial tachyarrhythmias usually occur between 6 to 10 years after Fontan completion. The most common tachyarrhythmia is right intraatrial reentrant tachycardia. Over time, episodic attacks of tachycardia become more frequent. Frequently, atrial fibrillation occurs, and the loss of AV synchrony results in decreased effort tolerance. The onset of atrial tachyarrhythmias mandates an evaluation of the Fontan pathway with attention turned to relieving any significant obstructions. In the setting of passive pulmonary blood flow, even small gradients can be very hemodynamically significant. Therapies for chronic atrial arrhythmias consist of medication, catheter ablation, and surgery. Given the complex anatomy, dilated atrium, and atrial scar with suture lines from prior surgeries, it is not surprising that atrial arrhythmias can become refractory to standard treatment in many patients. Catheter ablation typically has high initial success rates that are not maintained.

Bradyarrhythmias, caused by sinus node ischemia, are common. In a large cohort of patients with atriopulmonary connections, the incidence of bradyarrhythmias requiring pacemakers was 13%. Progressive fibrosis and scar around the sinus node, caused by prior surgical dissection, eventually leads to ischemia and clinical sinus node dysfunction. If accompanied by premature atrial contractions, sinus or junctional bradycardia can precipitate an intraatrial reentry tachycardia. Thus, sinus node dysfunction also serves as a risk factor for the development of atrial tachyarrhythmias. Clinically significant bradyarrhythmias require pacing. Pacemakers pose special problems in Fontan patients because the altered anatomy precludes transvenous placement. Thus, Fontan patients

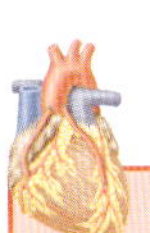

> **BOX 8.7** *Complications of Fontan Operation*
>
> - Atrial thrombus
> - Atrial arrhythmia (tachyarrhythmia or bradyarrhythmia)
> - Ventricular dysfunction
> - Chylothorax
> - Protein-losing enteropathy

who require pacing will have epicardial leads placed via repeat sternotomy with all the accompanying risks. Even though AV synchrony can be achieved with pacing, it is still not as desirable as intrinsic sinus rhythm. The incidence of sinus node dysfunction is less with a cavopulmonary versus an atriopulmonary connection.

The last major complication of Fontan physiology is protein-losing enteropathy (PLE), a condition as confounding as it is serious. The incidence is quoted to be as high as 15%, but a large international multicenter study found a rate of 3.7%. Clinically, there is an edematous state with ascites and pleural-pericardial effusions. Serum albumin is low, and the diagnosis is confirmed by finding enteric protein loss with elevated levels of stool α_1-antitrypsin. Most ominously, PLE is accompanied by 50% mortality rate 5 years from diagnosis despite treatment. It was believed that PLE constituted a straightforward situation of elevated portal pressures secondary to central venous hypertension. Elevated portal pressures lead to vascular congestion, lymphatic obstruction, and enteric protein loss from the gut. Unfortunately, there is not a good correlation between central venous pressures and PLE. This has led to a broader understanding of PLE as a multifactorial phenomenon caused by reduced mesenteric perfusion, chronic inflammation, and enterocyte dysfunction. Patients who present with PLE should have a complete hemodynamic evaluation. This is vital because interventions that improve cardiac output have proven successful in PLE. Any Fontan pathway obstruction should be treated and cardiac output optimized with medical therapy, fenestration, or pacing. In the absence of correctable obstructions, PLE portends a poor prognosis despite surgery or cardiac transplantation.

Modern Fontan Operation

The atriopulmonary connection proved an inefficient method of pulmonary blood flow. Colliding streams of blood from the superior and inferior vena cava resulted in energy loss and turbulence within the atrium. The energy required to propel blood forward into the pulmonary vasculature was lost as blood swirled sluggishly in the dilated atrium. The modern Fontan operation is a total cavopulmonary connection (Fig. 8.6). The lateral tunnel Fontan improved pulmonary blood flow, and only the lateral wall of the atrium was exposed to central venous hypertension. There was no dilated atrium to serve as a source of thrombus. The extensive atrial suture lines, however, remained a risk for arrhythmia. The extracardiac Fontan is a further modification of the total cavopulmonary connection. The extracardiac Fontan greatly reduces the number of atrial incisions and hopefully the long-term development of atrial arrhythmias. Reductions in arrhythmia and improvements in overall survival have been noted with the modern Fontan circulation. Results for the extracardiac Fontan are even better than those of the lateral tunnel Fontan but are limited by the shorter duration of follow-up. It is not yet certain if the development of long-term complications has been truly reduced or only delayed.

Preoperative Assessment

Patients with Fontan physiology are presenting in larger numbers for the entire array of noncardiac surgery, including obstetric procedures. Preoperative assessment begins with a directed history, concentrating on functional status and the presence of major complications. Heightened suspicion is clearly needed for patients with atriopulmonary connections and for those with a systemic right ventricle. Patients with Fontan circulation have a low cardiac output state. This low-output state exists despite the presence of good ventricular function, minimal AV valve regurgitation, and low PVR. A cohort of patients with an atriopulmonary Fontan performed at an older age showed striking reductions in anaerobic threshold (<50% of control participants), VO_2 max (<33% of control participants) and systemic ejection fraction both at rest and exercise. Further

186

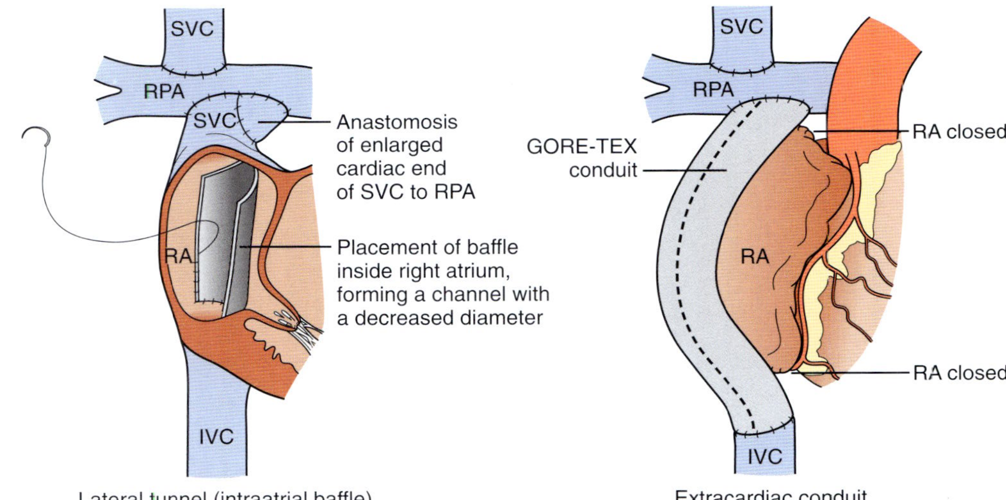

Fig. 8.6 Two variations of the modern Fontan operation: the lateral tunnel and extracardiac operations. *IVC*, Inferior vena cava; *RA*, right atrium; *RPA*, right pulmonary artery; *SVC*, superior vena cava. (From D'Udekem Y, Iyengar AJ, Cochrane AD, et al. The Fontan procedure: contemporary techniques have improved long-term outcomes. *Circulation*. 2007;116[11 suppl]:I157.)

compounding the issue is that patients' self-assessment grossly overestimates their objective exercise capacity. This places the anesthesiologist in a considerable dilemma when faced with a Fontan patient who rates his or her functional status as "good." The authors believe that transthoracic echocardiography should be the initial preoperative investigation and is mandatory except in cases of very minor surgery. Further testing is guided by the results of the echocardiogram and in consultation with a cardiologist experienced in caring for adults with CHD. Normal ventricular function on echocardiogram would stratify the patient as "low risk" only within the context of patients with Fontan circulation.

A term that should immediately get the attention of the anesthesiologist is *failing Fontan*. Specific reasons for failing may differ, but the common denominator in these patients is a marked limitation of functional status. They manifest some combination of refractory arrhythmias, PLE, liver dysfunction, hypoxemia, or congestive heart failure. Although PLE always signifies a failing Fontan, the converse is not always true. That is, patients can have severely limited function with elevated central venous pressures and even evidence of cirrhosis on liver biopsy without demonstrating PLE. Patients with a "failing Fontan" require a search for correctable lesions. First, any obstructions within the Fontan pathway should be treated, preferably with percutaneous techniques of dilation and stenting. Second, loss of sinus rhythm should be treated with pacing. If loss of sinus rhythm is accompanied by severe tachyarrhythmias, Fontan conversion surgery is indicated. Third, some patients develop collateral vessels. Aortopulmonary collaterals result in a progressive volume load on the single ventricle. Collaterals from the venous system to the systemic atrium or ventricle cause hypoxemia. In both cases, large collaterals should be coil occluded in the catheterization laboratory. Another option is the creation of a fenestration, which can improve cardiac output and lower central venous pressures but at the expense of a right-to-left shunt. Unfortunately, not all of these therapeutic options are indicated or successful in every patient. If no realistic hope of further improvement exists, the only option is cardiac transplantation.

The functional state of Fontan patients exists across a spectrum but generally falls into two groups. The first and largest group is made of those who report New York Heart Association (NYHA) I to II level of function but have been shown to possess much less cardiorespiratory reserve than age-matched two-ventricle control participants. These patients will tolerate most surgical procedures with an acceptably low risk. The second group is smaller but consists of patients who have manifested one of more of the "failing Fontan" criteria. Surgery in these patients carries much greater risk and should only be undertaken after careful consultation with physicians experienced in ACHD. When it comes to a discussion of anesthetic technique, the same lessons learned in caring for patients with acquired coronary artery disease apply. That is, there is no right drug for these patients nor is there a single "best" anesthetic technique. Rather, the critical issue is to gain a clear and comprehensive understanding of the patient's pathophysiology. The key is not which drugs are used but rather how they are used. Key principles for patients with Fontan physiology are addressed in Box 8.8.

Ventilatory Management

In an effort to minimize PVR, functional residual capacity should be maintained by the application of small amounts of positive end-expiratory pressure (PEEP) or continuous positive airway pressure (CPAP), and excessive lung volumes should be avoided. PEEP or CPAP will not significantly impede cardiac output if less than 6 cm H_2O. Spontaneous ventilation has been assumed to be optimal for these patients to minimize intrathoracic pressure and encourage forward flow into the pulmonary

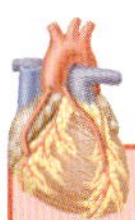

> **BOX 8.8** *Management Principles for Patients With Fontan Physiology*
>
> - Maintenance of preload is essential. A prolonged NPO (nothing by mouth) period without intravenous hydration should be avoided.
> - Regional and neuraxial techniques are attractive options, with appropriate attention to volume status. A neuraxial anesthetic is a poor choice if a high level of block is required. A slowly titrated epidural is preferable to a rapid-acting spinal anesthetic.
> - Airway management must be skilled to avoid hypercarbia and elevations in pulmonary vascular resistance.
> - Adequate levels of anesthesia must be established before stimulating events such as laryngoscopy. A surge of catecholamines may precipitate dangerous tachycardia.
> - Spontaneous ventilation that augments pulmonary blood flow is desirable but must not be pursued at all costs. Spontaneous ventilation under deep levels of anesthesia will result in significant hypercarbia. The benefit of spontaneous ventilation may be negated by the rise in pulmonary vascular resistance secondary to hypercarbia.
> - A plan must be in place to treat tachyarrhythmias.
> - Patients with pacemakers must have the device interrogated before surgery and a plan developed to avoid potential interference from electrocautery, particularly if the patient is pacemaker dependent.
> - If large volume shifts are anticipated, invasive monitoring with central catheters and transesophageal echocardiography is recommended.
> - An appropriate plan for postoperative pain management should be established. The need for anticoagulation in many Fontan patients may preclude the use of epidural analgesia.
> - A cardiologist experienced in caring for patients with congenital heart disease should be involved perioperatively.

circulation, but hard evidence for this approach is mostly lacking. Cardiac output should be optimized by limiting mean airway (intrathoracic) pressure, minimizing peak inspiratory pressure, limiting inspiratory time, using low respiratory rates, and applying judicious amounts of PEEP while using higher tidal volumes to maintain normocarbia. The benefits of very early postoperative tracheal extubation (in the operating room) have been considered particularly useful in these patients.

Pregnancy

It was inevitable that as some of the female Fontan patients reached childbearing age that they would become pregnant. Case reports first began appearing in 1989. Unfortunately, 20 years later, the body of knowledge on this important subject consists primarily of more case reports with no large registry documenting outcomes. The dilemma facing physicians caring for these patients is that Fontan patients are known to have decreased cardiac reserve, even those who report good functional status. Because pregnancy is a "stress test," how a particular Fontan patient will respond is variable, with the literature providing conflicting data. Some series demonstrate that women tolerated pregnancy, labor, and delivery well, but there was an increased risk of spontaneous abortion. More recent series found live birth pregnancies complicated by high rates of NYHA class deterioration, atrial arrhythmia, prematurity, and intrauterine growth retardation. Pregnancy is usually undertaken only in patients with relatively good functional status, thereby removing the highest risk patients.

Undoubtedly, most adult congenital cardiologists would counsel against pregnancy in any patient with evidence of failing Fontan circulation. In patients with good functional status, pregnancy can successfully be carried to term, albeit with increased risk of miscarriage and premature delivery. Epidural analgesia is well tolerated and indeed recommended for the first stage of labor. The cesarean section rate approaches 50%. Neuraxial anesthesia for cesarean section, in addition to its usual benefits, preserves spontaneous ventilation, which is desirable in Fontan patients. However, no increased risk from general anesthesia has been identified. Perioperative complications are low, and peripartum cardiac decompensation is rare.

Patient Ductus Arteriosus

Beyond the neonatal period, spontaneous closure of a PDA is uncommon. The risk of a long-standing moderate to large PDA is volume overloading of the left heart and the development of pulmonary vascular disease. The progression of pulmonary vascular disease is accelerated compared with patients with other types of right-to-left shunts with equivalent degrees of shunting. The development of pulmonary vascular disease is dependent on the volume and pressure of the right-to-left shunt. A PDA delivers blood at high shear stress (i.e., arterial pressure) to the pulmonary vasculature, and flow occurs continuously throughout the cardiac cycle. Over time, the ductus can become calcified or aneurysmally dilated with a risk of rupture. Ductal calcification or aneurysm increases the risk of surgery, which rarely requires CPB. Unrepaired, the natural history is for one-third of patients to die of heart failure, pulmonary hypertension, or endocarditis by 40 years of age and two-thirds by 60 years of age. Although small PDAs are of no hemodynamic consequence, even small PDAs carry a relatively high endocarditis risk. Therefore surgical closure should be considered for all adults with PDA. Transvascular closure by means of one of several devices is possible and is currently the treatment of choice unless excluded by atypical anatomy. If device closure is not practicable, it is possible to do a patch closure from inside the aorta or pulmonary artery.

Small PDAs do not carry a hemodynamic risk in pregnancy. However, the decrease in systemic vascular resistance accompanying pregnancy could lead to right-to-left shunting in a woman with a large PDA.

Pulmonary Valve Stenosis

Long-term asymptomatic survival is typical of patients, with the exception of neonates with critical stenosis. There is a 94% survival rate 20 years after diagnosis, and adults generally do not require surgical intervention. With aging, however, right ventricular fibrosis and failure can develop and represents the most common cause of death, usually in the fourth decade. Almost all patients who have relief of stenosis either surgically or by balloon valvuloplasty have normal right ventricular function postoperatively, although surgical reintervention may be required in a significant number in the long term. Percutaneous pulmonary valve implantation, done in the catheterization laboratory, is another option. However, abnormal ventricular function may not resolve after late surgical correction. Despite the volume overload that accompanies pregnancy, isolated pulmonic valve stenosis, even of a severe degree, is usually well tolerated during pregnancy.

In patients with significant right ventricular hypertension, right ventricular ischemia can occur if systemic hypotension and decreased coronary perfusion occur. Coronary ischemia resolves if coronary perfusion pressure is increased (e.g., with use of phenylephrine).

Tetralogy of Fallot

The classic description of tetralogy of Fallot includes (1) a large, nonrestrictive misaligned VSD with (2) an overriding aorta; (3) infundibular pulmonic stenosis; and (4) right ventricular hypertrophy that are derived from an embryonic antero-cephalad deviation of the outlet septum. However, there is a spectrum of the disease with more severe defects including stenosis of the pulmonic valve, stenosis of the pulmonary valve annulus, or stenosis and hypoplasia of the pulmonary arteries. Pentalogy of Fallot refers to the addition of an ASD. With advances in genetics, up to one-third or more of cases of tetralogy have been ascribed to one of several genetic abnormalities, including trisomy 21, the 22q11 microdeletion, and the genes *NKX 2-5*, *JAG1*, and *GATA4*. Tetralogy of Fallot is the most common cyanotic lesion encountered in the adult population. Unrepaired or nonpalliated, approximately 25% of patients survive to adolescence, after which the mortality rate is 6.6% per year. Only 3% survive to age 40 years. Unlike children, teenagers and adults with tetralogy do not develop "tet spells." Long-term survival with a good quality of life is expected after repair. The 32- to 36-year survival rate has been reported to be 85% to 86%. However, symptoms, primarily arrhythmias and decreased exercise tolerance, occur in 10% to 15% of patients 20 years after the primary repair. In the past, most children with tetralogy were managed with a preliminary palliation via an aortopulmonary shunt such as a Blalock-Taussig followed by complete correction. Essentially, all patients would eventually come for complete repair. Currently, most children are managed with a complete repair in infancy, without preceding palliation.

It is uncommon to encounter an adolescent or adult with an unrepaired tetralogy of Fallot. However, it can be encountered in immigrants or in patients whose anatomic variation was considered to be inoperable when they were children. In tetralogy, the right ventricle "sees" the obstruction from the pulmonic stenosis. PVR is typically normal to low. Right-to-left shunting is caused by obstruction at the level of the right ventricular outflow tract and is unaffected by attempts at modulating PVR. Shunting is minimized, however, by pharmacologically increasing systemic vascular resistance. In an unrepaired adult, systemic hypertension developing in adult life imposes an additional load on both ventricles because there is an unrestrictive VSD. The increase in systemic vascular resistance decreases right-to-left shunting and diminishes cyanosis but at the expense of right ventricular or biventricular failure. Increases in the inotropic state of the heart increase the dynamic obstruction at the right ventricular infundibulum and worsen right-to-left shunting. β-Blockers are often used to decrease inotropy. Halothane was the historic anesthetic of choice in children with tetralogy because of its myocardial depressant effects and ability to maintain systemic vascular resistance. Current practice is to use sevoflurane, without undue consequence from a reduction in systemic vascular resistance. Anesthetic induction in adults can easily be achieved with any of the available agents, keeping in mind the principles of maintenance of systemic blood pressure, avoidance of hypovolemia, and preventing increases in inotropy.

Sudden death or ventricular tachycardia requiring treatment can occur in up to 5.5% of postoperative patients after age 30 years, often years postoperatively. The foci for these arrhythmias are typically in the right ventricular outflow tract in the area of surgery, and they can be ablated in the catheterization laboratory. Older age at repair, severe left ventricular dysfunction, postoperative right ventricular hypertension from residual or recurrent outflow tract obstruction, wide-open pulmonary insufficiency, and prolongation of the QRS (to >180 ms) are all predictors of sudden death. Premature ventricular contractions and even nonsustained ventricular tachycardia are not rare and do not seem to be associated with sudden death, which makes appropriate treatment options difficult. QRS prolongation to longer than 180 ms, although highly sensitive, has a low positive predictive value.

Women with good surgical results without residual defects should tolerate pregnancy and delivery well with outcomes approximating those of the general population. However, there is a significant rate of CHD in the infant. Women with uncorrected tetralogy, particularly those with significant cyanosis, have a high incidence of fetal loss (80% with hematocrit >65%). The fall in systemic vascular resistance that accompanies pregnancy and delivery can worsen cyanosis, and the physiologic volume loading of pregnancy can exaggerate failure of both ventricles.

Transposition of the Great Arteries (D-Transposition)

In D-transposition of the great arteries, there is a discordant connection of the ventricles and the great arteries. The aorta (with the coronary arteries) arises from the right ventricle and the pulmonary artery arises from the left ventricle. Thus, the two circulations are separate. Postnatal survival requires interchange of blood between the two circulations, typically via a patent foramen ovale or a PDA or VSD. With a 1-year mortality rate approaching 100%, all adults with D-transposition have had some type of surgical intervention. Whereas older adults will have had atrial-type repairs (Mustard or Senning), children born after the mid-1980s will have had repair by arterial switch (the Jatene operation). Some will also have had repair of D-transposition with a moderate to large VSD by means of a Rastelli operation.

Atrial repairs function by redirecting systemic venous blood to the left ventricle (and thence to the transposed pulmonary artery) and pulmonary venous blood to the right ventricle (and thence to the aorta). Whereas the Mustard operation uses an intraatrial conduit of native pericardium (Fig. 8.7), the Senning operation uses native atrial tissue to fashion the conduit. The arterial switch operation transposes transected aorta and pulmonary artery such that they then arise above the appropriate ventricle. This operation also requires transposing the coronary arteries from the aorta to the pulmonary root, which after the procedure becomes the aortic root. The Rastelli procedure closes the VSD on a bias such that the left ventricle empties into the aorta and connects the right ventricle to the pulmonary artery by means of a valved conduit.

Atrial repairs result in a systemic right ventricle, and these patients consistently have abnormal right ventricular function that can be progressive with a right ventricular ejection fraction of about 40%. Mild tricuspid insufficiency is common, but severe tricuspid insufficiency suggests the development of severe right ventricular dysfunction. There is an 85% to 90% 10-year survival rate with these operations, but by 20 years, the survival rate is less than 80%. Over 25 years, about half develop moderate right ventricular dysfunction, and one-third develop severe tricuspid insufficiency. Although function always remains abnormal, it has been suggested that earlier surgery minimizes right ventricular dysfunction. Because of the incidence of right ventricular dysfunction, some patients with atrial repairs have been converted to an arterial switch after preparation of the left ventricle by a pulmonary artery band to prepare the ventricle for systemic arterial pressure.

Atrial repairs bring an incidence of late electrophysiologic sequelae, including sinus node dysfunction (bradycardia), junctional escape rhythms, AV block, and supraventricular arrhythmias. Atrial flutter occurs in 20% of patients by age 20 years, with half of them having progressive sinus node dysfunction by that time. On occasion, these tachyarrhythmias can result in sudden death, presumably from 1:1 conduction

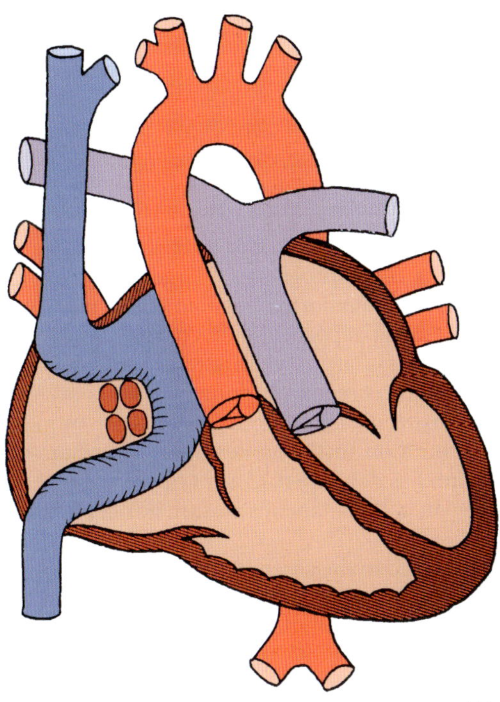

Fig. 8.7 Mustard operation. An intraatrial baffle has directed vena caval blood across the excised atrial septum to the mitral valve and pulmonary venous blood to the tricuspid valve. The right ventricle remains as the systemic ventricle and the left ventricle as the subpulmonary ventricle. (Reprinted with permission from Mullins C, Mayer D. *Congenital Heart Disease: A Diagrammatic Atlas*. New York: Wiley-Liss; 1988.)

producing ventricular fibrillation. The loss of sinus rhythm in the face of right ventricular (the systemic ventricle) dysfunction can also contribute to late sudden death. The risk of late death after an atrial repair is almost three times higher if there is an associated VSD. The incidence of tachyarrhythmias does decrease, however, after the 10th postoperative year.

Survival after an arterial switch operation is approximately 90% at 10 years. Very-long-term outcome after the arterial switch procedure is still not known. It does appear that the mortality rate is essentially 0% after 5 years postoperatively, and late surgical reintervention is mostly due to supravalvular pulmonic stenosis. Neoaortic root dilation, although only rarely requiring repair, has been noted as a long-term problem. Although many of these children have abnormal resting myocardial perfusion, up to 9% can show evidence of exercise-induced myocardial ischemia. The implication for the development of premature coronary artery disease in adulthood is not known, and there is also some concern about the ultimate function of the neoaortic valve. Patients who have had a Rastelli repair will require episodic reoperation for replacement of the prosthetic conduit valve.

After an atrial or a Rastelli repair, pregnancy and delivery are generally well tolerated; however, right ventricular failure and deterioration in functional capacity can occur. Women with an atrial repair in particular have an increased incidence of complications (e.g., prematurity and small-for-date infants).

Ventricular Septal Defects

More than 75% of small and moderate VSDs close spontaneously during childhood by a gradual ingrowth of surrounding septum. Of those that close spontaneously, almost all have closed by 10 years of age. Other mechanisms for natural closure include closure by tricuspid valve tissue, closure by prolapsed aortic leaflet, and closure by endocarditis. Some VSDs result in the development of aortic insufficiency in adults from prolapse of the aortic valve into the defect. Although the risk of endocarditis is ongoing, there is no hemodynamic risk of a small VSD in the adult. If pulmonary vascular disease is present, it can progress if a large VSD is left unrepaired.

Although some studies have reported possible ventricular dysfunction years after surgical repair, these are older reports and by current standard patients were operated on later. It does appear that the ventricle successfully remodels from chronic volume overload if surgical correction is done by 5 years of age and perhaps up to 10 to 12 years of age. Iatrogenic heart block is a possible surgical complication, but this was much more common in the earlier days of cardiac surgery. If significant pulmonary hypertension has developed, closure can sometimes be done by means of a unidirectional valve patch. Percutaneous closure devices for use with certain VSDs are available.

Pregnancy is well tolerated in the absence of preexisting heart failure or pulmonary hypertension. Pregnancy with a naturally or surgically closed defect carries with it no additional risk in the absence of additional cardiac problems.

CONCLUSION

Patients with ACHD pose unique challenges to anesthesiologists when undergoing noncardiac surgery. Understanding the patients' specific CHD, history of palliative or corrective surgeries, and current functional status is imperative to the proper care of such patients. If at all possible, noncardiac surgery on adult patients with moderate to complex CHD should be performed at an adult congenital heart center with the consultation of an anesthesiologist experienced with adult CHD.

SUGGESTED READING

Baumgartner H, Bonhoeffer P, De Groot NM, et al. ESC guidelines for the management of grown-up congenital heart disease (new version 2010). *Eur Heart J.* 2010;31:2915.

Bennett JM, Ehrenfeld JM, Markham L, Eagle SS. Anesthetic management and outcomes for patients with pulmonary hypertension and intracardiac shunts and Eisenmenger syndrome: a review of institutional experience. *J Clin Anesth.* 2014;26:286.

Cannesson M, Earing MG, Collange V, et al. Anesthesia for noncardiac surgery in adults with congenital heart disease. *Anesthesiology.* 2009;111:432–440.

d'Udekem Y, Iyengar AJ, Cochrane AD, et al. The Fontan procedure: contemporary techniques have improved long-term outcomes. *Circulation.* 2007;116:I157.

Diller GP, Dimopoulos K, Broberg CS, et al. Presentation, survival prospects, and predictors of death in Eisenmenger syndrome: a combined retrospective and case-control study. *Eur Heart J.* 2006;27:1737.

Diller GP, Gatzoulis MA. Pulmonary vascular disease in adults with congenital heart disease. *Circulation.* 2007;115:1039.

Gottlieb EA, Andropolous DB. Anesthesia for the patient with congenital heart disease presenting for noncardiac surgery. *Curr Opin Anaesthesiol.* 2013;26(3):318–326.

Hornung TS, Calder L. Congenitally corrected transposition of the great arteries. *Heart.* 2010;96:1154.

Howard-Quijano K, Smith M, Schwarzenberger JC. Perioperative care of adults with congenital heart disease for non-cardiac surgery. *Curr Anesthesiol Rep.* 2013;3:144–150.

Jooste EH, Haft WA, Ames WA, et al. Anesthetic carte of parturients with single ventricle physiology. *J Clin Anesth.* 2013;25:417.

Maxwell BG, Wong JK, Kin C, et al. Perioperative outcomes of major noncardiac surgery in adults with congenital heart disease. *Anesthesiology*. 2013;119:762.

Maxwell BG, Wong JK, Lobato RL. Perioperative morbidity and mortality after noncardiac surgery in young adults with congenital or early acquired heart disease: a retrospective cohort analysis of the National Surgical Quality Improvement Program database. *Am Surg*. 2014;80:321.

Metz TD, Jackson GM, Yetman AT. Pregnancy outcomes in women who have undergone an atrial switch repair for congenital d-transposition of the great arteries. *Am J Obstet Gynecol*. 2011;205:273.e1.

Momenah TS, El Oakley R, Al Najashi K, et al. Extended application of percutaneous pulmonary valve implantation. *J Am Coll Cardiol*. 2009;53:1859.

Mossad EB, Motta P, Vener DF. Anesthetic considerations for adults undergoing Fontan conversion surgery. *Anesthesiol Clin*. 2013;31:405.

O'Leary JM, Siddiqi OK, de Ferranti S, et al. The changing demographics of congenital heart disease hospitalizations in the United States, 1998 through 2010. *JAMA*. 2013;309:984.

Pedersen LM, Pedersen TA, Ravn HB, Hjortdal VE. Outcomes of pregnancy in women with tetralogy of Fallot. *Cardiol Young*. 2008;18:423.

Tempe DK, Virmani S. Coagulation abnormalities in patients with cyanotic congenital heart disease. *J Cardiothorac Vasc Anesth*. 2002;16:752.

Wang LH, Qioa C, Zhang X, et al. Evaluation of different minimally invasive techniques in the surgical treatment of atrial septal defect. *J Thorac Cardiovasc Surg*. 2014;148:188.

Warnes CA, Williams RG, Bashore TM, et al. ACC/AHA 2008 guidelines for the management of adults with congenital heart disease: a report of the American College of Cardiology/American Heart Association Task Force on Practice Guidelines (Writing Committee to Develop Guidelines on the Management of Adults With Congenital Heart Disease). Developed in collaboration with the American Society of Echocardiography, Heart Rhythm Society, International Society for Adult Congenital Heart Disease, Society for Cardiovascular Angiography and Interventions, and Society of Thoracic Surgeons. *J Am Coll Cardiol*. 2008;52:e143.

Williams RG, Pearson GD, Barst RJ, et al. Report of the National Heart, Lung, and Blood Institute Working Group on research in adult congenital heart disease. *J Am Coll Cardiol*. 2006;47:701.

Anesthesia for Noncardiac Surgery

Chapter 9

Cardiovascular Monitoring in Noncardiac Surgery

Gerard R. Manecke Jr, MD • Timothy M. Maus, MD

Key Points

1. Excellent cardiac and hemodynamic management is essential to achieving good outcomes in patients with cardiovascular disease, particularly those undergoing high-risk noncardiac surgery.
2. Much cardiovascular information can be obtained from the standard American Society of Anesthesiologists monitors, including those usually associated with evaluation of respiratory function (pulse oximetry, capnography). The pulse oximeter plethysmograph can be used to assess adequacy of the peripheral circulation; expired capnography reflects pulmonary blood flow and cardiac output.
3. The five-electrode electrocardiographic system commonly used perioperatively allows rapid diagnosis of a wide variety of cardiac abnormalities, including rhythm disturbances, conduction abnormalities, myocardial ischemia, myocardial infarction, and electrolyte abnormalities.
4. Although often unreliable as an intravascular volume monitor, invasive monitoring of the central venous pressure (CVP) can be useful in the management of cardiac patients. CVP provides information about the systolic and diastolic performance of the heart in response to fluid administration, as well as waveform information that can aid in the diagnosis of abnormalities such as tricuspid regurgitation and junctional rhythms.
5. The pulmonary artery catheter is a very powerful monitor, providing a wide array of data that include right-sided pressures, cardiac performance, and a surrogate for left atrial pressure (pulmonary capillary wedge pressure). Although its use has declined in noncardiac surgery, it is still very useful in select patients such as those with pulmonary hypertension or right ventricular failure. It is also useful for monitoring left ventricular function and solving hemodynamic problems when transesophageal echocardiography is unavailable.
6. Minimally invasive and noninvasive means of continuously monitoring arterial blood pressure, as well as cardiac output and dynamic parameters such as stroke volume variation, are now widely used. They are particularly useful in cardiac patients undergoing high-risk surgery. They facilitate perioperative goal-directed therapy (PGDT), enhanced recovery from surgery, and rapid diagnosis of hemodynamic problems.
7. Noninvasive monitors that assess tissue oxygenation, pH, and perfusion are likely to be further developed and used. Because the purpose of circulation is tissue perfusion, it is logical to quantify tissue perfusion and oxygenation. Somatic near-infrared spectroscopy is currently used for this purpose in PGDT algorithms.

Perioperative care includes effective cardiac, hemodynamic, and fluid management. Excellent cardiovascular management is particularly important in patients undergoing major noncardiac surgery and those with preexisting cardiovascular disease. It is only with meaningful, accurate monitoring that appropriate cardiac, hemodynamic, and fluid therapy can be provided. This chapter focuses on the various means by which the cardiac and hemodynamic status can be monitored, ranging from noninvasive to highly invasive techniques. Other indicators of cardiovascular function, such as urine output, are discussed as well. Echocardiography is not discussed here; it is presented in Chapter 10.

STANDARD AMERICAN SOCIETY OF ANESTHESIOLOGISTS MONITORS

Most of the standard American Society of Anesthesiologists (ASA) monitors provide information about the cardiovascular system (Box 9.1). Electrocardiogram (ECG), arterial blood pressure, heart rate, and intraarterial pressure tracings are obviously useful, but those used to monitor respiratory function, such as end-tidal carbon dioxide ($ETCO_2$) and pulse oximetry with its plethysmograph tracing, can also provide valuable cardiovascular information. The standard ASA monitors are listed in Table 9.1.

Electrocardiogram

The ECG is a mainstay for monitoring cardiac status. Continuously monitoring cardiac electrical activity, it provides heart rate and rhythm data, as well as assessment of cardiac conduction (PR interval, QRS duration) and repolarization (ST segment, T-wave morphology, and QT interval). The normal morphologies of the ECG signal and the ECG intervals are shown in Fig. 9.1.

A three-lead system, using three or four electrodes (right arm, left arm, left leg, ground), allows monitoring of limb leads I, II, or III, providing primarily rhythm and conduction data. This can suffice for healthy patients, but a five-electrode system (right arm, left arm, left leg, precordial, ground) is usually used perioperatively and in intensive care units. This system allows simultaneous monitoring of a limb lead (usually lead II) and a precordial "V" lead that enhances the detection of myocardial ischemia. The sensitivity for detecting myocardial ischemia when using a combination of leads II and V_5 has been reported to be 80%. The V lead can be placed according

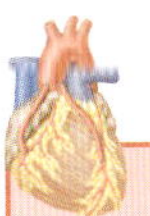

> **BOX 9.1** *Basic Perioperative Monitors of Cardiovascular Function*
>
> - Electrocardiogram
> - Heart rate
> - Noninvasive blood pressure
> - Pulse oximetry with plethysmograph analysis
>   - Perfusion index
>   - Pleth variability index
> - End-tidal carbon dioxide
>   - Pulmonary blood flow
> - Auscultation of heart sounds
>   - Amplitude and frequency of S_1 for inotropic state
>   - Amplitude and frequency of S_2 for systemic blood pressure

Table 9.1 Standard American Society of Anesthesiologists Monitoring

Category	Monitor	Frequency
Circulation	Electrocardiogram[a]	Continual
	Arterial blood pressure[a]	Every 5 min (minimum)
	Heart rate[a]	Every 5 min (minimum)
	Circulatory function (one of the following)[a]:	
	• Auscultation of heart sounds[a]	
	• Intraarterial pressure tracing[a]	Continual
	• Ultrasound of peripheral pulse[a]	
	• Pulse plethysmography or oximetry[a]	
Ventilation	End-tidal carbon dioxide[a]	Continual
Oxygenation	Inspired gas	Continual
	Pulse oximetry[a]	Continual
	Patient color[a]	
Temperature	Temperature probe	Immediately available, when changes in body temperature are anticipated

[a]Parameters that are useful in cardiovascular monitoring.
From American Society of Anesthesiologists Standards for Basic Monitoring, http://www.asahq.org.

to the particular area of interest, ranging from anterior (V_1) to lateral (V_6) (Fig. 9.2), with V_3 to V_5 generally being the most sensitive for anterior-lateral myocardial ischemia (lead II is used for inferior wall ischemia).

Myocardial ischemia most often manifests as ST-segment depression, although elevated ST segments, change in T-wave morphology, new conduction defects, or frequent premature ventricular contractions may also be signs of myocardial ischemia. ECG monitoring systems have automated digital signal processing to continuously display heart rate, QT interval, and ST-segment depression or elevation, as well as alarm systems for these parameters.

Abnormal rhythms, such as sinus bradycardia and tachycardia, junctional rhythms, atrial fibrillation, right and left bundle branch blocks, and heart block, are not uncommon in cardiac patients. All these abnormalities can be detected using a five-electrode system (Tables 9.2 and 9.3). Whereas a limb lead such as lead II is preferred for conduction and rhythm detection, the precordial leads are preferred for diagnosis of myocardial ischemia, infarction, and bundle branch blocks.

Cardiac patients often present with cardiac implantable electrical devices (CIEDs). Paced rhythms (pacing spikes) can be detected best in a limb lead such as lead II, and the timing and number can often allow identification of the type of pacing. CIEDs are discussed in Chapter 4.

Electrolyte abnormalities can cause various conduction and repolarization changes in the heart, with examples being peaked, high T waves in hyperkalemia and U waves in hypokalemia. Leads II and precordial leads are sufficient for detecting these abnormalities.

Electrocardiographic abnormalities more likely represent pathology in patients with cardiac disease than in healthy patients, so understanding and close monitoring of the ECG waveform is particularly important in cardiac patients.

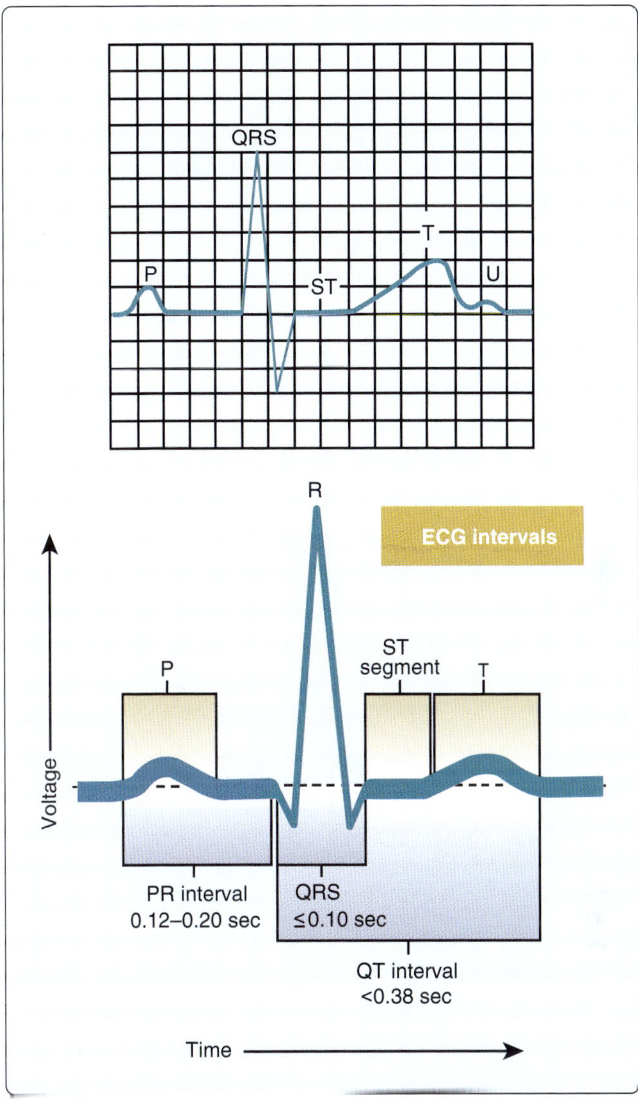

Fig. 9.1 Electrocardiographic morphology of one cardiac cycle and intervals.

Arterial Blood Pressure Monitoring

Intermittent noninvasive arterial blood pressure (NBP) monitoring is typically provided using an automated cuff that detects arterial pulsations using oscillometry. Close monitoring of blood pressure is often required in cardiac patients, and the frequency of measurements can be adjusted to as often as every minute. Care should be exercised, however, because pressure injury can result from prolonged, frequent NBP measurements. An emerging practical alternative is continuous noninvasive blood pressure monitoring, with examples being the Edwards Clearsight and the LiDCO Rapid devices. These systems consist of a finger cuff with mild inflation ("volume clamp method") with a high-resolution bladder and sensor system to detect pulsatile

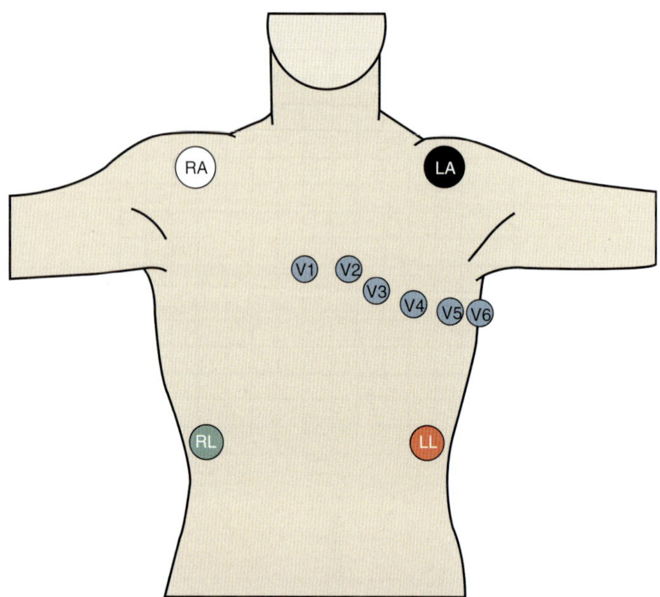

Fig. 9.2 Placement of the five-electrode system commonly used in operating rooms and intensive care units. The precordial lead (V) can be placed according to the area of interest, with the V_3 to V_5 positions generally being the most sensitive for myocardial ischemia.

Table 9.2	Common Perioperative Cardiac Electrical Abnormalities and Their Preferred Lead for Detection	
Cardiac Abnormality	**Preferred Lead**	**Common Characteristics**
Sinus bradycardia	II	HR <60 beats/min, with normal P wave and narrow QRS
Sinus tachycardia	II	HR >100 beats/min, with normal P wave and narrow QRS
Supraventricular tachycardia	II	HR >100 beats/min, narrow QRS
Ventricular tachycardia	II	HR >100 beats/min, wide QRS complex
Junctional (AV nodal) rhythm	II	P waves absent; CVP shows "canon" waves; may be slow
First-degree AV block	II	PR interval >200 ms
Second-degree AV block Mobitz I	II	Progressive lengthening of PR interval culminating in nonconducted P wave
Second-degree AV block Mobitz II	II	Occasional nonconducted P waves
Complete AV block	II	P waves not associated with QRS
Premature ventricular contractions	II	Wide QRS, premature with compensatory pause
Premature atrial contractions	II	Narrow QRS without compensatory pause
Right bundle branch block	Precordial	P wave followed by wide QRS in V_1 and V_2; may be a normal variant

Table 9.2 Common Perioperative Cardiac Electrical Abnormalities and Their Preferred Lead for Detection—cont'd

Cardiac Abnormality	Preferred Lead	Common Characteristics
Left bundle branch block	Precordial	P wave followed by wide QRS in V_5 and V_6; if old, may indicate old conduction system injury; if new, may indicate myocardial ischemia
Myocardial ischemia	Precordial	ST-segment depression
Myocardial infarction	Precordial	ST-segment elevation

AV, Atrioventricular; *CVP,* central venous pressure; *HR,* heart rate.

Table 9.3 Electrocardiographic Morphology of Common Abnormalities Encountered Perioperatively in Cardiac Patients

ECG Diagnosis	Example	Comments
Atrial fibrillation	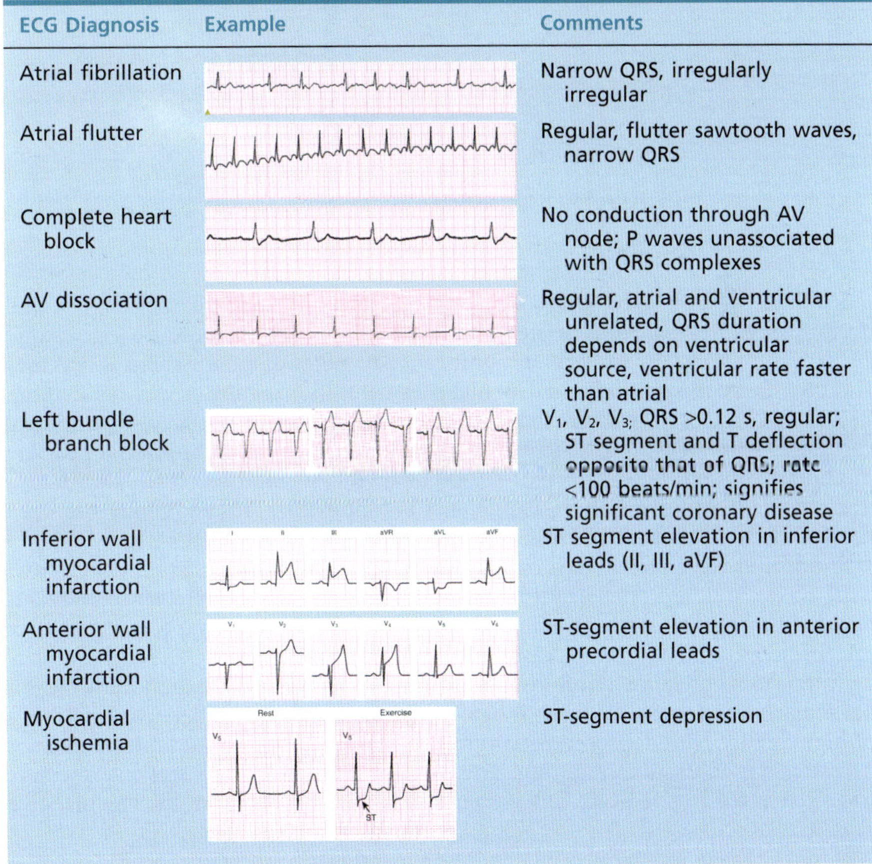	Narrow QRS, irregularly irregular
Atrial flutter		Regular, flutter sawtooth waves, narrow QRS
Complete heart block		No conduction through AV node; P waves unassociated with QRS complexes
AV dissociation		Regular, atrial and ventricular unrelated, QRS duration depends on ventricular source, ventricular rate faster than atrial
Left bundle branch block		V_1, V_2, V_3; QRS >0.12 s, regular; ST segment and T deflection opposite that of QRS; rate <100 beats/min; signifies significant coronary disease
Inferior wall myocardial infarction		ST segment elevation in inferior leads (II, III, aVF)
Anterior wall myocardial infarction		ST-segment elevation in anterior precordial leads
Myocardial ischemia		ST-segment depression

Continued

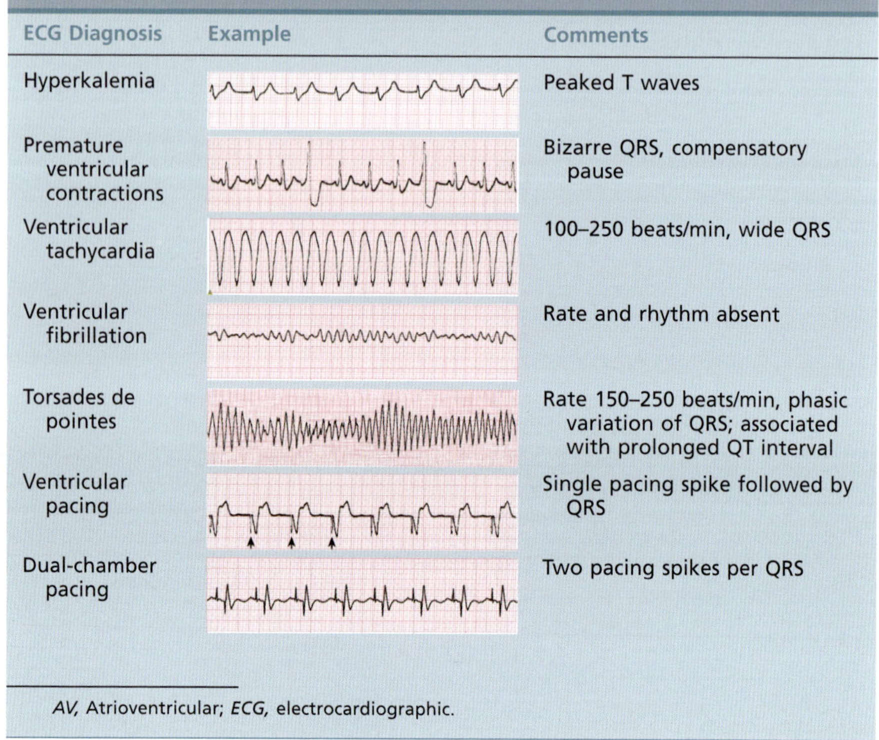

Table 9.3	Electrocardiographic Morphology of Common Abnormalities Encountered Perioperatively in Cardiac Patients—cont'd	
ECG Diagnosis	**Example**	**Comments**
Hyperkalemia		Peaked T waves
Premature ventricular contractions		Bizarre QRS, compensatory pause
Ventricular tachycardia		100–250 beats/min, wide QRS
Ventricular fibrillation		Rate and rhythm absent
Torsades de pointes		Rate 150–250 beats/min, phasic variation of QRS; associated with prolonged QT interval
Ventricular pacing		Single pacing spike followed by QRS
Dual-chamber pacing		Two pacing spikes per QRS

AV, Atrioventricular; *ECG,* electrocardiographic.

pressure. Because they provide a continuous measurement, they are particularly useful during procedures that are associated with rapid changes in blood pressure (e.g., carotid endarterectomy, airway surgery). A significant advantage of these systems is that they also provide cardiac output and dynamic parameter information as well (vide infra). Because the cuff is very distal, they may be inaccurate in cases of severe peripheral vascular disease or vasoconstriction. In those cases, invasive, intra-arterial pressure monitoring should be considered. Another possible method to obtain continuous noninvasive blood pressure measurements is tonometry. This technique has been used at the wrist (Tensys TLine).

Promising experimental techniques include systems using pulse-wave velocity and pulse-wave transit time. In the near future, technology providing noninvasive continuous blood pressure monitoring will almost certainly be widely adopted, supplanting invasive arterial measurement in many cases.

Intraarterial pressure monitoring is indicated for high-risk patients and surgeries, particularly when periodic arterial blood samples will be desired. An arterial wave of high fidelity, with appropriate damping, frequency response, and morphology, is necessary for accurate monitoring. The waveform results from a sine-like pressure wave generated by the heart, with superimposed reflections from the vascular tree (Fig. 9.3).

Arterial access is typically obtained with a catheter in the radial artery, brachial artery, or femoral artery. The dorsalis pedis, ulnar, and axillary arteries have also

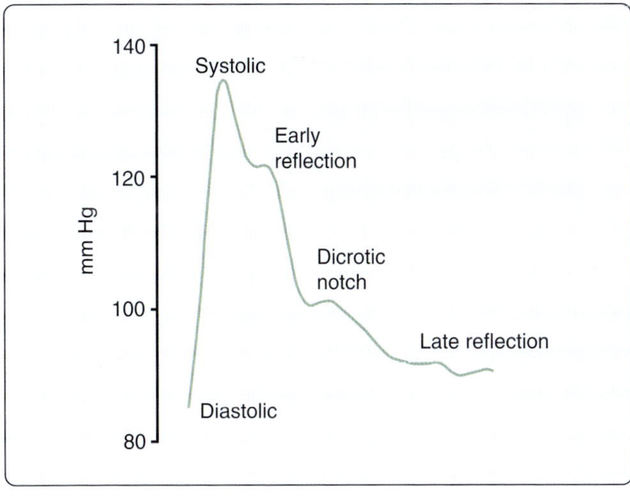

Fig. 9.3 Normal morphology of the radial artery pressure wave is the result of summation of a sine-like wave created by cardiac contraction and reflections from branch points in the vascular tree. The dicrotic notch results from the closure of the aortic valve.

been used. The radial artery is generally preferred because of easy access and the low incidence of complications. Brachial artery catheterization can usually be performed when radial artery attempts are unsuccessful and likewise has a low incidence of complications. Ulnar artery catheterization has been reported to be safe, but it may be ill-advised because in most cases, it provides the bulk of blood flow to the hand. It should not be used if there have been previous unsuccessful attempts at the ipsilateral radial artery or if an Allen text contraindicates its use. If central arterial pressure is required, as in cases in which there is a large central–to–peripheral arterial pressure gradient, the femoral artery can be used. Complications of femoral arterial catheterization include increased risk of infection and retroperitoneal hematoma. Femoral catheterization should be done under strict sterile conditions. When femoral catheterization is performed, surface ultrasound is recommended so as to avoid nearby nerve damage and deep injuries leading to retroperitoneal hematoma.

Pulse Oximetry

Pulse oximetry not only provides arterial oxygen saturation but also heart rate, an index of peripheral perfusion, and a dynamic parameter (pleth variability index [PVI]). These can be useful in assessing circulatory status and potential response to fluid challenge. Like other dynamic parameters such as pulse pressure variation (PPV), stroke volume variation (SVV), and systolic pressure variation (SPV), PVI results from cyclical changes in left ventricular filling associated with the respiratory cycle. Large changes indicate the likelihood that volume infusion will increase the cardiac output. Dynamic parameters such as PVI, when used during positive-pressure ventilation with tidal volumes of 8 mL/kg or greater and in the absence of frequent arrhythmias, are far more sensitive for potential volume responsiveness than any other clinically available metric, including central venous pressure (CVP) and pulmonary artery pressure. The primary mechanism for dynamic fluctuations in cardiac output is depicted in Fig. 9.4.

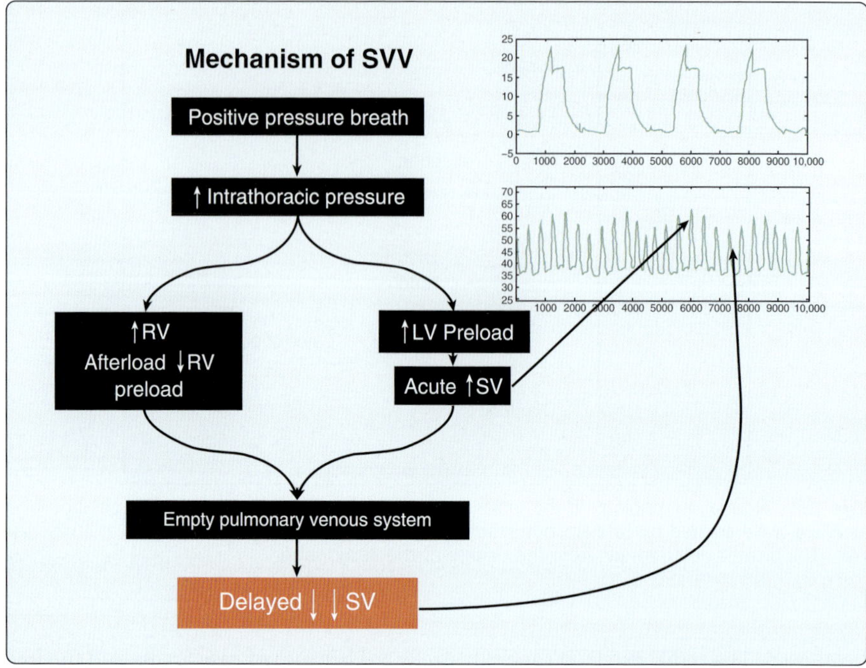

Fig. 9.4 Primary mechanism for dynamic changes in left ventricular (LV) stroke volume (SV) induced by positive-pressure ventilation. Positive pressure initially increases LV venous return by compressing the pulmonary veins, but this intrathoracic pressure decreases right-sided venous return, resulting in a delayed decrease in LV stroke volume. *RV,* Right ventricular; *SVV,* stroke volume variation.

Expired Carbon Dioxide

End-tidal carbon dioxide monitoring has revolutionized airway management, being an immensely valuable tool to confirm adequate ventilation. In addition to being a respiratory monitor, however, it also serves as a valuable adjunct in assessing the circulation. Expiration of CO_2 *from* the lungs requires delivery of CO_2 *to* the lungs *via* the pulmonary circulation. Therefore decreased blood flow to the lungs results in a decrease in $ETCO_2$ (Table 9.4). Indeed, cardiac output monitoring has been performed using expired carbon dioxide and a modification of the Fick equation, and expired CO_2 is now used as a metric in advanced cardiac life support to confirm adequate chest compressions and resuscitation.

URINE OUTPUT, pH, BASE DEFICIT, AND LACTATE

Urine output can be used as an index of cardiovascular stability, but in the perioperative period, it is neither sensitive nor specific. Oliguria and polyuria can be multifactorial, with a plethora of potential causes for each. Oliguria may result from hypovolemia, azotemia, heart failure, perioperative stress hormone release, patient positioning (e.g., Trendelenburg), mechanical obstruction, and surgical interruption of the urinary tract. Polyuria can result from osmotic diuretic administration, hyperglycemia, and diabetes insipidus. Thus urine output must be interpreted in the context of all other

Table 9.4 Common Circulatory Conditions That Result in Decreased Pulmonary Blood Flow and Thus Decreased Expired Carbon Dioxide

Circulatory Conditions Causing ↓ ETCO$_2$	Common Mechanisms
Pulmonary embolus	Mechanical obstruction of pulmonary blood flow by thrombus, fat, or air
RV failure	RV myocardial failure with decreased pulmonary blood flow may result from pulmonary hypertension, pneumothorax, cardiac tamponade, tricuspid regurgitation, myocardial ischemia, and myocardial infarction
↓ Left-sided CO	Hypovolemia, tamponade, LV failure can decrease overall CO and right-sided output, resulting in decreased pulmonary blood flow

CO, Cardiac output; *ETCO$_2$,* end-tidal carbon dioxide; *LV,* left ventricular; *RV,* right ventricular.

events occurring in the perioperative period, not as a primary index of cardiovascular performance or volume status. Similarly, blood pH, base deficit, and serum lactate require interpretation using other clinical parameters. There are many potential reasons for acidosis, high base deficit, and accumulating lactate, and their presence should prompt further investigation. Their presence should not, however, cause the provider to assume that hypovolemia is their cause. Like urine output, they should be used as adjuncts in understanding the patients' circulatory condition.

INVASIVE MONITORING

Central Venous Catheterization

Central venous pressure has long been used as a surrogate for intravascular volume (Table 9.5). It is typically obtained by placing a catheter in the internal jugular, subclavian, external jugular, or femoral veins. Placement should be done under strict sterile conditions using ultrasound guidance so as to improve first-pass success and decrease complications.

In individual patients, CVP can be used to trend the response of the right heart to volume, but it may be unreliable as a guide to fluid management. Its unreliability stems from the multifactorial nature of its genesis. Although fluid administration may increase CVP and hypovolemia decreases CVP, other factors, such as right heart diastolic and systolic function, right atrial compliance, central venous compliance, patient position, surgical pressure on the inferior vena cava, and minor changes in transducer height, confound its meaning. In addition, emergencies such as tension pneumothorax, hemothorax, and cardiac tamponade render CVP of little use in volume resuscitation (although high CVP may aid in making those diagnoses). In the absence of these confounders, CVP can be useful for trending, but as an index of how the heart is handling the amount of volume it is receiving, not as an index of volume status per se.

Table 9.5	Types of Cardiovascular Monitoring		
Cardiac		**Hemodynamic**	**Tissue Perfusion**
ECG Cardiac output • Thermodilution • Arterial pulse • Esophageal Doppler • Bioimpedance Inotropic state • Doppler peak velocity • Doppler maximum acceleration		Arterial BP • Noninvasive intermittent • Noninvasive continuous • Invasive continuous Cardiac output Central pressures • CVP • PAP	NIRS Mixed venous O_2 saturation Central venous O_2 saturation, U/O, pH, base deficit, lactate

BP, Blood pressure; *CVP,* central venous pressure; *ECG,* electrocardiogram; *NIRS,* near-infrared spectroscopy; *PAP,* pulmonary artery pressure; *U/O,* urinary output.

There are CVP waveform characteristics that can be useful for diagnosis. For example, large C-V waves may indicate tricuspid regurgitation, and "canon waves" may confirm a junctional rhythm. The CVP, together with mean arterial pressure, can be used to determine perfusion of the brain and other organs, and these parameters can be manipulated for the patient's benefit. For example, cerebral perfusion pressure can be augmented by lowering the CVP with a venodilator such as nitroglycerin or patient positioning while maintaining or raising mean arterial pressure using an arterial vasoconstrictor:

$$\text{Cerebral perfusion pressure} = \text{Mean arterial pressure} - \text{CVP}$$

A central venous catheter can have added benefits: secure, central venous access for administration of drugs and fluids and as a port for blood sampling. Central venous PO_2 and saturation can be determined, aiding in the assessment of adequacy of cardiac output. Central venous catheters with continuous oximetry are commercially available for monitoring of central venous oxygen saturation and can aid in management of critically ill patients, as well as perioperative goal-directed therapy (PGDT) (see Chapter 19).

Pulmonary Artery Catheterization

The pulmonary artery catheter is an extremely powerful device, capable of providing an impressive amount of hemodynamic information (Table 9.6). Lately, in the absence of large randomized trials showing its benefit, its use has declined in noncardiac surgery. It still, however, can be very useful in certain patients, particularly those with pulmonary hypertension or right ventricular failure. Pulmonary vascular resistance can be very useful in tracking response to pulmonary vasodilators, such as inhaled nitric oxide, and CVP or right atrial pressure measurement provides valuable insight into the function of the right heart.

In very-high-risk noncardiac surgical patients, particularly those with right-sided cardiovascular pathology, pulmonary artery catheterization should be strongly considered. For example, pulmonary artery catheterization is still commonly used in liver transplantation because of the large fluid shifts and blood loss associated

Table 9.6   **Capabilities of the Pulmonary Artery Catheter**

Physiologic Data Provided by the Pulmonary Artery Catheter	Circulation, Method, Utilization
Pulmonary artery pressure, pulmonary vascular resistance	PVR = (mPAP − PCWP/CO) × 80
Systemic vascular resistance	SVR = ([MAP − CVP]/CO) × 80
Pulmonary capillary wedge pressure	May be a surrogate for left atrial pressure and intravascular volume status; waveform can indicate myocardial ischemia or mitral regurgitation (C-V waves)
Central venous pressure	Right ventricular performance; may be surrogate for intravascular volume status
Right-side cardiac output	Thermodilution
Mixed venous oxygenation	PO_2 or saturation at distal port; indicator of adequacy of tissue perfusion; may be used for calculation of cardiac output and shunt
Central venous oxygenation	PO_2 or saturation at central venous port; indicator of adequacy of tissue perfusion
Diagnosis and management of VSD with left-to-right shunt	Blood gases: "step up" in oxygenation between right atrium and right ventricle

CO, Cardiac output; *MAP,* mean arterial pressure; *mPAP,* mean pulmonary artery pressure; *PCWP,* pulmonary capillary wedge pressure; *PVR,* pulmonary vascular resistance; *SVR,* systemic vascular resistance.

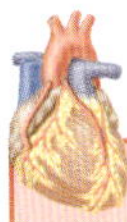

9

BOX 9.2   *Complications of Central Monitoring*

- Central venous access
  - Pneumothorax
  - Hemothorax
  - Arterial puncture leading to stroke, hematoma, bleeding
  - Thoracic duct trauma (left internal jugular approach)
  - Embolism
  - Sepsis
- PA catheterization
  - PA rupture
  - PA occlusion, thrombosis

PA, Pulmonary artery.

with the operation and the pulmonary hypertension that liver failure patients often demonstrate. Pulmonary artery catheterization facilitates complex hemodynamic problem solving, particularly when transesophageal echocardiography is unavailable.

Central venous and pulmonary artery catheterization are associated with potentially devastating complications, including pneumothorax, hemothorax, pulmonary artery rupture, thoracic duct damage, embolism, and sepsis (Box 9.2). Thus they should be used only by experienced personnel and only in patients likely to benefit.

MINIMALLY INVASIVE AND NONINVASIVE HEMODYNAMIC MONITORING

The importance of careful fluid management and optimization of hemodynamics during surgery is now widely appreciated. Tools that facilitate PGDT have thus become popular. Minimally invasive ways to assess the cardiac output and dynamic parameters using arterial pressure waves and esophageal Doppler (ED) have undergone multiple generations of development such that they are now accurate in most circumstances. Thoughtful, informed use of these monitors with associated appropriate therapy decreases hospital length of stay, complications, morbidity, and mortality in high-risk surgical patients. Careful fluid and hemodynamic management is integral to enhanced recovery after surgery (ERAS) programs. Cardiac output monitors not only allow the provider to optimize cardiac performance and peripheral perfusion, but they also facilitate quick problem solving when adverse hemodynamic events occur. For example, in the case of arterial hypotension, knowing the patients' cardiac output and SVV quickly allows clinicians to determine if the problem is decreased preload, afterload, or contractility. With only standard monitors such as heart rate and blood pressure, such immediate, definitive determinations are impossible. Hemodynamic monitoring for ERAS programs, PGDT, and the use of a four-quadrant approach to hemodynamic problem solving are discussed in Chapter 19.

Arterial Pulse Wave

It has been long known that in the absence of changes in vascular tone, the stroke volume and resulting pulse wave are proportional to one another. They are related to one another by a proportionality constant K:

$$\text{Stroke volume} = \text{Pulsatility} \times \text{K}$$

Pulsatility can be expressed as pulse pressure, area under the pulse curve, or other proprietary pulse indices. Classically, K (calibration constant) would be determined using a different, separate cardiac output determination, such as thermodilution (calibration to another method). Self-calibrating methods have now become available using characteristics of the arterial wave (e.g., Edwards FloTrac). This has allowed easy use, requiring only an arterial catheter. The LiDCO Rapid system can self-calibrate and can also be calibrated to another method. Both of these systems can now be used noninvasively (no arterial catheter required), with the finger cuff "volume clamp" method. The arterial pulse wave cardiac output, along with the dynamic parameters provided, such as PPV and SVV, have been successfully used in PGDT algorithms, helping to improve outcome.

Esophageal Doppler

Esophageal Doppler (ED) has been the most studied, preferred method of minimally invasive monitoring for PGDT. It is performed by placing a small, disposable ultrasound probe in the esophagus, adjusted such that the ultrasound beam faces the descending aorta (Fig. 9.5). The Doppler equation:

$$V = \frac{C(Fs - Ft)}{2Ft(\cos\theta)}$$

is applied to the returning signal, allowing calculation of the blood flow velocity in the descending aorta. The Doppler equation calculates the velocity of blood motion from the resulting change in frequency of a transmitted ultrasound wave. V is blood

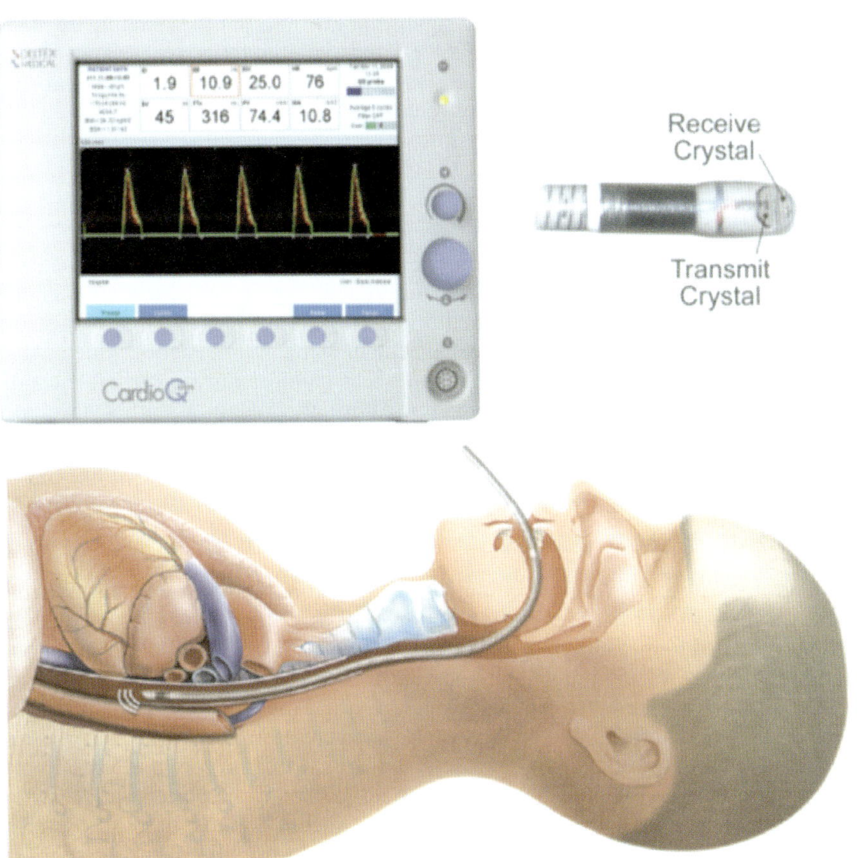

Fig. 9.5 Configuration of the esophageal Doppler system.

Table 9.7	Esophageal Doppler Parameters for Cardiovascular Assessment	
Parameter	**Significance**	**Goal**
Stroke volume index	Cardiac performance	>35 mL/m²
Cardiac index	Cardiac performance	>2.5 L/min/m²
Flow time (corrected)	Preload	>350 ms
Peak velocity	Cardiac contractility	>50 cm/s
Mean acceleration	Cardiac contractility	>10 cm/s²

flow velocity, C is the speed of sound, Ft is the transmitted frequency, Fs is the sensed frequency, and θ is the angle of incidence of the Doppler beam on the moving blood. The area under the velocity wave is calculated (velocity time integral [VTI], stroke distance). This value is then multiplied by the area of the descending aorta, as estimated by the patient's body characteristics, yielding stroke volume:

$$\text{Stroke volume} = \text{VTI} \times \text{Area}$$

Various ED parameters can be useful for hemodynamic assessment (Table 9.7).

Placement and use of the ED requires significant learning, but the resulting increased understanding of cardiovascular physiology and patient status are well worth the effort. With experience, the probe can be positioned quickly, and the real-time hemodynamic parameters and velocity waveform can be very valuable.

Bioimpedance and Cardiac Velocitometry

Progress in electrical signal acquisition and processing has led to improvements in bioimpedance technology and a related approach, cardiac velocitometry. Highly sensitive electrodes record changes in thoracic impedance related to cardiac stroke volumes. Cardiac velocitometry is an enhancement using bioimpedance, which makes use of the fact that the orientation of blood cells changes during cardiac ejection, resulting in changes in thoracic impedance. Although validation studies have been encouraging, application of bioimpedance to surgical patients has been limited by the effects of abdominal and thoracic surgery on thoracic impedance.

Near-Infrared Spectroscopy

Circulation exists to provide one thing: tissue perfusion. Near-infrared spectroscopy (NIRS), a surrogate for tissue perfusion, is now used as a "target" in PGDT algorithms. NIRS is designed to measure oxygen saturation of pulsatile and nonpulsatile (venous) blood, thereby providing an estimate of overall tissue oxygenation. A near-infrared light beam is transmitted into the tissue of interest, and the returning beam undergoes spectroscopy for determination of hemoglobin oxygen saturation. NIRS has primarily been used for cerebral oxygenation assessment in cardiac surgery and critical care but may also be used for assessment of peripheral perfusion via placement of sensors on the abdomen (somatic NIRS) and the thenar eminence. Hemodynamic monitoring ultimately will involve direct indices of tissue perfusion with spectroscopy, local biomarkers, or imaging.

CONCLUSION

Careful hemodynamic and fluid management is essential in the care of cardiac patients, particularly those undergoing high-risk noncardiac surgery. Many tools can be used to assess the circulation, ranging from the standard ASA monitors to those that assess cardiac output and dynamic parameters. The choice of monitors should be based on the individual situation, with the goals of preserving cardiac function and providing good tissue perfusion.

SUGGESTED READING

American Society of Anesthesiologists. Standards for Basic Monitoring. http://www.asahq.org/quality-and-practice-management/practice-guidance-resource-documents/standards-for-basic-anesthetic-monitoring.

Bednarczyk JM, Fridfinnson JA, Kumar A, et al. Incorporating dynamic assessment of fluid responsiveness into goal-directed therapy: a systemic review and meta-analysis. *Crit Care Med.* 2017;45:1538–1545.

Butler E, Chin M, Aneman A. Peripheral near-infrared spectroscopy: methodologic aspects and a sytematic review. *J Cardiothorac Vasc Anesth.* 2017;31:1407–1416.

Cronin B. Pulmonary artery catheter placement using transesophageal echocardiography. *J Cardiothorac Vasc Anesth.* 2016;31:178–183.

Hattori K, Maeda T, Masubuchi T, et al. Accuracy and trending ability of the fourth generation FloTrac/Vigileo system in patients with low cardiac index. *J Cardiothorac Vasc Anesth*. 2017;31:99–104.

Landesberg G, Mosseri M, Wolf Y, Vesselov Y, Weissman C. Perioperative myocardial ischemia and infarction: identification by continuous 12-lead electrocardiogram with online ST-segment monitoring. *Anesthesiology*. 2002;96(2):264–270.

Maus T, Lee D. Arterial-based cardiac output assessment. *J Cardiothorac Vasc Anesth*. 2008;22(3):468–473.

Meng L, Heerdt PM. Perioperative goal-directed haemodynamic therapy based on flow parameters: a concept in evolution. *Br J Anaesth*. 2016;117(S3):iii3–iii17.

Monnet T, Robert J-M, et al. Assessment of changes in left ventricular systolic function with oesophageal Doppler. *Br J Anaesth*. 2013;111(5):743–749.

Ollila A, Virolainen J, Vanhatalo J, et al. Postoperative cardiac ischemia detection by continuous 12 lead electrocardiographic monitoring in vascular surgery. *J Cardiothorac Vasc Anesth*. 2017;31:50–956.

Pearse RM, Harrison DA, MacDonald N, et al. Effect of a perioperative, cardiac output-guided hemodynamic therapy algorithm on outcomes following major gastrointestinal surgery: a randomized clinical trial and systemic review. *JAMA*. 2014;311:2181–2190.

Peter L, Noury N, Cerny M. A review of methods for non-invasive and continuous blood pressure monitoring: pulse transit time method is promising? *IRBM*. 2014;35:271–282.

Romagnoli S, Franchi F, Ricci Z, et al. The pressure recording analytical method (PRAM): technical concepts and literature review. *J Cardiothorac Vasc Anesth*. 2017;31:1460–1470.

Song IK, Ro S, Lee JH, et al. Reference levels for central venous pressure and pulmonary artery occlusion pressure monitoring in the lateral position. *J Cardiothorac Vasc Anesth*. 2017;31:939–943.

Troianos CA, Hartmann GS, et al. Guidelines for performing ultrasound guided vascular cannulation: recommendations of the American Society of Echocardiography and the Society of Cardiovascular Anesthesiologists. *J Am Soc Echocardiogr*. 2011;24:1291–1318.

Weiner MM, Geldard P, Mittnacht AJ. Ultrasound-guided vascular access: a comprehensive review. *J Cardiothorac Vasc Anesth*. 2013;27:345–360.

Wiener RS, Welch HG. Trends in the use of pulmonary artery catheters in the United States, 1993-2004. *JAMA*. 2007;298:423–429.

Chapter 10

Echocardiography in Noncardiac Surgery

Byron Fergerson, MD • Joshua Zimmerman, MD, FASE • Timothy M. Maus, MD

Key Points

1. The portability, ease of use, and rapid diagnostic capability of transesophageal echocardiography (TEE) make it the diagnostic modality of choice during acute hemodynamic instability.
2. Qualitative analysis of a condensed TEE examination aids in efficiency during the rapid diagnostic demands required in the emergency setting.
3. Rescue echocardiography is a process, not an event, and thus requires continuous reevaluation when treating hemodynamic instability.
4. Acute valvular insufficiency is evaluated in the same manner as chronic insufficiency, with a focus on new-onset regurgitation or a large change in chronic regurgitation.
5. An intimal flap visualized on TEE is the best method of determining the presence of aortic dissection.
6. TEE findings in cardiac tamponade include hypoechoic fluid around the heart, systolic collapse of the right atrium, and exaggerated respiratory variation in right and left ventricular (LV) inflow and outflow.
7. The complex geometry of the right ventricle makes quantitative assessment of function difficult. Qualitative evaluation of right ventricular free wall thickening, tricuspid annular excursion, and interventricular septal shape aid in diagnosis of dysfunction.
8. Although echocardiography is not the tool of choice for diagnosing pulmonary embolism (PE), it can help to guide management. The primary echocardiographic manifestations of PE are secondary to right heart failure.
9. LV dysfunction has multiple possible causes beyond ischemia. Qualitative assessment of function primarily through the LV short-axis view is a well-validated method of diagnosing dysfunction.
10. A hypercontractile left ventricle can lead to a dynamic outflow obstruction that is diagnosed by a dagger-shaped LV outflow pattern on Doppler imaging.
11. Alterations in the end-diastolic and end-systolic areas of the LV short-axis view help determine whether hemodynamic instability is caused by hypovolemia or low afterload.
12. Pulsed-wave Doppler interrogation of the LV outflow tract can yield a stroke distance from which the stroke volume (SV) can be calculated.
13. The ability to assess multiple cardiac parameters, including contractility, valvular function, and loading conditions, makes TEE a valuable tool in general hemodynamic monitoring and goal-directed therapy.
14. In conjunction with echocardiographic assessments of SV and contractility, Doppler-derived estimates of left atrial pressure can be used to evaluate the effectiveness of an intervention.
15. Transthoracic echocardiography can be very useful in the perioperative management of patients undergoing noncardiac surgical procedures. It can be substituted for TEE in many situations.

This chapter focuses on the applications of echocardiography to noncardiac surgical procedures. Echocardiography performed in the emergency setting, also known as rescue echocardiography, is discussed in detail. In addition, the utility of echocardiography as a hemodynamic monitor in general and the use of echocardiography in goal-directed fluid therapy are reviewed. Finally, the perioperative applications of transthoracic echocardiography (TTE) and instructions for performing a basic TTE examination are discussed.

RESCUE ECHOCARDIOGRAPHY

Echocardiography in general and transesophageal echocardiography (TEE) in particular are well suited for the rapid diagnostic demands of acute hemodynamic instability. The American Society of Echocardiography (ASE) recommends the use of TEE for acute, persistent, unexplained hypotension. Unexplained hypotension has multiple possible causes that potentially require a wide range of diagnostic modalities. Echocardiography encapsulates these modalities through its ability to reveal disturbances in contractility, valvular function, volume, and intracardiac and extracardiac pressures. Echocardiography not only provides a detailed, quantitative analysis but also allows for qualitative monitoring through rapid visual assessment. The ease and speed with which echocardiography can reveal diagnoses make it an ideal diagnostic modality in the emergency setting and one that is easily teachable.

Prospective data on the use of echocardiography in the emergency perioperative setting are sparse. Several reports have shown the benefit of using both TTE and TEE during hemodynamic instability, confirming the use of echocardiography in this role. It has been shown to be helpful in not only explaining the cause of the instability but also in guiding hemodynamic support or changes to surgical approach.

Inherent in the assessment of hemodynamic instability is urgency. The cause of the instability must be rapidly diagnosed and managed. To aid in efficiency, rescue echocardiography is best performed through a qualitative analysis of a condensed examination. The value of focusing on visual estimation of hemodynamic parameters instead of a detailed quantitative analysis is recognized by the ASE and the Society of Cardiovascular Anesthesiologists (SCA), which have created training pathways for basic TEE certification. The echocardiography literature is replete with examples of practitioners with limited training who accurately perform and evaluate echocardiographic examinations by using primarily qualitative analyses. The comprehensive TEE examination is effective but time consuming, and a condensed examination focusing only on the essential views significantly improves efficiency. The limited examination (Box 10.1) is a modification of the 11 cross-sectional views recommended by the ASE and SCA for the basic TEE examination and covers most clinically relevant disorders. Cardiac disturbances found on the limited examination can be further analyzed by using appropriate additional views. In agreement with the ASE and SCA, we suggest performing and storing the examination in its entirety before focusing on segments specific to the area of interest.

Rescue echocardiography is a process, not an event. The cardiovascular (CV) system is complex and dynamic, changing frequently based on loading conditions. What may be considered an appropriate intervention one minute may not be the next. As many as 14% of instances of hemodynamic instability may have no echocardiographic findings to explain their hemodynamic instability. In these scenarios, it is often difficult to discern the precise cause of the CV abnormality, particularly with regard to low afterload, hypovolemia, and right ventricular (RV) and left ventricular (LV) dysfunction. In addition, multiple abnormalities may be present. A best-guess approach to the

10

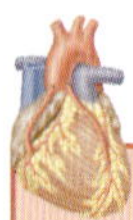

> **BOX 10.1** *Recommended Limited Transesophageal Echocardiographic Examination*
>
> 1. ME AV SAX view
> 2. ME AV LAX view
>   • Measurement of LVOT diameter
> 3. ME bicaval view
> 4. ME RV inflow–outflow view
> 5. ME four-chamber view
>   • With and without CFD on the TV and MV
>   • PWD of mitral Inflow
> 6. ME two-chamber view
>   • PWD of left upper pulmonary vein
> 7. ME LV LAX view
> 8. Midesophageal ascending aortic SAX
> 9. TG LV SAX view
> 10. Deep TG view
>   • PWD of LVOT
>   • Calculation of stroke volume
> 11. Descending aorta SAX view
>
> *AV,* Aortic valve; *CFD,* color-flow Doppler; *LAX,* long-axis; *LV,* left ventricular; *LVOT,* left ventricular outflow tract; *ME,* midesophageal; *MV,* mitral valve; *PWD,* pulsed-wave Doppler; *RV,* right ventricular; *SAX,* short-axis; *TG,* transgastric; *TV,* tricuspid valve.

Table 10.1 Causes of Acute Valvular Dysfunction

Aortic Valve Insufficiency	Mitral Valve Insufficiency
Endocarditis	Endocarditis
Aortic dissection	Chordal rupture
Chest trauma	Papillary muscle rupture
Iatrogenic causes	Ischemic cardiomyopathy
	Iatrogenic causes

abnormality is suggested followed by reevaluation after the proposed intervention. If parameters improve, the intervention should be continued. If they do not improve or worsen, an alternate diagnosis should be sought.

The most common causes of hemodynamic instability are acute valvular and aortic disease, cardiac tamponade, RV dysfunction, pulmonary embolism (PE), and LV hypocontractility and hypercontractility.

Acute Valvular Dysfunction

Although it must be considered in the differential diagnosis, acute new valvular insufficiency is an unlikely cause of hemodynamic instability. If it occurs, it is more likely to occur on left-sided valvular structures. Potential causes of acute aortic valve (AV) and mitral valve (MV) insufficiencies are listed in Table 10.1. The echocardiographic evaluation of valvular dysfunction is similar regardless of the acuity of the dysfunction. Assessment of valvular regurgitation with rescue echocardiography should be limited to a rapid, qualitative assessment. Quantitative measures such as effective regurgitant orifice area and regurgitant volume may be inaccurate in acute regurgitation. Visual assessment of the regurgitant jet with color-flow Doppler (CFD) focusing primarily on the vena contracta is the preferred approach. It is unlikely that any regurgitation that is less than moderate to severe would cause significant hemodynamic instability. The detection of new-onset severe mitral regurgitation intraoperatively should prompt an evaluation for myocardial ischemia (i.e., wall motion abnormalities). Because the papillary muscles originate from the underlying myocardial walls, wall motion abnormalities may lead to papillary muscle dysfunction with resultant leaflet tethering and mitral regurgitation (Fig. 10.1). One or both of the leaflets may be affected, so the determination of central versus eccentric jets does not include or exclude myocardial ischemia.

Because chronic regurgitation leads to myocardial remodeling, moderate to severe regurgitation in the setting of a normal ventricular size should alert the clinician to the high probability of new-onset dysfunction. Noting new-onset regurgitation or a large change in chronic regurgitation is more important than grading the severity of the regurgitation. Acute or subacute regurgitation in the setting of hemodynamic instability may be either the cause or a manifestation of changes in ventricular function and loading induced by another cardiac abnormality. Treatment of the underlying abnormality may improve the regurgitation.

Although new acute valvular pathology is a less likely intraoperative event, hemodynamic instability that results from an unrecognized presence of existing valvular disease is much more likely. For example, the induction of anesthesia in a patient with previously undiagnosed aortic stenosis may lead to hypotension with resultant myocardial ischemia. Prompt diagnosis and therapy are key to maintaining adequate coronary perfusion pressure and preventing a downward spiral of worsening hemodynamics. Again, the detection of aortic stenosis in the noncardiac operating room is more qualitative than quantitative. Calculating gradients is time consuming and may underestimate the severity in the setting of coexisting LV systolic dysfunction. Semiquantitatively, leaflet separation may be calculated or estimated in the mid-esophageal (ME) AV long-axis view (LAX). Leaflet separation greater than 15 mm denotes the lack of aortic stenosis, but leaflet separation of less than 8 mm carries a

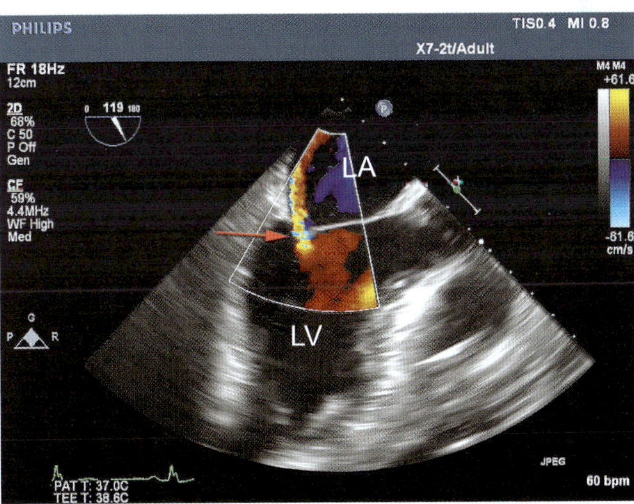

Fig. 10.1 Midesophageal four-chamber view in a patient with active ischemia and restricted posterior mitral valve leaflet *(red arrow)*. Note the posteriorly directed wall hugging (Coanda effect) mitral regurgitant jet. *LA,* Left atrium; *LV,* left ventricle.

97% positive predictive value of severe aortic stenosis (Fig. 10.2). Additionally, the ME AV short-axis (SAX) view may demonstrate significant calcium deposition and leaflet restriction and allow the estimation of AV area via planimetry (i.e., the tracing of the AV opening).

Acute Aortic Disease

The mortality rate is high in acute dissection of the thoracic aortic and increases with a delay in diagnosis. Helical computed tomography, magnetic resonance imaging (MRI), and TEE are equally reliable for diagnosing or ruling out a dissection, but TEE has the advantage of portability. The thoracic aorta may be visualized throughout the ME ascending aortic, upper esophageal aortic arch, and descending thoracic aortic views. Recognition of a blind spot preventing visualization with TEE of the distal ascending aorta and proximal aortic arch caused by the interposition of the trachea between the esophagus and aorta is essential to preventing a missed diagnosis.

The diagnosis of dissection is based on the detection of an intimal flap that divides the aorta into true and false lumina. The characteristics of the true and false lumens are summarized in Table 10.2. In general, the true lumen tends to be smaller and round in shape during systole, with systolic expansion and early laminar flow on

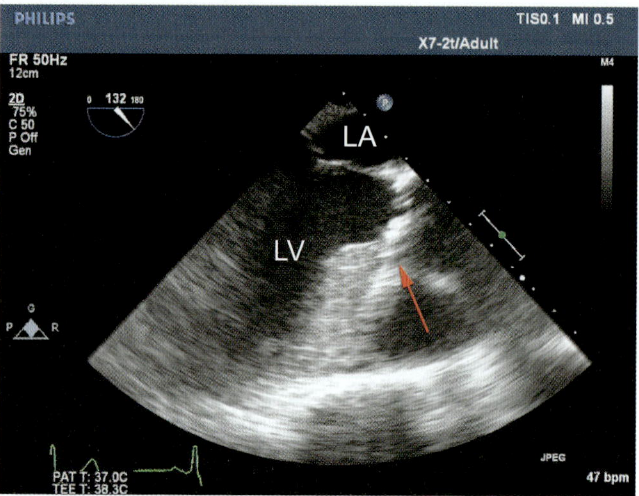

Fig. 10.2 Midesophageal long-axis view in a patient with significant aortic stenosis. Note the poor leaflet separation of the aortic valve indicating high positive predictive value of severe aortic stenosis. *LA,* Left atrium; *LV,* left ventricle.

Table 10.2	Differentiation of Aortic Dissection True and False Lumens	
True Lumen	**False Lumen**
Smaller size	Larger size
Round shape	Irregular or crescentic shape
Systolic expansion	Systolic compression
Early laminar flow	Late turbulent or sluggish flow
	± Spontaneous contrast
	± Thrombus

color-flow Doppler. The false lumen is typically larger and irregular or crescentic in shape with systolic compression and late turbulent flow (Fig. 10.3). On occasion, the false lumen contains spontaneous echo contrast or frank thrombus from the sluggish flow. TEE is also valuable in assessing for intimal tears, intramural hematomas, and penetrating ulcers. Equally important as identifying dissection is identification of associated complications such as acute aortic regurgitation and pericardial effusions with or without tamponade.

Cardiac Tamponade

Proper identification of pericardial tamponade is vital because the hemodynamic consequences can be devastating, and the treatment is specific: maintain contractility and preload and drain the pericardial fluid. The pericardium consists of two layers: visceral and parietal. The visceral layer adheres to the epicardium, and the parietal layer is the fibrous sac surrounding it. Five to 10 mL of pericardial fluid is normal. Potential causes of pathologic fluid accumulation are listed in Box 10.2. The pericardium is of limited size and distensibility, thereby restraining the four chambers and dampening the effects of changes in intrathoracic pressure. Acute effusions are most likely secondary to trauma (including iatrogenic or surgical) or myocardial infarction. Pericardial

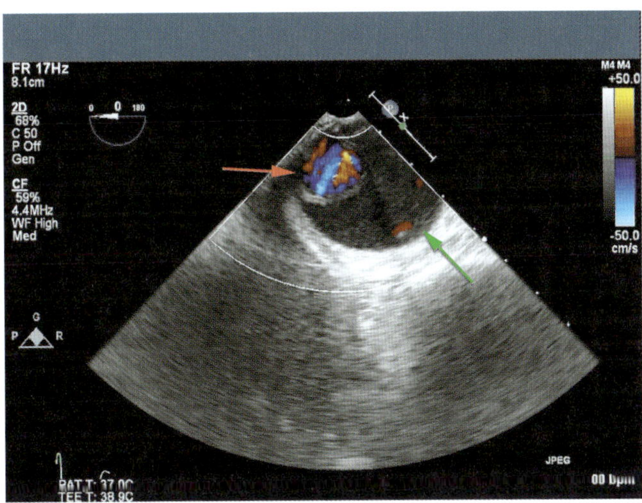

Fig. 10.3 Descending thoracic aorta short-axis view in a patient with an aortic dissection. The true lumen *(red arrow)* is round in shape with laminar flow in color-flow Doppler, and the false lumen *(green arrow)* is crescentic in shape with spontaneous echo contrast indicative of slow flow.

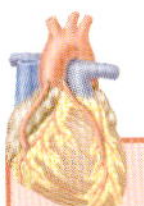

BOX 10.2   *Causes of Pericardial Effusions*

- Trauma
- Inflammation
- Infection
- Malignant disease
- Renal or hepatic failure
- Post–myocardial infarction status

tissue affected by chronic effusion tends to be more distensible and thus causes less hemodynamic instability. The effusion can envelop the space in a free-flowing fashion or may be loculated, affecting only a portion of the heart. Free-flowing effusions tend to accumulate in the dependent portion of the space. Pericardial fat is a relatively common finding in the anterior space and should not be confused with fluid accumulation. It tends to have a more granular appearance, rather than purely echolucent, and does not lead to chamber collapse.

Pressures within the pericardium and cardiac chambers during fluid accumulation follow a recognized pattern. Initially, fluid accumulation in the pericardial space compresses the right ventricle and causes the filling pressures to rise with little effect on the stroke volume (SV) of either ventricle. As the pericardial pressures rise, the right ventricle begins to collapse, but the thicker-walled left ventricle is unaffected. In the final stage, both the RV and LV SVs are significantly affected as the pericardial pressure determines passive flow. The external pressure on the cardiac chambers also exaggerates the normal respiratory variation in RV and LV SVs. In mechanically ventilated patients, elevated intrathoracic pressure compresses the superior vena cava (SVC) and inferior vena cava and thus reduces RV preload and SV. At the same time, LV preload and SV are enhanced by increasing return from the inflated lungs. Intrathoracic and pericardial pressures decrease on expiration, augment flow into the right ventricle, and push the interventricular septum into the left ventricle. Diastolic filling and LV SV are thus reduced. In a physiologically normal patient, these hemodynamic swings are minimal. Box 10.3 lists the values for normal respiratory variation in the right and left ventricles, and Table 10.3 summarizes the changes in SV associated with cardiac tamponade.

The limited TEE examination should be performed in its entirety because some hemodynamically significant effusions may be difficult to visualize. Pericardial effusions are viewed as darkened echolucent areas between the heart and the parietal pericardium.

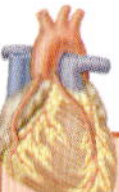

> **BOX 10.3** *Normal Respiratory Variation*
>
> - RV inflow <25%
> - LV inflow <15%
> - RV outflow <10%
> - LV outflow <10%
>
> *LV,* Left ventricular; *RV,* right ventricular.

Table 10.3 Respiratory Variation in Right and Left Ventricular Inflow in the Setting of Tamponade

	Mechanical Ventilation		Spontaneous Ventilation	
	Inspiration	Expiration	Inspiration	Expiration
Right ventricular inflow-outflow	↓	↑	↑	↓
Left ventricular inflow-outflow	↑	↓	↓	↑

↑, Increased; ↓, decreased.

No universally accepted rule exists for quantification, but effusions measuring less than 1 cm are considered small, effusions of 1 to 2 cm are considered moderate, and those larger than 2 cm are considered large (Fig. 10.4). Echogenic "stranding" in the pericardial space alerts the examiner to the possibility that the effusion is inflammatory or hemorrhagic. In the case of extreme hemodynamic instability, a large pericardial effusion should be considered to cause cardiac tamponade regardless of the results of the continuing study.

Pulsed-wave Doppler (PWD) interrogation of RV inflow or outflow may reveal exaggerated respiratory variations. These changes are the earliest signs of tamponade physiology and are followed by exaggerated variations in LV inflow and outflow. Because of the position and variable anatomy of the right ventricle, Doppler assessment of RV inflow and outflow can prove difficult, particularly within the time constraints of rescue echocardiography. LV inflow is best assessed in the ME four-chamber view with the PWD cursor placed at the MV leaflet tips (Table 10.4). LV outflow is best assessed by placing the PWD cursor in the LV outflow tract (LVOT) seen in the deep transgastric (TG) view (Fig. 10.5). The sweep speed should be 25 to 50 mm/s to view the variability most clearly.

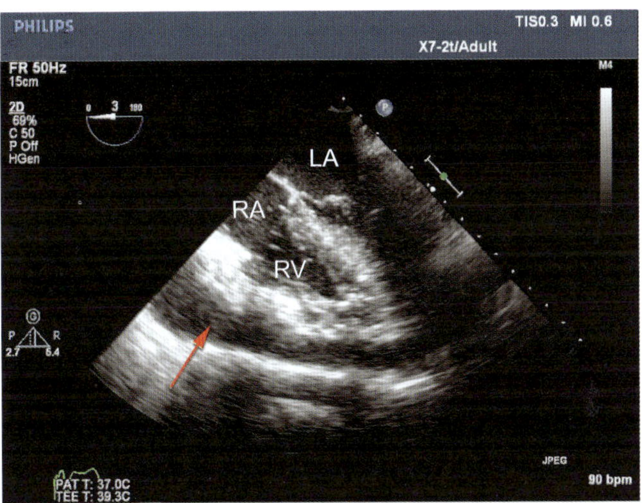

Fig. 10.4 Midesophageal four-chamber view in a patient with a large pericardial effusion *(red arrow). LA,* Left atrium; *RA,* right atrium; *RV,* right ventricle.

Table 10.4	Suggested Views for Doppler Interrogation of Ventricular Inflows and Outflows	
	View	**Pulsed-Wave Doppler Placement**
RV inflow	Modified bicaval	TV leaflet tips
RV outflow	TG RV inflow-outflow	RVOT
LV inflow	ME four chamber	MV leaflet tips
LV outflow	Deep TG	LVOT

LV, Left ventricular; *LVOT,* left ventricular outflow tract; *ME,* midesophageal; *MV,* mitral valve; *RV,* right ventricular; *RVOT,* right ventricular outflow tract; *TG,* transgastric; *TV,* tricuspid valve.

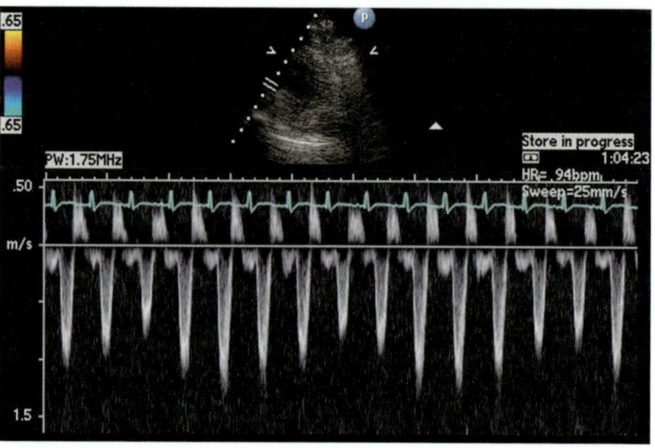

Fig. 10.5 Pulsed-wave echocardiographic interrogation of the left ventricular outflow tract by using the deep transgastric view in a patient with tamponade physiology showing respiratory variability. *HR,* Heart rate.

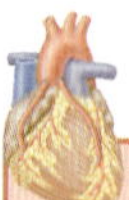

> **BOX 10.4** *Summary of Echocardiographic Findings in Pericardial Tamponade*
>
> - Pericardial effusion
> - Late diastolic or early systolic right atrial collapse
> - Diastolic right ventricular collapse
> - Increased respiratory variation in mitral inflow and left ventricular outflow tract

With increasing fluid accumulation, the pericardial pressure starts to exceed the right atrial (RA) pressure, thereby causing exaggerated atrial systolic (i.e., ventricular diastolic) contraction that extends into atrial diastole (i.e., ventricular systole). Assessment of this collapse is best performed in the ME RV inflow-outflow view or the ME four-chamber view. As the pericardial pressure increases further, the right ventricle begins to collapse in diastole. The RV outflow tract is most likely to collapse, and thus the preferred view is the RV inflow-outflow view (Box 10.4). A similar collapse of the thicker left-sided structures would indicate very high pericardial pressures. After the diagnosis is established, echocardiography can be a useful adjunct to guide needle placement during pericardiocentesis.

Right Ventricular Dysfunction

RV failure, defined as the inability of the right ventricle to provide adequate blood flow to the left ventricle in the setting of normal or elevated central venous pressure, is associated with a high mortality rate in both cardiac and noncardiac surgical procedures. Potential causes of RV failure are numerous and include RV contractile dysfunction as seen in ischemia, volume overload, sepsis, and nonischemic cardiomyopathy and the acute elevations in pulmonary artery pressures seen in hypoxia, acute respiratory distress syndrome, LV dysfunction, and PE. Abrupt, catastrophic RV dysfunction can result when the contractile reserve is reduced secondary to a feedback loop involving RV dysfunction, reduced cardiac output (CO), and decreased coronary perfusion causing worsening RV dysfunction.

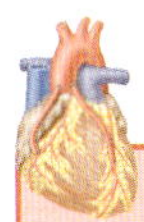

BOX 10.5   *Echocardiographic Parameters of Right Ventricular Dysfunction*

Dilated Right Ventricle

- Basal RVEDD >4.2 cm
- Mid-RVEDD >3.5 cm
- RVOT EDD >2.7 cm

Dilated Right Atrium

- RA area >18 cm^2
- RA length >5.3 cm
- RA diameter >4.4 cm
- Bowing into left atrium

Decreased RV Contraction

- TAPSE <16 mm
- RV FAC <35%

Evidence of Elevated PA Pressures

- Pulmonary artery diameter >21 mm
- "D-shaped" ventricular septum

Worsening TV Regurgitation

- Severe TV regurgitation noted by vena contracta >0.7 cm

EDD, End-diastolic diameter; *FAC*, fractional area change; *PA*, pulmonary artery; *RA*, right atrial; *RV*, right ventricular; *RVEDD*, right ventricular end-diastolic diameter; *RVOT*, right ventricular outflow tract; *TAPSE*, tricuspid annular-plane systolic excursion; *TV*, tricuspid valve.

Because the anatomy and function of the right ventricle are complex, geometric modeling and quantitative analysis are very difficult. For this reason, the echocardiographic assessment of RV function in the emergency setting should be qualitative, and this approach is as good as MRI at detecting dysfunction. Box 10.5 summarizes the echocardiographic manifestations of RV dysfunction. Visual assessment begins with inspection of right-sided chamber sizes to look for dilation of the right ventricle and right atrium. Encroachment into the left side with right-to-left bowing of the interatrial septum (seen best in the ME four-chamber and bicaval views) and a D-shaped intraventricular septum (seen best in the LV SAX view) indicates elevated right-sided pressures (Fig. 10.6). RV contractility can then be assessed by the fractional area change (FAC) or the tricuspid annular-plane systolic excursion (TAPSE) methods. The RV FAC is calculated by measuring the RV end-systolic and end-diastolic areas (RVESA and RVEDA, respectively) in the ME four-chamber view and using the following equation: [RVEDA − RVESA]/RVEDA. A reduced FAC has significant prognostic value in myocardial ischemia and PE.

The TAPSE method is best measured by placing the M-mode cursor on the tricuspid annulus in the modified bicaval or transgastric RV inflow-outflow views and measuring the distance the annulus moves from systole to diastole (Fig. 10.7). A distance of less than 17 cm is considered abnormal. For purposes of rescue echocardiography, a qualitative assessment of the TAPSE and the RV free wall in the ME RV inflow-outflow and four-chamber views is preferred.

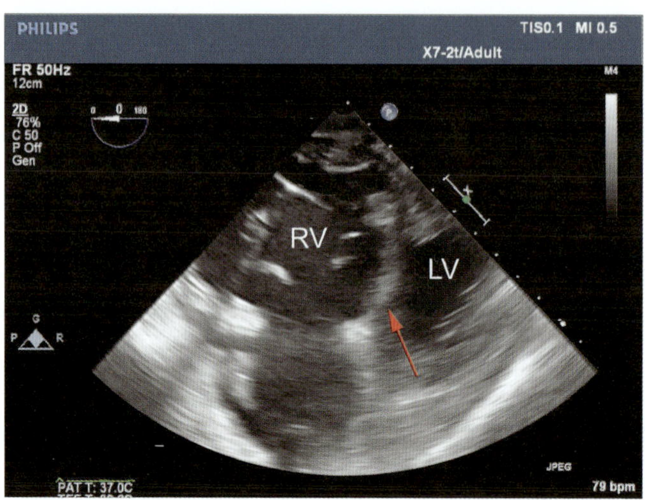

Fig. 10.6 Transgastric midpapillary short-axis view in a patient with massive right ventricular dilation and pressure overload. Note the deviated interventricular septum leading to a D-shaped left ventricle (LV) instead of the normal O-shaped orientation. *RV,* Right ventricle.

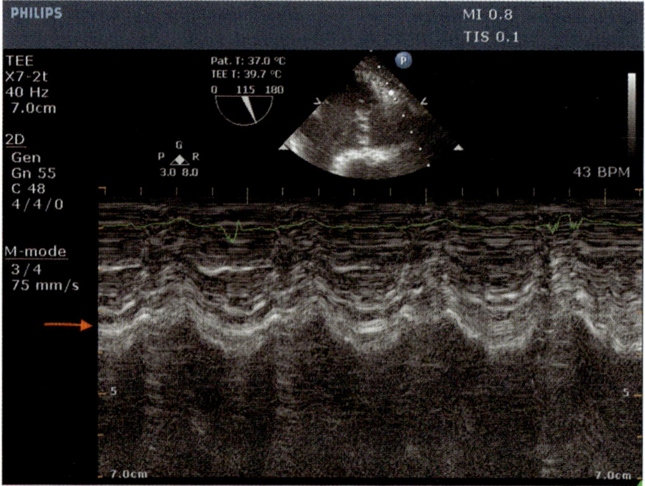

Fig. 10.7 An example of tricuspid annular plane excursion using M-mode echocardiography on the tricuspid annulus. The *red arrow* points to the tricuspid annulus. A visual estimation of the annular movement suggests good right ventricular function.

Pulmonary Embolism

The immobility and hypercoagulability associated with surgical procedures increase the risk of PE fivefold. This risk is only partially mitigated by prophylactic measures. Early diagnosis and treatment can reduce the overall mortality rate 10-fold. The examiner should have a high suspicion for PE in hemodynamically unstable patients with malignant disease, prolonged immobilization, obesity, or tobacco use, as well as in patients who use oral contraceptives, hormone replacement therapy, or antipsychotic drugs. The surgical procedures with the highest risks of PE are those associated with hip fractures, acute spinal cord injuries, and general trauma. The pathophysiology of PE begins with an abrupt increase in pulmonary artery pressures. Hypoxia and vasoconstriction worsen pulmonary vascular resistance. RV wall tension and oxygen demand increase, leading to subendocardial ischemia, RV dilation, and regional wall motion abnormalities (RWMAs). The intraventricular septum shifts left, and this shift reduces LV diastolic filling and SV. Overall, the cardiac pathophysiology of PE is complex, involving an interplay of wall tension, ischemia, structural damage, and inflammation.

Although TEE can help guide both diagnosis and management, it is not the gold standard. Echocardiography has high specificity and low sensitivity (90% and 56%, respectively). In fact, end-tidal carbon dioxide is a significantly better diagnostic tool. Although visualization of a clot, which can be found anywhere on the right side from the vena cava to the pulmonary artery, is pathognomonic of PE and can be seen in more than 80% of cases, the presence of a thrombus does not predict death. The ideal views to assess for thrombus include the ME bicaval, RV inflow–outflow, and ascending aorta SAX views. The main and right pulmonary arteries can be seen by withdrawal of the probe to the high esophagus until a cross-section of the ascending aorta is obtained. The left pulmonary artery is often obscured by the tracheobronchial tree. The most clinically useful echocardiographic findings in the setting of PE are those associated with acute RA and RV failure. Bowing of the interatrial septum to the left indicates high RA pressures, which can be particularly problematic in the setting of a patent foramen ovale. A patent foramen ovale in a patient with PE doubles the mortality rate and quintuples the rate of ischemic stroke, and aggressive thrombolytic treatment is therefore warranted. RV wall motion abnormalities are the most common echocardiographic findings in patients with PE. The extent of RV dysfunction correlates with the overall clot burden, with perfusion defects larger than 20% to 25% more likely to cause dysfunction and dilation. A reduced TAPSE correlates with mortality rates, and it can predict the extent of the clot burden as well as residual perfusion defects when the RV dilation has resolved.

Right ventricular dysfunction in the setting of PE predicts mortality rates, even in normotensive patients. The McConnell sign is suggested as a highly specific (94% specificity with 77% sensitivity) finding of a distinct pattern of RV RWMA in predicting PE. The sign consists of a hypokinetic free wall and a normal to hyperdynamic apex. This subsequently has been found to have reduced sensitivity and specificity, with some suggesting a "reverse" McConnell sign as an indication of PE. Therefore a particular array of RV RWMA does not accurately predict PE. RV pressure overload, however, does "flatten" the interventricular septum, thus reducing left-sided filling and CO. The subsequent reduction of coronary perfusion as well as the structural and inflammatory changes in the myocardium can additionally lead to LV dysfunction. A low ejection fraction (EF) is an independent predictor of death. In addition to the diagnosis of PE, echocardiography can aid in assessing the effectiveness of treatment. If a thrombus is visualized at presentation, continuous assessment of the thrombus during thrombolytic administration can show resolution of the clot and return of normal RV function. Echocardiography can also be useful in following the return of RV function over longer periods of time.

Left Ventricular Hypocontractility

Although LV dysfunction has many potential causes, the echocardiographic manifestations are similar. The SCA recommended a qualitative estimation of the LVEF when assessing candidates who may benefit from inotropic therapy. Visual estimation, or "eyeballing," has been validated with Simpson's biplane method, three-dimensional echocardiography, and radionuclide angiography. In addition, visual estimation of LV function can be accurately performed by noncardiologists and clinicians with only limited training. The primary method of visual estimation of LV contractility is through the FAC as seen in the TG LV midpapillary SAX view. The LV FAC is calculated by measuring the LV end-systolic and end-diastolic areas (LVESA and LVEDA, respectively) in the LV SAX view and using the following equation: [LVEDA – LVESA]/LVEDA. The normal values are similar to the normal values for EF. Initially, the calculation should be performed to assess contractile function. However, with more experience ($\approx \geq 20$ studies), a visual estimate is reliable. However, in patients with regional dysfunction, the TG LV midpapillary SAX view may miss some pathologic features. A brief, qualitative assessment of the left ventricle in the four-chamber, two-chamber, and LAX views to look for hypokinetic walls aids in the diagnosis. Particular attention should be paid to the apex because it contributes a significant portion of the overall EF.

When LV dysfunction is encountered, it is important to identify myocardial ischemia as the mechanism quickly because early revascularization improves outcomes. The echocardiographic manifestations of myocardial ischemia occur earlier and are more sensitive than the electrocardiogram (ECG), even in anesthetized patients. Segmental wall thickening of less than 30% suggests ischemia and can manifest within seconds. Distinguishing between new-onset RWMAs and hypokinesis from chronic ischemia can be difficult. Intraoperative pharmacologic stress testing is ideal, but it is often not practical in the urgent setting. Acute ischemia therefore must be diagnosed by a change in RWMA from baseline by two grades (e.g., from normal to severe hypokinesis) in two or more segments. Infarcted myocardium often appears thinner and brighter than surrounding tissue and is therefore easily distinguished from myocardium with acute ischemia. Complications of ischemia such as acute diastolic dysfunction, mitral regurgitation, and papillary muscle rupture can also aid in the diagnosis.

In addition to LV ischemia, the stress, inflammation, and catecholamine excess associated with acute illness can reduce LV contractility. Potentially reversible secondary cardiomyopathies can develop in patients with numerous noncardiac critical illnesses. Sepsis-induced cardiomyopathy, for example, may occur in more than half of patients, with sepsis as a result of inflammatory mediators, bacterial endotoxins, catecholamines, and microcirculatory dysfunction. LV and RV dysfunction ensues, with global and RWMAs, as well as worsening measures of diastolic function. The myocardial toxicity from excess catecholamines, whether through septic shock, drug administration, or stress, can also induce LV dysfunction. Stress-induced cardiomyopathy, also known as takotsubo cardiomyopathy, is a form of catecholamine-mediated ventricular dysfunction induced by physical or emotional stress. Takotsubo cardiomyopathy most often manifests with normal to hyperkinetic basal function and hypokinesis of the apex, likely secondary to an increased density of β-adrenergic receptors in the apex. The LV apex often appears to "balloon" out, and this is the most prominent feature found on echocardiography.

Left Ventricular Hypercontractility and Left Ventricular Outflow Tract Obstruction

An often overlooked consequence of a hyperdynamic left ventricle, whether secondary to low afterload, hypovolemia, or inotropic support, is dynamic LVOT obstruction (LVOTO). Although often associated with hypertrophic cardiomyopathy, LVOTO has been reported in the setting of hypertension, type 1 diabetes, myocardial ischemia, pheochromocytomas, takotsubo cardiomyopathy, valvular replacements and repairs, and catecholamine administration. The mechanism of LVOTO remains unclear and varies by cause. The primary mechanism likely results from localized increases in flow velocity during ejection that results from a narrow LVOT from LV thickening or hypovolemia. This change causes the anterior mitral leaflet and chordae to be drawn toward the septum through both a Venturi effect and a hydrodynamic "drag." This process distorts the mitral leaflet coaptation and results in middle to late systolic mitral regurgitation. Precipitating factors that further narrow the LVOT include hypovolemia, sepsis, inotropic agents, and diuretic agents. LVOTO should be considered in any hemodynamically unstable patient with risk factors for LVOT narrowing whose hemodynamic status worsens with inotropic support.

On echocardiographic examination, the left ventricle likely appears underfilled and hypercontractile. LV hypertrophy of varying degrees and morphologic features may be present. It is often possible to see movement of the anterior leaflet of the MV toward the upper septum in the ME LAX view (Fig. 10.8). CFD may show mitral regurgitation with an anteriorly directed jet that begins in middle to late systole. CFD may also show turbulent flow in the LVOT (Fig. 10.9). This finding is often the initial indicator of altered ejection dynamics in LVOTO. The hallmarks of LVOTO are a dagger-shaped spectral Doppler pattern in the LVOT and midsystolic closure of the AV. Early systolic ejection is usually normal because it takes time for the flow velocity to build. Obstruction occurs late in ventricular contraction, thus causing flow to diminish transiently and resulting in partial closure of the AV. M-mode interrogation of the AV in the ME LAX view shows a "notch" indicating midsystolic partial closure of the AV with a secondary opening. In addition, this dynamic property of the obstruction yields a late-peaking continuous-wave Doppler pattern as the gradient tends to develop in middle to end systole, producing a dagger shape (Fig. 10.10). The peak velocity of the wave is high, consistent with an elevated pressure gradient. The gradient can be measured by tracing the waveform.

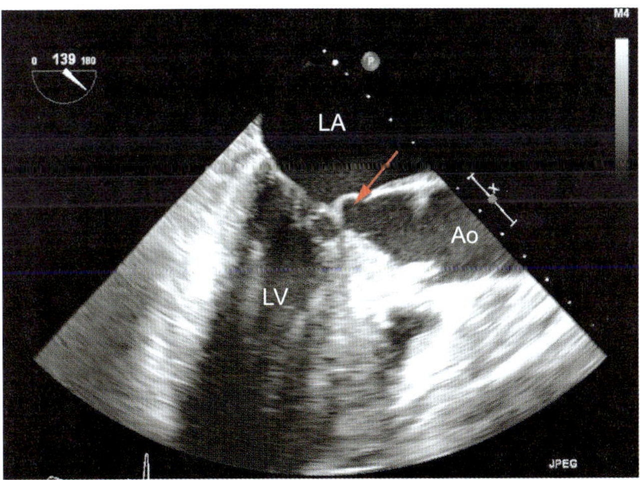

Fig. 10.8 Midesophageal long-axis view in a patient with hypertrophic cardiomyopathy demonstrating a narrowed left ventricular outflow tract and systolic anterior motion (*red arrow*). *Ao,* Ascending aorta; *LA,* left atrium; *LV,* left ventricle.

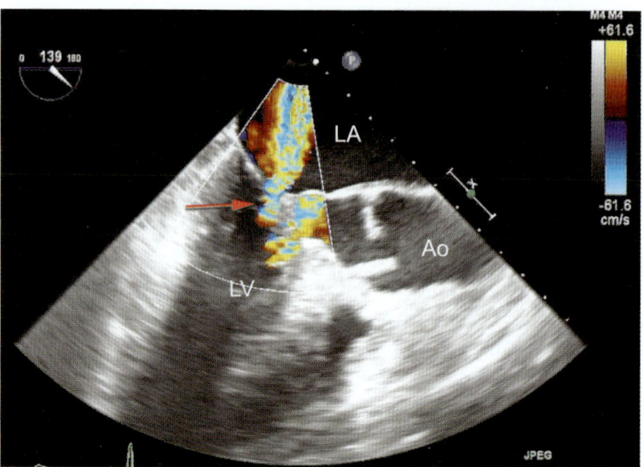

Fig. 10.9 Midesophageal long-axis view with color-flow Doppler in a patient with hypertrophic cardiomyopathy demonstrating systolic anterior motion and resultant mitral regurgitation *(red arrow)*. Note the aliasing in the left ventricular outflow tract indicating high velocities. *Ao,* Ascending aorta; *LA,* left atrium; *LV,* left ventricle.

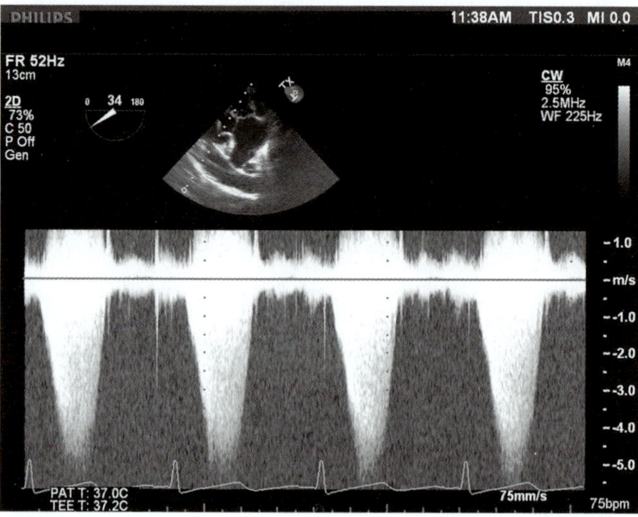

Fig. 10.10 Continuous-wave Doppler echocardiography in the left ventricular outflow tract of a patient with dynamic left ventricular outflow tract obstruction reveals a dagger-shaped waveform. *CW,* Continuous wave; *FR,* frequency.

Hypovolemia and Low Afterload

Cardiac tamponade, PE, and severe LV and RV dysfunction are relatively infrequent causes of hemodynamic instability. More commonly, reduced afterload or preload is encountered. A qualitative assessment of volume and afterload begins with LVEDA and LVESA in the TG SAX view, as well as Doppler quantification of SV. The LVEDA reflects the amount of fluid in the left ventricle. A euvolemic patient usually has a normal LVEDA. If the same patient also has reduced systemic vascular resistance, the

LVEDA usually remains normal because the preload is unchanged. Conversely, the LVEDA of a hypovolemic patient is often reduced. The LVESA, in contrast, should reflect the endpoint of the LVEF. A hypovolemic patient who starts off with a reduced LV diastolic volume (reduced LVEDA) ends with a reduced systolic volume (reduced LVESA). Alternatively, a patient with a normal LV diastolic volume (normal LVEDA) but an elevated EF secondary to reduced afterload also ends with a reduced end-systolic volume (reduced LVESA). As examples, consider the patients with varying LV end-diastolic volumes, EF, and systemic vascular resistance in Table 10.5. Normal values for LVEDA are 8 to 14 cm^2. These values may vary depending on multiple factors, including age, sex, FAC, and even the anesthetized state. LV SAX assessment by TEE has been shown to be a reasonable method of assessing ventricular volumes, and it is more accurate than pulmonary artery occlusion pressures. In addition, evidence indicates a correlation between LV volume and LVEDA in animals, pediatric patients after congenital heart defect repair, and anesthetized cardiac patients. LVEDA appears to decrease linearly at 0.3 cm per reduction in 1% of the estimated blood volume in cardiac patients. A correlation between a reduced LVESA and hypovolemia has also been established. A direct relationship between a low LVESA and low afterload, however, has not been well established in the literature. A qualitative assessment of the LVEDA and LVESA can therefore suggest hypovolemia, low afterload, or both, but it may require further evaluation through an estimation of SV to confirm the diagnosis.

Stroke Volume Assessment

A reduced LVESA likely represents either hypovolemia or low afterload. Whereas hypovolemia results in a reduction in SV, low afterload results in a high-CO state. SV can be calculated using the LVOT area and stroke distance. The LVOT diameter is usually measured in the LV ME LAX view (Fig. 10.11), but it can be measured in any image that allows for an unobstructed view of the LVOT. The measurement should be obtained at the same level as the PWD cursor, usually approximately 5 mm proximal to the AV, measured from endocardium to endocardium. Because the radius is squared, small inaccuracies in this measurement can introduce significant errors in the overall calculations. For this reason, it is important to use the baseline annular measurement for all calculations when performing serial SV measurements. The stroke distance, which is the average distance a red blood cell (RBC) travels during systolic ejection, can be calculated by measuring the RBC velocities in the LVOT with PWD. This parameter is best measured in the deep TG or TG LAX views because of the parallel alignment between the flow and the transducer. The PWD cursor should be placed just proximal to the insertion of the AV leaflets. The image obtained is of the velocities (i.e., speed

Table 10.5 Example of the Effects of Hypovolemia and Low Afterload on End-Diastolic and End-Systolic Volumes[a]

	EDV (mL)	SVR	EF (%)	ESV (mL)
Patient A	100	Normal	50	50
Patient B (hypovolemia)	50	Normal	50	25
Patient C (low afterload)	100	Low	75	25

[a]End-diastolic and end-systolic areas in the left ventricular short-axis view should reflect the changes in volume.

EDV, End-diastolic volume; *EF,* ejection fraction; *ESV,* end-systolic volume; *SVR,* systemic vascular resistance.

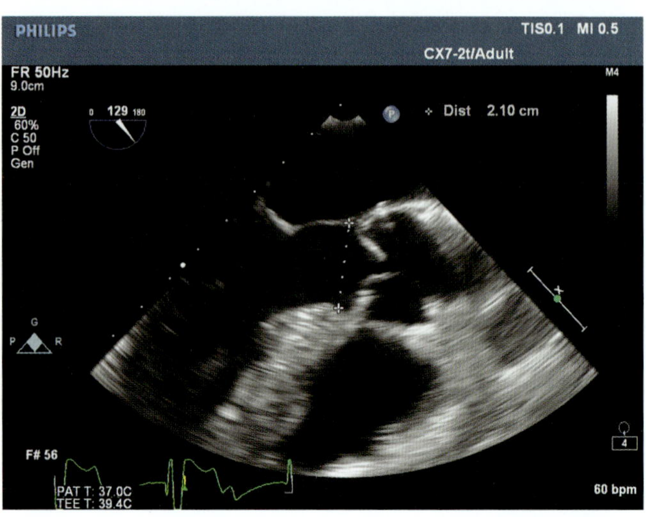

Fig. 10.11 Measurement of the left ventricular outflow diameter in the echocardiographic left ventricular long-axis view. *FR,* Frequency.

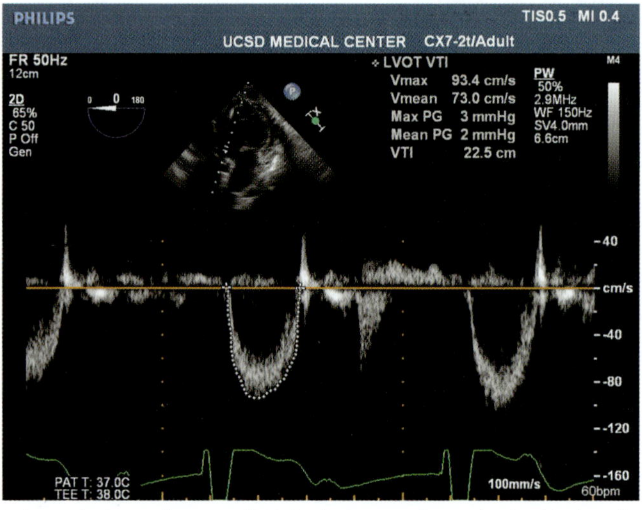

Fig. 10.12 Left ventricular outflow tract (LVOT) velocity waveforms obtained in the echocardiographic deep transgastric view. *FR,* Frequency; *PG,* pressure gradient; *PW,* pulsed-wave; *Vmax,* maximum velocity; *Vmean,* mean velocity; *VTI,* velocity-time integral.

and direction) of the RBCs in the LVOT over time (Fig. 10.12). The machine can then calculate the velocity-time integral (VTI) after tracing the outer border of one of the waveforms. The VTI is the calculated stroke distance. To understand this concept better, consider a car traveling 70 miles an hour for 2 hours. Fig. 10.13 shows this plotted on a graph with velocity on the y-axis and time on the x-axis. The area of the rectangle created by these measurements would yield a distance (i.e., 70 mph × 2 h = 140 miles). The VTI is similar to this calculation in that it is the area under the curve of RBC velocities over time. In this case, the velocities are represented by centimeters per second, the time by seconds, and the VTI by centimeters.

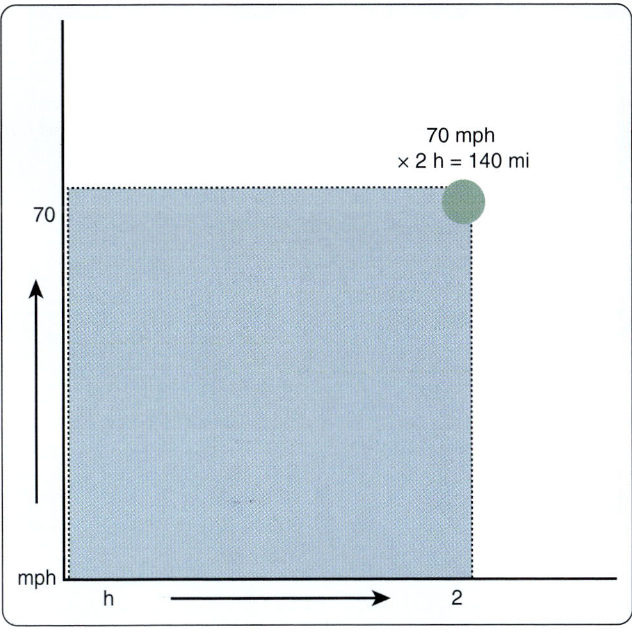

Fig. 10.13 Area under the curve for a velocity-time graph. If a car is going 70 miles per hour for 2 hours, the distance traveled (i.e., 140 miles) can be calculated by calculating the shaded area. The same principle applies to the velocity-time graph obtained through spectral Doppler echocardiography. The area under a curve obtained in the left ventricular outflow tract using pulsed-wave Doppler yields a distance (centimeters). This is called the velocity-time integral.

The calculation of SV assumes a cylindrical LVOT with the volume being the product of the area and the length. The area of a circle is $\pi \times radius^2$ or $diameter^2$ $(D^2) \times 0.785$. The length is represented by the VTI. SV is expressed in milliliters and can be calculated using the following equation:

$$SV = D^2 \times 0.785 \times VTI$$

Cardiac output can then be calculated by multiplying the SV by the heart rate. This method of SV calculation has been validated when compared with thermodilution, and it is the ASE-recommended method for determining CO.

Dynamic Indicators of Hypovolemia

Although changes in LVEDA and LVESA show that the cardiac chambers fill with volume administration, they do not predict whether volume administration improves SV (i.e., volume responsive). Dynamic indices, conversely, assess the effects of a change in preload on SV or its surrogate. Positive-pressure ventilation increases pleural and transpulmonary pressures, which reduce RV preload and increase RV afterload, respectively. This process reduces overall RV SV. At the same time, insufflation pushes blood out of the lungs into the left ventricle, thus augmenting LV SV. After several beats, the reduced RV SV results in reduced LV preload and hence reduced SV, which can be seen at end-expiration. These changes are exaggerated when the ventricles are on the steep part of the Frank-Starling curve. The magnitude of the variation has been shown to predict fluid responsiveness. Euvolemia puts the ventricles on the flatter portion of the curve and limits respiratory variability. PWD interrogation of the LVOT has been shown to assess these changes in SV accurately and thus predict

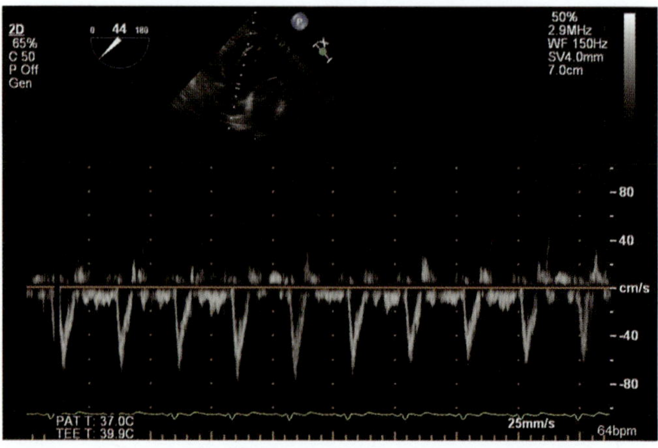

Fig. 10.14 Deep transgastric echocardiographic view with the pulsed-wave Doppler probe placed in the left ventricular outflow tract. The respiratory changes seen in the peak velocities indicate fluid responsiveness.

fluid responsiveness (Fig. 10.14). Analogous to SV variation from other CO methods, the following equation can be used with echocardiography in which V_{min} represents the minimum velocity in the LVOT, V_{max} is the maximum velocity, and Δ represents change:

$$\Delta V_{peak}\,(\%) = 100 \times (V_{max} - V_{min})/[V_{max} - V_{min})/2]$$

A ΔV_{peak} of 12% or greater indicates volume responsiveness with a sensitivity of 100% and a specificity of 89% (as indicated by an increase in cardiac index by $\geq$15%). ΔV_{peak} was found to decrease after fluid administration. In addition, with a negative predictive value of 100%, these data suggest that no patient with a ΔV_{peak} of less than 12% responds to fluid administration.

TRANSESOPHAGEAL ECHOCARDIOGRAPHY AS A MONITOR IN NONCARDIAC SURGICAL PROCEDURES

Argument for Use as a Monitor in Noncardiac Cases

The hemodynamic status of the intraoperative patient need not be acutely unstable for TEE monitoring to be effective. Although distinct entities such as PE and tamponade have been discussed, it is the effect of these processes on preload, afterload, contractility, and thus SV that is most important to diagnosis and treatment. It is well known that general anesthesia affects all these parameters. TEE is well suited to assess the more moderate changes in hemodynamic values that occur with surgical procedures and general anesthesia. Although evidence of the outcome benefits of intraoperative TEE as a monitor is currently lacking, evidence does indicate that echocardiography can change perioperative morbidity. In addition, a significant number of data indicate that the information gained from echocardiography can change perioperative management and management in the intensive care unit. The benefits are clear, and the complication rate is low, with an overall morbidity rate of 0.2% and a 0% mortality rate. The ASE and SCA currently recommend a noncomprehensive examination for intraoperative monitoring and state that it can "dramatically influence a patient's intraoperative management."

The data supporting the use of TEE as a monitor in noncardiac surgical procedures also apply to specific clinical situations. In addition to its use as a monitor for ischemia and volume in high-risk vascular surgical patients, TEE is valuable in assessing ventricular changes during aortic cross-clamping and in guiding endovascular stent placement and monitoring for complications. In fact, TEE is more sensitive and specific than angiography in detecting leaks and thrombi, and it can change the surgical procedure a significant amount of the time. Echocardiography is also useful in identifying traumatic cardiac and vascular injuries, including cardiac contusion, valvular disruption, and traumatic aortic injuries. Information derived from echocardiography reduced mortality rates in patients with penetrating cardiac injuries by more than 40%. TEE during hepatic resection and transplantation can have a major impact on intraoperative management, particularly when it is used to assess for PE and RV dysfunction, as well as changes in LV function. Regarding orthopedic procedures, aortic stenosis is frequently observed in the hip fracture population, accounting for more than one-third of patients. Not only can echocardiography aid in the diagnosis and management of this and similar coexisting cardiac diseases in orthopedic patients, but it can also aid in identifying and treating emboli associated with total hip arthroplasty with cement.

Given that one of the primary arguments against using echocardiography as a routine monitor is that outcome data are lacking, it is important to assess whether the monitors traditionally used have the same issues. Positive outcome data with the use of pulmonary artery catheters and central venous pressure monitoring are lacking. Pulmonary artery catheters do not affect outcome in several different patient groups confirmed in several systematic reviews, including high-risk surgical patients, patients with sepsis, cardiothoracic surgical patients, and vascular surgical patients. Moreover, neither central venous pressure nor pulmonary artery occlusion pressure correlates with ventricular preload. Evidence to support improved outcomes with the use of arterial catheters and pulse oximetry is similarly lacking. This observation is not meant as an indictment of traditional intraoperative monitors, nor does it suggest that seeking further outcome data on intraoperative echocardiography as a monitor is superfluous. This is simply to suggest that intraoperative echocardiography in noncardiac surgical procedures should not be discounted because of a lack of outcome data.

Transesophageal Echocardiography Goal-Directed Therapy

Transesophageal echocardiography is clearly a safe and valuable monitor in a multitude of intraoperative situations. The wide-ranging utility of TEE as a monitor is not solely the result of its accuracy in detecting singular cardiac events, but it also reflects the ability of TEE to provide a global view of cardiac function and the overall physiologic context within which the event occurs. This makes echocardiography the ideal monitor for goal-directed therapy (GDT). GDT is the optimization of a hemodynamic goal through fluid administration and/or inotropic or vasoactive support with the expectation that this treatment will optimize end-organ perfusion and oxygen delivery. Optimization involves assessment of the hemodynamic parameter before and after the intervention and then basing further intervention on the results. Such a concept is not foreign to anesthesiologists, who tend to use normal blood pressure and heart rate as standard hemodynamic goals. Unfortunately, these parameters are poor markers of end-organ perfusion, particularly when considering volume status. The hemodynamic parameters used for GDT are generally SV and CO or their surrogates. Although it remains controversial, a growing body of evidence indicates that in high-risk patients undergoing noncardiac surgical procedures, GDT reduces hospital length of stay, improves postoperative gastrointestinal function, decreases postoperative renal dysfunction, and improves short- and long-term survival.

The most obvious advantage of echocardiography over other monitors, such as the esophageal Doppler or pulse contour analyzer, is the ability to monitor contractility. LV systolic function is extremely complex, with multiple elements beyond EF. A normal preoperative EF may not predict intraoperative contractile performance, particularly as loading conditions change. Subtle systolic dysfunction can be unmasked by anesthesia, surgical procedures, or some other hemodynamic disturbance. Thus hypocontractility must remain on the differential diagnosis for hemodynamic instability regardless of initial assumptions. The TG LV midpapillary SAX view is an easy and effective way to estimate LV function qualitatively. In addition, it provides simultaneous information on contractile performance and loading conditions, which are interdependent. Frequent assessment of the TG LV midpapillary SAX allows for both a rapid estimation of preload, afterload, and contractility in the setting of hemodynamic instability, as well as the effects of any intervention performed to alleviate the disturbance.

Volume therapy in GDT focuses on changes in SV after volume administration. The method used to assess this change is similar to that used to monitor dynamic changes in SV with positive-pressure ventilation. Baseline values are obtained for LVOT, VTI, and LV SV. Volume is then administered, and these parameters are reassessed. An increase in SV of more than 10% indicates volume responsiveness, which warrants further volume loading and reassessment. An increase of less than 10% suggests that the patient will not benefit from further volume loading, and an alternate method to improve hemodynamics should be sought. Large volumes of fluid are not necessary. As little as 100 mL of colloid can be used, with a sensitivity of 95% and a specificity of 78%. Alternatively, passive leg raise can be used to test volume responsiveness by placing the bed at 45 degrees of semirecumbency and then tilting the bed so that the upper body is horizontal and the legs are at a 45-degree angle. Passive leg raise can achieve the same SV increase as a 300-mL volume bolus in fluid responders, with the advantage of being reversible.

Transesophageal echocardiography is not only able to identify improvements in forward flow, but it also can monitor intracardiac pressures, particularly left atrial pressure (LAP), to aid in preventing elevated filling pressures and pulmonary edema. Although LAP measurement may not reflect intravascular volume status, a large increase in LAP during fluid administration warns of impending edema that may be hastened by further volume. The echocardiographic assessment of LAP involves the use of spectral Doppler to assess diastolic compliance. Placement of the PWD cursor at the mitral leaflet tips during diastole yields two waves, E and A (Fig. 10.15). The E wave represents early diastolic filling as a result of a pressure gradient between the left atrium and the left ventricle. The A wave represents the gradient between the left atrium and left ventricle generated by atrial contraction. Simplifying the diastolic physiology for the sake of clarity, the pressure gradient during the E wave can be produced in one of two ways: (1) a normal LAP in the setting of a low LV end-diastolic pressure (LVEDP) in a compliant myocardium or (2) a high LAP generated by compensatory mechanisms to overcome a high LVEDP in a noncompliant myocardium. Because both mechanisms can generate the same pressure gradient, the E waves for both may look the same.

The velocity with which the mitral annulus ascends in diastole can help determine how the pressure gradient is established. PWD interrogation of the mitral annulus in the four-chamber view yields early and late diastolic waves termed E′ and A′ (Fig. 10.16). These waves are brighter (because of the high-density tissue) and slower

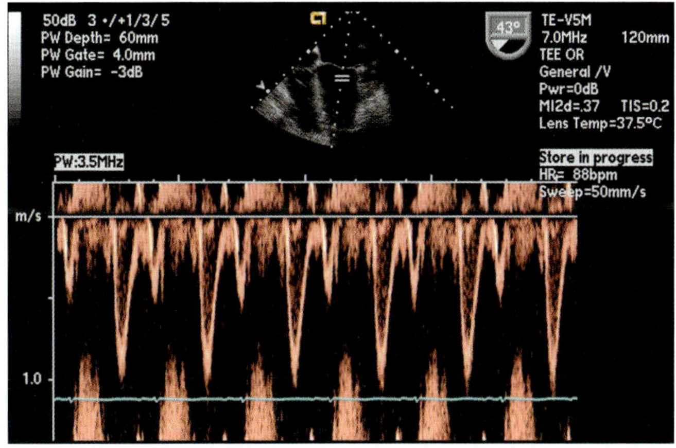

Fig. 10.15 Mitral inflow Doppler echocardiography with E and A waves. *HR,* Heart rate; *PW,* pulsed wave; *TEE,* transesophageal echocardiography.

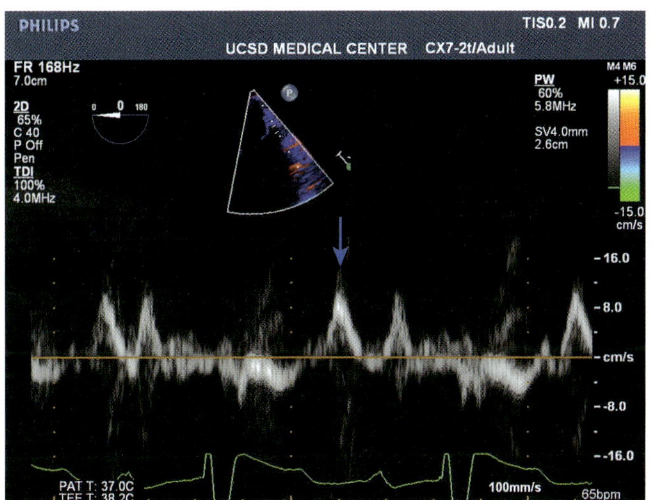

Fig. 10.16 Tissue Doppler echocardiographic imaging of the lateral side of mitral annulus in the four-chamber view. The *blue arrow* points to the E′ wave. *FR,* Frequency, *PW,* pulsed-wave; *TDI,* tissue Doppler image.

than the mitral inflow and require an adjustment of the gain and scale. The tissue Doppler function on the machine optimizes these parameters automatically. Whereas a relatively fast E′ is a marker for normal diastolic compliance, a slow E′ indicates poor diastolic compliance. Because the E wave is approximately the same for both low and high LVEDP and the E′ wave is reduced with a high LVEDP, the ratio of E to E′ increases as the LVEDP (and the LAP) increases. An elevated E/E′ ratio correlates with LAP in septic shock, heart failure, and ventilated patients in the intensive care unit, and it may be a better marker of high left heart pressures than brain natriuretic peptide. No universally accepted values for E/E′ and LAP have been established. However, based on the available data, whereas an E/E′ ratio greater than 18 is most likely associated with an elevated LAP, an E/E′ ratio of less than 12 most likely rules

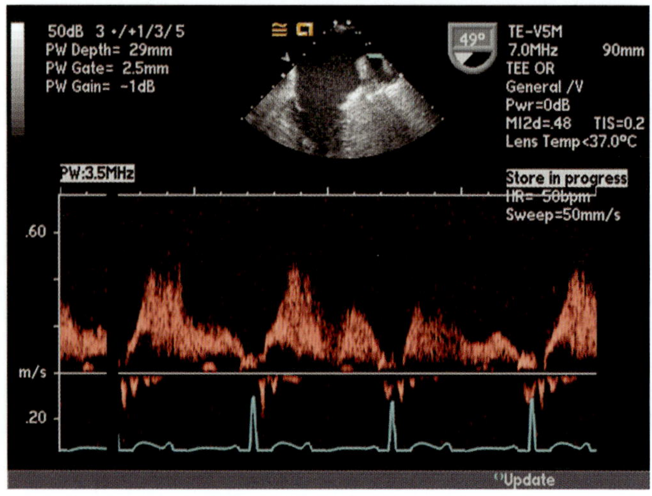

Fig. 10.17 Pulsed-wave Doppler echocardiography of the left upper pulmonary vein found in the midesophageal two-chamber view. *HR,* Heart rate; *PW,* pulsed wave; *TEE,* transesophageal echocardiography.

out elevated pressures. In addition, a statistical correlation has been demonstrated between pulmonary capillary wedge pressure (PCWP) and E/E′ by using the following formula: PCWP = 0.97 × E/E′ + 4.34. This formula allows an estimate of PCWP ≈ E/E′ + 4.

Pulsed-wave Doppler interrogation of the pulmonary venous inflow is another method to assess diastolic compliance and LAP. In a left ventricle with normal compliance, the LAP is lowest during systole because of the descent of the mitral annulus. The pressure gradient between the pulmonary vein (PV) and the left atrium is greatest during this period and generates the most blood flow. As the left atrium fills, the gradient decreases, and blood flow slows. The MV then opens, releasing the pressure in the left atrium and reestablishing a gradient between the PV and the left atrium. Blood flow from the PV to the left atrium resumes, although at a lower velocity and flow distance (i.e., VTI) as a result of a smaller gradient. PWD interrogation of a PV throughout the cardiac cycle yields waves in systole (PVs) and diastole (PVd), with the maximum velocity and VTI greater in systole than diastole in normal LAP (Fig. 10.17). In a left ventricle with poor diastolic compliance, the gradient between the PV and the left atrium is reduced in systole. The majority of blood flow therefore occurs in diastole after the MV opens, to yield a PVs with a lower maximum velocity and VTI than the PVd.

Suggested Method

For the purposes of general intraoperative hemodynamic monitoring and GDT, use of the limited examination mentioned earlier with the addition of spectral Doppler assessments of mitral inflow, mitral annular, and pulmonary venous inflow velocities is suggested (Box 10.6). At the start of the monitoring period, the entire limited examination should be performed. This should include baseline values for E, E′, PVs, and PVd, as well as an estimation of the LAP using an approximation of the equation noted:

$$PCWP = 0.97 \times E/E' + 4.34 \approx E/E' + 4$$

236

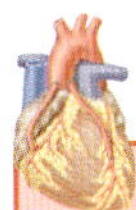

> **BOX 10.6** *Recommended Limited Examination for General Hemodynamic Monitoring and Goal-Directed Therapy Using Transesophageal Echocardiography*
>
> 1. ME AV SAX view
> 2. ME AV LAX view
>   - ME of LVOT diameter
> 3. ME bicaval view
>   - PWD of right upper PV
>   - Measurement of PVs, PVd, and DTd
> 4. ME RV inflow-outflow view
> 5. ME four-chamber view
>   - With and without CFD on the TV and MV
>   - Mitral inflow PWD for E wave
>   - Mitral annulus tissue Doppler for E′ wave
>   - Estimation of LAP ($\approx$E/E′ + 4)
> 6. ME two-chamber view
> 7. ME LV LAX view
> 8. TG LV SAX view
> 9. Deep TG view
>   - PWD of LVOT
>   - Calculation of stroke volume
>
> *AV*, Aortic valve; *CFD*, color-flow Doppler; *DTd*, deceleration time of the pulmonary vein in diastole; *LAP*, left atrial pressure; *LAX*, long-axis; *LV*, left ventricular; *LVOT*, left ventricular outflow tract; *ME*, midesophageal; *MV*, mitral valve; *PV*, pulmonary vein; *PVd*, pulmonary vein in diastole; *PVs*, pulmonary vein in systole; *PWD*, pulsed-wave Doppler; *RV*, right ventricular; *SAX*, short-axis; *TG*, transgastric; *TV*, tricuspid valve.

After this assessment, the focus of continued monitoring should be on the following views:

1. Four-chamber view for RV and LV systolic function and calculation of LAP
2. Transgastric SAX view for estimation of LV contractility, volume, and afterload
3. Deep transgastric view for spectral Doppler evaluation of the LVOT for SV and SV variation

Interventions to optimize SV should then be based on the TEE findings. For general hemodynamic monitoring, the main hemodynamic abnormalities encountered are poor contractility, hypovolemia, or low afterload. However, arrhythmias and high afterload must also be considered. Malignant arrhythmias obviously require emergency intervention to reestablish CO. Less acute arrhythmias, particularly sinus bradycardia and tachycardia, are far more common and can significantly compromise CO. Elevated afterload can also affect CO, even in the setting of high normal or only slightly elevated blood pressures. This finding highlights the interdependency of contractility and loading conditions. Mildly elevated afterload in a patient with normal systolic function may have little effect on CO, but it may have a significant effect in a patient with compromised systolic function. Table 10.6 lists the echocardiographic findings in the most commonly seen hemodynamic abnormalities.

The appropriate intervention should then be performed, and the foregoing parameters should be reevaluated by TEE. With the exception of pressor administration,

10

Table 10.6	Echocardiographic Findings in the Most Commonly Encountered Hemodynamic Abnormalities	
Abnormality	**Stroke Volume**	**Potential Other Findings**
↓ Contractility	↓	↓ Ejection fraction ↓ Segmental or global wall thickening
↓ Volume	↓	↓ End-diastolic area ↓ End-systolic area ↑ SV variability
↓ Afterload	↑	Hyperdynamic systolic function ↓ End-systolic area Normal end-diastolic area
↑ Afterload	↓	↑ End-systolic area ↓ Ejection fraction ↓ Segmental or global wall thickening ↑ Mitral or aortic valve regurgitation
Sinus bradycardia	↓	Bradycardia Normal end-diastolic area
Sinus tachycardia	↓	Tachycardia ↓ End-diastolic and end-systolic areas

↑, Increased; ↓, decreased.

all interventions should lead to an increase in SV. Although pressor administration reduces SV in a hyperdynamic left ventricle, a large reduction in SV may indicate that pharmacologic vasoconstriction is not the appropriate response. Echocardiographic parameters of LAP should also be assessed, particularly when volume or pressors have been given. An increase in E/E′ ratio or a reduction in PV systolic fraction suggests an acute increase in LAP. Further volume or pressor administration may result in pulmonary edema. RV and LV contractility, LV SAX assessment of preload and afterload, SV and SV variation, and LAP should be continuously monitored. Interventions should be tailored to the acute cardiac physiologic features, with the goals of maintaining perfusion pressure, improving SV, and preventing pulmonary edema. Additional TEE parameters suggesting that an intervention is appropriate or potentially inappropriate are listed in Table 10.7.

TRANSTHORACIC ECHOCARDIOGRAPHY

The preceding discussion focuses on the application of TEE to noncardiac surgical patients. TEE is safe and has repeatedly been shown to add value to intraoperative management. However, cardiac assessment does not begin and end in the operating room, even in the emergency setting. The utility of TEE in awake patients is obviously limited. TTE provides anesthesiologists with additional noninvasive windows to aid in cardiac diagnosis and monitoring. The images acquired from TTE are the same as those in TEE but at a different angle. Technically speaking, the "window" differs, but the "view" does not. The information and interpretation are the same. All the hemodynamic assessments listed earlier can be performed with TTE using similar views. The following discussion reviews the value and application of TTE by anesthesiologists, including how to perform a basic examination.

Table 10.7 **Echocardiographic Changes Following a Hemodynamic Intervention That Indicate the Success of the Intervention**

Intervention	Successful	Consider Alternative
Inotrope	↑ SV, CO ↑ EF ↑ RV, LV contractility	No change in SV or CO Arrhythmia, ischemia[a] ↑ LAP[b]
Volume	↑ SV, CO ↓ SV variation ↑ EDA, ESA	No change in SV or CO ↑ LAP[b] ↓ EF
Pressor	↑ ESA Normalized left ventricle	↓↓ SV, CO[c] ↑ LAP[b]
Vasodilator	↑ SV, CO ↓ ESA ↑ EF, contractility ↓ LAP[b]	No change in SV or CO Hyperdynamic right ventricle, left ventricle
(+) Chronotrope	↑ SV, CO	↓ SV, CO ↑ LAP ↓ EDA Arrhythmia, ischemia[a]
(–) Chronotrope	↑ SV, CO	↓ CO ↑ LAP[b]

[a]For echocardiographic signs of ischemia, see above.

[b]Echocardiographic parameters of ↑ LAP consist of ↑E/E′ wave ratio, ↓ pulmonary vein in systole velocity-time integral, and/or ↓ deceleration time of the pulmonary vein in diastole. Echocardiographic parameters of ↓ LAP would be the opposite.

[c]A reduction in SV is an appropriate response to pressor administration in the setting of low afterload. An excessive reduction, however, may mean that the increase in SVR with the pressor is too much for this particular contractile state.

CO, Cardiac output; *EDA,* end-diastolic area; *EF,* ejection fraction; *ESA,* end-systolic area; *LAP,* left atrial pressure; *LV,* left ventricular; *RV,* right ventricular; *SV,* stroke volume; ↑, increased; ↓, decreased.

Value of Perioperative Transthoracic Echocardiography

The American College of Cardiology (ACC) guidelines give a class I recommendation to preoperative echocardiography in patients "with clinically suspected moderate or greater degrees of valvular stenosis or regurgitation" and a class IIa recommendation in patients with dyspnea of unknown origin. Although these recommendations apply to a significant number of preoperative patients, the ASE also encourages the use of echocardiography in the following situations:

- When symptoms or conditions are potentially related to a cardiac disease
- When results from previous testing (e.g., chest radiograph, biomarkers) are concerning for heart disease
- To reevaluate known structural heart disease with a change in clinical status
- When pulmonary hypertension is suspected
- With diagnoses of atrial fibrillation
- When hypertensive heart disease is suspected

Given that preoperative patients frequently meet these criteria and the information obtained from TTE is recognized to add value to the long-term care of these patients, it seems reasonable to apply these broader criteria to preoperative echocardiography when feasible.

Preoperative cardiac assessment involves diagnosing CV dysfunction, predicting the effects of anesthesia on CV function, and attempting to mitigate the risks through preoperative optimization. Resting preoperative TTE predicts postoperative cardiac complications better than does clinical risk assessment alone, and it is as sensitive as but more specific than dipyridamole thallium scanning.

Equally important is how the information on cardiac pathophysiology obtained through echocardiographic studies can guide anesthetic care. Anesthesia encapsulates a wide range of care options, and perioperative CV risk cannot be assumed to be the same across all potential anesthetic cases. Physiologic optimization is an ongoing process that carries through the preoperative, intraoperative, and postoperative periods. In the immediate perioperative period, acute cardiac physiologic status guides this care. Cardiac physiology, from systolic and diastolic function to valvular regurgitation, depends on loading conditions that can quickly vary. A preoperative TTE examination is well suited to define the current CV state and allows the anesthesiologist to adjust care appropriately. Point-of-care TTE in the hands of anesthesiologists has been shown to alter intraoperative care. Preoperative point-of-care TTE has also been linked to improved outcomes including a reduction in mortality rates. The information obtained through echocardiography is beneficial above and beyond the history and physical examination. The sensitivity of symptoms of heart failure (including orthopnea, paroxysmal nocturnal dyspnea, and dyspnea with 4 metabolic equivalents of activity) is less than 35%, and even including physical findings of lower extremity edema, jugular venous distention, and an S_3 gallop, the sensitivity is still only approximately 50%.

The utility of TTE is not limited to the preoperative period. The advantages of TTE over TEE in awake postoperative patients are obvious. TTE also plays an important role intraoperatively. Twenty percent of the TTE examinations performed to assess hemodynamic instability in the perioperative patients in one study were performed in the operating room; in another study, more than 80% of the TTE examinations were performed intraoperatively. Intraoperative TTE is most commonly used when TEE is contraindicated, when a TEE probe cannot physically be placed, or when TEE images are not adequate as a result of technical difficulties.

How to Perform a Basic Transthoracic Echocardiography Examination

Investigators have repeatedly shown that noncardiologist providers can successfully be trained in bedside TTE. This group of providers includes medical students, internal medicine residents, emergency medicine physicians, critical care physicians, internists, and anesthesiology residents. First-year medical students using bedside ultrasonography to diagnose cardiac disease were shown to significantly more likely reach accurate diagnoses than were attending cardiologists who were not using ultrasonography. The teachability of point-of-care TTE is likely related to a paradigm shift with regard to image acquisition and interpretation. Because of the size and complexity of the original ultrasound machines, their use was limited to practitioners with specialized training. Current technology, conversely, has yielded small, easily portable units geared toward decision making in real time. A detailed analysis of the images is not required to make immediate decisions on prognosis and hemodynamic management. Similar to the echocardiographic assessment of hemodynamic emergencies with TEE, perioperative TTE requires only a qualitative analysis, thus reducing the training required for competency.

With adequate training, anesthesiologists can be credentialed to perform TEE and potentially bill for their studies. Although currently no standard exists for training or credentialing anesthesiologists to perform TTE, guidelines are in place for other specialties. The ACC guidelines on training in echocardiography suggest that cardiologists with level II training in TTE who want to incorporate TEE into their practice should perform at least 50 examinations before being considered competent. An argument could be made that similar criteria should apply to anesthesiologists with level II training in TEE when seeking proficiency in TTE. With training in basic image acquisition and interpretation and 50 supervised studies, an anesthesiologist should be considered competent to perform TTE examinations.

The following are instructions for acquiring TTE images; a limited examination should be performed, focusing on the pertinent images that aid in perioperative care.

1. Equipment: A phased-array probe is necessary for this examination. Any machine that is used to perform TEE should also have TTE capabilities. Point-of-care devices can also acquire adequate images for qualitative analysis.
2. Positioning: When imaging is done from the parasternal and apical windows, the patient should be in the full left lateral decubitus position with the left arm resting under the head to help spread the ribs. To access the LV apex, it is necessary to move the patient to the very edge of the bed or stretcher or to tilt the patient slightly back from a true left lateral position. Although the left lateral position is preferred, it is also possible to perform the entire examination with the patient supine. The subcostal window is accessed with the patient supine and the legs slightly bent to relax the abdominal muscles.
3. Basic technique and assessment
   a. Parasternal LAX view (Fig. 10.18):
      i. Technique: The probe should be positioned at the third or fourth intercostal space, just to the left of the sternum, with the "indicator" pointing toward the left shoulder (Fig. 10.19).
      ii. Assessment: This view is one of the easiest to perform, even in supine or morbidly obese patients. It provides information on RV size and function; AV function; left trial size; and LV function, size, and thickness.

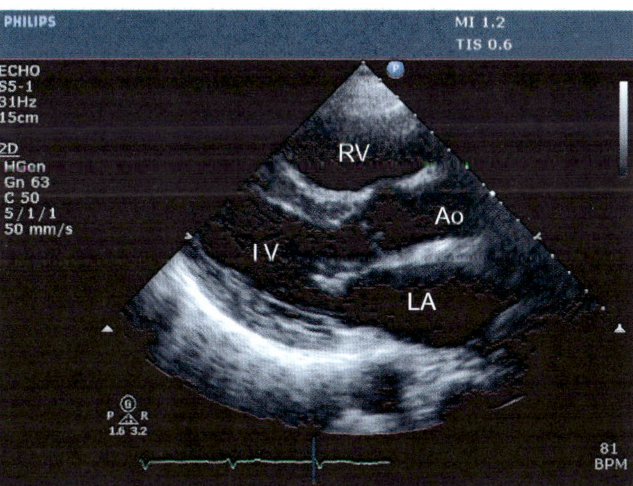

Fig. 10.18 Parasternal long-axis view allowing visualization of the left atrium (LA), mitral valve, left ventricle (LV), aortic valve, ascending aorta (Ao), and right ventricle (RV).

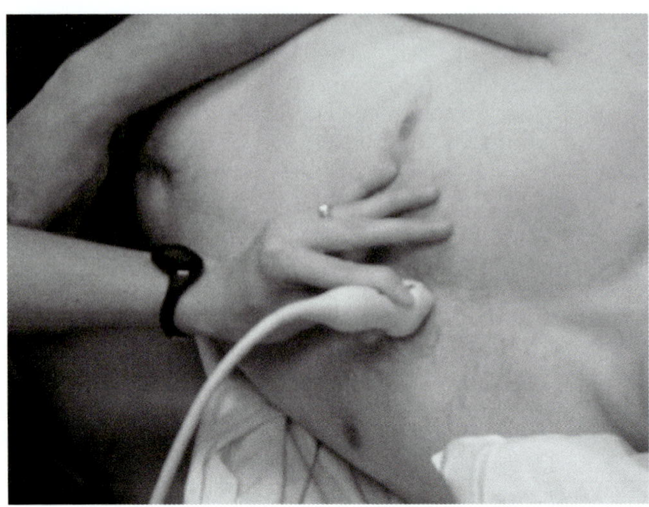

Fig. 10.19 How to obtain the parasternal long-axis echocardiographic view. The patient is in the left lateral decubitus position to position the heart on the chest wall. The probe is placed in the third or fourth intercostal space with the marker toward the right shoulder.

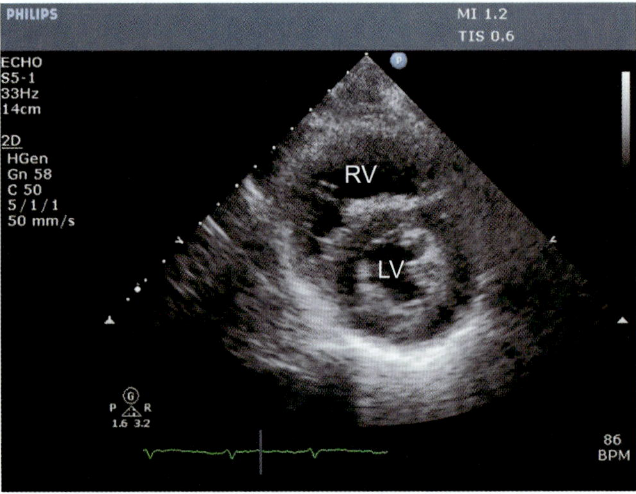

Fig. 10.20 Parasternal short-axis view allowing a cross-sectional view of the left ventricle (LV) and the right ventricle (RV).

   b. Parasternal SAX view (Fig. 10.20)

     i. Technique: From the LAX, the probe is rotated approximately 90 degrees clockwise until the indicator points toward the patient's right shoulder (Fig. 10.21). The probe should then be tilted until the appropriate LV cross-section is obtained.

     ii. Assessment: With angulation of the probe, the basal, middle, and apical cross-sections showing the 16 LV segments can be assessed for wall motion abnormalities. Global LV function and filling can be assessed as well. By angling the probe to look more anteriorly (angling the "tail" toward the apex), a SAX view of the AV can be seen.

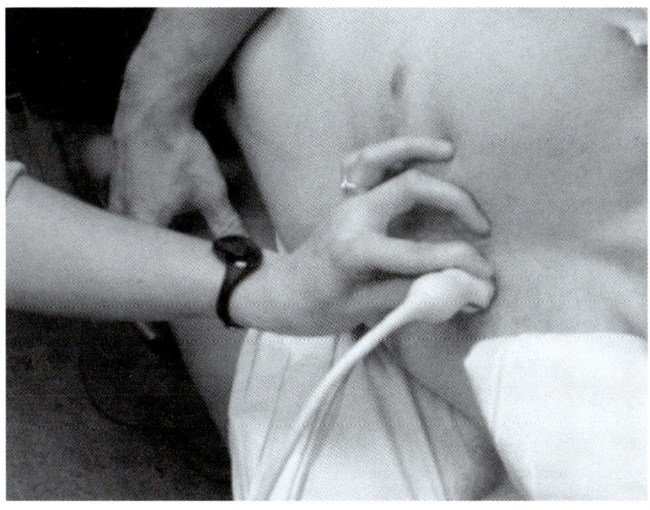

Fig. 10.21 How to obtain the parasternal left ventricular short-axis echocardiographic view. The probe is turned clockwise approximately 90 degrees.

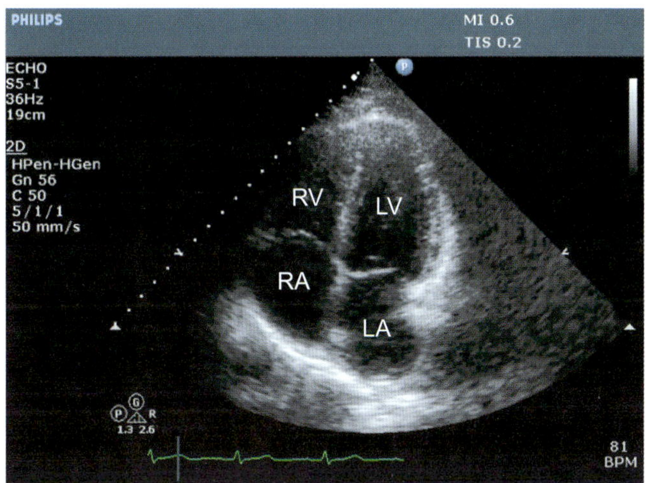

Fig. 10.22 Apical four-chamber view demonstrating the left ventricle (LV), right ventricle (RV), left atrium (LA), and right atrium (RA). This view allows evaluation of LV function, RV function, chamber sizes, interventricular and interatrial septal position, and interrogation of mitral inflow and lateral mitral annular tissue Doppler imaging.

c. Apical four-chamber (Fig. 10.22)

   i. Technique: The apical window can be found by placing the probe at the point of maximal impulse (Fig. 10.23). The indicator should point toward the patient's left. The apex of the left ventricle will appear directly under the probe with minimal foreshortening of the left ventricle and without showing the coronary sinus or LVOT.

   ii. Assessment: This view shows global and regional LV and RV function, chamber sizes, and mitral and tricuspid valve function. The valves can be interrogated with CFD. Spectral Doppler can be used to assess right-sided pressures with

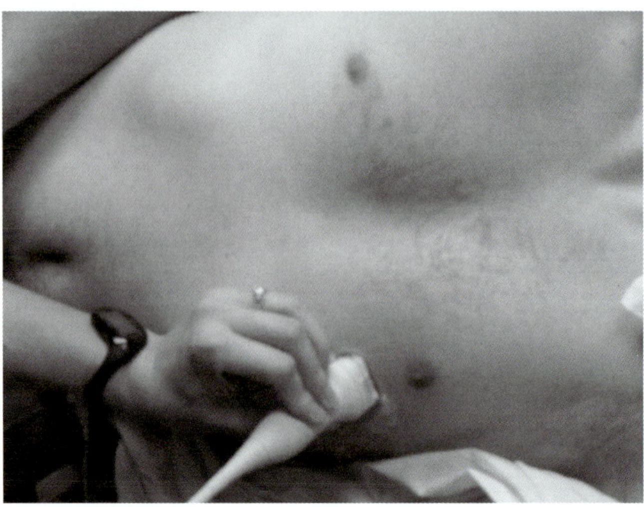

Fig. 10.23 How to obtain an apical four-chamber echocardiographic view. Ideally, the probe would be placed at the point of maximal impulse in the axilla with the marker pointing toward the floor. This placement is often difficult with the beds used in the preoperative period. Placement of the probe under or near the nipple often produces adequate images.

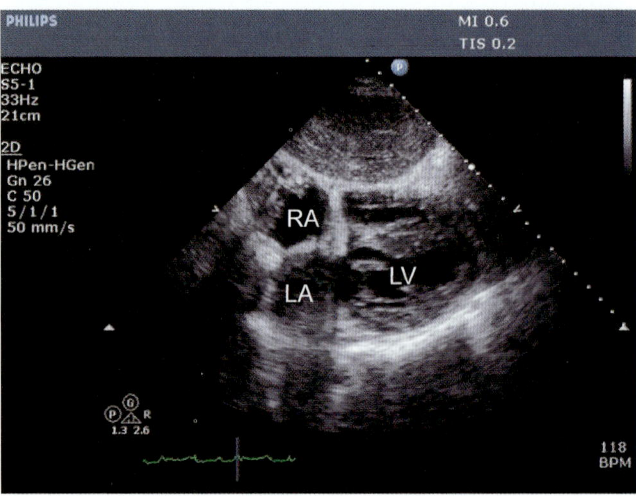

Fig. 10.24 Subcostal four-chamber view demonstrating all four chambers of the heart. This orientation allows excellent identification of the pericardium and potential pericardial effusions. *LA*, left atrium; *LV*, left ventricle; *RA*, right atrium.

continuous-wave Doppler through any tricuspid regurgitation. Assessment of diastolic function can be performed with a combination of PWD interrogation of mitral inflow and tissue Doppler evaluation of septal and lateral mitral annulus motion in diastole. Slight angling of the tail of the probe toward the feet will reveal the five-chamber view. PWD interrogation of the LVOT yields LVOT VTI and thus allows for SV calculation.

   d. Subcostal four-chamber (Fig. 10.24)

      i. Technique: The patient should be placed supine for these images. It is useful to have the patient bend the knees or place pillow under the knees to relax

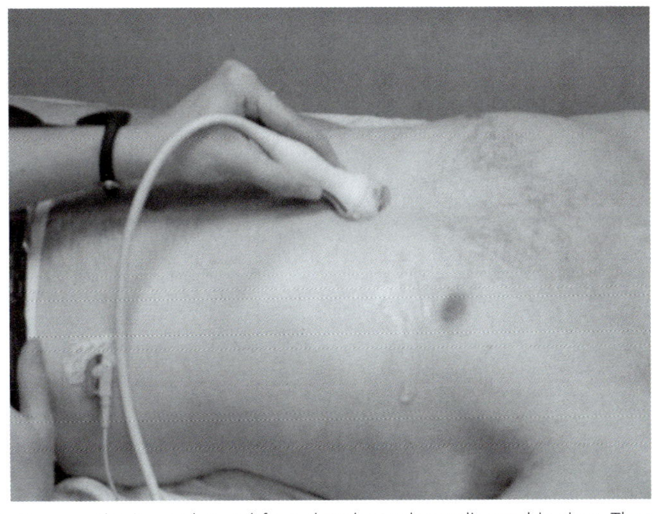

Fig. 10.25 How to obtain a subcostal four-chamber echocardiographic view. The probe should be positioned near the xyphoid process with the marker toward the left side of the patient's body.

the abdominal musculature. The probe is placed just below or slightly left of the xiphoid process, with the indicator pointed to the patient's left and with the probe nearly horizontal (Fig. 10.25).

ii. Assessment: The right ventricle is seen very well, allowing for evaluation of thickness, function, and size. Pericardial effusions can be seen here, as well as evidence of tamponade (i.e., compression of the right atrium or right ventricle). The left ventricle and atrioventricular valves can also be evaluated.

CONCLUSION

Echocardiography, using either TTE or TEE modalities, is extremely useful to perioperative physicians by aiding in both diagnosis and management. Because of its portability and ease of use, it is the diagnostic tool of choice in the setting of hemodynamic instability. Echocardiography is not limited to emergencies; it provides a significant amount of information as a general hemodynamic monitor. With numerous complementary tools at the examiner's disposal, echocardiography is also the ideal monitor for GDT. Finally, limited preoperative echocardiographic assessment, even in the hands of noncardiologists, significantly alters intraoperative and postoperative anesthetic management and may even reduce perioperative mortality rates.

SUGGESTED READING

American College of Cardiology Foundation Appropriate Use Criteria Task Force, American Society of Echocardiography, American Heart Association, et al. ACCF/ASE/AHA/ASNC/HFSA/HRS/SCAI/ SCCM/ SCCT/SCMR 2011 appropriate use criteria for echocardiography: a report of the American College of Cardiology Foundation Appropriate Use Criteria Task Force, American Society of Echocardiography, American Heart Association, American Society of Nuclear Cardiology, Heart Failure Society of America, Heart Rhythm Society, Society for Cardiovascular Angiography and Interventions, Society of Critical Care Medicine, Society of Cardiovascular Computed Tomography, Society for Cardiovascular Magnetic Resonance American College of Chest Physicians. *J Am Soc Echocardiogr.* 2011;24:229–267.

American Society of Anesthesiologists and Society of Cardiovascular Anesthesiologists Task Force on Transesophageal Echocardiography. Practice guidelines for perioperative transesophageal echocardiography: an updated report by the American Society of Anesthesiologists and the Society of Cardiovascular Anesthesiologists Task Force on Transesophageal Echocardiography. *Anesthesiology*. 2010;112:1084–1096.

Canty DJ, Royse CF, Kilpatrick D, et al. The impact of pre-operative focused transthoracic echocardiography in emergency non-cardiac surgery patients with known or risk of cardiac disease. *Anaesthesia*. 2012;67:714–720.

Canty DJ, Royse CF, Kilpatrick D, et al. The impact on cardiac diagnosis and mortality of focused transthoracic echocardiography in hip fracture surgery patients with increased risk of cardiac disease: a retrospective cohort study. *Anaesthesia*. 2012;67:1202–1209.

Cowie B. Focused transthoracic echocardiography predicts perioperative cardiovascular morbidity. *J Cardiothorac Vasc Anesth*. 2012;26(1–6):989–993.

Cowie B. Three years' experience of focused cardiovascular ultrasound in the peri-operative period. *Anaesthesia*. 2011;66:268–273.

Fayad A, Shillcutt S, Meineri M, et al. Comparative effectiveness and harms of intraoperative transesophageal echocardiography in noncardiac surgery. *Semin Cardiothorac Vasc Anesth*. 2018;22:122–126.

Fleisher LA, Fleischmann KE, Auerbach AD, et al. 2014 ACC/AHA guideline on perioperative cardiovascular evaluation and management of patients undergoing noncardiac surgery: a report of the American College of Cardiology/American Heart Association Task Force on Practice Guidelines. *J Am Coll Cardiol*. 2014;64:e77–e137.

Gudmundsson P, Rydberg E, Winter R, Willenheimer R. Visually estimated left ventricular ejection fraction by echocardiography is closely correlated with formal quantitative methods. *Int J Cardiol*. 2005;101:209–212.

Haji DL, Royse A, Royse CF. Review article: clinical impact of non-cardiologist-performed transthoracic echocardiography in emergency medicine, intensive care medicine and anaesthesia. *Emerg Med Australas*. 2012;25:4–12.

Hamilton MA, Cecconi M, Rhodes A. A systematic review and meta-analysis on the use of preemptive hemodynamic intervention to improve postoperative outcomes in moderate and high-risk surgical patients. *Anesth Analg*. 2011;112:1392–1402.

Lang RM, Bierig M, Devereux RB, et al. Recommendations for chamber quantification: a report from the American Society of Echocardiography's Guidelines and Standards Committee and the Chamber Quantification Writing Group, developed in conjunction with the European Association of Echocardiography, a branch of the European Society of Cardiology. *J Am Soc Echocardiogr*. 2005;18:1440–1463.

Loxdale SJ, Sneyd JR, Donovan A, et al. The role of routine pre-operative bedside echocardiography in detecting aortic stenosis in patients with a hip fracture. *Anaesthesia*. 2012;67:51–54.

Mingo S, Benedicto A, Jimenez MC, et al. Dynamic left ventricular outflow tract obstruction secondary to catecholamine excess in a normal ventricle. *Int J Cardiol*. 2006;112:393–396.

Rajaram SS, Desai NK, Kalra A, et al. Pulmonary artery catheters for adult patients in intensive care. *Cochrane Database Syst Rev*. 2013;(2):CD003408.

Reeves ST, Finley AC, Skubas NJ, et al. Basic perioperative transesophageal echocardiography examination: a consensus statement of the American Society of Echocardiography and the Society of Cardiovascular Anesthesiologists. *Anesth Analg*. 2013;117:543–558.

Rhodes A, Cecconi M, Hamilton M, et al. Goal-directed therapy in high-risk surgical patients: a 15-year follow-up study. *Intensive Care Med*. 2010;36:1327–1332.

Rudski LG, Lai WW, Afilalo J, et al. Guidelines for the echocardiographic assessment of the right heart in adults: a report from the American Society of Echocardiography. *J Am Soc Echocardiogr*. 2010;23:685–713.

Schulmeyer MC, Santelices E, Vega R, Schmied S. Impact of intraoperative transesophageal echocardiography during noncardiac surgery. *J Cardiothorac Vasc Anesth*. 2006;20:768–771.

Sheehan F, Redington A. The right ventricle: anatomy, physiology and clinical imaging. *Heart*. 2008;94:1510–1515.

Shillcutt SK, Markin NW, Montzingo CR, Brakke TR. Use of rapid 'rescue' perioperative echocardiography to improve outcomes after hemodynamic instability in noncardiac surgical patients. *J Cardiothorac Vasc Anesth*. 2012;26:362–370.

Tranter MH, Wright PT, Sikkel MB, Lyon AR. Takotsubo cardiomyopathy: the pathophysiology. *Heart Fail Clin*. 2013;9:187–196.

Chapter 11

Cardiovascular Pharmacology in Noncardiac Surgery

Liem P. Nguyen, MD • Neal S. Gerstein, MD, FASE

Key Points

1. Intraoperative hemodynamic instability may be associated with increased cardiovascular complications and represents one of the most common findings associated with mortality.
2. Phenylephrine can be used for the treatment of intraoperative hypotension through an increase in stroke volume and cardiac output in patients with preload-recruitable stroke work.
3. Binding of vasopressin to its cognate receptor (V_1) leads to potent vasoconstriction and an increase in systemic vascular resistance (SVR).
4. Methylene blue–mediated downregulation of the endothelial nitric oxide synthase and soluble guanylate cyclase pathways restores vascular tone in patients with vasopressor-refractory hypotension.
5. Epinephrine is an endogenous catecholamine that augments cardiac output and arterial pressure through its stimulation of both β-adrenergic and α-receptors, respectively.
6. Dobutamine is a synthetic catecholamine that displays a strong affinity for the β-receptor (β_1 and β_2), resulting in dose-dependent increases in cardiac output and heart rate and reductions in SVR.
7. The higher affinity of norepinephrine for the α-adrenergic receptor provides the basis for its powerful overall vasoconstrictor effect and less potent inotropic and chronotropic properties.
8. In addition to augmenting cardiac contractility, the lusitropic effects of milrinone on ventricular relaxation and compliance make it an attractive choice to improve diastolic filling parameters.
9. Acute perioperative hypertension is a risk factor for adverse cardiovascular outcome and is mainly a result of an increase in sympathetic activity.
10. Nitroglycerin reduces cardiac filling pressures with minimal effects on SVR because of its effect on venous capacitance.
11. Nitroprusside possesses a quick onset of action and great potency, making it a rational choice for management of intraoperative hypertension.
12. Clevidipine is an ultra-fast-acting and selective arterial dilator that reduces arterial pressure with minimal effects on cardiac filling pressures or heart rate.
13. In the intraoperative setting, β-blockers are considered first-line agents in the treatment of acute myocardial ischemia, supraventricular tachyarrhythmias, and hypertension related to tachycardia.
14. Smart infusion pumps offer significant advantages in the perioperative setting, mainly the ability to deliver very small volumes of fluids or drugs at precisely programmed rates.
15. The majority of sympathomimetic agents and commonly used inotropes in the perioperative period have short effective half-lives and are typically administered by intravenous continuous infusion, and their effects rapidly dissipate with cessation of their infusion.

16. Perioperative arrhythmias are clinically important because of the potential associated hemodynamic instability. Perioperative arrhythmia etiology is multifactorial; in addition to possible preexisting cardiac conduction defects or surgical-related contributions, anesthetic agents themselves may negatively affect normal cardiac electrical activity at various levels (e.g., sinoatrial [SA] node, atrioventricular node, His-Purkinje system).
17. Activation of the sympathetic nervous system and renin–angiotensin–aldosterone system is central to the pathophysiology of congestive heart failure, providing the pharmacologic targets for many of the currently available heart failure drugs.
18. The first in-class drug sacubitril-valsartan (Entresto) combines a neprilysin inhibitor (sacubitril), which blocks the degradation of natriuretic peptides, with an angiotensin receptor blocker (valsartan). The dual combination of neprilysin inhibitor–angiotensin receptor antagonist was developed to address two distinct pathophysiologic mechanisms underlying heart failure, activation of the renin–angiotensin axis and decreased natriuretic peptide activity.
19. Ivabradine is a specific heart rate–decreasing agent that selectively inhibits the funny (I_f) current in SA nodal tissue. Ivabradine reduces heart rate with minimal effects on myocardial contractility, blood pressure, and intracardiac conduction. This mechanism is distinct from other negative chronotropic agents and is the main advantage of this new class of heart failure agents.
20. The presence of perioperative pulmonary hypertension portends a poor prognosis because it carries a significant risk for mortality and associated complications.
21. Several pulmonary vasodilators are available for the management of pulmonary hypertension. The ideal perioperative pulmonary vasodilator reduces pulmonary vascular resistance by relaxing the pulmonary vasculature without causing a drop in SVR or systemic hypotension.

The intraoperative management of hemodynamics plays a critical role in the optimization of tissue perfusion under general anesthesia. The effects of general anesthesia predominantly lead to a reduction in cardiac output and arterial blood pressure, often jeopardizing tissue perfusion to vital organs. Intraoperative hemodynamic instability may be associated with increased cardiovascular complications in the perioperative period and represents one of the most common findings associated with intraoperative mortality during general anesthesia. The main thrust of this chapter is to review the pharmacology of inotropes and vasoactive agents as it pertains to the optimization of intraoperative hemodynamics. Three main pharmacologic classes of vasoactive agents are reviewed: (1) agents that increase mean arterial pressure (MAP), (2) agents that increase cardiac output, and (3) agents that reduce MAP. The main focus of this chapter is to discuss the pharmacology and perioperative use of vasoactive agents in the setting of noncardiac surgery.

VASOACTIVE AGENTS USED IN THE PERIOPERATIVE PERIOD (BOXES 11.1 TO 11.3)

Vasopressors

Phenylephrine

Phenylephrine is a widely used vasopressor in the operating room for the treatment of hypotension. The primary binding target of phenylephrine is the α-adrenergic receptor with the highest affinity for the α_1-receptor. Phenylephrine is an α_1 selective agonist but may affect β-receptors in high doses. It is equipotent to norepinephrine

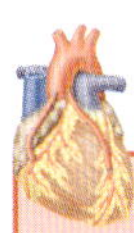

BOX 11.1　*Vasoconstrictor Agents That Increase Mean Arterial Blood Pressure*

- Phenylephrine is a widely used vasopressor in the operating room for the treatment of hypotension. On the arterial vasculature, α_1-receptor activation by phenylephrine leads to increases in arterial pressure, systemic vascular resistance, and ventricular afterload. On the venous side, α_1-adrenergic receptor stimulation leads to a reduction in venous capacitance, which may lead to increased venous return depending on the preload dependency or position of the heart on the Frank-Starling curve.
- Ephedrine is a short-acting indirect α- and β-adrenergic agonist that also enhances the endogenous release of norepinephrine from adrenergic nerve terminals. The overall hemodynamic effect is characterized by an elevation in mean arterial pressure through an increase in systemic vascular resistance and a rise in heart rate and cardiac output to varying degrees.
- Arginine vasopressin causes potent vasoconstriction throughout the circulation, leading to increases in systemic vascular resistance and arterial blood pressure. Vasopressin binding in the kidney mediates its antidiuretic effect and markedly increases renal concentrating ability to increase intravascular volume.
- Methylene blue is a heterocyclic aromatic molecule that blocks the nitric oxide synthase and soluble guanylate cyclase pathways, leading to the restoration of vascular tone and arterial pressure.

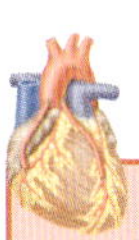

BOX 11.2　*Vasoactive Agents That Increase Cardiac Output*

- Epinephrine is an endogenous catecholamine that stimulates both α- and β-adrenergic receptors in a dose-dependent fashion. The β-selective pharmacology of epinephrine is characterized by a higher binding affinity for the β-receptor at lower doses (0.01–0.04 µg/kg/min) and a stronger preference for the α–receptor at higher doses (0.05–0.2 µg/kg/min). This provides the clinical basis for the biphasic response observed for epinephrine, in which at lower doses, the hemodynamic effects are predominated by increased inotropy and chronotropy of the heart (β effect), and at higher doses, a vasopressor effect (α effect) is primarily observed.
- Dobutamine is a synthetic catecholamine that displays a strong affinity for the β-receptor (β_1 and β_2), resulting in dose-dependent increases in cardiac output and heart rate and reductions in systemic vascular resistance and diastolic filling pressures. Dobutamine is a rational choice for patients with right or left ventricular dysfunction and afterload mismatch.
- Isoproterenol is a potent, nonselective β-adrenergic agonist devoid of α-adrenergic agonist activity. The potent chronotropic, inotropic, and vasodilatory effects of isoproterenol make it an excellent candidate for the treatment of acute bradyarrhythmias or atrioventricular heart block, pulmonary hypertension, and heart failure.
- Norepinephrine is an endogenous catecholamine exhibiting potent α-adrenergic activity with a mild to modest effect on the β-adrenergic receptor. The higher affinity for norepinephrine for the α-adrenergic receptor provides the basis for its powerful overall vasoconstrictor effect and less potent inotropic and chronotropic properties. The overall hemodynamic effects of norepinephrine are characterized by increases in systolic, diastolic, and pulse pressures, with minimal net impact on cardiac output and heart rate.
- Milrinone has a unique mechanism of action independent of the adrenergic receptor. Its inotropic effects are mediated primarily through an inhibition of the phosphodiesterase enzyme and not through β-receptor stimulation. As a result, the effectiveness of milrinone is not altered by previous β-blockade, nor is it reduced in patients who may experience β-receptor downregulation. Milrinone is also effective in improving diastolic relaxation and compliance.

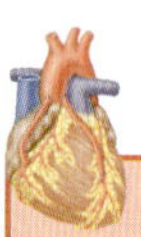

BOX 11.3　*Vasoactive Agents That Lower Arterial Blood Pressure*

- Nitroglycerin belongs to the nitrovasodilator group of drugs that exert their effect through the donation of nitric oxide (NO) and activation of the soluble guanylate cyclase pathway in smooth muscle. Nitroglycerin preferably dilates the venous capacitance vessels, resulting in decreases in right atrial, pulmonary artery, pulmonary capillary wedge, and ventricular end-diastolic pressures with minimal effects on systemic vascular resistance. Nitroglycerin also has a vasodilator effect on coronary arteries, reducing the resistance to blood flow.
- Nitroprusside is a potent nitrovasodilator that acts by releasing NO to induce both arterial and venous dilation. Nitroprusside possesses a quick onset of action and great potency, making it a rational choice for management of intraoperative hypertension and for afterload reduction during surgery.
- Clevidipine is an ultra-fast-acting, dihydropyridine L-type calcium channel blocker with a direct action on arteriolar resistance vessels and limited effects on venous capacitance vessels. Clevidipine inhibits the L-type calcium channel in arterial smooth muscle, causing potent vasodilation. Because of its rapid metabolism by circulating esterases, its effect is quickly terminated independent of hepatic or renal function. Hemodynamically, clevidipine reduces arterial pressure through direct action on the arterioles without affecting the filling pressures or causing reflex changes in heart rate.
- Nicardipine is a dihydropyridine L-type calcium channel blocker with a selective arterial vasodilator mode of action. Nicardipine has unique pharmacologic effects in that the drug selectively reduces systemic and coronary artery resistance, thereby decreasing left ventricular afterload and increasing coronary blood flow.
- The β-adrenergic antagonists reduce myocardial work and oxygen demand by decreasing heart rate, blood pressure, and myocardial contractility. β-Blocker–mediated heart rate reduction may also have a salient effect on increasing coronary blood flow.

but has a slightly longer duration of action. Binding of phenylephrine to the α_1 receptor leads to a number of pharmacologic effects. On the arterial vasculature, α_1-receptor activation by phenylephrine leads to increases in arterial pressure, systemic vascular resistance (SVR), and ventricular afterload. On the venous side, α_1-adrenergic receptor stimulation leads to a reduction in venous capacitance, which may lead to increased venous return depending on the preload dependency or position of the heart on the Frank-Starling curve. In patients with preload-recruitable stroke work, phenylephrine titration can lead to increased stroke volume and cardiac output. By contrast, patients who are operating on the plateau of the Frank-Starling relationship and are not preload dependent may exhibit a phenylephrine-induced decrease in stroke volume caused by a rise in SVR and reflex decreases in heart rate. Clinically, the biphasic response of phenylephrine mandates a careful determination of the patient's fluid or preload responsiveness to achieve the desired hemodynamic result.

Hemodynamically, the clinical effect of phenylephrine is complex and is essentially dose dependent. The initial starting dose for an infusion of phenylephrine typically ranges from 0.2 to 2.0 µg/kg per minute or 5 to 200 µg/min. Bolus administration of phenylephrine typically starts at 50 to 100 µg/dose. At the lower dose range, patients under the vasodilatory effects of general anesthesia typically respond to phenylephrine with an increase in preload return and concomitant augmentation of stroke volume. An increase in MAP may result as a consequence of increased recruitable stroke work as well as a modest rise in SVR. The effect of low-dose phenylephrine on pulmonary vascular resistance (PVR) is generally negligible. As the dose of phenylephrine is increased, a critical threshold is eventually reached, and reductions in stroke volume and heart rate, combined with rises in SVR and PVR, are generally observed. The dose that induces decreases in stroke volume and reflex bradycardia is complex and dependent on a myriad of factors, highlighting the careful individual titration of phenylephrine in each patient.

The clinical use of phenylephrine in the operating room is quite broad; therefore only a few clinical scenarios are highlighted in this section. The administration of phenylephrine is commonly used in the setting of hypotension to counter the vasodilatory effects of anesthetic agents. Indeed, phenylephrine may be used to treat hypotension after induction or during maintenance of anesthesia. In this setting, initial low doses of phenylephrine may increase preload and MAP through constriction of the venous and arterial beds, respectively. If the anesthesiologist increases the dose or administers a large initial bolus, reflex bradycardia may result with a detrimental effect on cardiac output. In patients who are more afterload sensitive because of poor contractile reserve, abrupt rises in preload and afterload may result in a more exaggerated decrease in cardiac output after phenylephrine administration. Phenylephrine is also appropriate for the treatment of hypotension in the setting of aortic stenosis. As the left ventricular (LV) afterload is relatively fixed by the stenotic valve, increases in diastolic blood pressure with phenylephrine therapy may increase coronary perfusion. Any phenylephrine-induced reductions in heart rate may also prove beneficial because lower heart rates may improve diastolic filling time and minimize myocardial oxygen consumption. Another important clinical use of phenylephrine is for the hemodynamic management of patients with hypertrophic subaortic stenosis or dynamic LV outflow obstruction from systolic anterior motion of the mitral valve. The dynamic nature of outflow obstructions is such that they worsen as ventricular volume decreases because of increased contractility. Increases in LV afterload may act to decrease contractility, thereby reducing the severity of the outflow obstruction.

Ephedrine

Ephedrine is a short-acting indirect α- and β-adrenergic agonist that also enhances the endogenous release of norepinephrine from adrenergic nerve terminals. Ephedrine, a plant alkaloid, has a duration of effect of approximately 10 to 15 minutes, is minimally metabolized, with an elimination half-life of 6 hours in urine. Repeated dosing may lead to tachyphylaxis because of intrinsic catecholamine depletion. The overall hemodynamic effect is characterized by an elevation in MAP through an increase in SVR and rises in heart rate and cardiac output to varying degrees. Initial intravenous (IV) bolus doses of ephedrine typically start at 5 to 10 mg (0.07–0.1 mg/kg) and is carefully titrated to prevent deleterious and unwanted effects such as tachycardia. At higher doses (0.15–0.2 mg/kg), unpredictable rises in heart rate and MAP may be observed as well as the potential for tachyphylaxis, especially with repetitive dosing. The mechanism governing the acute tolerance after repeat boluses of ephedrine may be caused by a depletion of endogenous norepinephrine levels and a decrease in adrenergic receptor density. In addition to the hemodynamic effects, ephedrine possesses bronchodilator properties through its stimulation of the β_2-receptor, leading to its use in patients with reactive airway disease and possibly in the treatment of anaphylaxis.

Clinically, ephedrine can be titrated cautiously to treat intraoperative hypotension during general anesthesia. It is particularly useful when a temporizing measure is needed to improve hemodynamics in the setting of relative bradycardia and hypotension. It has been recommended for the treatment of propofol-induced hypotension and bradycardia after induction of anesthesia. It may also be a rational choice for the treatment of hypotension and bradycardia following sympathectomy after epidural or spinal anesthesia.

Vasopressin

Arginine vasopressin (antidiuretic hormone) is a peptide hormone produced in the posterior pituitary that plays a crucial role in the regulation of vascular tone and circulating blood volume. The half-life of vasopressin is approximately 10 minutes with a range between 5 and 20 minutes. Exogenous vasopressin must be administered intravenously, and in bolus form, its effects are brief; hence, it is typically administered by continuous infusion. Activation of the vasopressin receptor (V_1) in the vasculature leads to potent vasoconstriction throughout the circulation, leading to increases in SVR and arterial blood pressure. Vasopressin (V_2) receptor activation in the kidney mediates its antidiuretic effect and markedly increases renal concentrating ability to promote volume avidity. Moreover, binding of vasopressin in the pulmonary vasculature may confer a vasodilatory effect through a nitric oxide (NO)-mediated pathway, resulting in a decrease in PVR in certain patients.

Vasopressin is often administered as an IV infusion, with dosing regimens starting at 0.01 to 0.04 U/min for the treatment of low SVR and hypotension. The pharmacology of vasopressin lends itself to be used in unique clinical scenarios. Because its vasoconstrictive effects are mediated through the V_1 receptor as opposed to the adrenergic receptor, vasopressin infusions may represent a rational strategy to decrease high doses of catecholamines such as norepinephrine or epinephrine to treat refractory vasodilation. In particular, vasopressin therapy has found great utility in the treatment of septic shock caused by vasopressin depletion, profound vasoplegia during cardiac surgery, and catecholamine-resistant hypotension from adrenergic receptor downregulation. The use of vasopressin may also be a rational choice for the treatment of low SVR and concomitant pulmonary hypertension. Because of the differential vasoconstricting and vasodilating effects on the systemic and pulmonary vasculature, respectively, vasopressin provides a means to manage hypotension in the setting of coexisting elevated PVR. Similarly, vasopressin therapy may find utility in patients with right ventricular (RV) dysfunction and systemic hypotension as the vasoconstricting effects of vasopressin may spare the pulmonary vasculature. Vasopressin is also an excellent adjunct in patients on vasodilatory inotropes such as milrinone, dobutamine, or isoproterenol. The addition of vasopressin may be used to augment arterial pressure in patients who have adequate cardiac output in the setting of low SVR.

Methylene Blue

Methylene blue is a heterocyclic aromatic molecule that blocks the nitric oxide synthase (NOS) and soluble guanylate cyclase (sGC) pathway that regulates smooth muscle function and vascular tone. IV methylene blue administration exhibits complex pharmacokinetics because of multiphasic distribution into various tissue compartments along with a slow terminal rate of disappearance. Methylene blue is excreted in the urine anywhere between 4 and 24 hours after administration with a half-life of 5 to 6.5 hours. Methylene blue–mediated downregulation of the endothelial NOS and sGC pathway restores vascular tone in patients with vasopressor-refractory hypotension. The hemodynamic effects of methylene blue are often observed with an initial single IV dose of 1.0 to 2 mg/kg. However, it is common for the effects to be transient, and some clinical scenarios may necessitate repeat dosing or maintenance with a continuous infusion at 0.25 to 2 mg/kg per hour to ameliorate the hypotension. Administration of methylene blue for the treatment of vasoplegic syndrome may be useful in a variety of clinical scenarios, including after cardiopulmonary bypass, congestive heart failure, anaphylaxis (including protamine reaction), sepsis, renal failure, and hepatic failure.

INOTROPES

Sympathomimetic Amines

Sympathomimetic drugs (i.e., catecholamines) are pharmacologic agents capable of providing diverse inotropic and vasoactive effects. Catecholamines exert positive inotropic action by stimulation of the β_1 and β_2 receptors (Table 11.1). The predominant hemodynamic effect of a specific catecholamine depends on the degree to which the various α, β, and dopaminergic receptors are stimulated. One of the primary indications for initiating inotropic support is for the treatment of ventricular dysfunction or low cardiac output states. Although β-agonists improve contractility and tissue perfusion, their effects may increase myocardial oxygen consumption (Mvo_2) and reduce coronary perfusion pressure (CPP) (Table 11.2). However, if the factor most responsible for decreased cardiac function is hypotension with concomitantly reduced CPP, infusion of α-adrenergic agonists can increase blood pressure and improve diastolic coronary perfusion.

Catecholamines also are effective for treating primary RV contractile dysfunction, with all of the β_1-adrenergic agonists augmenting RV contractility. The efficacy of epinephrine, norepinephrine, dobutamine, isoproterenol, dopamine, and phospho-diesterase III (PDE III) inhibitors in managing RV contractile dysfunction has been well described. When decreased RV contractility is combined with increased afterload, a combination of agents that exert both pulmonary vasodilator and positive inotropic effects may be used, including low-dose epinephrine, isoproterenol, dobutamine, PDE III inhibitors, and inhaled NO or prostaglandins.

Most sympathomimetic agents and inotropes have short effective half-lives, are rapidly metabolized, and are typically administered by continuous infusion, and their effects rapidly dissipate with cessation of their infusion. Hence, in most regards, these vasoactive agents are all pharmacokinetically similar and selection of a given agent is not based on specific pharmacokinetic differences (with levosimendan an exception [see later]).

The sympathomimetic catecholamines (epinephrine, norepinephrine, dopamine, dobutamine, isoproterenol) are all metabolized by monoamine oxidase (MAO) and catechol-O-methyltransferase (COMT), and all have a plasma half-life of approximately 2 minutes. Significant concentrations of MAO and COMT are present in both the liver and kidney, which are the sites of metabolism for the majority of intravenously administered catecholamines. MAO is also present in the intestinal mucosa as well as in peripheral and central nerve endings. COMT is present in the adrenal medulla and tumors arising from chromaffin tissue, but not in sympathetic nerves. Synthetic sympathomimetic drugs (e.g., fenoldopam) may have a longer duration of action because of their resistance to metabolism by MAO or COMT.

Epinephrine

Epinephrine is an endogenous catecholamine that stimulates both α- and β-adrenergic receptors in a dose-dependent fashion (see Tables 11.1 and 11.2). The pharmacology of epinephrine is characterized by a higher binding affinity for the β-receptor at lower doses (0.01–0.04 µg/kg per minute) and a stronger preference for the α receptor at higher doses (0.05–0.2 µg/kg per minute). This provides the clinical basis for the biphasic response observed for epinephrine; at lower doses, the hemodynamic effects are predominated by increased inotropy and chronotropy of the heart (β effect), and at higher doses, a vasopressor effect (α effect) is primarily observed. Epinephrine infusion in the lower dose range of 0.01 to 0.04 µg/kg per minute may be used to increase stroke volume, with mild elevations in heart rate in patients requiring

Table 11.1 Inotropic Agents

| Drug | Dosage | | Site of Action | | Mechanism of Action | Indications |
	Intravenous Bolus	Infusion	α	β		
Dobutamine	—	2–20 µg/kg/min	+	++++	Direct and indirect	Right heart dysfunction, heart transplantation, CHF, cardiogenic shock
Dopamine	—	1–10 µg/kg/min	++	+++	Direct	Renal insufficiency
Epinephrine	2–16 µg	2–10 µg/min or 0.01–0.4 µg/kg/min	+++	+++	Direct and indirect	Left heart dysfunction, hypotension from low cardiac output, heart transplantation, shock
Ephedrine	5–25 mg	—	+	++	Indirect	Intraoperative hypotension, hypotension with bradycardia
Isoproterenol	1–4 µg	0.5–10 µg/min or 0.01–0.10 µg/kg/min		++++	Direct	Heart transplantation, severe bradycardia
Norepinephrine	—	2–16 µg/min or 0.01–0.3 µg/kg/min	++++	+++	Direct	Low SVR states, combination with inodilators, shock
Milrinone	50 µg/kg	0.375–0.75 µg/kg/min	–	–	PDE-5 inhibition	Diastolic dysfunction, right heart dysfunction, pulmonary hypertension, β-receptor desensitization

CHF, Congestive heart failure; *PDE,* phosphodiesterase.

Table 11.2 Hemodynamic Effects of Inotropes

Drug	CO	dP/dt	HR	SVR	PVR	PCWP	MvO$_2$
Dobutamine							
2–20 µg/kg/min[a]	↑↑↑	↑	↑↑	↓	↓	↓ or ↔	↑
Dopamine							
0–3 µg/kg/min	↑	↑	↑	↓	↓	↑	↑
3–8 µg/kg/min	↑↑	↑	↑	↓	↓	↑	↑
>8 µg/kg/min	↑↑	↑	↑↑	↑	(↑)	↑ or	↑↑
Isoproterenol							
0.5–10 µg/min	↑↑	↑↑	↑↑	↓↓	↓	↓	↑↑
Epinephrine							
0.01–0.4 µg/kg/min	↑↑	↑	↑	↑ (↓)	(↑)	↑ or ↔	↑↑
Norepinephrine							
0.01–0.3 µg/kg/min	↑	↑	↔ (↑↓)	↑↑	↔	↔	↑
Milrinone[b]							
0.375–0.75 µg/kg/min	↑↑	↑	↑	↓↓	↓↓	↓↓	↓

[a]Indicated dosages represent the most common dosage ranges. For the individual patient, a deviation from these recommended doses might be indicated.
[b]Phosphodiesterase inhibitors are usually given as a loading dose followed by a continuous infusion: milrinone: 50 µg/kg loading dose, 0.375–0.75 µg/kg/min continuous infusion.
CO, Cardiac output; *dP/dt*, myocardial contractility; *HR*, heart rate; *MvO$_2$*, myocardial oxygen consumption; *PCWP*, pulmonary capillary wedge pressure; *PVR*, pulmonary vascular resistance; *SVR*, systemic vascular resistance.
Modified from Lehmann A, Boldt J. New pharmacologic approaches for the perioperative treatment of ischemic cardiogenic shock. *J Cardiothorac Vasc Anesth*. 2005;19:97-108.

augmentation of myocardial contractility. As the dose of epinephrine is increased to the range of 0.05 to 0.2 µg/kg per minute, the physiologic effects of both the α-receptor and β-receptor activation are combined as rises in SVR and heart rate are observed, respectively (see Tables 11.1 and 11.2). The biphasic hemodynamic response makes epinephrine an excellent choice for clinical situations that simultaneously mandate an increase in myocardial contractility and augmentation of arterial blood pressure. Under the vasodilatory effects of anesthetic agents, the titration of epinephrine may prove useful in the patient with hypotension secondary to a combination of systemic vasodilation and poor ventricular performance. In this instance, careful titration of epinephrine to achieve the desired effect is crucial to prevent untoward tachycardia or arrhythmias. Compared with dobutamine, epinephrine may exhibit less tachycardia and vasodilation, which may improve hemodynamics in patients with poor ejection fraction under general anesthesia.

Dobutamine

Dobutamine is a synthetic catecholamine that displays a strong affinity for the β receptor (β_1 and β_2), resulting in dose-dependent increases in cardiac output and heart rate and reductions in SVR and diastolic filling pressures (see Tables 11.1 and 11.2). Dobutamine has a half-life of 2 minutes, a rapid onset of effect, and steady-state concentrations reached within 10 minutes. Tachyphylaxis may occur with dobutamine infusions longer than 72 hours. In patients with a low cardiac output syndrome, dobutamine often increases the heart rate, and depending on the patient, it may induce an increase or decrease in the SVR and MAP. However, under the effects of general anesthesia, a rise in SVR with dobutamine is generally not observed, and the overall effect is a negligible or mild decrease in SVR. The starting low dose range for dobutamine is 3 to 5 μg/kg per minute. At this dose, dobutamine may be associated with higher incidences of tachycardia and atrial or ventricular arrhythmias compared with low-dose epinephrine infusions at 0.01 to 0.03 μg/kg per minute. Moreover, because of its primary selectivity for the β receptor, dobutamine is a rational choice for patients with right or LV dysfunction and afterload mismatch. Because of a minimal effect on PVR, dobutamine can be used to augment RV stroke volume, especially in the setting of pulmonary hypertension. Similarly, patients who are sensitive to LV afterload mismatch may find dobutamine to be an appropriate drug to increase contractility while unloading the left ventricle. Additionally, dobutamine may be a useful inotrope for the patient with a previously transplanted heart. Because a newly denervated heart relies primarily on β-receptor stimulation to control myocardial contractility and heart rate, dobutamine therapy may provide the necessary chronotropic and inotropic support required for the hemodynamic management of heart transplant recipients.

Isoproterenol

Isoproterenol is a potent, nonselective β-adrenergic agonist, devoid of α-adrenergic agonist activity. Compared with other catecholamines, isoproterenol is a poorer substrate for MAO and has less uptake by sympathetic neurons; hence, its duration of action may be slightly longer than that of epinephrine, but it still is brief. Isoproterenol dilates skeletal, renal, and mesenteric vascular beds and decreases diastolic blood pressure (see Tables 11.1 and 11.2). The potent chronotropic, inotropic, and vasodilatory effects of isoproterenol make it an excellent candidate for the treatment of bradycardia (especially after orthotopic heart transplantation), pulmonary hypertension, and heart failure. Isoproterenol remains the inotrope of choice for stimulation of cardiac pacemaker cells in the management of acute bradyarrhythmias or atrioventricular (AV) heart block. It reduces refractoriness to conduction and increases automaticity in myocardial tissues. The tachycardia seen with isoproterenol is a result of direct effects of the drug on the sinoatrial (SA) and AV nodes and reflex effects caused by peripheral vasodilation. It is routinely used in the setting of cardiac transplantation for increasing automaticity and inotropy, as well as for its vasodilatory effect on the pulmonary arteries. To normalize arterial blood pressure, it may be necessary to combine isoproterenol with vasopressin to counter the potent vasodilatory effects of β_2-receptor agonism. The recommended dose range of isoproterenol is 0.5 to 10 μg/ min or 0.01 to 0.10 μg/kg per minute.

Dopamine

Dopamine is an endogenous catecholamine and an immediate precursor of norepinephrine and epinephrine (see Tables 11.1 and 11.2). Its actions are mediated by stimulation of both adrenergic (α and β) and dopaminergic receptors (D_1 receptors). The dose response of dopamine is characterized by the D_1 and β effects predominating at lower doses and α effects at higher doses. Dopamine is unique in comparison with other endogenous catecholamines because of its effects on the kidneys. It has been shown to increase renal artery blood flow by vasodilating the afferent arteries and indirect vasoconstriction of the efferent arteries through D_1-receptor activation. At the lower dose range (0.5–3.0 µg/kg per minute), dopamine predominantly stimulates the dopaminergic receptors; at doses ranging from 3 to 7 µg/kg per minute, it activates most adrenergic receptors in a nonselective fashion; and at higher doses (>10 µg/kg per minute), dopamine behaves as a vasoconstrictor. But it is important to highlight that the dose-dependent effects of dopamine can be very unpredictable because of a large degree of inter- and intraindividual variability. There is also significant overlap between the dose ranges, in that titration at the lower dose range of 2.5 and 5.0 µg/kg per minute may still exert a positive effect on the β, α, and D_1 receptors, resulting in increases in cardiac index, heart rate, and SVR, as well as mild increases in renal blood flow, respectively. Nevertheless, the dopaminergic effect may be useful in patients with preexisting renal disease or in the setting of oliguria. As the dose increases above 5 µg/kg per minute, significant increases in MAP and PVR without increasing cardiac output may result. Compared with dobutamine and epinephrine, dopamine may be inferior with respect to improving stroke volume and cardiac output. In addition, dopamine may cause more frequent and less predictable degrees of tachycardia than dobutamine or epinephrine at doses that produce comparable improvement in contractile function. The propensity of dopamine to increase heart rate and induce tachyarrhythmias may therefore limit its utility in clinical practice.

Norepinephrine

Norepinephrine is an endogenous catecholamine exhibiting potent α-adrenergic activity with a mild to modest effect on the β-adrenergic receptor (see Tables 11.1 and 11.2). The higher affinity for norepinephrine of the α-adrenergic receptor provides the basis for its powerful overall vasoconstrictor effect and less potent inotropic and chronotropic properties. The overall hemodynamic effects of norepinephrine are characterized by increases in systolic and diastolic blood pressure and MAP, with minimal net impact on cardiac output and heart rate. In this regard, norepinephrine is used primarily as a vasopressor to manage low SVR caused by vasodilation. For instance, norepinephrine has been used effectively in combination with milrinone or dobutamine to counteract the vasodilatory effects of inodilators and maintain arterial pressure. Norepinephrine also plays a prominent role in the management of septic shock. As a potent vasoconstrictor, it is important to highlight that in certain patients, norepinephrine may produce reflex reductions in heart rate by increasing SVR and arterial pressure. Infusion of norepinephrine in patients with poor ventricular function should therefore be used with caution. Recommended starting doses of norepinephrine are in the range of 2 to 16 µg/min or 0.01 to 0.3 µg/kg per minute.

Phosphodiesterase III Inhibitors

Milrinone

The PDE III milrinone has a unique mechanism of action independent of the adrenergic receptor. Its inotropic effects are mediated primarily through an inhibition of the phosphodiesterase enzyme (PDE III) and not through β-receptor stimulation (see Tables 11.1 and 11.2). As a result, the effectiveness of milrinone is not altered by previous β-blockade, nor is it reduced in patients who may experience β-receptor downregulation. With IV administration, milrinone has an elimination half-life of 1 hour, is 80% protein bound, has a volume of distribution (Vd) of 0.3 L/kg, and has a clearance rate of 6.1 mL/kg per minute. In patients with chronic heart failure, clearance and elimination are at least doubled compared with healthy patients. Moreover, significant renal insufficiency prolongs milrinone's plasma half-life in proportion to the decrement in creatinine clearance. Milrinone dosing should be reduced in patients with reduced creatinine clearance.

In addition to the positive inotropic effects, milrinone has been shown to improve myocardial diastolic relaxation and compliance (i.e., positive "lusitropic" effect) while augmenting coronary perfusion. The proposed mechanism for this effect on diastolic performance is that by decreasing LV wall tension, ventricular filling is enhanced, and myocardial blood flow and oxygen delivery are optimized. Milrinone dosing is unique in that the drug can be loaded at 50 µg/kg over 10 minutes followed by a maintenance infusion of 0.375 to 0.75 µg/kg per minute. Significant increases in stroke volume and cardiac index are observed with significant decreases in pulmonary capillary wedge (PCW) pressure, central venous pressure, pulmonary artery pressure (PAP), and SVR. A major advantage of milrinone is the marked afterload reduction of both the PVR and SVRs as the dose of milrinone is increased. The pulmonary and systemic vasodilatory effects of milrinone render it an excellent choice for patients with RV dysfunction and pulmonary hypertension and LV dysfunction and elevated SVR, respectively. The lusitropic effects of milrinone on ventricular relaxation and compliance make it an attractive choice to improve the diastolic filling parameters of a stiff, noncompliant heart. Caution is necessary when milrinone doses above 0.75 µg/kg per minute are used because this is associated with more severe degrees of hypotension. The combination of milrinone with vasopressin may be useful in patients who do not respond to catecholamines secondary to adrenergic receptor downregulation. The combination of vasopressin, which spares the pulmonary vasculature and an inodilator, may be an attractive choice for the hemodynamic management of RV dysfunction in the presence of elevated PVR.

Levosimendan

Levosimendan is a calcium-sensitizing drug that exerts positive inotropic properties by sensitizing myofilaments to calcium and vasodilatation by opening adenosine triphosphate–dependent potassium channels on vascular smooth muscles. This inodilator usually increases cardiac output and decreases preload.

Pharmacokinetics and pharmacodynamics of levosimendan are unique in that an active metabolite is formed with potency and efficacy similar to those of the parent compound. After a loading dose, steady-state levels are reached at approximately 4 hours after drug infusion. However, an active metabolite known as OR-1986 peaks at 48 hours and remains active for more than 300 hours (12–14 days after the end of infusion). This leads to clinical effects for up to 7 days after the discontinuation of a levosimendan infusion.

The active metabolite, OR-1986, is primarily responsible for the sustained increase in stroke volume index, decrease in cardiac workload, and improved coronary and renal blood flow in patients with low cardiac output after cardiac surgical procedures. The formation of an intermediate- or long-acting metabolite may allow for earlier pharmacologic weaning without fear of losing the beneficial inotropic and hemodynamic effects as a result of drug discontinuation.

VASODILATORS

Acute perioperative hypertension is a risk factor for adverse cardiovascular outcome and is mainly a result of an increase in sympathetic activity, resulting in arteriolar vasoconstriction and increased SVR. Episodes of intraoperative hypertension can present a great challenge in that the timing of such events may be extremely sudden and unpredictable, mandating the need for rapid-acting antihypertensive drugs. The indications for using rapid-onset vasodilators such as nitroglycerin, nitroprusside, nicardipine, and clevidipine include management of perioperative systemic or pulmonary hypertension, myocardial ischemia, and ventricular dysfunction complicated by excessive pressure or volume overload. Specific to the intraoperative period, nitroglycerin, nitroprusside, or clevidipine may be more appropriate choices because of their shared features such as rapid onset, ultra-short half-lives, and easy titratability. This section reviews the pharmacology of the vasodilator class of drugs and highlights the important pharmacologic differences among the various vasodilators as they pertain to perioperative hemodynamic management (Table 11.3). See Table 11.4 for the pharmacokinetics of common antihypertensive and vasodilator agents.

Nitroglycerin

Nitroglycerin belongs to the nitrovasodilator group of drugs that exert their effect through the donation of NO and activation of the sGC pathway in smooth muscle (see Table 11.3). Nitroglycerin is a NO donor, a class of drugs that activates guanylate cyclase, resulting in cyclic guanosine monophosphate (cGMP) production, causing reuptake of calcium by the sarcoplasmic reticulum with resultant vasodilation.

The Vd of nitroglycerin is 3 L/kg, and it is cleared from this volume at extremely rapid rates, with a resulting serum half-life of about 3 minutes. The observed clearance rates (0.5–1 L/kg per minute) exceed hepatic blood flow. Nitroglycerin is enzymatically denitrated in the liver, erythrocytes, and vascular endothelium. Renal insufficiency has no impact on its pharmacokinetics. The first products in the metabolism of nitroglycerin are inorganic nitrate and the 1,2- and 1,3-dinitroglycerols. The dinitrates are less effective vasodilators than the parent compound, but they are longer lived in the serum, and their overall contribution to the effect of chronic nitroglycerin regimens is not known. The dinitrates are further metabolized to nonvasoactive mononitrates and, finally, to glycerol and carbon dioxide.

The hemodynamic effects of nitroglycerin mainly stem from the NO-mediated smooth muscle relaxation. Low-dose nitroglycerin preferably dilates the venous capacitance vessels compared with arteriole dilation. The resultant venodilation reduces right atrial, pulmonary artery, PCW, and ventricular end-diastolic pressures with minimal effects on SVR. Nitroglycerin also exerts important effects on the coronary circulation, with a vasodilator effect on coronary arteries reducing the resistance to blood flow. As the vasodilator of choice for the treatment of ischemia, nitroglycerin-mediated dilation of coronary arteries in combination with decreases in ventricular end-diastolic pressure may overall improve the blood flow to the subendocardium, especially with the addition of phenylephrine to maintain CPP. Similarly, in the management of ventricular volume overload, use of nitroglycerin is advantageous because of its predominant influence on the venous bed; preload can be reduced without significantly compromising systemic arterial pressure. Initial IV doses of nitroglycerin start at 5 to 10 µg/min and can range up to 75 to 150 µg/min for the treatment of myocardial ischemia. At doses above 150 µg/min, arterial dilation may become clinically evident.

Nitroprusside

Nitroprusside is a potent nitrovasodilator that acts by releasing NO to induce both arterial and venous dilation (see Table 11.3). The hemodynamic response is a function of a combination of venous pooling and reduced arterial impedance. Sodium nitroprusside (SNP) is rapidly distributed to a volume that is approximately coextensive with the extracellular space. The drug is cleared from this volume by intraerythrocytic

Table 11.3 Vasodilators and Adrenergic Antagonists

Drug	Dose	Onset of Action	Duration of Action	Mechanism of Action	Comments and Indications
Nicardipine hydrochloride	5–15 mg/h IV	5–10 min	15–30 min; may exceed 4 h	CCB, arterial dilator, coronary vasodilator	Treatment of coronary vasospasm, improves coronary blood flow, afterload reduction, cardiac output increases
Clevidipine	1–2 mg/h IV	2–4 min	5–15 min	CCB, arterial dilator	Organ independent of metabolic clearance, ultra-fast onset and offset, lipid emulsion, afterload reduction
Sodium nitroprusside	0.25–10 µg/kg/min as IV infusion	Immediate	1–2 min	NO donor, balanced venodilator and arterial dilator	Hypertensive crisis, balanced afterload and preload reduction, cyanide toxicity
Nitroglycerin	5–100 µg/min as IV infusion	1–5 min	5–10 min	NO dilator, venodilator, weak arterial dilator	Treatment of myocardial ischemia, preload reduction
Metoprolol	1–2 mg IV every 5 min	5–15 min	2–4 h	β_1-Selective blockade	Tachycardia, myocardial ischemia
Labetalol	5–20 mg IV bolus every 10 min 0.5–2.0 mg/min IV infusion	5–15 min	3–6 h	α_1, β_1, β_2 blockade	Hypertension, aortic dissection
Esmolol	250–500 µg/kg/min IV bolus; then 50–100 µg/kg/min by infusion; may repeat bolus after 5 min or increase infusion to 300 µg/min	1–2 min	2–10 min	β_1-Selective blockade	Tachycardia, hypertension, aortic dissection, supraventricular tachyarrhythmias
Propranolol	0.5–1 mg	1–5 min	3–6 h	β_1 and β_2 blockade	Tachycardia, hypertension, aortic dissection, supraventricular tachyarrhythmias

CCB, Calcium channel blocker; IV, intravenous; NO, nitric oxide.

Table 11.4   Common Antihypertensive and Vasodilator Agent Pharmacokinetics

Drug	Onset of Effect	Duration of Effect	Distribution Half-Life (Initial Phase)	Terminal Half-Life (Terminal Phase)	Volume of Distribution (L/kg)	Plasma Clearance (mL/min/kg)	Protein Binding
Nitroprusside	1 min	1–10 min	20 min	72 h for SCN metabolite	Matches extracellular space volume	Proportional to CrCl	NR
Nitroglycerin	1–5 min	5–10 min	NR	1–3 min	3.3	500–1000	60%
Nicardipine	1 min	3 h	2.7 min	14.4 h	8.3	400	>95%
Clevidipine	2–4 min	5–15 min	1 min	15 min	0.17	140	>99.5%
Labetalol	5–20 min	3–6 h	NR	6–8 h	9.4	25	50%
Esmolol	1–5 min	10–30 min	2 min	8 min	3.43	20,000	55%
Metoprolol	5 min	5–7 h	NR	4–7 h	3.2–5.6	54,100–75,400	10%
Fenoldopam	5–15 min	10–13 min	NR	10 min	0.23–0.66	1490–2290	88%
Enalaprilat	30 min	6 h	NR	11 h	1.7	proportional to CrCl	60%

CrCl, Creatinine clearance; *NR*, not reported; *SCN*, thiocyanate.

reaction with hemoglobin and SNP's resulting circulatory half-life is 2 minutes. SNP is unstable and decomposes when exposed to light. SNP metabolites are hemodynamically inactive but toxic. Hence, infusions exceeding 5 µg/kg per minute for longer than 24 hours may generate the production of the toxic metabolites cyanide and thiocyanate. SNP vasodilatory effects occur within 30 seconds of IV administration; cessation of effects occurs within 3 minutes of infusion termination. Renal elimination of SNP is 3 days; however, accumulation occurs with renal insufficiency. The cyanide byproduct is converted to thiocyanate by hepatic rhodanese; liver disease can lead to cyanide toxicity and resultant lactic acidosis.

Nitroprusside possesses a quick onset of action and great potency, making it a rational choice for management of intraoperative hypertension and for afterload reduction during surgery. In patients with impaired ventricular function, nitroprusside-mediated afterload reduction may yield improvements in cardiac output. Although SNP is an effective venous and arterial vasodilator during surgery, it has notable limitations. Nitroprusside use is associated with reflex tachycardia, tachyphylaxis, inhibition of hypoxic pulmonary vasoconstriction, increases in intracranial pressure, and reduced renal blood flow. The potential for cyanide toxicity is also an important consideration when administering SNP, especially in patients receiving high doses or prolonged infusions. Furthermore, SNP may be difficult to titrate and often causes hypotension because of overshoot. It is therefore prudent to start infusion rates at 0.1 to 0.3 µg/kg per minute with careful titration to maximum doses near 2.0 to 5 µg/kg per minute. Intraoperatively, SNP has been used during surgery to induce controlled hypotension to minimize bleeding complications. Nitroprusside in combination with a β-antagonist has also found use in controlling the rate of pressure rise in the aorta during acute dissection.

Clevidipine

Clevidipine is an ultra-fast-acting, dihydropyridine L-type calcium channel blocker (CCB) with a direct action on arteriolar resistance vessels and limited effects on venous capacitance vessels (see Table 11.3). Clevidipine is similar in structure to other dihydropyridine calcium channel antagonists, with the exception of an additional ester linkage, which enables its rapid metabolism (mean [standard deviation], 5.8 [1.1] minutes). In healthy subjects, clevidipine has a linear dose and steady-state blood concentration relationship.

Because clevidipine is metabolized by blood and tissue esterases, neither renal nor hepatic impairment has an impact on elimination, and there is no need for dose adjustment. Clevidipine's mechanism of action is not affected by inhibitors or activators of the cytochrome P450 metabolic pathway. Moreover, there is no indication that tolerance develops to prolonged infusions, although there is some evidence of rebound hypertension after discontinuation in patients not transitioned to alternative antihypertensive therapies. Because of its high lipid solubility, it is prepared in a lipid emulsion for IV infusion. The extremely fast onset and offset of about 1 to 3 minutes allow clevidipine to be especially suited for intraoperative management of acute hypertension. Clevidipine inhibits the L-type calcium channel in arterial smooth muscle, causing potent vasodilation. Because of its rapid metabolism by circulating esterases, its effect is quickly terminated independent of hepatic or renal function. Hemodynamically, clevidipine reduces arterial pressure through direct action on the arterioles without affecting the filling pressures or causing reflex changes in heart rate. Stroke volume and cardiac output typically increase. Because of its potency and rapid onset, it is an effective drug for the intraoperative management of hypertension. Clevidipine may be more effective at achieving blood pressure targets within a prespecified range than nitroglycerin or SNP in the intraoperative period.

The initial recommended starting dosage is 1 to 2 mg/h with a maximum dose of 32 mg/h. In most cases, the target hemodynamic goals of clevidipine are reached within a dose range of 4 to 6 mg/h. Because of the relatively high lipid content, it is recommended that no more than 1000 mL of clevidipine be administered in the first 24-hour period.

Nicardipine

Nicardipine is also a dihydropyridine L-type CCB with a selective arterial vasodilator mode of action (see Table 11.3). Nicardipine achieves rapid dose-related increases in plasma concentrations during the first 2 hours after the start of an infusion, approaching steady-state levels by 24 to 48 hours. After infusion termination, nicardipine concentrations decrease rapidly, with at least a 50% decrease during the first 2 hours after infusion. Nicardipine is highly protein bound (>95%) over a wide concentration range. Upon infusion cessation, nicardipine plasma concentrations decline triexponentially, with a rapid early distribution phase (α-half-life, 2.7 minutes), an intermediate phase (β-half-life, 44.8 minutes), and a slow terminal phase (γ-half-life, 14.4 hours) that can only be detected after long-term infusions. Plasma clearance is 0.4 L/kg per hour, and the Vd using a noncompartment model is 8.3 L/kg. The pharmacokinetics of IV nicardipine are linear over the dosage range of 0.5 to 40.0 mg/h.

Nicardipine has unique pharmacologic effects in that the drug selectively reduces systemic and coronary artery resistance, thereby decreasing LV afterload and increasing coronary blood flow. Nicardipine infusion in patients with impaired cardiac function or coronary artery disease may lead to increases in stroke volume and a favorable effect on myocardial oxygen tension. However, its use may be limited to the postoperative setting because of its longer half-life and slower offset of action compared with clevidipine or nitroprusside. The recommended starting dose of nicardipine is 5 mg/h, with titration in increments of 2.5 mg/h to a maximum 15 mg/h every 5 to 15 minutes until hemodynamic goals are reached. One of the main indications for the use of nicardipine is in the treatment of postoperative hypertension in which it may be just as effective as nitroprusside in reaching blood pressure goals. Control of hypertension with nicardipine may be particularly beneficial in patients with coexisting coronary artery disease or systolic dysfunction in which cardiac index, stroke volume, and coronary blood flow may increase compared to the hemodynamic effects of nitroprusside treatment. The beneficial effects on stroke volume and coronary flow may stem from the vasodilatory selectivity of nicardipine on the arterial and coronary beds as opposed to venodilation. Accordingly, nicardipine infusion may be used in the treatment or prevention of vasospasm in patients with coronary artery lesions or aortocoronary bypass grafts.

β-Adrenergic Blockers

The physiologic response to surgical stress is characterized by activation of the sympathetic nervous system, resulting in a spike in circulating levels of catecholamines. The stress response may adversely affect the cardiovascular system, resulting in hemodynamic instability, myocardial ischemia, and possibly an increased mortality rate. Among the strategies to reduce the stress response, the β-adrenergic antagonists play a major role in providing a pharmacologic means of blunting the rise in sympathetic activity. In the intraoperative setting, the β-adrenergic blockers are considered first-line agents in the treatment of acute myocardial ischemia, supraventricular tachyarrhythmias (including atrial fibrillation [AF]), and hypertension related to tachycardia.

The β-adrenergic antagonists exert a multitude of effects to achieve the therapeutic efficacy observed in a broad range of perioperative applications. These agents effectively reduce myocardial work and oxygen demand by decreasing heart rate, blood pressure, and myocardial contractility. β-Blocker–mediated heart rate reduction may have a salient effect on increasing coronary blood flow. Increased collateral blood flow and redistribution of blood to ischemic areas may occur with β-blockade. Microcirculatory oxygen delivery improves, and oxygen dissociates more easily from hemoglobin after β-adrenergic blockade. The electrophysiologic effects of β-receptor blockade are broad and typically result in reduction in AV node conduction, slowing of the sinus rate, and decreases in the rate of depolarization of ectopic pacemakers.

The perioperative administration of β-adrenergic blockers may prove beneficial in select high-risk patients undergoing noncardiac surgery. However, the benefits of β-blocker administration must be tempered by the significant risk of severe complications such as increased rate of stroke and death if administered in the perioperative period. Indeed, increased rates of stroke and death may be associated with initial preoperative β-blocker administration on the day of surgery. Furthermore, clinically significant hypotension and bradycardia related to β-blocker use may explain the higher rates of stroke in the postoperative period. These findings highlight the importance of carefully titrating β-blocker dosage for several days or weeks in advance of surgery. The following β-blockers are among the most useful agents in the anesthesiologist's armamentarium because of their well-characterized pharmacologic effects and availability in IV form.

Propranolol

Propranolol is the prototype β-blocker demonstrating equal affinity for β_1 and β_2 receptors and lacking any clinically significant α-adrenergic receptor activity (see Table 11.3). The serum half-life of the drug after IV dosing is about 3 to 6 hours. Arterial blood pressure is lowered by a decrease in myocardial contractility and slowing of the heart rate. Overall, cardiac output and myocardial oxygen demand are decreased. Reductions in heart rate with propranolol occur at serum levels lower than the concentrations that depress myocardial contractility. As drug levels decrease after discontinuation of therapy, reductions in the chronotropic response last much longer than reductions in inotropy. This is an important concept in treating tachycardias in patients with significant ventricular dysfunction.

Clinically, propranolol can be useful in the setting of decreasing the force of contraction in patients with hypertrophic obstructive cardiomyopathy or aortic aneurysm. Propranolol is also particularly effective in slowing the ventricular response to supraventricular tachyarrhythmias and possibly ventricular tachyarrhythmias. The usual IV dose of propranolol initially is 0.5 to 1.0 mg titrated to effect. A titrated dose resulting in maximal pharmacologic serum levels is 0.1 mg/kg. A continuous infusion of 1 to 3 mg/h can prevent tachycardia and hypertension but must be used cautiously because of the potential of cumulative effects. Discontinuation of an infusion may lead to a rebound effect and precipitate tachycardia and hypertension.

Metoprolol

Metoprolol is a cardioselective β_1-receptor antagonist that possesses a serum half-life of 2 to 4 hours (see Table 11.3); when administered intravenously, maximal receptor blockade occurs within approximately 20 minutes. Equivalent maximal β-blocking effect is achieved with oral and IV doses in the ratio of approximately 2.5 to 1. There is a linear relationship between the log of plasma levels and reduction of exercise heart rate. Metoprolol is extensively distributed, with a reported Vd of 3.2 to 5.6 L/kg. About 10% of metoprolol in plasma is bound to serum albumin. Metoprolol is rapidly and efficiently absorbed after oral administration, but its first-pass extraction by the liver is lower, and 40% of the administered dose reaches the systemic circulation.

Plasma half-life after oral administration is approximately 3 hours. Metoprolol is 90% metabolized; hydroxylation and O-demethylation are the primary pathways. The metabolites lack β-receptor effects. The rate of hydroxylation of metoprolol is genetically determined. Elimination of metoprolol is mainly by biotransformation in the liver, with a mean elimination half-life of 3 to 4 hours; in poor CYP2D6 metabolizers (slow hydroxylators), the half-life may be 7 to 9 hours.

Metoprolol is administered intravenously in 1- to 2-mg doses, titrated to effect. The potency of metoprolol is approximately half that of propranolol. Maximal β-blocker effect is achieved with 0.2 mg/kg given intravenously. The main perioperative use of metoprolol is for the management of myocardial ischemia, hypertension, and the stress response of surgery. Perioperative administration of metoprolol may reduce adverse cardiac-related events but at the expense of increased risk of intraoperative bradycardia, prolonged hypotension, stroke, and all-cause mortality. Careful individualized titration of metoprolol is therefore warranted. Increased vigilance to the side effects of metoprolol, namely prolonged hypotension and bradycardia, may be crucial for minimizing the risk of stroke and death.

Esmolol

Esmolol is a unique cardioselective β_1-receptor blocking agent with a rapid onset on the order of 5 to 10 minutes and short duration of action of 2 to 10 minutes (see Table 11.3). The unique chemical structure of esmolol renders it susceptible to hydrolysis by esterases, providing the basis for its quick termination of action. Esmolol's peak effects occur within 6 to 10 minutes of its administration and has a half-life of 8 minutes. Total body clearance is 20 L/kg per hour, which is greater than cardiac output; hence, esmolol's metabolism is not limited by the rate of blood flow to metabolizing tissues such as the liver or affected by hepatic or renal blood flow. Through its selective antagonism of the β_1-receptor, esmolol produces significant reductions in blood pressure, heart rate, and myocardial contractility. Esmolol is often recommended to be given as a loading dose of 500 µg/kg over 1 minute followed by an infusion rate at 25 to 300 µg/kg per minute. However, a test dose of 20 mg or a lower loading dose may be preferable under the effects of anesthesia. The efficacy of esmolol has been established in a variety of patients, including those with unstable angina, myocardial ischemia, supraventricular arrhythmias, and perioperative tachycardia and hypertension. Esmolol can also be used effectively in patients with congestive heart failure and reactive airway disease because of its unique short t ½ and β_1 selectivity. Hypotension is the most commonly reported adverse reaction, which may be minimized with low dose infusions without a loading dose.

In the perioperative setting, esmolol is the ideal agent to minimize the risk of β-blocker–related hypotension and bradycardia based on its ultra-short-acting properties. Under the dynamic setting of the operating room, titration of esmolol can be safe and effective, resulting in dose-dependent decreases in heart rate and blood pressure. It has been effective for blunting the sympathetic response to intubation, surgical stimuli, and emergence. In patients with coronary artery disease, infusion of esmolol may reduce episodes of myocardial ischemia and undesirable tachycardia. For patients in supraventricular tachycardia (SVT), including AF or sinus tachycardia, esmolol achieves rapid ventricular rate control. The efficacy of esmolol in the treatment of supraventricular tachyarrhythmias is comparable to the longer acting nonselective β-antagonist propranolol. Compared with diltiazem, esmolol may have a greater rate of conversion to sinus rhythm in the short term. In patients with aortic dissection, esmolol can be effective in combination with an arterial dilator such as nicardipine, nitroprusside, or clevidipine to reduce myocardial contractile forces and stress on the aorta.

Labetalol

Labetalol belongs to the class of drugs that serve as competitive antagonists at both the α_1-adrenergic and β-adrenergic receptors (see Table 11.3). In contrast to metoprolol and esmolol (β_1-selective antagonists), labetalol acts as competitive antagonist at α_1 and β receptors. Labetalol has a maximal onset time of 20 minutes and no active metabolites, and the elimination half-life is approximately 6 hours. The selective α_1-receptor and nonselective β-receptor antagonist can be delivered by bolus or continuous infusion. The potency of β-adrenergic blockade is 5- to 10-fold greater than α_1-adrenergic blockade. Labetalol also has partial β_2-agonist effects that promote vasodilation. In contrast to other β-blockers, labetalol should be considered a peripheral vasodilator that does not cause a reflex tachycardia. The dual action of labetalol on both the α_1 and β receptors contributes to the decline in blood pressure and systemic vascular resistance. The onset of action is observed within 2 to 15 minutes after IV administration of labetalol and may last for about 2 to 6 hours. The longer duration of action and variability in pharmacokinetics may make labetalol extremely difficult to titrate as a continuous infusion.

Hemodynamically, stroke volume and cardiac output remain unchanged, with the heart rate remaining essentially unchanged or decreasing slightly. Labetalol reduces the SVR without reducing total peripheral blood flow. The reduction in blood pressure is dose dependent, and acutely hypertensive patients usually respond after a bolus dose of 100 to 250 μg/kg. The duration of hypotension may be unpredictable because it may last as long as 6 hours after IV dosing. Unlike pure β-adrenergic blocking agents that decrease cardiac output, labetalol does not have a significant negative effect on cardiac output. Labetalol may be administered at a loading dose of 5 to 20 mg followed by incremental doses of 10 to 80 mg at repeated 10-minute intervals until the desired hemodynamic response is achieved. Alternatively, after the initial loading dose, an infusion can be started at 1 to 2 mg/min and titrated up until the desired hemodynamic endpoints are met. Larger bolus boluses may precipitate severe hypotension and should be avoided. Labetalol is an effective drug for the management of acute aortic dissection and hypertensive emergencies in the perioperative period.

VASOACTIVE DRUG ADMINISTRATION USING INFUSION PUMPS

Smart infusion pumps (Fig. 11.1) have become increasingly prevalent in the perioperative setting, and they offer significant advantages, including the ability to deliver very small volumes of fluids or many of the drugs discussed at precisely programmed rates. They are not, however, a panacea for medication errors. From 2005 through 2009, the U.S. Food and Drug Administration (FDA) received approximately 56,000 reports of adverse events associated with the use of infusion pumps, including numerous injuries and deaths. Adverse events were related to hardware issues (battery failures, sparking, and fires), as well as software issues (error messages, double recording a single key strike such that 10 becomes 100), some of which were related to poor user interface design or human factors issues. In addition to issues with pump hardware or software, user error is common. Compliance with the drug library is critical for prevention of error, but a systematic review found numerous studies showing high rates of user override of soft alerts, as well as a variable compliance rate with drug library use.

Although no comprehensive assessment of the incidence and nature of errors related to infusion pumps has been made, it is clear from the available evidence that

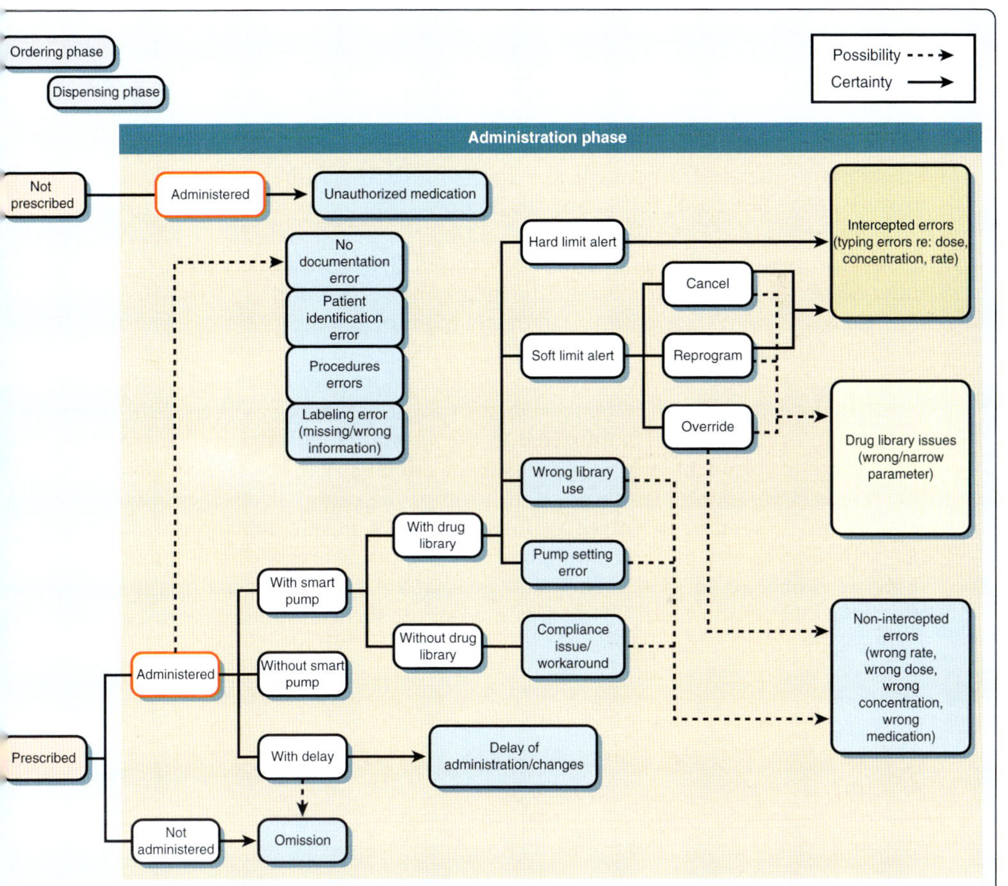

Fig. 11.1 Processes of intravenous medication administration with smart pumps and potential errors or intercepted errors in the prescribing phase to the administration phase. (Modified from Ohashi K, Dalleur O, Dykes PC, Bates DW. Benefits and risks of using smart pumps to reduce medication error rates: a systematic review. *Drug Saf*. 2014;37:1011–1120.)

programming errors are significant sources of error. Infusion pumps play a major role in drug administration in surgical patients, so errors related to infusion pumps are of significant concern to anesthesiologists. Some infusion pumps use drug libraries with predefined dosing limits and warn the practitioner if the dosing parameters entered will result in a dose that is outside the predefined dosing limits. Infusion pumps have been shown to intercept and prevent errors, primarily wrong rate and dose. A properly functioning and properly programmed pump can potentially intercept errors during multiple steps in the medication delivery process. Most intercepted errors represented a low level of harm, but some studies included examples of many-fold errors of high-alert drugs (100 times the intended dose of norepinephrine) or more than 100-fold underdoses.

However, the evidence for the effectiveness of pumps with drug libraries is mixed, with some studies suggesting benefit and others not. Lack of compliance with "soft alerts" that warn users but do not prevent drug administration may limit effectiveness. Pumps that allow for bar code identification of medications and that interact with the electronic medical record or anesthesia information system may prove more effective. Smart pump technology alone may not solve a problem; close attention to the details of implementing the pump technology and making it work properly are essential. One study found that tested smart pumps prevent only 4% of the adverse drug events in the intensive care unit (ICU). Many errors are related to bolus dosing and failure to monitor and respond to drug-related problems adequately.

Although smart pumps can alert to programming errors that may result in an incorrect dose, they do not recognize that a wrong drug has been placed in the pump or that the drug is being administered to the wrong patient. Bar coding may be a solution to this problem. A bar code on a medication bag can be scanned, along with the patient's bar-coded identification, to prompt the pump electronically with the appropriate drug and concentration, thus preventing misidentification of the drug or the patient, as well as preventing pump programming errors. Furthermore, if the pump is connected to the electronic medical record, the dosing information from the pump can be automatically documented in the record. Application of bar code scanning to infusion pumps is a relatively new and evolving technology.

ANTIARRHYTHMIC DRUGS USED IN THE PERIOPERATIVE PERIOD (BOXES 11.4 AND 11.5)

Arrhythmias are some of the most common cardiovascular complications in the perioperative period. General anesthesia for a variety of surgical procedures is associated with intraoperative arrhythmias with a reported overall incidence of 70%. Perioperative arrhythmia etiology is multifactorial; in addition to preexisting cardiac conduction defects and surgery-related contributions, anesthetic agents may negatively affect normal cardiac electrical activity at various levels (e.g., SA node, AV node, His-Purkinje system). Intraoperative arrhythmias are clinically important because of the potential associated hemodynamic instability. Hence, the following section describes commonly used antiarrhythmic agents needed to appropriately manage a variety of intraoperative arrhythmias.

The most widely used electrophysiologic and pharmacologic classification of antiarrhythmic drugs is that proposed by Vaughan Williams (Table 11.5). There is, however, substantial overlap in pharmacologic and electrophysiologic effects of specific agents among the classes, and the linkage between observed electrophysiologic effects

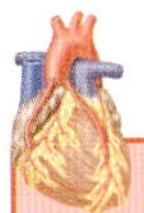

BOX 11.4 *Intravenous Supraventricular Antiarrhythmic Therapy*

Class I Drugs

- Procainamide (IA): converts acute atrial fibrillation, suppresses PACs and precipitation of atrial fibrillation or flutter, converts accessory pathway SVT; 100 mg IV loading dose every 5 min until arrhythmia subsides or total dose of 15 mg/kg (rarely needed) with continuous infusion of 2 to 6 mg/min.

Class II Drugs

- Esmolol: converts or maintains slow ventricular response in acute atrial fibrillation; 0.5 to 1 mg/kg loading dose with each 50 μg/kg/min increase in infusion, with infusions of 50 to 300 μg/kg/min. Hypotension and bradycardia are limiting factors.

Class III Drugs

- Amiodarone: converts acute atrial fibrillation to sinus rhythm; 5 mg/kg IV over 15 min.
- Ibutilide (Convert): converts acute atrial fibrillation and flutter.
  - Adults (>60 kg): 1 mg IV given over 10 min; may repeat once
  - Adults (<60 kg) and children: 0.01 mg/kg IV given over 10 min; may repeat once
- Vernakalant: 3 mg/kg over 10 min in acute-onset atrial fibrillation; if no conversion; wait 15 min and then repeat with 2 mg/kg over 10 min. Hypotension may occur in a few patients.

Class IV Drugs

- Verapamil: slow ventricular response to acute atrial fibrillation; converts AV node reentry SVT; 75–150 mg/kg IV bolus.
- Diltiazem: slow ventricular response in acute atrial fibrillation; converts AV node reentry SVT; 0.25 mg/kg bolus, then 100–300 μg/kg/h infusion.

Other Therapy

- Adenosine: converts AV node reentry SVT and accessory pathway SVT; aids in diagnosis of atrial fibrillation and flutter. Increased dosage required with methylxanthines, decreased use required with dipyridamole.
  - Adults: 3–6 mg IV bolus, repeat with 6–12 mg bolus
  - Children: 100 μg/kg bolus, repeat with 200 μg/kg bolus
- Digoxin: maintenance IV therapy for atrial fibrillation and flutter; slows ventricular response.
  - Adults: 0.25 mg IV bolus followed by 0.125 mg every 1–2 h until rate is controlled; not to exceed 10 μg/kg in 24 h
  - Children (<10 years): 10–30 μg/kg load given in divided doses over 24 h
  - Maintenance: 25% of loading dose

AV, Atrioventricular; *IV,* intravenous; *PACs,* premature atrial contractions; *SVT,* supraventricular tachycardia.

and the clinical antiarrhythmic effect is often tenuous. Likewise, especially in class I, there may be considerable diversity within a single class. The commonly used antiarrhythmic agents are discussed in this chapter; a more exhaustive discussion is beyond the scope of this text and can be found in *Kaplan's Cardiac Anesthesia,* 7th edition.

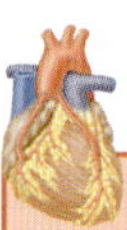

Class I Drugs

- Procainamide (IA): 100 mg IV loading dose every 5 min until arrhythmia subsides or total dose of 15 mg/kg (rarely needed) with continuous infusion of 2–6 mg/min.
- Lidocaine (IB): 1.5 mg/kg in divided doses given twice over 20 min with continuous infusion of 1–4 mg/min.

Class II Drugs

- Propranolol: 0.5–1 mg given slowly up to a total β-blocking dose of 0.1 mg/kg; repeat bolus as needed.
- Metoprolol: 2.5 mg given slowly up to a total β-blocking dose of 0.2 mg/kg; repeat bolus as needed.
- Esmolol: 0.5–1.0 mg/kg loading dose with each 50 μg/kg/min increase in infusion, with infusions of 50–300 μg/kg/min. Hypotension and bradycardia are limiting factors.

Class III Drugs

- Bretylium: 5 mg/kg loading dose given slowly with a continuous infusion of 1–5 mg/min. Hypotension may be a limiting factor.
- Amiodarone: 150 mg over 10 min IV; then 1 mg/min for 6 h; then 0.5 mg/min for the next 18 h. Repeat bolus as needed.

Other Therapy

- Magnesium: 2 g of $MgSO_4$ over 5 min; then continuous infusion of 1 g/h for 6–10 h to restore intracellular magnesium levels.

From Royster RL. *Diagnosis and management of cardiac disorders. ASA Refresher Course Lectures.* Park Ridge, IL: American Society of Anesthesiologists; 1996.

Table 11.5 Classification of Antiarrhythmic Drugs

Effects	Type of Antiarrhythmic Drug			
	I (Membrane Stabilizers)	II (β-Adrenergic Receptor Antagonists)	III (Drugs Prolonging Repolarization)	IV (Calcium Antagonists)
Pharmacologic	Fast channel (Na^+) blockade	β-Adrenergic receptor blockade	Uncertain: possible interference with Na^+ and Ca^{2+} exchange	Decreased slow–channel calcium conductance
Electrophysiologic	Decreased rate of V_{max}	Decreased V_{max}, increased APD, increased ERP, and increased ERP:APD ratio	Increased APD, increased ERP, increased ERP:ADP ratio	Decreased slow–channel depolarization; decreased ADP

ADP, Adenosine diphosphate; *APD,* atrial premature depolarization; *ERP,* effective refractory period; V_{max}, maximum velocity.

Class I Antiarrhythmic Drugs: Sodium Channel Blockers (Membrane Stabilizers)

Class I drugs inhibit the fast inward depolarizing current carried by sodium ions. Because of the diversity of other effects of the class I drugs, subgroups of class I drugs have been proposed (IA, IB, and IC) (Table 11.6).

Procainamide (Class IA)

Procainamide is used to treat ventricular arrhythmias, and to suppress atrial premature beats to prevent the occurrence of AF and atrial flutter. It has been useful for chronic suppression of premature ventricular contractions (PVCs), but it may be supplanted for this use by class IB drugs such as mexiletine. Procainamide converts acute-onset AF, suppresses premature atrial contractions (PACs) and precipitation of AF or flutter, and converts accessory pathway SVT; a 100-mg IV loading dose is given every 5 minutes until arrhythmia subsides or total dose of 15 mg/kg (rarely needed) is given with a continuous infusion of 2 to 6 mg/min. Procainamide is an effective emergency treatment for ventricular arrhythmias, especially after lidocaine failure, but amiodarone has become a more popular drug for IV suppression of ventricular arrhythmias.

Lidocaine (Class IB)

Lidocaine is the clinical standard for the acute IV treatment of ventricular arrhythmias except those precipitated by an abnormally prolonged QT interval. Lidocaine may be one of the most useful drugs in clinical anesthesia because it has local and general anesthetic properties in addition to an antiarrhythmic effect. The direct electrophysiologic effects of lidocaine produce virtually all of its antiarrhythmic action. Hepatic extraction of lidocaine is about 60% to 70%, and essentially all lidocaine is metabolized. In patients with impaired hepatic function or blood flow (e.g., those with heart failure), the dose requirement is approximately 50% of that for healthy persons.

Table 11.6 Subgroup of Class I Antiarrhythmic Drugs

Electrophysiologic Activity	Subgroup		
	IA	IB	IC
Phase 0	Decreased	Slight effect	Marked decrease
Depolarization	Prolonged	Slight effect	Slight effect
Conduction	Decreased	Slight effect	Markedly slowed
ERP	Increased	Slight effect	Slight prolongation
APD	Increased	Decreased	Slight effect
ERP:APD ratio	Increased	Decreased	Slight effect
QRS duration	Increased	No effect during sinus rhythm	Marked increase
Prototype drugs	Quinidine, procainamide, disopyramide, diphenylhydantoin	Lidocaine, mexiletine, tocainide	Lorcainide, encainide, flecainide, aprindine

APD, Atrial premature depolarization; *ERP,* effective refractory period; V_{max}, maximum volume.

Various IV dosages can be used, but the important factor is to rapidly achieve steady-state therapeutic plasma concentrations. An initial bolus dose of 1 to 1.5 mg/kg should be followed immediately by a continuous infusion of 20 to 50 µg/kg per minute or 1 to 4 mg/min to prevent the therapeutic hiatus produced by the rapid redistribution half-life of lidocaine.

The major toxic effect of lidocaine is associated with the central nervous system (CNS) and manifests as drowsiness and disorientation, which progress to agitation, muscle twitching, and hearing abnormalities and culminate in seizures. Lidocaine can be an effective general anesthetic agent, and cases of coma with electroencephalographic silence similar to brain death patterns have been produced by an overdose of lidocaine and have resolved completely on discontinuation of the drug. Local anesthetic–induced seizures do not produce permanent damage to the CNS as long as cardiovascular and respiratory complications of the seizure are prevented. Pharmacologically, benzodiazepines are superior to barbiturates (e.g., thiopental) for stopping local anesthetic–induced seizure activity. Drug therapy alone is insufficient, and airway control, ventilation, and especially oxygenation are paramount to prevent CNS morbidity.

Class II Drugs: β-Adrenergic Receptor Antagonists

β-Adrenergic receptor blockers are effective antiarrhythmics in patients during the perioperative period or in patients who are critically ill because many of their arrhythmias are adrenergically mediated.

Metoprolol

Metoprolol is a relatively selective β_1-receptor antagonist. The potency of metoprolol for β_1-receptor blockade is equal to that of propranolol, but metoprolol exhibits only 1% to 2% of the effect of propranolol at β_2 receptors. Metoprolol is useful for treating supraventricular and ventricular arrhythmias that are adrenergically driven. The primary advantage of metoprolol is its relative lack of most of the bronchoconstrictive effects in patients with chronic obstructive pulmonary disease. The acute IV dose is 1 to 2 mg titrated to therapeutic effect up to 0.1 to 0.2 mg/kg.

Esmolol

Esmolol is a cardioselective β_1-receptor antagonist with an extremely brief duration of action. Electrophysiologic effects of esmolol are those of β-adrenergic receptor antagonism. Esmolol is rapidly metabolized in blood by hydrolysis of its methyl ester linkage with a half-life of 8 to 10 minutes. Esmolol is not affected by plasma cholinesterase; the esterase responsible is located in erythrocytes and is not inhibited by cholinesterase inhibitors. Of importance to clinical anesthesia, no metabolic interactions between esmolol and other ester molecules are known. Esmolol dosages up to 500 µg/kg per minute have not modified neuromuscular effects of succinylcholine. In patients with asthma, esmolol (300 µg/kg per minute) only slightly increases airway resistance.

Esmolol has become a useful agent in controlling sinus tachycardia in the perioperative period, a time when a titratable and brief β-blockade is highly desirable. Dosing begins at 25 µg/kg per minute and is titrated to effect up to 250 µg/kg per minute. Doses greater than this may cause significant hypotension because of reduced cardiac output. Esmolol is especially effective in treating acute-onset AF or flutter perioperatively, and it results in acute control of the ventricular response and conversion of the arrhythmia to sinus rhythm.

Class III Drugs: Potassium Channel Blockers and Agents That Prolong Repolarization

Amiodarone

Amiodarone is a benzofuran derivative that was initially introduced as an antianginal drug and was subsequently found to have antiarrhythmic effects. The drug has a wide spectrum of effectiveness, including supraventricular, ventricular, and preexcitation arrhythmias. It also may be effective against ventricular tachycardia (VT) and ventricular fibrillation (VF) refractory to other treatment. Amiodarone has been approved by the American Heart Association as the first-line antiarrhythmic in cardiopulmonary resuscitation (CPR). Amiodarone may be effective prophylactically in preventing AF after surgery. It also can decrease the number of shocks in patients who have implantable cardioverter-defibrillators compared with other antiarrhythmic drugs. Amiodarone prolongs repolarization and refractoriness in the SA node, in atrial and ventricular myocardium, in the AV node, and in the His-Purkinje system.

The electrophysiologic effects of chronic amiodarone treatment mimic those of thyroid ablation. Moreover, the repolarization effects of the drug are reversed by triiodothyronine (T_3) administration. This suggests that among the basic effects of amiodarone is the blockade of the cardiac effect of T_3. This mechanism has been proposed as an alternative to the active metabolite accumulation theory to account for the slow onset of the antiarrhythmic effect of amiodarone.

Amiodarone increases the amount of electric current required to elicit VF (i.e., increase in the VF threshold). In most patients, refractory VT is suppressed by acute IV use of amiodarone. Amiodarone also has an adrenergic-receptor (α and β) antagonistic effect produced by a noncompetitive mechanism; the contribution of this effect to the antiarrhythmic action of the drug is unknown.

Hemodynamic effects of IV amiodarone (10 mg/kg) include decreased LV dP/dt, maximal negative dP/dt, mean aortic pressure, heart rate, and peak LV pressure after coronary artery occlusion in dogs. Cardiac output is increased despite the negative inotropic effect as a result of the marked decrease in LV afterload.

Because steady-state plasma levels are achieved slowly, loading techniques have been developed. In acute situations with stable patients, a 150-mg IV bolus is followed by a 1.0-mg/min infusion for 6 hours and then 0.5 mg/min thereafter. In CPR, a 300-mg IV bolus is given and repeated with multiple boluses as needed if defibrillation is unsuccessful.

Adverse reactions to chronic oral amiodarone are numerous. Photosensitivity of the skin occurs in 57% of patients without apparent relation to dose or plasma level. Other skin manifestations include abnormal pigmentation (i.e., slate gray) and an erythematous, pruritic rash. Corneal microdeposits occur in most patients taking amiodarone chronically, although visual symptoms are uncommon.

Pulmonary side effects are more severe. Clinical features include exertional dyspnea, cough, and weight loss. Hypoxia may occur; pulmonary function studies show decreased total lung capacity and diffusion rate. Chest radiographic findings are diffuse bilateral interstitial infiltrates, which histologically may be fibrosing alveolitis. Pulmonary effects may resolve with discontinuation of treatment or with dose reduction. The pathophysiologic mechanism of these pulmonary effects is unknown but may be related to abnormal production of phospholipid. The overall incidence rate of pulmonary toxicity is up to 6%, with a mortality rate among affected patients of 20% to 25%.

Thyroid abnormalities are associated with amiodarone. The frequencies of hyperthyroidism and hypothyroidism range from 1% to 5% and 1% to 2%, respectively.

Amiodarone contains two iodine atoms per molecule, or 75 mg of organic iodide per 200 mg of drug, and 10% of that amount may become free iodine. The iodine alone does not account for the thyroid abnormalities because intake of an amount of inorganic iodine equivalent to that ingested with chronic amiodarone intake does not have the same effect. Amiodarone therapy increases thyroxine (T_4) and reverse T_3, but it only slightly decreases T_3. Hyperthyroidism may develop in patients with underlying thyroid disease with a single amiodarone dose, and it may develop months after discontinuation of amiodarone therapy.

Despite relatively widespread use of amiodarone, anesthetic complications infrequently have been reported, including bradycardia and hypotension. Reports have described profound resistance to the vasoconstrictive effects of β-adrenergic agonists. The slow decay of amiodarone in plasma and tissue makes such adverse reactions possible long after discontinuing its administration. Because T_3 can reverse the electrophysiologic effects of amiodarone, T_3 possibly could be used to reverse hemodynamic abnormalities, although this theory has not been tested. Epinephrine is more effective than dobutamine or isoproterenol in reversing amiodarone-induced cardiac depression.

Class IV Drugs: Calcium Channel Blockers

Although the principal direct electrophysiologic effects of the three main chemical groups of CCBs (i.e., verapamil, a benzoacetonitrite; nifedipine, a dihydropyridine; and diltiazem, a benzothiazepine) are similar, verapamil and diltiazem are the primary antiarrhythmics. The drugs commonly classified as CCBs, typified by verapamil, diltiazem, nifedipine, and nicardipine, exhibit specificity for vascular smooth muscle and cardiac tissues, but within the group, specificity for these tissues varies. Whereas nifedipine and nicardipine (and other dihydropyridines) are more potent in smooth muscle than cardiac tissue, verapamil and diltiazem are more potent in cardiac tissue.

Verapamil and Diltiazem

Verapamil and diltiazem have been used extensively in the treatment of supraventricular arrhythmias, AF, and atrial flutter. They are especially effective at preventing or terminating paroxysmal supraventricular tachycardia (PSVT) by blocking impulse transmission through the AV node and prolonging AV nodal conduction and refractoriness. They are also useful in the treatment of AF and atrial flutter by slowing AV nodal conduction and decreasing the ventricular response.

A significant precaution in the use of verapamil and diltiazem to treat PSVT involves preexcitation of the AV node in Wolff-Parkinson-White syndrome. If PSVT is orthodromic (i.e., anterograde conduction through the AV node and retrograde over the accessory pathway) with a narrow or normal QRS complex, verapamil has a high success rate by blocking anterograde AV nodal conduction. If the PSVT is antidromic (i.e., anterograde conduction through accessory pathway and retrograde over the AV node) with a widened QRS complex, successful blockade with verapamil is unlikely because it has little effect on refractoriness or conduction in accessory pathways.

Another adverse effect of verapamil is the potentiation of neuromuscular blockade. At clinically relevant doses of verapamil, the effect is slight, but the clinical potential for synergistic interaction with residual muscle relaxants seems substantial. Cautious clinical attention to neuromuscular function is necessary to safely use verapamil in patients who are receiving or have recently received muscle relaxants. Verapamil dosage for acute IV treatment of PSVT is 0.07 to 0.15 mg/kg over 1 minute, with the same dose repeated after 30 minutes if the initial response is inadequate (10 mg maximum). Because the cardiovascular depressant effects of the inhalation anesthetics involve inhibition of calcium-related intracellular processes, the interaction of verapamil and these anesthetics is synergistic. AV block can occur and may be refractory, especially when verapamil is combined with β-blockers.

Diltiazem in doses of 0.25 to 0.30 mg/kg IV followed by a titratable IV infusion of 100 to 300 μg/kg per hour infusion is rapid acting and efficacious in controlling ventricular response rate in new-onset AF and atrial flutter.

Other Antiarrhythmic Agents

Adenosine

Adenosine is a virtually ubiquitous endogenous nucleoside that has potent electrophysiologic effects in addition to having a major physiologic role in regulation of vasomotor tone. Adenosine is unique in that it is produced as an intermediate metabolite of adenosine monophosphate. It has an extremely short half-life in plasma (1.5–2 seconds) because of metabolism by adenosine deaminase to inosine or by adenosine kinase to adenosine monophosphate. Both enzymes are contained within the intracellular cytosolic compartment, indicating a rapid transmembrane transport system for adenosine. Inhibition of this transport system by dipyridamole markedly enhances the cardiac effects of adenosine.

The important cardiac electrophysiologic effects of adenosine are mediated by the A_1 receptor and consist of negative chronotropic, dromotropic, and inotropic actions. Adenosine decreases SA node activity, AV node conductivity, and ventricular automaticity. In many ways, these effects mimic those of acetylcholine. The primary antiarrhythmic effect of adenosine is to interrupt reentrant AV nodal tachycardia, and this effect most likely is related to the potassium current effects.

For clinical use, adenosine must be administered by a rapid IV bolus in a dose of 100 to 200 μg/kg, although continuous IV infusions of 150 to 300 μg/kg per minute have been used to produce controlled hypotension. For practical purposes, in adults, a dose of 3 to 6 mg is given by IV bolus followed by a second dose of 6 to 12 mg after 1 minute if the first dose was not effective. This therapy rapidly interrupts narrow-complex tachycardia caused by AV nodal reentry.

Comparison with verapamil has shown adenosine to be equally effective as an antiarrhythmic, but with the advantages of fewer adverse hemodynamic effects, a faster onset of action, and a more rapid elimination so that undesired effects are short-lived.

Potassium

Because of the close relationship between extracellular pH and potassium, the primary mechanism of pH-induced arrhythmias may be alteration of potassium concentration. Hypokalemia and hyperkalemia are associated with cardiac arrhythmias, but hypokalemia is more common perioperatively in surgical patients and is associated with arrhythmias. Decreasing the extracellular potassium concentration increases the peak negative diastolic potential, which appears to decrease the likelihood of spontaneous depolarization. However, because the permeability of the myocardial cell membrane to potassium is directly related to extracellular potassium concentration, hypokalemia decreases cellular permeability to potassium. This prolongs the action potential duration (APD) by slowing repolarization, which slows conduction, increases the dispersion of recovery of excitability, and predisposes to the development of arrhythmias.

Electrocardiographic (ECG) correlates of hypokalemia include appearance of a U wave and increased P-wave amplitude. The arrhythmias most commonly associated with hypokalemia are premature atrial contractions, atrial tachycardia, and SVT. Hypokalemia also accentuates the toxicity of cardiac glycosides.

Moderate hyperkalemia, in contrast, increases membrane permeability to potassium, which increases the speed of repolarization and decreases APD, reducing the tendency to arrhythmias. An increased potassium concentration also affects pacemaker activity. The increased potassium permeability caused by hyperkalemia decreases the rate of spontaneous diastolic depolarization, which slows heart rate, and, in the extreme case, can produce asystole. The repolarization abnormalities of hyperkalemia lead to the characteristic ECG findings of T-wave peaking, a prolonged PR interval, decreased QRS amplitude, and a widened QRS complex. AV and intraventricular conduction abnormalities result from the slowed conduction and uneven repolarization.

Treatment of hyperkalemia is based on its magnitude and on the clinical presentation. For life-threatening, hyperkalemia-induced arrhythmias, the principle is rapid reduction of extracellular potassium concentration with a treatment that does not acutely decrease total-body potassium content. Calcium chloride (10–20 mg/kg IV) directly antagonizes the effects of potassium on the cardiac cell membranes. Sodium bicarbonate in dose of 1 to 2 mEq/kg or a dose calculated from acid–base measurements to produce moderate alkalinity (pH $\approx$7.45–7.50) will shift potassium intracellularly. A change in pH of 0.1 unit produces a 0.5- to 1.5-mEq/L change of potassium concentration in the opposite direction. An IV infusion of glucose and insulin has a similar effect; glucose at a dose of 0.5 to 2.0 g/kg with insulin in the ratio of 1 unit to 4 g of glucose is appropriate. Sequential measurement of serum potassium levels is important with this treatment because marked hypokalemia can result. Loop diuretics and potassium-binding resins promote excretion of potassium, although the effects are less rapid than with the previously mentioned modalities.

With chronic potassium deficiency, the plasma level poorly reflects the total-body deficit. Because only 2% of total-body potassium is in plasma and total-body potassium stores may be 2000 to 3000 mEq, a 25% decline in serum potassium from 4 to 3 mEq/L indicates an equilibrium total-body deficiency of 500 to 800 mEq, replacement of which should be undertaken slowly.

Acute hypokalemia frequently occurs as a result of hemodilution, urinary losses, and intracellular shifts. With frequent assessment of serum potassium concentrations and continuous ECG monitoring, potassium infusion at rates of up to 10 to 15 mEq/h may be administered to treat serious hypokalemia.

Magnesium

Magnesium deficiency is a relatively common electrolyte abnormality in critically ill patients, especially in chronic situations. Hypomagnesemia is associated with a variety of cardiovascular disturbances, including arrhythmias. Sudden death from coronary artery disease, alcoholic cardiomyopathy, and heart failure may involve magnesium deficiency.

Functionally, magnesium is required for the membrane-bound Na^+/K^+-ATPase, which is the principal enzyme that maintains normal intracellular potassium concentration. Not surprisingly, the ECG findings seen with magnesium deficiency mimic those seen with hypokalemia: prolonged PR and QT intervals, increased QRS duration, and ST-segment abnormalities. As with hypokalemia, magnesium deficiency predisposes to the development of the arrhythmias produced by cardiac glycosides. Magnesium is effective as an adjuvant in the treatment of patients with a prolonged QT syndrome and torsades de pointes.

Arrhythmias induced by magnesium deficiency may be refractory to treatment with antiarrhythmic drugs and electrical cardioversion or defibrillation. Adjunctive

276

treatment of refractory arrhythmias with magnesium has been advocated even when magnesium deficiency has not been documented. Magnesium deficiency is common in cardiac patients because of the diuretic agents these patients are often receiving. Magnesium lacks a counterregulatory hormone to increase magnesium levels, in contrast to hypocalcemia, which is corrected by parathyroid hormone.

Magnesium has been studied alone and in combination with other drugs in the prophylaxis and treatment of perioperative arrhythmias. A protocol using magnesium as first-line therapy and amiodarone as backup therapy appears effective in management of arrhythmias after surgery, as well as in critically ill patients. Magnesium dosing is 2 g of MgSO over 4 to 5 minutes followed by a continuous infusion of 1 g/h for 6 to 10 hours to restore intracellular magnesium levels.

PHARMACOLOGIC MANAGEMENT OF CHRONIC HEART FAILURE

Neuroendocrine-mediated activation of the sympathetic nervous system and renin–angiotensin–aldosterone system (RAAS) marked by increases in plasma catecholamines, renin, angiotensin I and II, and aldosterone have been well characterized in patients with heart failure with reduced ejection fraction (HFrEF) as an adaptation to decreased systemic perfusion. The compensatory response leads to a net increase in SVR, circulating blood volume, and cardiac output. One of the central themes in the management of chronic HFrEF is the pharmacologic regulation of excessive neuroendocrine activation. Accordingly, pharmacologic agents directed at modulating the RAAS such as angiotensin-converting enzyme (ACE) inhibitors and angiotensin receptor blockers (ARBs) have improved outcomes in patients with chronic heart failure.

Renin-Angiotensin Blockers

Angiotensin-Converting Enzyme Inhibitors

Angiotensin-converting enzyme inhibitors comprise a class of agents that directly inhibit the conversion of angiotensin I to the potent vasoconstrictor, angiotensin II. Inhibition of angiotensin II in the kidney promotes natriuresis and diuresis, thereby reducing circulating blood volume. The action of ACE inhibitors also extends to the promotion of bradykinin levels, a potent vasodilator of both arteries and veins. The overall combined action of ACE inhibitors results in the reduction of both preload and afterload on the heart. In patients with LV dysfunction, those receiving enalapril versus placebo, or hydralazine–isosorbide dinitrate, conferred a survival benefit providing the clinical evidence for the use of ACE inhibitors as first-line therapy to reduce mortality.

One of the main side effects of ACE inhibitor therapy is symptomatic hypotension. In the perioperative period, this could present as profound hypotension or, in rare cases, vasoplegic syndrome. Several studies have implicated ACE inhibitor therapy as a risk factor for vasoplegic syndrome in cardiac surgery. However, very few studies have demonstrated any direct association of vasoplegic syndrome and ACE inhibitors in noncardiac surgery. Nevertheless, vasoplegic syndrome has been reported in a variety of clinical scenarios during noncardiac surgery, including, but not limited to, liver transplantation, trauma surgery, during massive transfusion of blood components, ischemia-reperfusion, neuroendocrine tumor removal, sepsis, and anaphylaxis. The perioperative use of ACE inhibitors in clinical situations associated with increased risk of hypotension therefore warrants extreme caution because it may contribute to the development of vasoplegic syndrome and an increased mortality rate.

Angiotensin Receptor Blockers

Angiotensin receptor blockers prevent the vasoconstrictive and sodium-retaining effects of angiotensin II binding to its receptor. In clinical practice, ARBs play a central role in providing a pharmacologic alternative to blocking the renin–angiotensin pathway in patients who are intolerant of ACE inhibitors for the treatment of heart failure. ARBs exert a similar hemodynamic effect to ACE inhibitors in that reductions in right atrial pressure, wedge pressure, and SVR are observed. Similar to patients receiving ACE inhibitors, the potential for profound hypotension is also present in patients receiving ARBs, especially during the perioperative period. Furthermore, it is important to highlight the markedly increased potential for vasoplegic syndrome in patients taking both ACE inhibitors and ARBs in combination presenting for surgery. The combination of both antihypertensive drugs may prove to be life threatening in the perioperative period and is therefore not recommended. The direct-acting renin inhibitor aliskiren should also be avoided in patients receiving either an ACE inhibitor or ARB.

Recent Advancements in the Treatment of Heart Failure

Angiotensin Receptor–Neprilysin Inhibitors

Continued efforts to further improve outcomes in patients with HFrEF have led to the recent introduction of the first in-class drug sacubitril-valsartan (Entresto). Sacubitril-valsartan combines a neprilysin inhibitor, sacubitril, that blocks the degradation of natriuretic peptides with an ARB, valsartan (Fig. 11.2). The dual combination of neprilysin inhibitor–angiotensin receptor antagonist was developed to address two distinct pathophysiologic mechanisms underlying heart failure, activation of the renin-angiotensin axis and decreased natriuretic peptide activity. Combined inhibition of the renin-angiotensin system and neprilysin-mediated breakdown of atrial and brain-derived natriuretic peptides had effects that were superior in patients receiving monotherapy consisting of either drug alone. In patients with chronic HFrEF, the inhibition of both the renin-angiotensin pathway and neprilysin-mediated degradation of natriuretic peptides with sacubitril-valsartan was superior in reducing the risk of death from cardiovascular causes or hospitalization for heart failure than was ACE inhibitor monotherapy with enalapril. With regard to safety data, sacubitril-valsartan may cause significant hypotension through its potent vasodilatory effects. Similar to ACE inhibitors, sacubitril-valsartan may cause elevations in serum creatinine and potassium from impairment of renal function. However, it should be noted that the degree of renal impairment was less severe in patients receiving sacubitril-valsartan versus enalapril.

Ivabradine

Ivabradine (Corlanor) is a specific heart rate–decreasing agent, similar to the phenylalkylamine CCB verapamil. It acts on the SA node by selectively inhibiting the funny (I_f) current in SA nodal tissue, resulting in decreases in the rates of diastolic depolarization and heart rate. In contrast to β-blockers, ivabradine reduces heart rate both at rest as well as during exercise, with minimal effects on myocardial contractility, blood pressure, and intracardiac conduction. The reduction in heart rate and increased diastolic filling time also bestow a beneficial effect on myocardial relaxation. This mechanism is distinct from other negative chronotropic agents and is the main advantage of this new class of heart failure agents. In patients with HFrEF, ivabradine therapy has been shown to result in improvement of functional parameters and exercise capacity. In addition, the improvement in clinical symptoms also correlates

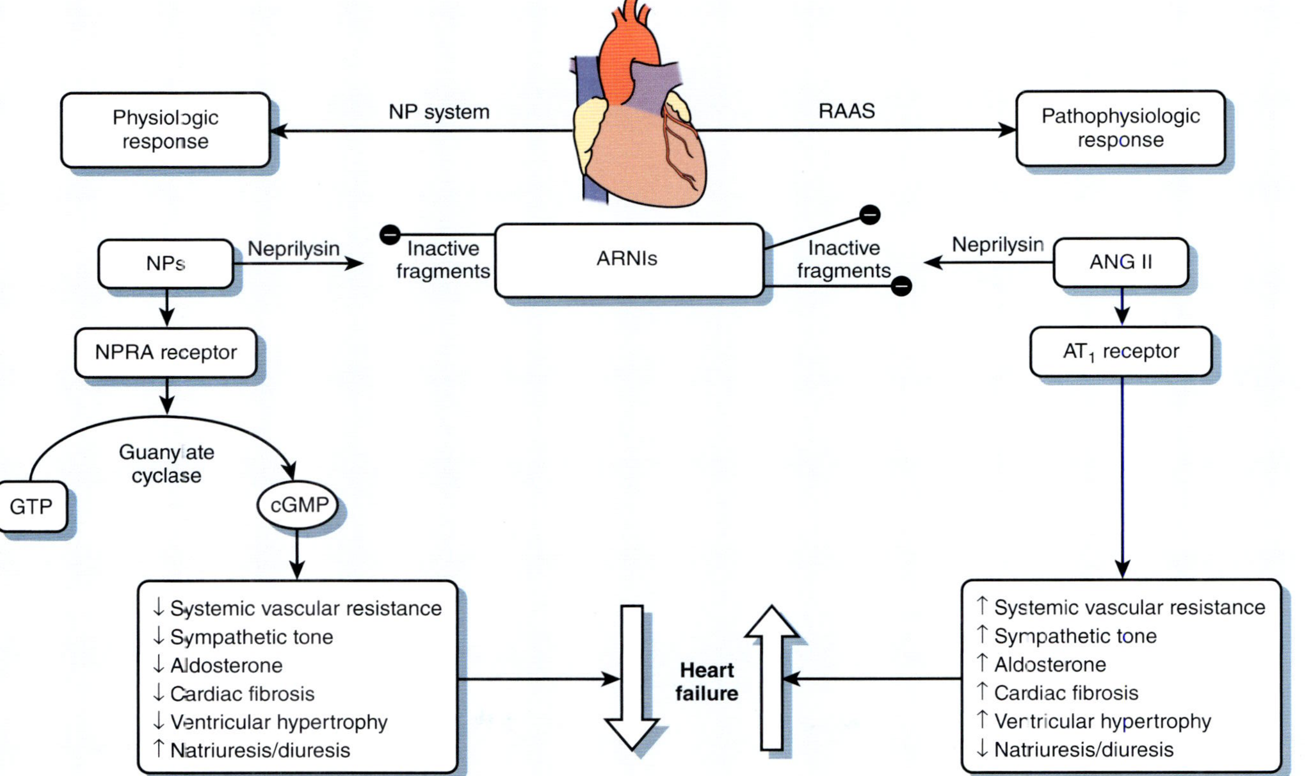

Fig. 11.2 Angiotensin receptor–neprilysin inhibitors (ARNIs) independently modulate distinct neuroendocrine systems central to heart failure: the renin-angiotensin-a dosterone system (RAAS) and the natriuretic peptide (NP) system. *ANG,* Angiotensin; *cGMP,* cyclic guanosine monophosphate; *GTP,* guanosine triphosphate; *NPRA,* natriuretic peptide receptor A; NPs, natriuretic peptides.

with a significant increase in LV function and a reduction in N-terminal pro–brain natriuretic peptide (NT-proBNP). It should also be highlighted that use of ivabradine significantly improves exercise capacity, quality of life, and neurohormonal modulation in patients with ischemic heart failure. Ivabradine monotherapy or in combination with carvedilol was more effective than carvedilol alone in improving exercise capacity and quality of life in HFrEF patients. Ivabradine is recommended in symptomatic HFrEF patients who are in sinus rhythm with a heart rate greater than 70 beats/min despite treatment with maximally tolerated doses of β-blockers. This treatment regimen is effective in reducing the risk of heart failure hospitalization and cardiovascular death. In addition, for patients who are unable to tolerate or have contraindications to β-blocker therapy, ivabradine is an excellent alternative. Ivabradine is also recommended for the treatment of stable angina pectoris with symptomatic heart failure (New York Heart Association class II–IV). It is important to note that the beneficial effects of ivabradine therapy in patients with heart failure are mainly driven by a significant reduction in heart rate because patients with higher baseline heart rates had a greater reduction in cardiovascular-related mortality. The beneficial effect of ivabradine is less pronounced in patients with lower baseline heart rates. Similarly, ivabradine reduces the rate of both myocardial infarction and coronary revascularization in patients with coronary artery disease with LV dysfunction and baseline heart rate greater than 70 beats/min. This effect is analogous to the association between the magnitude of heart rate reduction and outcome with β-blocker therapy. Ivabradine is generally well tolerated, with few notable adverse effects, including bradycardia, AF, and visual disturbances.

PHARMACOLOGIC MANAGEMENT OF PULMONARY HYPERTENSION (BOX 11.6)

The presence of perioperative heart failure with pulmonary hypertension portends a poor prognosis because it carries a significant risk for associated complications and death. Patients with pulmonary hypertension presenting for surgery often develop varying degrees of right heart dysfunction as a consequence of afterload mismatch or RV ischemia secondary to hypotension. Because the development of perioperative acute right heart failure is associated with a marked increase in mortality rate, the

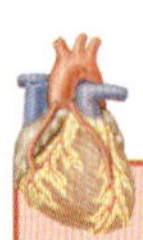

BOX 11.6   *Perioperative Management of Pulmonary Hypertension*

- Hypoxia, hypercarbia, hypothermia, high airway pressures, PEEP, and acidosis can all exacerbate pulmonary hypertension.
- In the presence of pulmonary hypertension, augmentation of right heart performance with selective inotropes that lower PVR can be useful in optimizing hemodynamics.
- The use of selective pulmonary vasodilators may be useful in lowering PVR without deleteriously decreasing SVR.
- iNO is an effective selective pulmonary vasodilator that can be used to reduce PVR without causing systemic hypotension.
- Inhaled prostacyclins may represent an excellent alternative to iNO in the future.

iNO, Inhaled nitric oxide; *PEEP,* positive end-expiratory pressure; *PVR,* pulmonary vascular resistance; *SVR,* systemic vascular resistance.

management of pulmonary hypertension in this setting is of paramount importance (see Chapter 7). This section focuses on the pharmacology of pulmonary vasodilators in the perioperative period when the surgical stress response may cause unavoidable and abrupt changes in preload, afterload, and PVR. The main goal of perioperative management of pulmonary hypertension is the reduction in PVR without any concomitant decreases in SVR and blood pressure.

Inhaled Nitric Oxide

Nitric oxide is produced by the endothelium of the vasculature by NOS, which plays a crucial role in regulating pulmonary vasculature tone. The site of action of NO resides in the adjacent smooth muscle, where it binds to the enzyme, sGC, leading to a marked increase in the levels of cGMP and relaxation of smooth muscles adjacent to the vasculature endothelium. Inhaled delivery of nitric oxide (iNO) has the major advantage of exerting local effects and thus serves as a selective pulmonary vasodilator, minimizing any systemic effects on hemodynamics. When NO diffuses from the smooth muscle into the bloodstream, it binds to hemoglobin and is rapidly inactivated, corresponding to a half-life of approximately 2 to 6 seconds.

The main role for iNO in the perioperative setting is the treatment of pulmonary hypertension and in the management of ventilated patients with hypoxia. iNO may be used to reduce pulmonary pressures and RV afterload while avoiding systemic hypotension at concentrations of 5 to 20 ppm. In patients who have elevated pulmonary pressures secondary to hypoxia, iNO may also be used to improve oxygenation by increasing blood flow to more ventilated pulmonary segments. In the setting of right heart dysfunction and afterload mismatch, iNO may improve right heart performance and mixed venous oxygen saturation while preserving systemic arterial and CPP. Although a specific dosage regimen for iNO is not clearly defined, there are data to support the lack of additional improvement in pulmonary pressures after escalating doses greater than 10 to 20 parts ppm. However, it is important to highlight the potential detrimental effects of iNO in specific clinical scenarios. iNO may reverse the beneficial effects of hypoxic pulmonary vasoconstriction and paradoxically worsen hypoxia in certain patients. Similarly, in patients with LV dysfunction, iNO may further increase pulmonary venous return to the left heart and precipitate acute heart failure.

The major concern for the use of iNO is the potential for toxicity of NO and its associated toxic metabolites, methemoglobin and nitrate. Extreme concentrations of iNO are associated with acute lung injury with resultant inflammation interstitial edema. Nitrate accumulation has been implicated as a direct irritant causing bronchospasm and possibly pulmonary edema. The use of iNO also poses additional complications during withdrawal, when patients can experience rebound pulmonary hypertension and abrupt RV failure and hypoxia. It is therefore prudent to carefully wean the delivery of iNO, especially in patients with poor RV reserve.

Prostacyclin and Analogs

Prostacyclin is an endogenous prostaglandin synthesized from arachidonic acid, which induces a cyclic adenosine monophosphate (cAMP)-mediated relaxation of vascular smooth muscle and pulmonary vasodilation. There are three main prostacyclin analogs (Tables 11.7 and 11.8) approved by the FDA for treatment of pulmonary hypertension: epoprostenol (Flolan), iloprost (Ventavis), and treprostinil (Remodulin). Epoprostenol was the first prostaglandin developed and displays a very short half-life

Table 11.7	Inhaled Pulmonary Vasodilators		
Pulmonary Vasodilator	**Mechanism of Action**	**Common Dose**	**Key Characteristics**
Nitric oxide	Prostacyclin receptor agonist; activates intracellular adenylate cyclase, which increases concentrations of cAMP	1–20 ppm via continuous inhalation	Short half-life Can cause methemoglobinemia Expensive Limited systemic exposure
Epoprostenol (Flolan)	Prostacyclin analog; activates intracellular adenylate cyclase, which increases concentrations of cAMP	25–50 at ng/kg/min IV *or* fixed volume of 8 mL/h	Complicated nebulized administration Mostly used when patient is intubated Some systemic exposure Potential for platelet inhibition and bleeding Potential hypotension
Iloprost (Ventavis)	Prostacyclin analog; activates intracellular adenylate cyclase, which increases concentrations of cAMP	5–10 μg inhaled 6 to 9 times/day	Ease of administration Easy to use when patient is extubated Expensive Some systemic exposure Potential for platelet inhibition and bleeding Potential hypotension May cause bronchospasm, cough, headache, and flushing
Treprostinil (Remodulin)	Prostacyclin analog activates intracellular adenylate cyclase, which increases concentrations of cAMP	3 breaths (18 μg) inhaled 4 times a day; titrate to target of 9 breaths (54 μg) 4 times a day	May cause flushing, headache, jaw pain, and diarrhea Long half-life Easy dosing schedule
Milrinone	Inhibits PDE III, which increases concentrations of cAMP	6 mg/h continuous inhalation	Less evidence of clinical efficacy Patient must be intubated Less expensive Systemic exposure Potential hypotension Potential arrhythmia

cAMP, Cyclic adenosine monophosphate; *PDE,* phosphodiesterase.

Table 11.6   Oral and Intravenous Pulmonary Vasodilators

Pulmonary Vasodilator	Mechanism of Action	Common Dose and Route of Administration	Key Characteristics
Sildenafil (Viagra)	PDE inhibitor; increases NO production by inhibiting breakdown of cGMP, thereby increasing NO-mediated pulmonary vasodilation	20 mg orally 3 times a day	Headache, flushing, epistaxis Profound hypotension when combined with nitrates Improves hemodynamic parameters and symptoms of pulmonary hypertension
Tacalafil (Cialis)	PDE inhibitor; increases NO production by inhibiting breakdown of cGMP, thereby increasing NO-mediated pulmonary vasodilation	2.5, 10, 20, 40 mg orally once a day	Headache, flushing, myalgias Profound hypotension when combined with nitrates Improves hemodynamic parameters and symptoms of pulmonary hypertension
Bosentan (Tracleer)	Competitive inhibitor of ET-A and ET-B receptor	62.5 mg orally twice a day for 4 weeks, then titrate up to 125 mg twice a day	May cause liver transaminitis, syncope, anemia, edema, flushing
Ambrisentan (Letairis)	Competitive inhibitor of ET-A	5–10 mg orally daily	Edema, headache, syncope, teratogenic, anemia
Epoprostenol (Flolan)	Prostacyclin analog; activates intracellular adenylate cyclase, which increases concentrations of cAMP	IV initial dose of 2 ng/kg/min and titrate every 15 min to maximum tolerated dose of 25–40 ng/kg/min	Easy to use when patient is extubated May cause rebound pulmonary hypertension when infusion stopped Flushing, nausea, headache, jaw pain Potential for platelet inhibition and bleeding Potential hypotension
Treprostinil (Remodulin)	Prostacyclin analog; activates intracellular adenylate cyclase, which increases concentrations of cAMP	IV initial dose of 1.25 ng/kg/min; titrate at increments of 1.25 ng/kg/min per week for the first 4 weeks of treatment; later 2.5 ng/kg/min per week	May cause liver dysfunction, flushing, headache, jaw pain, and diarrhea
Selexipag (Uptravi)	Prostacyclin receptor agonist; activates intracellular adenylate cyclase, which increases concentrations of cAMP	Starting dose of 200 μg twice daily; increase dose by 200 μg twice daily at weekly intervals to maximum tolerated dose up to 1600 μg twice daily	Moderate hepatic impairment, headache, jaw pain, diarrhea Rare occurrences of hyperthyroidism
Riociguat (Adempas)	Stimulates guanylate cyclase, increases sensitivity of guanylate cyclase to NO	1 mg orally 3 times a day; increase dose by 0.5 mg every 2 weeks to maximum dose of 2.5 mg orally 3 times a day	Syncope, liver transaminitis, bleeding

cAMP, Cyclic adenosine monophosphate; *ET-A,* endothelin receptor A; *ET-B,* endothelin receptor B; *NO,* nitric oxide; *PDE,* phosphodiesterase.

of 3 to 6 minutes. IV epoprostenol has been demonstrated to improve pulmonary hemodynamics, RV function, and exercise tolerance in patients receiving the vasodilator over several months. Initial starting doses of epoprostenol start at 1 to 2 ng/kg per minute with uptitration in increments of 1 to 2 ng/kg per minute to a maximum of 50 ng/kg per minute. Systemically administered epoprostenol is hindered by development of hypotension and nonselective pulmonary vasodilation, which can worsen ventilation–perfusion matching. In the perioperative setting, IV epoprostenol has not been studied as a rescue medication for the reduction of pulmonary pressures in the operating room. However, patients with pulmonary hypertension may present for noncardiac surgery under chronic maintenance IV epoprostenol therapy. In these patients, maintenance of the infusion may be prudent to prevent any abrupt rebound in pulmonary hypertension.

Inhaled epoprostenol (iEPO) in the perioperative setting has been shown to provide similar effect on hemodynamics and oxygenation to iNO. It is important to highlight that these data were obtained from small-sample-sized studies conducted in cardiac surgical patients. No studies are available on the use of iEPO in the noncardiac setting. Furthermore, one of the main drawbacks to the use of iEPO is the potential for platelet dysfunction and increased bleeding risk, which has been shown in a small number of trials. In addition, there is a need for a specialized delivery system consisting of a syringe pump and a jet nebulizer to deliver the drug to the inspiratory limb of the breathing circuit. There is also a modest degree of uncertainty regarding the concentration of iEPO reaching the alveoli and the possibility for the ventilator valves to malfunction from the special buffering agent. Nevertheless, there are several potential advantages of iEPO over iNO, such as the reduced risk of methemoglobinemia and toxic metabolites, ease of administration, and reduced cost. For these reasons, iEPO has replaced iNO as the preferred agent for the treatment of acute pulmonary hypertension in the ICU at some institutions.

Aerosolized iloprost provides an alternative method for delivery of prostacyclin analog therapy for patients with pulmonary hypertension. Iloprost is a more stable prostacyclin analog than epoprostenol, displaying a longer half-life of 20 to 30 minutes, which obviates the need for continuous nebulization, but the frequency of administration (6 to 9 times/day) is a concern for patient compliance. After administration of inhaled iloprost, the plasma concentration peaks at 100 to 200 pg/mL, which declines to undetectable (<25 pg/mL) within 30 minutes. The use of iloprost is generally indicated as an alternative to iNO. Iloprost has the advantage of being devoid of rebound pulmonary hypertension after its discontinuation and is also more stable than other inhaled vasodilators, allowing for administration in repeated doses using a nebulizer device without the need for a continuous infusion or ventilator. The latter makes it suitable for further administration after the extubation of the patient. The simplicity in the administration of inhaled iloprost makes it an ideal alternative to the tightly fitting facemask required to continue iNO in awake and extubated patients. Both inhaled and IV iloprost have been shown to reduce PVR, mean PAP, and with minimal systemic effects. The data on iloprost in the noncardiac surgical setting are scarce, with studies only limited to patients undergoing cardiac surgery. Inhaled iloprost has been successfully used for the management of intraoperative pulmonary hypertension and RV dysfunction during heart transplantation, improving global hemodynamics. IV iloprost is typically administered after failed treatment with inhaled iloprost, which in some patients may lead to improved efficacy. The recommended administration schedule for inhaled iloprost is six to nine doses (inhalations) per day with a minimum of 2 hours between doses and a target maintenance dose of 5 μg per administration. Although inhaled iloprost provides an alternative to parenteral prostacyclin therapy, the relatively short half-life of the compound requires a frequent dosing schedule, potentially limiting compliance and perhaps efficacy.

Conversely, inhaled treprostinil (Remodulin) is a prostacyclin analog approved for the treatment of pulmonary arterial hypertension (PAH) that may provide a more convenient treatment option for patients receiving inhaled iloprost while maintaining the clinical benefit of inhaled prostacyclin therapy. With an elimination half-life of approximately 4.5 hours, the recommended dosing of inhaled treprostinil is four times per day with approximately 4 hours between doses and a target maintenance dose of 9 breaths per treatment session. Given the more favorable administration schedule of inhaled treprostinil compared with inhaled iloprost, treprostinil has been recently developed as a viable alternative with a less frequent dosing schedule, which is typically administered via ultrasonic nebulizer four times a day. In patients with symptomatic pulmonary hypertension, inhaled treprostinil increases exercise tolerance and quality of life while decreasing mean PAP and PVR after treatment for over 12 weeks. Currently, there are no studies to guide therapy for the use of inhaled treprostinil in the perioperative setting as a rescue therapy.

Selexipag (Uptravi) is the newest of the oral prostacyclin derivatives and represents a highly selective, high-affinity agonist of the prostacyclin receptor. Oral selexipag has been shown to increase cardiac index and significantly reduce PVR in patients who were already receiving treatment for pulmonary hypertension. Patients receiving oral selexipag benefited from a reduction of all-cause mortality and complications related to pulmonary hypertension compared to the placebo arm. The beneficial effects of selexipag were similar in treatment for both naïve patients and patients on a background treatment for pulmonary hypertension, highlighting the potential for selexipag to be used as combination therapy with other currently available oral treatments. Selexipag administration is initiated at a dose of 200 μg twice daily and is increased weekly in twice-daily increments of 200 μg as tolerated with a maximum dose of 1600 μg twice daily. The most frequent adverse events reported with selexipag are headache, diarrhea, jaw pain, flushing, myalgias, and extremity pain. There have been rare cases of hyperthyroidism associated with selexipag therapy.

Phosphodiesterase Inhibitors

The synthesis of cGMP by sGC is a central step in the activation of endothelial smooth muscle relaxation in the lung. The endogenous PDE enzyme serves to regulate the levels of circulating cGMP by cleaving the second messenger, providing a means for controlling pulmonary vasodilation. The PDE class of inhibitors prevents the enzymatic breakdown of cGMP and enhances cGMP-mediated pulmonary vasodilation. The selective PDE enzyme isoform 5 (PDE-5) inhibitors primarily consists of sildenafil (Viagra) and tadalafil (Cialis), which are generally recommended for patients with mild to moderate pulmonary hypertension. In addition to the beneficial effects of pulmonary vasodilation, PDE-5 inhibitors may also improve ventilation/perfusion matching by increasing blood flow to more ventilated lung segments. This has been observed in patients with pulmonary hypertension and pulmonary fibrosis receiving the first-in-class PDE-5 inhibitor, sildenafil. Sildenafil treatment improves pulmonary hemodynamics, functional class, and exercise tolerance. In the perioperative setting, oral sildenafil has been used in patients to bridge the discontinuation of iNO, demonstrating effective decreases in pulmonary pressures without major concerns for concomitant systemic hypotension, pulmonary hypertensive crises, or rebound pulmonary hypertension. Moreover, sildenafil has also been used in combination with other agents to augment their vasodilatory effects or to limit the impact of their withdrawal. Combination therapy with oral sildenafil and inhaled iloprost was more effective than either agent alone in treating severe pulmonary hypertension in patients presenting for cardiac surgery. Similarly, sildenafil has also been effective as adjunctive therapy in managing persistent pulmonary hypertension despite treatment with isoproterenol, milrinone, nitroprusside, or nitroglycerin in the perioperative period when pulmonary hemodynamics improved further after addition of sildenafil administration. Associated adverse effects can include headache, flushing, and epistaxis. Profound hypotension may result if sildenafil is combined with nitrate use. The newer PDE-5 inhibitor tadalafil has been approved for its clinical use in pulmonary hypertension. Tadalafil is unique in that it exhibits a very long half-life ($\approx$17–18 hours), providing a more simple once-a-day daily dosing regimen as opposed to the three-times-a-day schedule of sildenafil. Despite being less well studied than sildenafil, the longer acting tadalafil has been shown to reduce pulmonary pressures and improve clinical symptoms in patients with pulmonary hypertension.

Endothelin Receptor Antagonists

Endothelin-1 is an endogenous hormone that binds to the endothelin receptors A (ET-A) and B (ET-B), inducing potent pulmonary vasoconstriction, smooth muscle proliferation, fibrosis, and inflammation. Endothelin receptor antagonists (ERAs) competitively inhibit action of endothelin-1. Bosentan (Tracleer) is the first approved blocker of both ET-A and ET-B receptors for the treatment of mild to moderate pulmonary hypertension. Oral bosentan has been shown to lower PAP and PVR and improve cardiac hemodynamics without significant systemic effects in patients with pulmonary hypertension. Bosentan has also been used in combination with prostacyclins or PDE-5 inhibitors, resulting in improved hemodynamics, RV function, exercise tolerance, quality of life, and mortality. One major advantage of combination therapy is the facilitation of dose reduction. Currently, ERAs play an important role in the medical management of chronic pulmonary hypertension, especially for functional class III or IV patients. However, their use in the perioperative setting is currently limited by the long half-life. Overall, bosentan is well tolerated with the exception of dose-dependent hepatic transaminitis observed in a small group of patients receiving bosentan.

Ambrisentan (Letairis) is a distinct ERA that displays a high selectivity for the ET-A receptor subtype. Distinct from bosentan, which blocks both the ET-A and ET-B receptors, ambrisentan preferentially binds to the ET-A receptor with a sufficiently long half-life to allow once-daily dosing. Patients treated with ambrisentan benefit from sustained improvements in exercise capacity and a reduced risk of clinical worsening and death. Other benefits such as improvements in mean pulmonary arterial pressure, cardiac output, PVR, and RV ejection fraction have also been reported. In direct comparison with bosentan, ambrisentan may offer several important advantages. Because of its longer half-life, ambrisentan is administered only once daily as opposed to twice daily in the case of bosentan. The other main advantage of ambrisentan is that the selective ET-A antagonism has been shown to be less hepatotoxic in clinical trials. In fact, the FDA no longer requires monthly monitoring of liver function in patients receiving ambrisentan. A change from bosentan to ambrisentan is often indicated in patients who experience a rise in liver enzymes with the former. No head-to-head study comparing the relative efficacy of ambrisentan versus bosentan has been undertaken. Accordingly, it is unknown whether selective ET-A receptor blockade with ambrisentan confers greater clinical benefit than dual-ET receptor blockade with bosentan.

Riociguat (Adempas)

Riociguat (Adempas) is a first-in-class activator of the soluble form of the enzyme sGC. Administered as an oral agent (maximum dosing of 2.5 mg three times daily), riociguat exhibits a dual mechanism of action on the NO–guanylate cyclase pathway: direct stimulation of sGC and increasing the sensitivity of sGC to endogenous NO. Riociguat is approved as an effective oral pulmonary vasodilator, significantly improving exercise capacity, PVR, and systemic hemodynamic parameters in patients with symptomatic pulmonary hypertension compared with placebo. In patients with pulmonary hypertension associated with systolic LV dysfunction, patients receiving oral riociguat showed significant improvements in PVR, SVR, cardiac index, and stroke volume index without changes in heart rate or systolic blood pressure compared with the placebo group. Analogous results were observed with riociguat therapy in patients with pulmonary hypertension secondary to diastolic heart failure in whom an increase in stroke volume and cardiac index were significantly improved, without deleterious increases in heart rate. Parallel improvements in RV end-diastolic area and left atrial area by echocardiographic assessments were seen as well in the group receiving oral riociguat compared with placebo. With respect to safety data, riociguat is generally well tolerated with the only serious adverse effects reported being syncope, hemoptysis from pulmonary hemorrhage, bleeding, and hepatic transaminitis.

SUGGESTED READING

Aronson S, Dyke CM, Stierer KA, et al. The ECLIPSE trials: comparative studies of clevidipine to nitroglycerin, sodium nitroprusside, and nicardipine for acute hypertension treatment in cardiac surgery patients. *Anesth Analg.* 2008;107(4):1110–1121.

Bangash MN, Kong ML, Pearse RM. Use of inotropes and vasopressor agents in critically ill patients. *Br J Pharmacol.* 2012;165(7):2015–2033.

Brooke BS. Perioperative beta-blockers for vascular surgery patients. *J Vasc Surg.* 2010;51(2):515–519.

Cheng JW, Tonelli AR, Pettersson G, Krasuski RA. Pharmacologic management of perioperative pulmonary hypertension. *J Cardiovasc Pharmacol.* 2014;63(4):375–384.

Dua N, Kumra VP. Management of perioperative arrhythmias. *Indian J Anaesth.* 2007;51:310–323.

Fox DL, Stream AR, Bull T. Perioperative management of the patient with pulmonary hypertension. *Semin Cardiothorac Vasc Anesth.* 2014;18(4):310–318.

Gordon C, Collard CD, Pan W. Intraoperative management of pulmonary hypertension and associated right heart failure. *Curr Opin Anaesthesiol.* 2010;23(1):49–56.

Hoeper MM, McLaughlin VV, Dalaan AM, Satoh T, Galiè N. Treatment of pulmonary hypertension. *Lancet Respir Med.* 2016;4(4):323–336.

Hubers SA, Brown NJ. Combined angiotensin receptor antagonism and neprilysin inhibition. *Circulation.* 2016;133(11):1115–1124.

Jentzer JC, Coons JC, Link CB, Schmidhofer M. Pharmacotherapy update on the use of vasopressors and inotropes in the intensive care unit. *J Cardiovasc Pharmacol Ther.* 2015;20(3):249–260.

Kirsten R, Nelson K, Kirsten D, Heintz B. Clinical pharmacokinetics of vasodilators. Part II. *Clin Pharmacokinet.* 1998;35:9–36.

Marik PE, Varon J. Perioperative hypertension: a review of current and emerging therapeutic agents. *J Clin Anesth.* 2009;21(3):220–229.

Minai OA, Yared JP, Kaw R, Subramaniam K, Hill NS. Perioperative risk and management in patients with pulmonary hypertension. *Chest.* 2013;144(1):329–340.

Nuckols TK, Bower AG, Paddock SM, et al. Programmable infusion pumps in ICUs: an analysis of corresponding adverse drug events. *J Gen Intern Med.* 2008;23:41–45.

Ohashi K, Dalleur O, Dykes PC, Bates DW. Benefits and risks of using smart pumps to reduce medication error rates: a systematic review. *Drug Saf.* 2014;37:1011–1120.

Overgaard CB, Dzavík V. Inotropes and vasopressors: review of physiology and clinical use in cardiovascular disease. *Circulation.* 2008;118(10):1047–1056.

Owens AT, Brozena SC, Jessup M. New management strategies in heart failure. *Circ Res.* 2016;118(3):480–495.

Pilkington SA, Taboada D, Martinez G. Pulmonary hypertension and its management in patients undergoing non-cardiac surgery. *Anaesthesia.* 2015;70(1):56–70.

Price LC, Wort SJ, Finney SJ, Marino PS, Brett SJ. Pulmonary vascular and right ventricular dysfunction in adult critical care: current and emerging options for management: a systematic literature review. *Crit Care.* 2010;14(5):R169.

Rothschild JM, Keohane CA, Cook EF, et al. A controlled trial of smart infusion pumps to improve medication safety in critically ill patients. *Crit Care Med.* 2005;33:533–540.

Subramaniam K, Yared JP. Management of pulmonary hypertension in the operating room. *Semin Cardiothorac Vasc Anesth.* 2007;11(2):119–136.

Thunberg CA, Morozowich ST, Ramakrishna H. Inhaled therapy for the management of perioperative pulmonary hypertension. *Ann Card Anaesth.* 2015;18(3):394–402.

Weeda ER, Nguyen E, White CM. Role of ivabradine in the treatment of patients with cardiovascular disease. *Ann Pharmacother.* 2016;50(6):475–485.

Chapter 12

General, Regional, or Monitored Anesthesia Care for the Cardiac Patient Undergoing Noncardiac Surgery

Brian Frugoni, MD • K. Annette Mizuguchi, MD, PhD, MMSc

Key Points

1. With monitored anesthesia care, the stress response to surgery may not be adequately blocked, and the resulting tachycardia may aggravate the patient's underlying cardiac disease.
2. A decrease in minute ventilation and increase in carbon dioxide associated with sedation can have deleterious effects on patients with right heart dysfunction.
3. The recommended dose of epinephrine is reduced to less than 1 µg/kg in the treatment of local anesthetic toxicity; lipid emulsions are preferable.
4. Neuraxial and regional anesthesia may decrease the surgical stress response and can obviate or supplement a general anesthetic, although chronic anticoagulation can impact the safety of these techniques.
5. Epidural anesthesia is often favored over spinal anesthesia for cardiac patients undergoing noncardiac surgery because the level of anesthesia can be incrementally adjusted.
6. Subarachnoid neuraxial catheter placement may permit a safe spinal anesthetic in patients at high risk for complications, with both general anesthesia and traditional spinal anesthesia, by allowing careful titration of the block level.
7. All volatile inhalation agents cause dose-dependent decreases in contractile function, induce arterial and venovasodilation, decrease cardiac myocardial oxygen consumption (Mvo_2), and may induce protective myocardial preconditioning.
8. The anesthetic technique for a cardiac patient undergoing noncardiac surgery is dependent on (1) the type of surgery or procedure, (2) the extent of cardiac disease, and (3) the presence of other comorbidities.

Given the increasing prevalence of heart disease, the frequency of patients with significant cardiac disease presenting for noncardiac surgery will likely increase in the future. The anesthetic technique selected for these patients depends on a number of factors, including the type of surgery or procedure, the type and severity of the underlying cardiac disease, and the presence of other comorbidities. Factors influencing the selection of an anesthetic technique (i.e., general, regional, neuraxial, or monitored anesthesia care [MAC]) for cardiac patients undergoing noncardiac surgery are discussed in this chapter.

Patients with cardiac disease undergoing noncardiac surgery are at higher risk of developing perioperative complications. Both surgery and anesthesia can result in adverse cardiac events via sympathetic nervous system stimulation, inflammation, and hypercoagulability that may be induced. Intraoperatively, practitioners caring for the cardiac patient may also encounter hemodynamic instability, acute blood loss, and hypothermia. Therefore choosing the anesthetic technique that will maintain the desired hemodynamic goals (Table 12.1); improve operating conditions; and provide the patient with amnesia, analgesia, or both is crucial.

MONITORED ANESTHESIA CARE

Monitored anesthesia care, as defined by the American Society of Anesthesiologists (ASA), involves the preoperative evaluation, intraoperative monitoring and management, and postoperative care of a patient undergoing a surgical procedure without general anesthesia. Intrinsic to MAC is the ability to identify and manage intraoperative physiologic derangements while providing sedation, analgesia, or both to the patient. Sedation and analgesia are often provided during MAC, but they are not required components. However, the practitioner providing MAC must have the ability to convert to a general anesthetic if necessitated by patient or procedural factors.

Monitored anesthesia care, including local anesthesia with or without sedation, is a useful and often successful anesthetic technique for appropriately selected cases. Although MAC may be deemed by some individuals to be the least invasive of all anesthetic techniques because of its association with minor procedures and minimal hemodynamic changes, it is important to acknowledge the challenges, limitations, and potential dangers of MAC. For example, the stress response to surgery may not be adequately attenuated, and the resulting sympathetic stimulation may aggravate the patient's underlying cardiac disease. Patients undergoing procedures under MAC are often pharmacologically sedated; however, because they are not under general anesthesia, they may be aware of their surroundings and will respond to an inadequately blocked surgical stimulus or a stressful operating room (OR) environment. In addition, local anesthetic toxicity can occur with local infiltration of the surgical field and at very high blood levels can lead to cardiovascular collapse. Furthermore, tachycardia induced by the intravascular or subcutaneous injection of local anesthetic with epinephrine can be detrimental for patients with coronary artery disease.

Under MAC, tissue oxygen demand is not significantly decreased from the normal awake state and in fact may be significantly increased if a stress response leads to increased sympathetic tone. Alternatively, hypoxia from excessive sedation and hypoventilation may adversely affect myocardial oxygen supply. Further complicating the scenario, surgeons often request a motionless field to safely complete the procedure. In general, patient movement is more common under MAC and may be even more prevalent in the cardiac population because their physiology may not permit adequate sedation. Close communication with the surgical team is essential for a successful procedure under MAC because it may help prevent or mitigate some of these potential adverse events.

That being said, MAC also has theoretic benefits in patients with underlying cardiac disease. Avoiding the hemodynamic changes often associated with the induction of and emergence from general anesthesia, as well as positive-pressure ventilation, may be desirable in this population. Furthermore, adequate local anesthesia not only minimizes stimulation during a procedure but also can provide for postoperative analgesia and mitigate undesirable increases in sympathetic tone (Box 12.1).

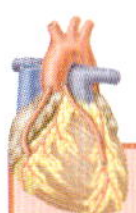

> ### BOX 12.1   *Monitored Anesthesia Care and Myocardial Oxygen Demand and Delivery*
>
> - Tissue oxygen demand is not significantly decreased from the normal awake state.
> - Hypoxia from sedation and hypoventilation may adversely affect myocardial oxygen supply.
> - Avoidance of the hemodynamic perturbations associated with induction and emergence from general anesthesia may help optimize myocardial supply in select cases.

Unfortunately, no randomized controlled trials have compared outcomes of MAC with outcomes of general anesthesia in cardiac patients. However, the overall goals of MAC and general anesthesia remain the same—minimization of hemodynamic perturbations. Therefore if the adequate administration of local anesthesia, analgesia, or sedatives can mitigate patient stress and hemodynamic perturbations, then MAC may be an optimal anesthetic plan for the cardiac patient undergoing noncardiac surgery.

Monitoring During Monitored Anesthesia Care

As with general anesthesia, standard ASA monitors are required for MAC. Depending on the surgical procedure, expected duration, chance of conversion to general anesthesia, and the potential for hemodynamic fluctuation, more invasive monitors may be indicated. The placement of an arterial catheter may be unnecessary for short, simple procedures. However, in patients with critical valvular heart disease, pulmonary hypertension, severe cardiomyopathy, or other critical cardiac illnesses, an arterial catheter may be indicated. Similarly, the need for invasive arterial monitoring may be determined by the need for deep sedation or a high likelihood of conversion to a general anesthetic. Central venous pressure monitoring is rarely necessary for a planned MAC unless peripheral intravenous (IV) access is unobtainable. Given a lack of airway instrumentation, transesophageal echocardiography (TEE) is often not feasible. However, intermittent TEE examinations are occasionally done for specific procedures (e.g., transcatheter aortic valve replacement done under MAC). Intermittent transthoracic echocardiography may be helpful for challenging cases done under MAC if the windows are accessible.

Sedation

Patients undergoing procedures with MAC commonly receive some form of sedation, analgesia, or both, with the goal being the relief of pain and anxiety during the procedure. Modulation of pain and anxiety during a procedure is especially important in patients with underlying cardiac disease given the risks posed by any increase in sympathetic tone. Most medications commonly used for sedation during routine anesthetics may be used safely and effectively in patients with cardiac disease, provided potential side effects are monitored for and managed appropriately (Table 12.2).

12

Table 12.1 Hemodynamic Goals for Common Adult Cardiac Disease

Cardiac Disease	HR	Preload	Afterload (SVR)	PVR	Contractility	Avoid	Goal
AS	Sinus rhythm; 60–80 beats/min	Increased or adequate	Increased	Maintain	Maintain	• Hypotension • Tachycardia (decreases diastolic filling time and CO) • Bradycardia (can result in decreased CO and hypotension)	• Sinus rhythm
AR	Fast: 80–100 beats/min	Increased	Decreased	Maintain	Maintain	• Bradycardia	• Decreasing regurgitant volume and maximizing effective forward flow and CO • Augmentation of forward flow
MS	Sinus rhythm, slower HR to increase diastolic filling time and improve ventricular filling	Normal or increased	Normal	Maintain	Decreased	• Tachycardia (can lead to increased LAP and PAP and induce pulmonary edema and right heart failure) • Pulmonary vasoconstriction	• Maintain LV diastolic filling and optimizing right heart function • Tight control of vascular tone and intravascular volume to avoid decreases in SV and pulmonary edema

MR	Increased (normal to increased)	Increased (in some with dilated LA and LV, increased preload can increase regurgitant fraction)	Decreased	Decreased	Maintain	• Myocardial depression	• Mild tachycardia • Vasodilation for maximizing true LV output (volume ejected across the AV) and minimizing regurgitant flow (volume ejected across MV)
TS	Maintain (depends on sinus rhythm)	Increased	Increased	Maintain	Maintain		
TR	Increased or maintain	Increased	Maintain	Decreased	Maintain		
PS	Increased	Increased	Maintain	Decreased or maintain	Maintain		• Similar to AS but the RV is much more sensitive to increases in afterload
CAD	Slow: 50–80 beats/min	Decreased	Increased	Maintain	Maintain		• Maximize coronary supply and demand • Demand: (1) HR, (2) wall tension, and (3) contractility • Supply: (1) coronary blood flow, (2) diastolic time, (2) arterial oxygen content, (4) release of oxygen, and (5) oxygen extraction
HCM	Normal	Increased	Increased		Decrease	• Tachycardia • Inotropes • Vasodilators	• Myocardial depression

AR, Aortic regurgitation; *AS,* aortic stenosis; *AV,* aortic valve; *CAD,* coronary artery disease; *CO,* cardiac output; *HCM,* hypertrophic cardiomyopathy; *HR,* heart rate; *LA,* left atrium, *LAP,* left atrial pressure; *LV,* left ventricle; *MR,* mitral regurgitation; *MS,* mitral stenosis; *MV,* mitral valve; *PAP,* pulmonary artery pressure; *PS,* pulmonic stenosis; *PVR,* pulmonary vascular resistance; *RV,* right ventricle; *SV,* stroke volume; *SVR,* systemic vascular resistance; *TR,* tricuspid regurgitation; *TS,* tricuspid stenosis.

Table 12.2 Sedatives and Analgesics for Monitored Anesthesia Care

Drug	Dose
Propofol	Bolus: 0.25–1 mg/kg Infusion: 25–75 µg/kg/min
Midazolam	Bolus: 0.02–0.1 mg/kg
Fentanyl	Bolus: 25–100 µg
Remifentanil	Infusion: 0.02–0.05 µg/kg/min
Dexmedetomidine	Bolus: 0.5–1 µg/kg over 10 min Infusion: 0.3–1 µg/kg/h

Propofol

Propofol is a lipid-soluble alkylphenol derivative that has become widely used for the induction and maintenance of sedation because of its rapid onset and redistribution, titratability, potential for amnesia, and antiemetic properties. It is rapidly redistributed after bolus administration, with an initial distribution half-life of 2 to 8 minutes and is rapidly metabolized by the liver. Because of lipid solubility, prolonged use via infusion increases the context-sensitive half-time; however, the decline in serum levels remains relatively rapid compared with other IV anesthetics. Sedation with propofol may be accomplished via several techniques: (1) single bolus dose (or titrated bolus doses) for short procedures, (2) bolus followed by infusion or repeated boluses for longer procedures, and (3) infusion alone without bolus.

Although it has many beneficial properties, propofol has significant effects on the cardiovascular system that should be considered in patients with underlying cardiac disease. Although the direct action of propofol on the myocardium is controversial, it likely has some direct myocardial depressant effects via L-type Ca^{2+} channels or sarcolemma calcium release modulation. This depressant effect may be more pronounced in the failing myocardium and may result in a significant reduction in cardiac output. Propofol also causes reliable decreases in preload and systemic vascular resistance (SVR) by a multifactorial process that includes decreased sympathetic tone, decreased calcium mobilization in smooth muscle, and inhibition of prostacyclin synthesis. The net result is decreases in arterial blood pressure, SVR, and potentially cardiac output that may be more pronounced in patients with cardiac disease. Heart rate is reported to be relatively unchanged.

Despite the aforementioned effects, propofol sedation during MAC can be safely accomplished in patients with cardiac disease as long as these cardiovascular effects are carefully considered. Patients with poor left ventricular (LV) function and slow circulation times take longer to show an effect from a propofol bolus or change in infusion rate. Therefore a cumulative overdose may occur in this patient population if adequate dosing intervals are not maintained. Further compounding this issue, older adult patients who frequently have cardiac disease also require lower doses for the same clinical effect. Given these characteristics and propofol's narrow therapeutic index, it is possible to transition rapidly from light sedation to general anesthesia and apnea. The risk of hypoventilation and apnea must be considered in patients who are sensitive to changes in partial pressure of CO_2 (e.g., severe pulmonary hypertension).

Patients with valvular disease who are sensitive to changes in SVR (e.g., aortic stenosis) must be treated with extreme caution, and in severe cases, propofol may be best avoided. However, propofol may be safely used for patients with valvular heart disease if reduced doses are used and the drug is carefully titrated to effect. In higher risk patients, sedation with an infusion only rather than a bolus followed by an infusion may lead to greater hemodynamic stability at the expense of longer time to an adequate sedation depth.

Fentanyl

Fentanyl is a synthetic opioid that is 50 to 100 times more potent than morphine and significantly more lipid soluble. It is a common component of MAC and general anesthesia because of its rapid onset, short half-life, and minimal systemic side effects (e.g., histamine release, venodilation) compared with morphine. After IV administration, fentanyl demonstrates an initial effect in 1 to 2 minutes and maximum effect at 6 minutes, with an expected duration of action of 30 to 60 minutes. Termination of action is due to redistribution from the central nervous system (CNS) to the muscle and fat compartments. These properties make it useful for procedures under MAC; however, it has no amnestic properties, and if amnesia is desired, it must be combined with another agent.

Fentanyl provides excellent pain control during invasive procedures and can be used via intermittent bolus with titration to the desired effect. Alternatively, it may be administered as an infusion, but this is rarely indicated for procedures under MAC. Redistribution to secondary compartments and a terminal half-life of 2 to 4 hours lead to progressively increasing serum concentration during a continuous infusion and increase the chance of adverse events.

In general, opiates have a favorable cardiovascular profile and have been used successfully in cardiac surgery for decades. The major hemodynamic effects of bradycardia and decreases in arterial blood pressure, which are usually mild, are attributed to decreased sympathetic tone. The main problems associated with opioid use during MAC are related to hypoventilation and apnea. Careful monitoring is indicated, especially in at-risk populations (e.g., older adults) that will respond poorly to elevated CO_2 and atelectasis.

Remifentanil

Although remifentanil is a synthetic opioid like fentanyl, it is structurally unique in that it contains ester linkages. It is therefore metabolized by blood- and tissue-nonspecific esterases, resulting in a very short half-life of 5 to 20 minutes. It is not affected by liver or kidney dysfunction, nor is the half-life prolonged in pseudocholinesterase deficiency.

Remifentanil has been used successfully in MAC anesthesia, including procedures done in the cardiac catheterization suite. The most common technique for remifentanil-based MAC is a low-dose infusion that is titrated to analgesia and sedation. Bolus administration is possible, but infusion is often preferred because of the rapid onset and short duration of action. It has been administered in intermittent bolus form for short painful events such as uterine contractions during labor, but for procedures with relatively constant stimulation levels, an infusion provides more stable analgesia.

Major side effects include intense pruritus, dizziness, and respiratory depression. Otherwise, the cardiovascular profile is similar to that of other opiates (e.g., fentanyl), and as with other opiates, dose-related side effects such as respiratory depression may be more common in elderly patients.

Dexmedetomidine

Dexmedetomidine is a highly specific α_2 agonist useful for both procedural and intensive care unit (ICU) sedation. It produces a sedative–hypnotic effect with associated analgesia and sympatholysis via agonism at central presynaptic α_2 receptors. It redistributes rapidly after short-term administration, with a context-sensitive half-time of 4 minutes after a 10-minute infusion. However, it demonstrates a prolonged duration of action with longer infusions because of an elimination half-life of 2 to 3 hours.

Dexmedetomidine may be administered as a bolus or as an infusion with or without a loading dose for procedural sedation during MAC. The method of administration determines the hemodynamic effects, with bolus administration producing a biphasic cardiovascular profile. After a bolus, there is an initial increase in blood pressure and decrease in heart rate that are likely due to stimulation of peripheral postsynaptic α_2 receptors. After 15 minutes, the heart rate returns to baseline, and arterial blood pressure decreases to approximately 15% below baseline. Avoiding a loading dose and relying solely on an infusion may avoid this biphasic response.

The overall cardiovascular effects of dexmedetomidine are generally well tolerated by patients with cardiac disease. However, there is some indirect decrease in contractility and reduction in SVR caused by sympatholysis, which may have adverse consequences for critically ill patients. Compared with propofol, dexmedetomidine has a slower onset and offset, making it more difficult to titrate during MAC anesthesia. However, it has minimal respiratory depressant effects, which is a significant advantage compared with propofol. In addition, dexmedetomidine has analgesic properties. Dexmedetomidine does not appear to be as amnestic as propofol, and patients are more easily arousable, which may be an advantage or disadvantage depending on the surgical procedure.

Midazolam

A water-soluble benzodiazepine, midazolam has a long history of use in patients with cardiac disease. As a γ-aminobutyric acid type A (GABA$_A$) agonist, benzodiazepines such as midazolam have hypnotic, amnestic, anxiolytic, and anticonvulsant effects that make them very useful for a variety of surgical procedures. There are also minimal hemodynamic changes associated with the administration of midazolam, the most significant being a small decrease in blood pressure with an unchanged cardiac index. It has been used safely in patients with ischemic heart disease, as well as valvular heart disease.

Because it has no analgesic properties, midazolam is often combined with an opiate for procedural sedation. Given as a bolus, it has an effect within 2 to 3 minutes and lasts 1 to 6 hours. Infusions may be used for prolonged sedation or as part of a general anesthetic but are rarely indicated for MAC.

Midazolam with or without fentanyl remains a valuable tool for procedures under MAC, especially minimally invasive procedures. Low doses of midazolam and fentanyl titrated to effect generally produce little hemodynamic change and are well tolerated by patients with severe cardiac disease or other significant comorbidities. However, patients receiving benzodiazepines typically remain sedated longer after completion of the procedure than those given propofol. Therefore undesirable prolonged postoperative amnesia or sedation is a potential adverse effect of midazolam. In addition, adverse effects are more common and may persist for a longer period of time in the older adult patient population.

Local Anesthesia

Local anesthetics are membrane-stabilizing drugs that inhibit sodium influx through voltage-gated sodium channels in the neuron cell membrane and decrease the rate of depolarization, thus inhibiting the generation of action potentials. They are divided into two classes (amides and esters), with amides being used most commonly for

Table 12.3 Commonly Used Local Anesthetics

Drug	Maximum Dose	Duration of Action
Lidocaine	Without epinephrine: 4.5 mg/kg (maximum, 300 mg) With epinephrine: 7 mg/kg (maximum, 500 mg)	90–200 min
Mepivacaine	Without epinephrine: 5 mg/kg (maximum, 400 mg) With epinephrine: 7 mg/kg (maximum, 550 mg)	120–240 min
Chloroprocaine	Without epinephrine: 15 mg/kg With epinephrine: 20 mg/kg	30–60 min
Bupivacaine	Without epinephrine: 2 mg/kg (maximum, 175 mg) With epinephrine: 3 mg/kg (maximum, 225 mg)	180–360 min
Ropivacaine	2–3 mg/kg (maximum, 250 mg)	180–360 min
Tetracaine	Without epinephrine: 1.5 mg/kg With epinephrine: 2.5 mg/kg	180–600 min

surgical local anesthesia. Commonly used drugs include lidocaine, mepivacaine, bupivacaine, or ropivacaine with or without epinephrine (Table 12.3). These medications can provide excellent pain control in appropriate procedures as long as the surgical field is adequately blocked.

Cardiac patients presenting for noncardiac surgery under MAC may be at higher risk of developing local anesthetic systemic toxicity given that they often have multiple known risk factors (e.g., advanced age, heart failure, ischemic cardiomyopathy, conduction abnormalities, or concurrent medications that inhibit sodium channels) (Table 12.4). Local anesthetic toxicity is related to elevated plasma concentrations of unbound drug. Risk factors for increased plasma levels include intravascular injection, excessive dose or rate of administration, delayed clearance, and injection in highly vascular tissue. Amide local anesthetics are hepatically metabolized and may have decreased clearance in patients with liver disease, including liver disease secondary to cardiac dysfunction (e.g., hepatic congestion from right-sided heart failure). Liver disease also results in a decrease in production of proteins that bind local anesthetics, which leads to an increased unbound drug fraction. Acidosis, which may be present in patients with severe cardiac disease and reduced oxygen delivery, also lead to an increase in unbound drug fraction caused by dissociation from binding proteins. Furthermore, patients with very low ejection fractions are more likely to receive higher total doses of local anesthetic because of "stacked" injections. This is because of their slow circulation time and the delayed clinical effect or signs of toxicity.

Another consideration is the inclusion of epinephrine in the local anesthetic solution. For example, for every 20 mL of local anesthetic with epinephrine 1:200,000, a patient will receive 100 μg of subcutaneous epinephrine. If large volumes of local anesthetic with epinephrine are used, the total epinephrine dose administered may be enough to cause hypertension and tachycardia. This may even occur without accidental IV injection. As previously stated, hypertension and tachycardia may be problematic in patients with ischemic heart disease or pulmonary hypertension. Therefore it is important to remain vigilant and closely monitor these patients during and after injections (Box 12.2).

Table 12.4 Medications That Inhibit Sodium Channels

Drug	Uses
Class IA Antiarrhythmics	
Quinidine	AF, atrial flutter, SVT, and VT
Procainamide	
Disopyramide	
Class IB Antiarrhythmics	
Lidocaine	Ventricular tachyarrhythmias
Tocainide	
Mexiletine	
Class IC Antiarrhythmics	
Flecainide	Life-threatening SVT and VT
Propafenone	
Moricizine	
Anticonvulsants	
Phenytoin	
Carbamazepine	
Oxcarbazepine	
Lamotrigine	
Valproic acid	
Felbamate	
Topiramate	

AF, Atrial fibrillation; *SVT,* supraventricular tachycardia; *VT,* ventricular tachycardia.

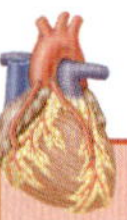

BOX 12.2 *Risk Factors for Local Anesthetic Systemic Toxicity*

- Advanced age, heart failure, ischemic cardiomyopathy, conduction abnormalities, and medications that inhibit sodium channels
- The total epinephrine dose should be considered when epinephrine-containing local anesthetics are administered to patients who may poorly tolerate tachycardia.

Local Anesthetic Systemic Toxicity

Signs and symptoms (e.g., CNS) may be delayed or subtle or absent in this patient population, with cardiovascular signs often being the only clinical manifestation of local anesthetic toxicity (Box 12.3). Treatment of local anesthetic toxicity depends on the severity of the reaction (Box 12.4). The first course of action is to secure the airway and administer 100% oxygen to mitigate acidosis and hypoxia. Seizure prevention or termination is also important to prevent or reduce the associated metabolic acidosis. According to the American Society of Regional Anesthesia and Pain Medicine (ASRA) guidelines, benzodiazepines are the preferred antiepileptic medication. ASRA guidelines specifically state to avoid propofol for treating seizures in patients with signs of cardiovascular instability or patients at risk of progressing to cardiovascular collapse. This recommendation is based on animal studies showing that benzodiazepines adequately prevented local anesthetic-induced seizures by raising the seizure threshold and the fact that propofol can exacerbate or accelerate the progression to cardiac arrest.

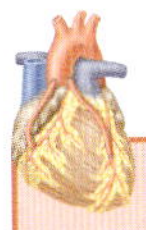

> **BOX 12.3   *Signs and Symptoms of Local Anesthetic Toxicity***
>
> ### Central Nervous System Signs
>
> - Early symptoms (nonspecific symptoms): metallic taste, circumoral tongue paresthesia, numbness, diplopia, tinnitus, dizziness
> - Excitation: agitation, nervousness, confusion, muscle twitching, feeling of "impending doom," grand mal seizure
> - Depression: coma or respiratory arrest
>
> ### Cardiovascular Signs
>
> - Initial signs: hyperdynamic in nature, including hypertension, tachycardia, and ventricular arrhythmias
> - Progressive hypotension
> - Conduction block, bradycardia, or asystole
> - Ventricular arrhythmias: VT, torsades de pointes, VF
>
> *VF*, Ventricular fibrillation; *VT*, ventricular tachycardia.
> Modified from the American Society of Regional Anesthesia and Pain Medicine Guidelines.

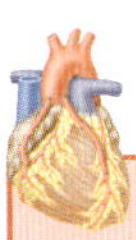

> **BOX 12.4   *Treatment of Local Anesthetic Systemic Toxicity***
>
> - Get help.
> - Ventilate with 100% oxygen.
> - Antiepileptics: benzodiazepines preferred; avoid propofol in patients with signs of cardiovascular instability
> - Alert the nearest facility with cardiopulmonary bypass capability.
> - Management of cardiac arrhythmias
>   - Basic and advanced life support require adjustment of medications and prolonged resuscitation efforts.
>   - Avoid vasopressin, calcium channel blockers, β-blockers, and local anesthetics.
>   - Reduce individual epinephrine doses to <1 µg/kg.
> - Lipid emulsion (20%) therapy (based on a 70-kg patient)
>   - Bolus 1.5 mL/kg (lean body mass) over 1 min.
>   - Start a continuous infusion at 0.25 mL/kg/min.
>   - Repeat bolus once or twice for persistent cardiovascular collapse.
>   - Double the infusion rate to 0.5 mL/kg/min if hypotension persists.
>   - Continue the infusion for at least 10 min after circulatory stability is attained.
>   - The recommended upper limit for lipid emulsion is approximately 10 mL/kg over the first 30 min.
>
> Resource: Weinberg G. Treatment regimens: lipid rescue resuscitation. Squarespace; 2012. www.lipidrescue.org.

Lipid emulsion (20%) therapy with a bolus followed by continuous infusion has successfully treated patients in cardiac arrest. Unfortunately, the timing of lipid therapy is controversial. Waiting to start a lipid infusion only after unsuccessful advanced cardiac life support (ACLS) is unreasonable. However, starting a lipid infusion at the earliest sign of local anesthetic toxicity can result in unnecessary treatment because not all patients progress to severe cardiac toxicity. Even though some in vitro studies have shown attenuation of bupivacaine toxicity with propofol as the lipid source, the use of propofol is strongly discouraged. This is because the lipid content is low at clinically administered volumes, and the associated hypotension is detrimental to resuscitation. Because cardiovascular depression from local anesthetics can persist or recur after treatment, it is recommended that patients be monitored for more than 12 hours after treatment with lipid emulsion.

Although all local anesthetics block the cardiac conduction system via sodium channels, the more potent local anesthetics (e.g., bupivacaine) present a greater risk for severe cardiac toxicity. This risk can be attributed to bupivacaine's higher affinity for sodium channels compared with lidocaine. Additionally, it dissociates from the sodium channel much more slowly than lidocaine. Therefore in severe cases of local anesthetic-induced cardiac toxicity, establishing cardiopulmonary bypass to provide circulatory support provides superior resuscitation to closed chest cardiac compressions by improving tissue perfusion and minimizing metabolic acidosis. Ultimately, this leads to a decrease in the amount of local anesthetic bound to myocardial sodium channel receptors. Cardiopulmonary bypass can also help maintain the hepatic blood flow that is necessary for metabolism of circulating local anesthetics. Therefore the ASRA recommendations for the treatment of local anesthetic systemic toxicity include "alert[ing] the nearest facility having cardiopulmonary bypass capability" as part of the initial focus in treatment. Of note, patients who survive after cardiopulmonary bypass do not seem to have permanent cardiac injury from the local anesthetic.

The ASRA guidelines also specifically recommend avoiding vasopressin, calcium channel blockers or local anesthetic antiarrhythmics (e.g., lidocaine) when managing cardiac arrhythmias secondary to local anesthetic systemic toxicity. Vasopressin is not recommended by the ASRA because animal studies showed that vasopressin was associated with poor hemodynamic and metabolic parameters and resulted in pulmonary hemorrhage in all animals studied. Finally, the recommended dose of epinephrine is reduced to less than 1 μg/kg because epinephrine can provoke severe arrhythmias and was associated with poor recovery of hemodynamic and metabolic parameters. Epinephrine was also found to impair resuscitation from local anesthetic toxicity and reduced the efficacy of lipid rescue.

Special Considerations

During MAC with sedation, there remains an ever-present risk of airway obstruction or respiratory compromise. With the development of short-acting potent IV anesthetic agents (e.g., remifentanil and propofol), patients under MAC can be quickly sedated to an anesthetic depth equivalent to a general anesthetic without a protected airway. Furthermore, a decrease in minute ventilation and the associated increase in carbon dioxide can have deleterious effects on patients with right heart dysfunction. These potential complications mandate vigilance, appropriate titration, and careful selection of patients by the anesthesiologist. Consideration must be given to patient position and the ease of access to the airway. In patients who do not tolerate elevations in CO_2 or those at risk from low oxygen tension, there must be no delay in the treatment of hypoventilation, apnea, and hypoxia.

Finally, MAC may not be suitable for patients who cannot lie flat or remain still for lengthy procedures. Extremely anxious patients or those with a persistent cough may also require a general anesthetic as opposed to MAC.

Conclusion

Monitored anesthesia care is often a viable anesthetic choice for patients with cardiac disease undergoing minor procedures. A number of sedation and analgesic choices may be safely used in these patients, provided sufficient care is taken to match the agent to the patient's particular cardiac disease. For MAC to be successful, the expectations of the patient, surgeon, and anesthesiologist need to be aligned. The surgeon may need to allow time for an appropriate plane of sedation to be achieved with slowly titrated agents, pause the procedure, or provide additional local anesthesia if needed, and the patient will need to understand that the anesthetic care plan may change intraoperatively. Communication among the care team is crucial. In particular, in remote locations where conditions are suboptimal for the anesthesia team (e.g., poor lighting, obstructed views, limited resources or personnel), communication may be the key to preventing complications and to successful resuscitation if it is required.

REGIONAL AND NEURAXIAL ANESTHESIA

Regional anesthesia may be the sole anesthetic or supplement a MAC or general anesthetic for cardiac patients undergoing noncardiac surgery. The type of regional anesthetic technique recommended will depend on the planned procedure, the coagulation status of the patient, the compressibility of the regional site, and the underlying cardiac disease. In general, regional anesthesia may be differentiated into central (neuraxial) blocks and peripheral nerve blocks (PNBs). Neuraxial anesthesia involves blockade of the nerves at the level of the CNS, either within the cerebrospinal fluid (CSF) (spinal) or at the level of the nerve root (epidural). Peripheral nerve blocks, conversely, are any nerve block beyond the level of the epidural space. As previously discussed, the provider should remain vigilant for signs and symptoms of local anesthetic toxicity in this at-risk population.

Neuraxial Anesthesia

The choice between spinal and epidural anesthesia in patients with cardiac disease stems from the expected physiologic changes associated with each block. Spinal anesthesia results from depositing a local anesthetic in the lumbar CSF. Movement of the local anesthetic depends on patient positioning and medication baricity, with a hyperbaric local anesthetic (typically 0.75% bupivacaine with dextrose) moving to the dependent portions of the subarachnoid space. In a supine patient, this typically results in extension of the block to the upper mid thoracic region. Because of relative sensitivities of the different nerve types to local anesthetic, the sympathetic block in a spinal anesthetic may extend one or two spinal levels above the sensory block. This can result in a total sympathectomy and associated 15% to 25% decrease in SVR, as well as a decrease in heart rate from blockade of the cardioaccelerator fibers from T1 to T4. Significant hypotension may result, and this may have profound implications for patients with cardiac disease. Use of isobaric 0.5% bupivacaine may avoid this sympathectomy by preventing local anesthetic from spreading to the thoracic region. However, because isobaric medication will remain near the spinal level where it is injected, its use is limited to procedures at or below the low thoracic dermatomal level.

Epidural anesthesia involves injection of local anesthetic into the space between the ligamentum flavum and the dura mater, which contains the nerve roots exiting the subarachnoid space. The level of block depends largely on the volume of local anesthetic injected, with larger volumes causing a higher block in a relatively linear fashion. Onset is slower than with subarachnoid block, and the block may be less dense. Similarly, the sympathectomy and changes in SVR are often (although not always) less profound.

Epidural anesthesia is often favored over spinal anesthesia for cardiac patients undergoing noncardiac surgery because the dermatome level can be incrementally adjusted. By titrating the level of sensory and therefore sympathetic blockade, changes in vasomotor tone (reflected by changes in blood pressure and heart rate) can be attenuated and less dramatic than those associated with spinal anesthesia. However, in certain situations, spinal anesthesia may be more appropriate. Subarachnoid blocks are technically easier and often faster to place, have a higher success rate, and provide profound analgesia. This dense block may be beneficial because it will successfully eliminate any sympathetic response to surgery on the lower extremities or abdomen. Epidural blocks, on the other hand, provide an option for continuous postoperative analgesia. Regardless, it is important to understand that both spinal and epidural anesthesia can cause sympathetic blockade and result in hypotension and bradycardia. Patients with ischemic heart disease may develop myocardial oxygen supply-demand imbalance if hypotension is not addressed rapidly. Also, patients with obstructive left-sided heart lesions (e.g., severe aortic stenosis, hypertrophic obstructive cardiomyopathy [HOCM]) may decompensate rapidly if faced with any decrease in SVR and hypotension. Conversely, patients with left heart failure may benefit from a reduction in SVR, provided coronary perfusion is maintained.

In addition to traditional subarachnoid and epidural blocks, placement of a subarachnoid catheter may be performed to provide a continuous spinal. A continuous spinal catheter permits for the careful and precise titration of neuraxial blockade while also providing the density and profound muscle relaxation of the subarachnoid block. Small incremental doses of local anesthetic (e.g., 0.75% hyperbaric bupivacaine or 0.5% isobaric bupivacaine given 0.5–1 mL at a time) may be titrated to effect. In addition, the subarachnoid dose may be repeated via the catheter during the procedure, which allows for longer duration procedures under a spinal technique. Potential downsides include a higher risk of postdural puncture headache (because a Touhy needle is typically used for the dural puncture) and greater risk of meningitis (Box 12.5). In published case series, both of these risks appear to be rare. Anecdotally, continuous spinals have been used successfully for lower extremity surgery in patients with lesions classically deemed high risk for general anesthesia (e.g., critical aortic stenosis).

Anticoagulation and Neuraxial Anesthesia

When considering neuraxial anesthesia in a cardiac patient undergoing noncardiac surgery, it is important to review the patient's medication history. Antithrombotic therapy places patients at an increased risk of surgical bleeding, as well as formation of an epidural or spinal hematoma, and the discontinuation or reversal of anticoagulation

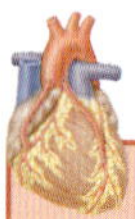

BOX 12.5   *Continuous Spinal Anesthetics*

- Benefits: dense blockade, titration of block height, sympatholysis; repeat administration for longer procedures
- Risks: postdural puncture headache or meningitis, undesirable hemodynamic effects of sympatholysis

therapy to proceed with neuraxial anesthesia places these patients at increased risk for perioperative thrombotic events. In particular, the discontinuation of dual-antiplatelet therapy (i.e., aspirin plus a $P2Y_{12}$ inhibitor) in a patient with a recently placed coronary artery stent can result in stent thrombosis during the perioperative period. Therefore before proceeding with a neuraxial or regional technique in these patients, careful consideration and management of their anticoagulation are imperative. The risk of perioperative thrombosis must be weighed against the risk of a general anesthetic and bleeding during the procedure.

ASRA publishes guidelines on the recommended interval between the discontinuation of anticoagulation and initiating a neuraxial procedure, which varies based on the anticoagulant. Aspirin as a sole agent is not a contraindication for a neuraxial procedure. Other antiplatelet agents carry a higher risk for epidural hematoma and must be held before placement of the block. Patients on warfarin should have a normal international normalized ratio (INR) before a neuraxial block. Heparin and low-molecular-weight heparin (LMWH) must be held until the anticoagulant effect has resolved, which depends on the dosing regimen. There has been a recent expansion in the number of new or novel oral anticoagulants available for patients with cardiac disease (see Table 12.5 for a partial list). It is recommended that ASRA guidelines be reviewed before invasive procedures if the provider is not familiar with the patient's anticoagulation regimen.

Reversal of Anticoagulation

There are circumstances in which patients with cardiac disease on anticoagulation may suffer life-threatening consequences if anticoagulation is held or reversed for surgical procedures (e.g., ventricular assist device thrombosis). However, there are other cases (e.g., emergency surgery, catastrophic bleeding) in which reversal of anticoagulants may be necessary. Furthermore, for some anticoagulated patients, the risks posed by a general anesthetic may be too great. Before the rapid development of novel oral anticoagulants in recent years, the routes of anticoagulation and their reversal were relatively few. Unfractionated heparin, used routinely in the OR, is reversed with protamine. Protamine also may be of use in antagonizing LMWH products (e.g., enoxaparin), although the efficacy may be limited. Warfarin was classically reversed by the administration of vitamin K, which is both slow to antagonize warfarin and makes reestablishment of anticoagulation more difficult. As an alternative to vitamin K, fresh-frozen plasma (FFP) has a faster onset of reversal but may require large fluid volumes. Additionally, it is difficult or impossible to achieve full INR normalization with FFP alone. Development of prothrombin complex concentrates (PCCs), available as three-factor PCC (II, IX, X; Profilnine SD) and four-factor PCC (II, VII, IX, X; 4F-PCC [Kcentra, Octaplex] with nonactivated factor VII or 4F-aPCC [FEIBA] with activated factor VII) forms allow rapid INR normalization with much lower volume administration and is quickly becoming the preferred method of urgent warfarin reversal.

Other novel oral anticoagulants (i.e., factor Xa inhibitors and direct thrombin inhibitors) previously had few options for urgent reversal. The direct thrombin inhibitor dabigatran now has a unique monoclonal antibody reversal agent, idarucizumab, which is effective in restoring normal coagulation parameters. Dabigatran is also removed with hemodialysis and can be reversed with PCC (activated form preferred, FEIBA). Factor Xa inhibitors may be reversed with PCC as well (nonactivated form preferred, Kcentra), but they are not amenable to hemodialysis because of protein binding. A unique reversal agent (andexanet alfa [Andexxa]) for factor Xa inhibitors received Food and Drug Administration approval in 2018.

Table 12.5 Commonly Used Anticoagulants and Reversal Agents

Drug	Parameter or Minimum Time Between Last Dose and Neuraxial Block	Potential Reversal Agent(s)
Traditional Anticoagulants		
Heparin IV infusion	aPTT <40	Protamine sulfate: 1 mg per 100 U/heparin
Heparin BID prophylaxis	4–6 h	
Heparin TID prophylaxis	4–6 h	
Enoxaparin full treatment dose (1 mg/kg BID or 1.5 mg/kg/d)	24 h	Protamine sulfate: 1 mg/mg enoxaparin if dose <8 h 0.5 mg/mg enoxaparin if dose >8 h
Enoxaparin prophylactic dose (daily or BID)	12 h	
Warfarin	INR <1.5	4F-PCC: 25–50 U/kg depending on INR FFP rFVIIa Vitamin K (not usually recommended)
Direct Thrombin Inhibitors		
Dabigatran	5 days	Idarucizumab (Praxbind): 5 g (2.5 g × 2, 15 min apart) 4F-aPCC (activated form preferred, FEIBA): 25 U/kg IV Hemodialysis
Argatroban and bivalirudin	Avoid	
Factor Xa Inhibitors		
Apixaban	3 d	Andexanet alfa (Andexxa): 400 mg bolus plus infusion of 4 mg/min 4F-PCC (nonactivated form preferred) 25–50 U/kg IV
Rivaroxaban	3 d	
Antiplatelet Agents		
Aspirin	No contraindication	Desmopressin Platelet transfusion
Clopidogrel	7 d	
Prasugrel	7–10 d	
Ticlopidine	14 d	
Ticagrelor	5–7 d	

aPTT, Activated partial thromboplastin time; *BID,* twice daily; *FFP,* fresh-frozen plasma; *4F-aPCC,* four-factor activated prothrombin complex concentrate; *4F-PCC,* four-factor prothrombin complex concentrate; *INR,* international normalized ratio; *IV,* intravenous; *rFVIIa,* recombinant factor VIIa; *TID,* three times daily.

Administration of PCC (especially activoated PCC) can create a prothrombotic state, which may be especially problematic for the cardiac patient (e.g., risk of myocardial infarction, stent thrombosis). PCC formulations also contain some heparin and are therefore contraindicated in patients with heparin-induced thrombocytopenia. The decision to reverse anticoagulation must include a risk-to-benefit analysis taking into account the patient's physiology, cardiac lesion, indication for anticoagulation, and risks of both bleeding and reversal (Box 12.6; see also Table 12.5).

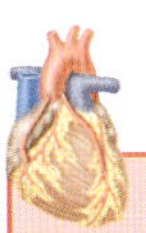

> **BOX 12.6** *Anticoagulation Reversal*
>
> - More options are now available for reversal of chronic anticoagulation, which may allow regional or neuraxial techniques to be safely performed on cardiac patients. However, the risk of thrombosis must be carefully considered before reversal.

Peripheral Nerve Block

A broad category encompassing all regional anesthesia performed distal to the CNS, PNBs have many potential benefits for cardiac patients. A PNB may be performed as the sole anesthetic for an extremity surgery or a component of MAC with sedation or may provide intraoperative and postoperative pain control for a general anesthetic.

Compared with neuraxial anesthesia, a PNB will not create a systemic sympathectomy (although it will inhibit sympathetic tone to the region affected by the block) and may be better tolerated by patients with lesions that require maintenance of SVR. The duration of block will typically be longer than a spinal anesthetic, and if a regional catheter is placed, it may provide postoperative pain control of the same potential duration as an epidural catheter. Although the ASRA recommends neuraxial guidelines be followed in regard to coagulation status requirements to perform a deep PNB, the risks of a block on an anticoagulated patient (e.g., bleeding, hematoma) are potentially less catastrophic in a PNB compared with a neuraxial block (e.g., epidural hematoma). On the other hand, neuraxial blocks are able to provide dense anesthesia to a larger area of the body with tolerable local anesthetic doses. Because of the dose of local anesthetic required to surgically anesthetize a large peripheral nerve, there is a limit to the number of blocks at a given time. It is generally not feasible to surgically block more than one extremity at a time, although more limited blocks for postoperative pain control may be successfully done. Also, extremity PNBs are often unable to completely eliminate tourniquet pain, especially as the duration of the procedure increases. This stimulation may cause increases in sympathetic tone and lead to unwanted tachycardia and increased SVR.

The type of block performed will, of course, depend on the proposed procedure. Operations involving the chest wall, such as a thoracotomy or video-assisted thoracoscopic surgery, may benefit from paravertebral nerve blocks, which effectively anesthetize the spinal nerve in one root distribution for each level blocked (with potential for spread to adjacent dermatomes). The paravertebral block is done lateral to the spinal column in a triangular space bounded by the superior costotransverse ligament, parietal pleura, and the vertebral body. Theoretically, the sympathectomy is limited to the single spinal nerve blocked, making this block useful for patients with stenotic lesions. However, it is necessary to exercise caution because there is potential for local anesthetic to spread to the epidural space and cause a systemic sympathectomy. There is also a risk of pneumothorax given the position of the nerve adjacent to the parietal pleura. Several levels may be blocked for surgeries in larger areas, and continuous infusion catheters may also be placed.

For lower extremity surgery below the knee (commonly needed for patients with vascular and cardiac disease), blockade of the femoral and sciatic nerve is relatively easy to accomplish and may spare a neuraxial or general anesthesia. Procedures above the knee require four separate nerve blocks and are more difficult to reliably accomplish.

Procedures on the upper extremities may be done under supraclavicular, infraclavicular, or axillary block. Finally, pain after minor lower abdominal procedures may be partially mitigated by unilateral or bilateral transverse abdominis plane (TAP) blocks. In general, any procedure that can improve postoperative pain, decrease opiate consumption, and limit pain-related tachycardia and hypertension is advisable as long as the risk-to-benefit ratio is favorable.

Epidural anesthesia and PNBs, compared with subarachnoid blocks, often require large doses of local anesthetic to achieve adequate effect. Consideration must be paid to the maximum allowable dose of the particular agent used, keeping in mind the aforementioned risks of local anesthetics in patients with cardiac disease. Local anesthetic with epinephrine is frequently used in PNBs because lidocaine is a vasodilator, and epinephrine will not only prolong the duration of action but also identify accidental IV injection. In patients with significant coronary artery disease, arrhythmias, or pulmonary hypertension, the epinephrine dose may need to be reduced or eliminated. As with all management issues in cardiac patients, a risk-to-benefit analysis is critical when making these decisions.

General Anesthesia

Indications for general anesthesia are the same for cardiac patients undergoing noncardiac surgery as healthy patients undergoing the surgery. Frequently the planned procedure and patient preference will dictate whether the patient requires a general anesthetic or not. General anesthesia has both advantages and disadvantages compared with MAC or regional anesthesia in cardiac patients. Volatile anesthetic used in the maintenance of general anesthesia produces a decrease in myocardial oxygen demand caused by decreases in contractility, afterload, and preload. It also provides some myocardial preconditioning, which may be protective against ischemic injury, although this has been most extensively evaluated in cardiac surgery. General anesthesia also may decrease psychological stress compared with MAC or regional anesthesia. These characteristics may provide for a better myocardial oxygen balance in patients with coronary artery disease. In addition, patient movement is reduced under general anesthesia, which provides a more stable surgical field, and the inherent risks of MAC and regional are potentially avoided (e.g., local anesthetic toxicity, epidural hematoma, pneumothorax). Finally, patient comfort during the procedure is often easier to maintain, and the risks posed by intraoperative conversion to a general anesthetic are eliminated (Box 12.7).

Although general anesthesia is commonly used for cardiac patients undergoing noncardiac surgery, several modifiable key risk factors can have an impact on the outcome and may not be present during MAC or regional anesthesia. These key points in the perioperative period are associated with increased cardiac work secondary to stress

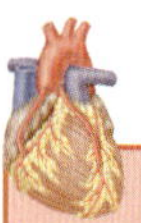

BOX 12.7	***Advantages of General Anesthesia in Cardiac Patients for Noncardiac Surgery***

- Decrease in myocardial oxygen demand (volatile gases)
- Ischemic preconditioning (volatile gases)
- Reduced psychological stress
- Limitation of patient movement

and include the induction of anesthesia, intubation, surgical stimulation, extubation, and postoperative care management. In cardiac patients, attenuation of the stress response requires the prompt treatment of tachycardia, bradycardia, hypertension, and hypotension to prevent exacerbation of any underlying cardiac disease.

Induction of anesthesia and intubation can be carried out using a variety of agents. Anesthesiologists commonly use a combination of medications (e.g., benzodiazepines, narcotics, propofol, etomidate, or ketamine) with the goal of inducing unconsciousness and obtaining a depth of anesthesia that will mitigate any increase in sympathetic tone (i.e., hypertension and tachycardia) associated with laryngoscopy and intubation. When hemodynamic parameters need to be maintained within very strict parameters, it is prudent to have vasopressors as well as vasodilators available. In some patients, especially those with poor right ventricular function or known severe pulmonary hypertension, small doses of IV epinephrine (e.g., 5–10 μg) may be required to support the right heart during induction and intubation.

The muscle relaxant used to facilitate intubation mainly depends on the patient's kidney and liver function as well as the surgical procedure. Although various muscle relaxants have been reported to exert varying degrees of effect on the heart rate and rhythm, for the most part, the clinical effect of currently available agents is minimal.

Anesthetic Agents

The choice of an inhalation agent or a total IV anesthetic will again depend on the surgery and the patient's comorbidities. Several agents used for induction and maintenance of general anesthesia are described above in the section on MAC.

Propofol, commonly used for the induction of general anesthesia, produces a reliable decrease in mean arterial pressure (MAP) with bolus administration because of a decrease in preload and SVR as well as a questionable decrease in contractility. Although it may be safely used for induction of certain cardiac patients, extreme care must be used in patients reliant on SVR (e.g., stenotic lesions) and MAP (e.g., coronary artery disease). Propofol may also be used as a continuous infusion, either as part of a balanced anesthetic or as a total intravenous anesthetic (TIVA). The higher infusion rates of propofol required for TIVA compared with MAC sedation frequently result in hypotension in patients with vascular disease or systolic dysfunction. These patients may require pressors or inotropes to maintain acceptable MAP and cardiac output. Benzodiazepines and narcotics, also commonly used during induction, have mild sympatholytic effects that may cause small decreases in MAP. They are routinely used safely in cardiac patients.

Volatile Anesthetics

Volatile anesthetics are frequently used for maintenance of general anesthesia. They are able to reliably provide amnesia and prevent patient movement in response to surgical stimulation, and they may produce bronchodilation at clinical concentrations. They have multiple effects on the cardiovascular system that are relevant to patients with cardiac disease. All volatile anesthetics cause some degree of decrease in myocardial contractility, with older agents (e.g., halothane) causing a larger impairment of contractility than the newer agents (e.g., sevoflurane, isoflurane, and desflurane). This is mediated through an alteration in intracellular Ca^{2+} homeostasis at several myocardial targets. The effect on contractility is more pronounced on failing myocardium. Volatile anesthetics also produce a dose-dependent prolongation of LV isovolumic relaxation, which is likely related to their effect on myocardial contractility rather than a direct effect on lusitropy.

Modern volatile anesthetics also produce a dose-dependent decrease in MAP, in large part because of their effect on SVR. This contrasts to halothane, which maintained SVR and instead caused a decrease in MAP because of a decrease in cardiac output. All volatile agents cause an increase in heart rate, although classically, sevoflurane increases heart rate only at high concentrations (>1.5 minimum alveolar concentration). Desflurane causes sympathetic stimulation with rapid increases in concentration, which transiently increases both the heart rate and MAP. This effect may be attenuated with β-blockers, opiates, or clonidine. Because of the modern volatile anesthetics' tendency to decrease SVR more than contractility, cardiac output is generally maintained with these agents in a healthy heart. However, with a failing heart, the predominant vascular effect may be venodilation rather than a beneficial decrease in LV afterload. This effect combined with a decrease in preload and contractility may cause a significant decrease in cardiac output in patients with cardiomyopathies who are administered volatile anesthetics.

Volatile anesthetics produce coronary artery vasodilation in vitro. However, in vivo, the effect is more complicated. Cardiac myocardial oxygen consumption (Mvo_2) is decreased because of reductions in heart rate, afterload, and contractility. Therefore autoregulation may cause coronary vasoconstriction in vivo. Earlier concerns that isoflurane-induced coronary vasodilation may cause "steal" in at-risk vasculature have not borne out in recent literature.

Volatile anesthetics may also be beneficial to patients with cardiac disease by inducing a phenomenon similar to ischemic preconditioning. This characteristic of myocardial cells reduces the extent of ischemic injury after a preceding brief ischemic episode. Volatile anesthetics have been shown to activate similar pathways via mitochondrial adenosine triphosphate–dependent potassium channels and the inhibition of mitochondrial permeability transition pores. Early (1–2 hours) and late (over 2–3 days) effects are seen. Controversy exists regarding the ideal technique (i.e., volatile anesthetic exposure) to maximize the effect and whether propofol possesses similar characteristics. Regardless, there is some evidence that obesity and hyperglycemia may mitigate the benefit of preconditioning.

Nitrous Oxide

Nitrous oxide has unique cardiovascular effects. In subanesthetic doses, it augments sympathetic tone and usually leads to a stable or an increased cardiac output, heart rate, and stroke volume. However, it may have direct myocardial depressant effects, which may be unmasked in the presence of sympatholytics.

Recent data on a large number of patients with known or presumed coronary artery disease demonstrated no increased cardiovascular risk from the use of nitrous oxide in major noncardiac surgery. Some caveats exist, however, including the suggestion that nitrous oxide may increase pulmonary vascular resistance in patients with pulmonary hypertension. Nitrous oxide can also contribute to the enlargement of intravascular air bubbles and the deleterious effects of air emboli. This is especially important for patients with intraatrial (e.g., patent foramen ovale or atrial septal defects) or intraventricular connections. Similarly, for procedures in which an iatrogenic puncture of the intraatrial septum is required (e.g., atrial fibrillation ablation therapy or the placement of a percutaneous LV assist device), nitrous oxide should be avoided.

Etomidate

A structurally unique induction agent, etomidate depresses the CNS via GABA receptors. It has minimal cardiovascular and respiratory effects with only some slight myocardial depression that may be expressed in patients with severe disease. Overall, it is perceived as the most hemodynamically stable induction agent. Downsides include postoperative nausea, myoclonic movements with induction, and the potential for adrenal suppression. It has no analgesic properties and has a short duration of action because of redistribution. Therefore it must be supplemented with other agents to maintain general anesthesia soon after its administration. Because of maintenance of SVR and MAP, it is useful in cardiac patients sensitive to drops in perfusion pressure and afterload.

Ketamine

As an agonist at the N-methyl-D-aspartate (NMDA) receptor, ketamine is distinct from other general anesthetics. Able to induce a dissociative anesthesia, it also has useful analgesic effects. It induces sympathetic stimulation, thereby often increasing heart rate, MAP, and catecholamine levels. However, its direct myocardial depressant effects may be unmasked in patients who are catecholamine depleted. It has potential utility in the induction of patients who will not tolerate decreases in MAP and SVR, but the associated tachycardia is undesirable in patients with coronary artery disease. The dissociated state also may cause psychological distress in some patients, which may be mitigated by coadministration with a benzodiazepine.

Maintenance of General Anesthesia

As with surgery on healthy patients, patients with cardiac disease benefit from a balanced approach to the maintenance of anesthesia. Even though all volatile inhalation agents cause dose-dependent decreases in contractile function, as well as arterial and some venous vasodilation, inhalation agents can be used as the sole anesthetic agent or part of a balanced technique in cardiac patients undergoing noncardiac surgery. However, as previously mentioned, some patients may require intermittent boluses or continuous IV infusions of a vasopressor or inotrope during the procedure to offset side effects of anesthetics and support cardiac output and blood pressure.

Advantages of volatile anesthesia include the ability to titrate anesthetic depth relatively quickly compared with prolonged infusions of propofol, benzodiazepines, or narcotics other than remifentanil, as well as the availability of end-tidal agent monitoring to gauge the depth of anesthesia and likelihood of amnesia. Volatile anesthetic effect and half-life are relatively unaffected by other organ dysfunction such as liver or kidney disease, which may be present in patients with cardiac disease. Disadvantages include an increased incidence of postoperative nausea and vomiting (which may lead to tachycardia and increased oxygen demand) and airway irritation that may result in coughing upon emergence.

Selection of specific agents depends on both surgical and patient factors. There may be certain instances in which specific patients may benefit from partial or total IV anesthesia. For instance, patients with severe obstructive pulmonary disease may benefit from TIVA because gas trapping and ventilation/perfusion mismatch may delay emergence from volatile anesthesia. However, these patients also may benefit from the bronchodilation properties of volatile anesthetics. Patients with severe obstructive lesions such as critical aortic stenosis may not tolerate the afterload reduction associated with propofol or volatile anesthetics and therefore may require a narcotic and/or benzodiazepine-heavy regimen for induction and maintenance. Conversely, patients with dynamic outflow tract obstruction (e.g., HOCM) may benefit from the myocardial depression of a volatile anesthetic that can lessen the obstruction, presuming preload and afterload are maintained.

When general anesthesia is planned, airway instrumentation is often required. There are several advantages to placement of an endotracheal tube in patients with cardiac disease. Hypoxia associated with hypoventilation during MAC sedation without an advanced airway can adversely affect myocardial oxygen supply. Hypercarbia may increase sympathetic output and cause tachycardia and hypertension and will cause an increase in pulmonary vascular resistance. Avoidance of these risks with endotracheal intubation and mechanical ventilation may be beneficial. Although positive-pressure ventilation may induce hypotension through a number of mechanisms, including a reduction in preload to the right heart; intrathoracic positive pressure also reduces LV wall tension and may be beneficial in left heart failure. Finally, having definitive airway control can remove one patient variable if an intraoperative crisis occurs whether it is surgical or patient related.

On the other hand, the process of endotracheal intubation is stimulating and can cause unwanted tachycardia and hypertension. The balance during induction between avoiding medication-related hypotension and providing enough anesthetic depth to avoid sympathetic stimulation in patients with cardiac disease is delicate and must be undertaken with care and planning. Also, the greater depth of anesthesia required to permit patients to tolerate an endotracheal tube may necessitate more pressor or inotrope support. Finally, the process of emergence and extubation carry similar risks to induction with regard to tachycardia, hypertension, and potential for hypoxia and hypercapnia. Patients with severe cardiac disease or other severe comorbidities may not qualify for extubation at the end of a procedure, leading to an ICU stay with all the inherent associated risks and benefits.

SPECIAL SITUATIONS

Eye Surgery

Patients requiring ophthalmic procedures such as cataract surgery are often older, and the incidence of cardiac disease in this population is high. Fortunately, many of these cases are amenable to topical or regional anesthesia and therefore may be done under MAC with light or moderate sedation. Because surgical stimulation is minimal after the local anesthetic has taken effect, often a low dose of benzodiazepine and fentanyl are adequate to ensure patient comfort, which are well tolerated by patients with even severe cardiac disease. Limitations may include patients with severe heart failure who are unable to lie flat because of orthopnea, those with a chronic cough who cannot remain still for 1 to 2 hours, and more complex procedures with longer surgical times.

Surgical eye blocks (e.g., retrobulbar and peribulbar blocks) may be performed in cardiac patients not on anticoagulation. There is a risk of central spread of local anesthetic during a retrobulbar block with resultant neuraxial anesthesia, which may cause a problematic sympathectomy for patients with obstructive cardiac lesions. The oculocardiac reflex, caused by increased vagal tone due to pressure on the eye or traction on the extraocular muscles, may cause symptomatic hemodynamic compromise from bradycardia. Although it may be prevented with atropine, this can induce an unwanted tachycardia. It also may be prevented by a retrobulbar block, although placement of the block itself may trigger the reflex because of the pressure of the local anesthetic injected or as a result of a retrobulbar hemorrhage. Deep general anesthesia may limit the oculocardiac reflex but, as previously stated, has obvious downsides in the cardiac patient.

Ambulatory Surgery

Patients with cardiac disease frequently present for procedures that are routinely done on an outpatient basis. These include same-day surgical procedures, as well

310

as gastrointestinal endoscopies and invasive cardiac examinations. Deciding which patients may be discharged after an anesthetic and by extension which patients may safely undergo procedures at an ambulatory surgery center rather than a hospital-based OR must be influenced by the type and severity of cardiac disease, as well as any comorbidities and the proposed surgical procedure. Recent data suggest that there are several risk factors for morbidity and mortality after ambulatory surgeries, including overweight or obese body mass index, previous percutaneous cardiac intervention or cardiac surgery, history of transient ischemic attack or cerebrovascular accident, prolonged operative time, hypertension, and chronic obstructive pulmonary disease. Although these risk factors are not necessarily contraindications to procedures in an ambulatory setting, they do suggest caution in patients with cardiac risk factors.

In general, patients with critical valvular disease, decompensated heart failure, or unstable angina should not undergo elective surgical procedures. Urgent or emergent procedures would typically occur on an inpatient basis with subsequent hospital observation. Patients with stable, well-managed cardiac disease, including coronary artery disease, heart failure, and valvular disease, may have low-risk procedures done as outpatients assuming there are no perioperative complications that require observation. These procedures typically include endoscopies, eye procedures, and simple extremity procedures. Patients with cardiac disease who are to undergo longer, moderate-risk procedures, such as intraabdominal operations or more significant orthopedic procedures, may benefit from planned overnight observation postoperatively.

In summary, the choice of anesthetic technique in the cardiac patient undergoing noncardiac surgery depends on (1) the type of surgery or procedure, (2) the severity of cardiac disease, and (3) the presence of other comorbidities. Careful attention to hemodynamic goals during the perioperative period, as well as excellent communication with the healthcare providers involved in the patient's care will ultimately determine the patient's perioperative experience.

SUGGESTED READING

Christos S, Naples R. Anticoagulation reversal and treatment strategies in major bleeding: update 2016. *West J Emerg Med*. 2016;17(3):264–270.

Devereaux PJ, Sessler DI. Cardiac complications in patients undergoing major noncardiac surgery. *N Engl J Med*. 2015;373:2258–2269.

Duceppe E, Parlow J, MacDonald P, et al. Canadian Cardiovascular Society guidelines on perioperative cardiac risk assessment and management for patients who undergo noncardiac surgery. *Can J Cardiol*. 2017;33:17–32.

Fleisher LA, Fleischmann KE, Auerbach AD, et al. 2014 ACC/AHA guideline on perioperative cardiovascular evaluation and management of patients undergoing noncardiac surgery: a report of the American College of Cardiology/American Heart Association Task Force on Practice Guidelines. *J Am Coll Cardiol*. 2014;64:e77–e137.

Frogel J, Galusca D. Anesthetic considerations for patients with advanced valvular heart disease undergoing noncardiac surgery. *Anesthesiol Clin*. 2010;28:67–85.

Hofer CK, Mizuguchi AK, Popescu WM. Monitoring the patient at risk of hemodynamic instability in remote locations. *Int Anesthesiol Clin*. 2012;50:141–172.

Horlocker TT, Wedel DJ, Rowlingson JC, Enneking FK. Executive summary: regional anesthesia in the patient receiving antithrombotic or thrombolytic therapy: American Society of Regional Anesthesia and Pain Medicine Evidence-Based Guidelines (Third Edition). *Reg Anesth Pain Med*. 2010;35:102–105.

Kunst G, Klein AA. Peri-operative anaesthetic myocardial preconditioning and protection—cellular mechanisms and clinical relevance in cardiac anaesthesia. *Anaesthesia*. 2015;70(4):467–482.

Long WB, Rosenblum S, Grady IP. Successful resuscitation of bupivacaine-induced cardiac arrest using cardiopulmonary bypass. *Anesth Analg*. 1989;69:403–406.

Mathis MR, Naughton NN, Shanks AM, et al. Patient selection for day case-eligible surgery: identifying those at high risk for major complications. *Anesthesiology*. 2013;119:1310–1321.

Mercado P, Weinberg GL. Local anesthetic systemic toxicity: prevention and treatment. *Anesthesiol Clin*. 2011;29:233–242.

Myles PS, Leslie K, Chan MTV, et al. The safety of addition of nitrous oxide to general anesthesia in at-risk patients having major non-cardiac surgery (ENIGMA-II): a randomized, single-blind trial. *Lancet.* 2014;384:1446–1454.

Nishimura RA, Otto CM, Bonow RO, et al. 2017 AHA/ACC focused update of the 2014 AHA/ACC guideline for the management of patients with valvular heart disease: a report of the American College of Cardiology/American Heart Association Task Force on Clinical Practice Guidelines. *J Am Coll Cardiol.* 2017;70:252–289.

Nishimura RA, Otto CM, Bonow RO, et al. 2014 AHA/ACC guideline for the management of patients with valvular heart disease: a report of the American College of Cardiology/American Heart Association Task Force on Practice Guidelines. *Circulation.* 2014;129:e521–e643.

Pislaru SV, Abel MD, Schaff HV, Pellikka PA. Aortic stenosis and noncardiac surgery: managing the risk. *Curr Probl Cardiol.* 2015;40:483–503.

Priebe HJ. Preoperative cardiac management of the patient for non-cardiac surgery: an individualized and evidence-based approach. *Br J Anaesth.* 2011;107:83–96.

Raval AN, Cigarroa JE, Chung MK, et al. Management of patients on non-vitamin K antagonist oral anticoagulants in the acute care and periprocedural setting: a scientific statement from the American Heart Association. *Circulation.* 2017;135:e604–e633.

Siegal D, Curnutte J, Connolly S, et al. Andexanet alfa for the reversal of factor Xa inhibitor activity. *N Engl J Med.* 2015;373:2413–2424.

Soltesz EG, van Pelt F, Byrne JG. Emergent cardiopulmonary bypass for bupivacaine cardiotoxicity. *J Cardiothorac Vasc Anesth.* 2003;17:357–358.

Yurttas T, Wanner PM, Filipovic M. Perioperative management of antithrombotic therapies. *Curr Opin Anaesthesiol.* 2017;30:466–473.

Chapter 13

Vascular Surgery: Endovascular and Open Surgery

Elizabeth A. Valentine, MD • E. Andrew Ochroch, MD, MSCE

Key Points

1. Patients who present for cerebrovascular, aortic, or peripheral arterial interventions are at elevated risk for concomitant coronary artery disease.
2. A thorough preoperative assessment for cardiovascular disease and medical optimization of any comorbid conditions are essential before elective vascular surgery. This preoperative process is typically not possible for emergency vascular procedures. For urgent but not truly emergent procedures, an expedited workup and targeted medical optimization may aid in perioperative management.
3. The most significant risk factor for future stroke in the setting of carotid stenosis is the presence of recent symptomatic neurologic symptoms. Symptomatic high-grade carotid stenosis should undergo repair. The benefit of intervention for patients with symptomatic but moderate stenosis or in asymptomatic patients with high-grade stenosis is statistically significant, although less robust.
4. Because of the high mortality and morbidity associated with emergent repair, abdominal aortic aneurysms should be repaired if increasingly symptomatic or if rapidly expanding or the aneurysm diameter exceeds 5 cm.
5. With aggressive medical management and lifestyle modifications, the natural history of claudication related to peripheral arterial disease is generally indolent and relatively benign. A small subset will progress to critical disease. In general, critical limb ischemia mandates surgical intervention. Timing for intervention in intermittent claudication should take into account the severity and tolerability of the symptoms as well as patient-specific risk factors.
6. Endovascular interventions have become a mainstay of treatment for vascular disease. In general, short-term morbidity and mortality are improved with endovascular repair, although the early preoperative benefit is not always maintained in long-term follow-up.
7. Endovascular interventions have their own unique complication profile and often warrant repeat intervention and life-time surveillance.

Cardiovascular disease (CVD) is the leading cause of death both in the United States and worldwide. The lifetime risk of developing CVD in the Framingham Heart Study has been estimated to be greater than 50% in men and nearly 40% in women. Although the total number of deaths attributable to CV events has declined over the past decade, CVD still accounts for nearly one in every three deaths in the United States.

Among the various disease processes that can lead to CVD, atherosclerosis is the most common. The process of atherosclerotic plaque formation is both complex and dynamic, involving lipid deposition, smooth muscle proliferation, and an inflammatory milieu (Fig. 13.1). These lesions progress into fibrous plaques prone to rupture, erosion,

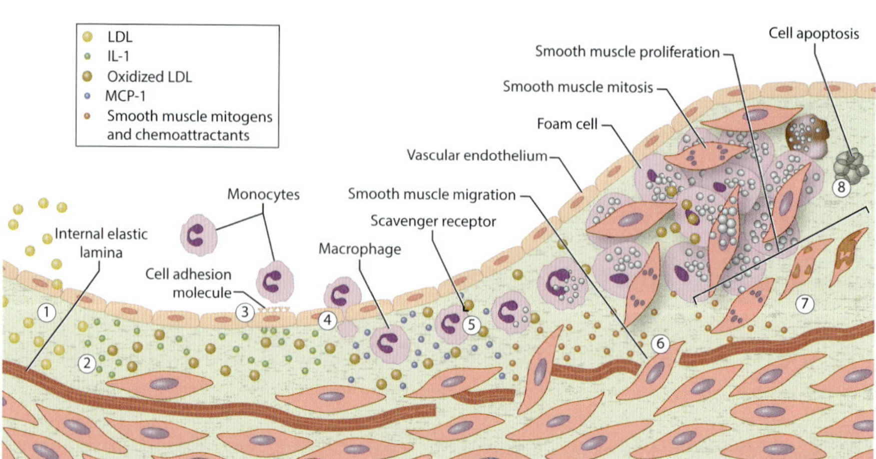

Fig. 13.1 Evolution of atherosclerotic plaque formation. *1,* Accumulation of lipoprotein in the intimal layer; *2,* oxidative stress; *3,* cytokine induction with expression of adhesion molecules; *4,* infiltration of inflammatory cells; *5,* development of foam cells and propagation of inflammatory mediators; *6,* smooth muscle migration; *7,* smooth muscle proliferation; and *8,* calcification. apoptosis, and fibrosis. *IL-1,* Interleukin-1; *LDL,* low-density lipoprotein; *MCP-1,* monocyte chemoattractant protein 1. (Modified from Libby P. The vascular biology of atherosclerosis. In: Mann DL, Zipes DP, Libby P, et al, eds. *Braunwald's Heart Disease: A Textbook of Cardiovascular Medicine.* 10th ed. Philadelphia: Elsevier; 2015:873–890.)

and hemorrhage. The end result is a narrowed intravascular lumen that creates the potential for downstream ischemia caused by mismatch between oxygen supply and demand. Some risk factors for CVD, such as age, gender, ethnicity, and family history, are not modifiable. Others are controllable by lifestyle and pharmacologic measures. A large, international study identified nine potentially modifiable risk factors that contributed to greater than 90% of the patient-attributable risk of a cardiovascular event: hypertension, dyslipidemia, diabetes, smoking, abdominal obesity, regular physical activity, daily consumption of fruits and vegetables, regular alcohol consumption, and psychosocial factors.

Cardiovascular disease can be grouped into four major categories: coronary artery disease (CAD), cerebrovascular disease, aortic disease, and peripheral arterial disease (PAD). Depending on the location of the lesion, this can result in ischemia or infarction of the heart, brain, abdominal viscera, or limbs. Patients with atherosclerotic disease in one area are at increased risk of vascular disease in other major vascular beds (Table 13.1). Noncoronary atherosclerotic disease is considered a CAD equivalent and confers a risk of a major adverse cardiac event equivalent to CAD. The 10-year risk of developing CAD in patients with noncoronary atherosclerotic disease is greater than 20%. Thus it is common to see significant CAD in patients undergoing major noncardiac vascular surgery and vice versa.

GENERAL CONSIDERATIONS FOR PERIOPERATIVE MANAGEMENT FOR VASCULAR SURGERY

Preoperative Assessment and Management

The goal of the preoperative assessment of the patient is to delineate the extent of underlying cardiac and noncardiac disease and medically optimize any underlying

Table 13.1 Concomitant Rates of Atherosclerotic Disease in Major Vascular Beds

	Cerebrovascular Disease	Abdominal Aortic Disease	Peripheral Artery Disease
Coronary artery disease	8–40%	30–40%	4–40%
Cerebrovascular disease	—	9–13%	17–50%
	—	—	7–12%

Significant overlap exists in risk factors for coronary, cerebrovascular, aortic, and peripheral arterial disease. As many as 50% of patients with atherosclerotic disease in one vascular bed will have concomitant disease present in at least one other vascular distribution.

Data from Beck AW, Goodney PP, Nolan BW, et al. Predicting 1-year mortality after elective abdominal aortic aneurysm repair. *J Vasc Surg.* 2009;49:838–843; Nathan DP, Brinster CJ, Woo EY, et al. Predictors of early and late mortality following open extent IV thoracoabdominal aortic aneurysm repair in a large contemporary single-center experience. *J Vasc Surg.* 2011;53:299–306; and Fransen GA, Desgranges P, Laheij RJ, et al. Frequency, predictive factors, and consequences of stent-graft kink following endovascular AAA repair. *J Endovasc Ther.* 2003;10:913–918.

conditions. Because of the significant association of CAD, cerebrovascular disease, aortic degenerative disease, and PAD, a major focus of the preoperative assessment is to detect, evaluate, and optimize preexisting vascular comorbidities. Perioperative management must be tailored to the individual patient to protect any at-risk organ system. The association of smoking with CVD means that many patients have pulmonary comorbidities that may also increase their risk with surgery and anesthesia.

It is incumbent upon the anesthesiologist to work with the patient's surgical and medical teams to ensure medical optimization before surgery, including appropriate management of preoperative medications. As such, it is critical that the anesthesiologist recognize the potential benefits and risks of maintaining, stopping, or initiating medications in the perioperative period. As a general rule, most antihypertensive medications should be continued in the perioperative period. The preponderance of evidence suggests that patients on chronic β-blockers should be continued on the medication in the perioperative period, although β-blockers should not be instituted as new therapy on the day of surgery because of an increased risk of stroke and death. Current guidelines recommend that statin therapy should be continued in the perioperative setting, and perioperative statin therapy has been associated with the reduction of perioperative cardiac morbidity and mortality in vascular surgical patients. Management of antiplatelet agents must balance the risk of stopping medications versus the risk of bleeding in the perioperative period, particularly in the setting of recent percutaneous intervention with coronary stents. Although most recent clinical guidelines suggest that earlier discontinuation of dual-antiplatelet therapy may be considered in some cases, decisions about the duration of dual-antiplatelet therapy are best made on an individual basis based on an assessment of risk versus benefit and with input from a multidisciplinary team (surgery, anesthesiology, and cardiology).

Because of the risk of anemia, as well as a significant risk for blood loss, a complete blood count to assess starting hemoglobin and hematocrit should be obtained before vascular surgery. An active type and screen should be available, with blood products cross-matched as appropriate. A metabolic panel to assess baseline renal function is reasonable because of the likelihood of underlying renal insufficiency as well as risk

315

for postoperative renal dysfunction. Coagulation studies should be considered for any patient who has been on anticoagulation and are mandatory if considering neuraxial manipulation either for anesthesia (e.g., spinal or epidural) or therapeutic intervention (e.g., spinal drain). A preoperative electrocardiogram (ECG) is often useful to serve as a baseline for evaluation of a perioperative insult. A preoperative echocardiogram is reasonable to assess baseline function for any patient with cardiovascular risk factors undergoing vascular surgery, particularly if there are new or worsening symptoms.

The American College of Cardiology (ACC) and American Heart Association (AHA) have released well-known guidelines regarding the perioperative cardiovascular evaluation and management of patients undergoing noncardiac surgery. The most recent recommendations from these guidelines simplify previous risk stratification before elective surgery (Fig. 13.2; also see Chapter 1). The first step is to evaluate whether a clinical emergency exists; if so, the patient should proceed to surgery without delay with best medical optimization. The second step evaluates whether the patient has an acute coronary syndrome, which should be evaluated and optimized according to guideline-directed medical therapy before nonemergent surgery. Subsequent steps use a combination of surgical risk calculators, patient functional capacity, and clinical decision making to determine if further cardiac evaluation is warranted before surgery. In general, patients undergoing vascular surgery represent at least an intermediate (>1%) risk for an adverse perioperative cardiac event and may benefit from additional testing if it will change perioperative management (see Chapter 1 for further details).

Several observational studies previously suggested that preoperative cardiac revascularization improves patient outcomes before high-risk noncardiac surgery. The Coronary Artery Revascularization Prophylaxis (CARP) study was the first and only randomized controlled trial to evaluate outcomes following prophylactic cardiac revascularization before major vascular surgery. This study found no difference in outcomes in patients undergoing major vascular surgery who underwent routine revascularization by either coronary artery bypass grafting or percutaneous coronary intervention versus medical management. A subsequent analysis found that patients with unprotected left main disease may be the only subset of patients who benefits from prophylactic revascularization. In large part because of the CARP trial, cardiac revascularization is not typically recommended before surgery unless otherwise indicated according to current practice guidelines.

In general, most patients undergoing elective vascular surgery warrant cardiac evaluation because of their multiple comorbidities, high likelihood of concomitant CAD, and often difficult-to-quantity functional capacity related to vague symptomology (e.g., shortness of breath may be an anginal equivalent, related to concomitant pulmonary disease, or simple deconditioning) or other limiting factors (e.g., claudication before reaching 4 METs; previous amputations limiting exertion). Many vascular procedures are performed on an emergent basis, with little time for extensive workup. For urgent, but not emergent, procedures (e.g., peripheral intervention for critical limb ischemia), there may be time for limited workup and optimization. For true emergencies (e.g., ruptured aortic aneurysm), the case should proceed with best mitigation of perioperative risk (Box 13.1).

Intraoperative Anesthetic Management

The primary anesthetic used during vascular surgery will depend on factors such as patient comorbidities, surgeon skill and comfort level, anatomic considerations, and the invasiveness of the surgical procedure. As such, anesthetic techniques for specific procedures are discussed in subsequent sections. Upon arrival to the

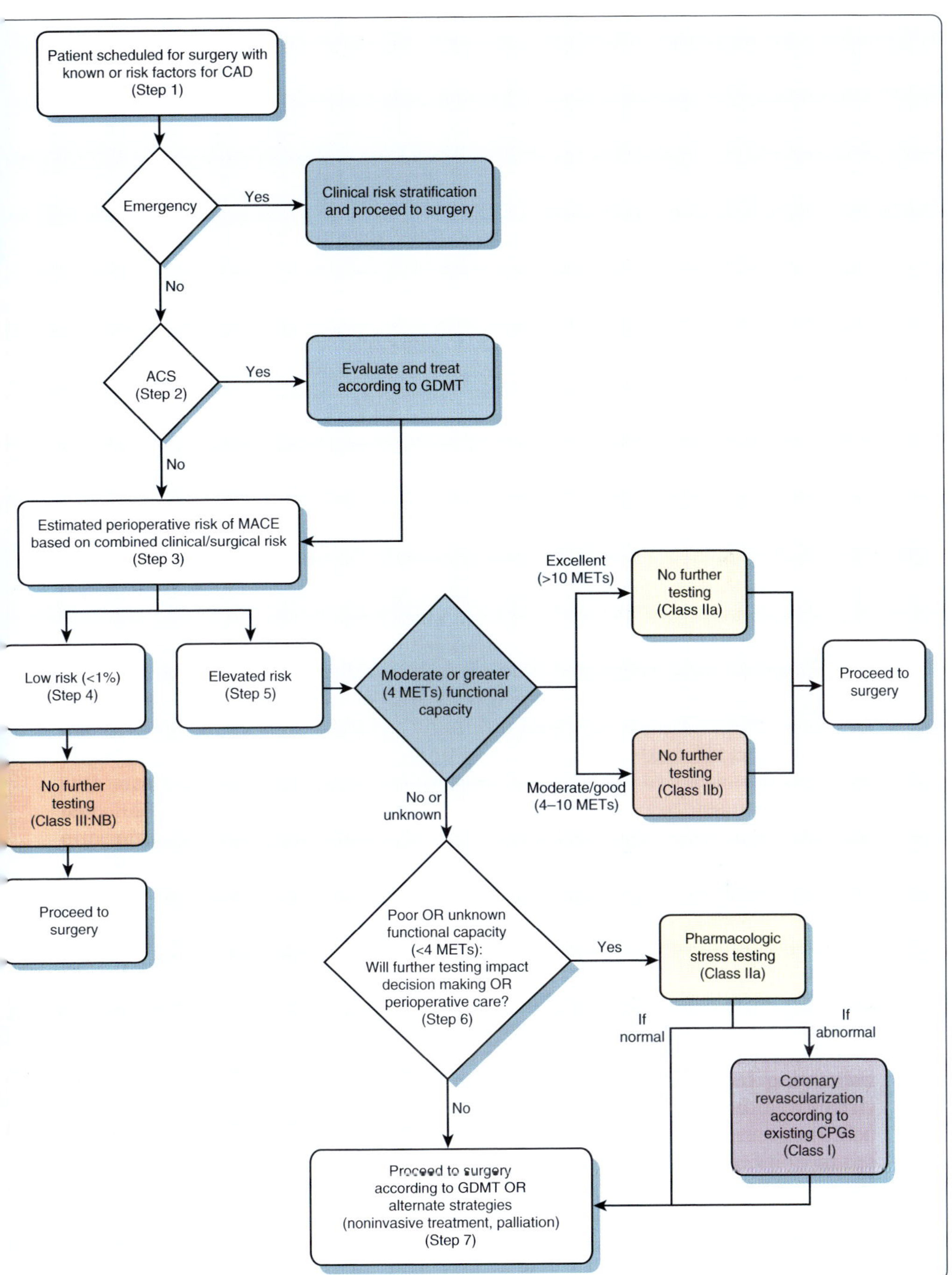

Fig. 13.2 The 2014 American College of Cardiology/American Heart Association guideline algorithm depicting the stepwise approach to perioperative cardiac assessment for coronary artery disease. *ACS,* Acute coronary syndrome; *CABG,* coronary artery bypass graft; *CAD,* coronary artery disease; *CPG,* clinical practice guideline; *DASI,* Duke Activity Status Index; *GDMT,* guideline-directed medical therapy; *HF,* heart failure; *MACE,* major adverse cardiac event; *MET,* metabolic equivalent; *NB,* no benefit; *NSQIP,* National Surgical Quality Improvement Program; *PCI,* percutaneous coronary intervention; *RCRI,* Revised Cardiac Risk Index; *STEMI,* ST-segment elevation myocardial infarction; *UA/NSTEMI,* unstable angina/non–ST elevation myocardial infarction; *VHD,* valvular heart disease. (From Fleisher LA, Fleischmann KE, Auerbach AD, et al. 2014 ACC/AHA guideline on perioperative cardiovascular evaluation and management of patients undergoing noncardiac surgery: a report of the American College of Cardiology/American Heart Association Task Force on Practice Guidelines. *J Am Coll Cardiol.* 2014;64[22]:014, e77–e137.)

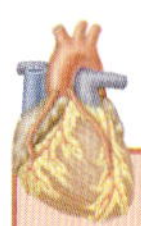

BOX 13.1   *Strategies for Perioperative Management of Emergent Vascular Surgery Procedures*

- Rapidly evaluate patient for signs and symptoms of acute coronary syndrome or equivalent (e.g., crackles or peripheral edema suggestive of decompensated heart failure; harsh systolic murmur suggestive of undiagnosed or worsened stenotic valvular disease) and treat accordingly.
- Maintain patient on preoperative antiplatelet therapy if not contraindicated, particularly if a recent coronary stent is present.
- Avoid tachycardia (will increase myocardial oxygen demand while decreasing supply). Continue preoperative β-blocker, if applicable, if hemodynamically stable.
- Avoid extremes of both hypertension (increases left ventricular wall stress) and hypotension (may compromise perfusion to vital organs).
- Avoid anemia, particularly if there is evidence of end-organ compromise.
- Assure adequate pain control to minimize sympathetic stimulation.
- Maintain normothermia.

operating room (OR), all patients should be placed on standard American Society of Anesthesiologists (ASA) monitors, including regular noninvasive blood pressure measurement, pulse oximetry, and continuous ECG. It is prudent to place an arterial catheter for invasive blood pressure monitoring for all but the most minor of vascular procedures because of the inherent risk for rapid hemodynamic changes and major blood loss. Patient comorbidities, cross-clamping on major vascular structures, and potential for hemorrhage all contribute to the hemodynamic instability frequently observed during these procedures. Invasive arterial monitoring also allows for frequent blood sampling to assess ventilation and oxygenation, ongoing blood loss and resuscitation needs, and overall metabolic milieu. Because induction of general anesthesia and endotracheal intubation are among the more hemodynamically labile periods, placing the arterial monitoring before induction of general anesthesia is wise.

Invasive monitoring with central venous or pulmonary arterial cannulation is not routine for most vascular procedures. Common exceptions include open aortic procedures or when patient comorbidities dictate utility. Large-bore intravenous (IV) access, either peripheral or central, is mandatory for any major vascular procedure because of the inherent risk of blood loss and need for resuscitation. An active type and screen and adequate blood product availability should be confirmed before undertaking any major vascular procedure.

Although transesophageal echocardiography (TEE) is the most sensitive method for detecting intraoperative myocardial ischemia, it has not supplanted clinical assessment and routine ECG for determination of patients at risk for myocardial ischemia during noncardiac surgery. The ASA, in conjunction with the Society of Cardiovascular Anesthesiologists, has released practice guidelines for the intraoperative use of TEE. In general, expert opinion has recommended that TEE should be considered in noncardiac surgery in the following circumstances: when the patient has CV pathology that may result in significant clinical compromise, when life-threatening hypotension is anticipated, and when persistent unexplained hypotension or hypoxia occurs. Furthermore, these practice guidelines recommended TEE should be strongly considered for major open abdominal aortic procedures, and TEE does not have a routine role during endovascular aortic and distal procedures.

Postoperative Management

In general, patients can undergo tracheal extubation uneventfully in the OR and recover in the postanesthesia care unit after most vascular surgical procedures. Patients undergoing major abdominal aortic procedures may benefit from close surveillance and management in an intensive care unit setting where mechanical ventilation is frequently continued after initial admission to the unit. In this case, sedation and analgesia should be provided with short-acting agents to facilitate rapid emergence and serial neurologic assessments. Common complications after major vascular surgery include myocardial ischemia, hemodynamic lability, stroke, coagulopathy, renal failure, respiratory failure, coagulopathy, hemorrhage, hypothermia, delirium, and metabolic disturbances.

CAROTID ARTERY AND CEREBROVASCULAR DISEASE

An imbalance between blood supply and demand to the brain can result in permanent cerebral infarction (stroke) or transient ischemic attack (TIA), conventionally defined as focalized neurologic deficit lasting less than 24 hours with no evidence of permanent infarction. Although TIAs resolve, they are clinically important because they strongly predict for clinical stroke in the near future. Strokes can be defined as ischemic, caused by disruption of blood flow through a vessel, or hemorrhagic, caused by bleeding into the brain parenchyma or surrounding spaces. Approximately 87% of strokes in the United States are ischemic in origin, and at least 20% of ischemic strokes are related to extracranial atherosclerotic disease, such as carotid stenosis. The prevalence of carotid artery disease rises with age, male gender, and racial minorities.

Considerations for Intervention

The determination of when and how to intervene for carotid atherosclerotic disease is complex (Box 13.2). The stroke risk related to the disease itself must be balanced with the inherent stroke risk due to intervention. Furthermore, surgical decision making must also take into consideration patient-specific risk factors and risk factors for open (carotid endarterectomy [CEA]) versus endovascular carotid artery angioplasty and stenting (CAS) management. Revascularization is achieved in CEA by opening the lumen of the cervical segment of the extracranial carotid artery and removing the atherosclerotic plaque (typically at the carotid bifurcation). CAS is a minimally invasive alternative, during which a stent is deployed across the atherosclerotic plaque to restore the patency of the vessel lumen.

Symptomatic carotid disease is defined as the onset of sudden and focal neurologic symptoms, either temporary or permanent, that are ipsilateral to the carotid pathology. The most important indicator of future stroke risk is the presence of symptoms within the previous 6 months. Several landmark trials have evaluated the benefit of CEA versus medical management for patients with symptomatic carotid disease. Pooled analyses of these trials found a consistent benefit was demonstrated for patients with greater than 70% stenosis, with a number needed to treat (NNT) of 6.3 to prevent one stroke over 5 years. A benefit was also demonstrated in patients with moderate (50%–69%) stenosis, although this benefit was less robust with an NNT of 22. CEA was not beneficial below 50% carotid stenosis and was found to be harmful for patients with less than 30% stenosis. There was no significant benefit of CEA with near-total occlusion of the internal carotid artery.

The role of CEA in asymptomatic carotid artery disease has also been extensively studied. A meta-analysis of the literature found a small absolute risk reduction of

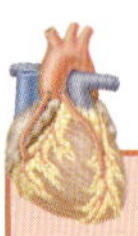

> ### BOX 13.2 · *Considerations for Carotid Revascularization for Stroke Prevention*
>
> - All patients should be aggressively treated with antiplatelet therapy, statins, and β-blockade, and should receive management of comorbid conditions per current clinical practice guidelines.
> - Revascularization should occur within 2 weeks of stroke or TIA for further stroke prevention.
> - Revascularization is recommended for patients with symptomatic stenosis greater than 50%. The more significant the stenosis, the stronger the indication for surgical intervention.
> - CEA is preferred over CAS unless there are contraindications to CEA (e.g., decompensated heart disease, previous neck surgery or radiation, contralateral vocal cord paralysis from previous surgery or an atypical and/or surgically inaccessible lesion).
> - In asymptomatic stenosis greater than 60%, CEA may be considered in acceptable risk candidates (i.e., predicted combined stroke and death rates <3%) in addition to best medical therapy.
> - Symptomatic patients with stenosis of <50% and asymptomatic patients with stenosis of <60% should be treated with best medical therapy and should not undergo intervention.
> - Intervention is not indicated for patients with chronic total occlusion or patients with severe neurologic disability that precludes preservation of useful function.
>
> *CAS,* Carotid artery angioplasty and stenting; *CEA,* carotid endarterectomy; *TIA,* transient ischemic attack.

about 1% per year for the outcome of any stroke for patients with asymptomatic carotid disease who underwent CEA. The NNT to prevent one stroke at 3 years was approximately 33. The net benefit to CEA in asymptomatic patients is delayed because of perioperative morbidity; the early perioperative morbidity outweighs the modest reduction in stroke risk until 2 years or more after surgery. Thus asymptomatic patients must be carefully selected to have at least a 5-year expected survival to benefit from surgical intervention.

Carotid artery angioplasty and stenting is an alternative to open surgical intervention for patients with carotid atherosclerotic disease, particularly for patients considered to be poor candidates for surgery or anesthesia. Endovascular treatment of carotid disease has been extensively studied and compared to traditional CEA. The preponderance of evidence suggests similar long-term results in preventing disabling or fatal strokes between CEA and CAS; however, significant differences in short-term morbidity and mortality have been found between the two procedures, with a higher periprocedural stroke rate in patients undergoing CAS but a higher myocardial infarction (MI) rate in patients undergoing CEA. Examples of patients who are generally considered favorable candidates for CAS include those at a prohibitively elevated medical risk (e.g., contralateral occlusion, severe medical comorbidities) or surgical risk (e.g., previous radiation to the neck, history of previous neck dissection, intracranial or high extracranial location) to undergo open repair. Alternatively, severe aortic arch atheroma or significant carotid tortuosity typically increase the complication rate for CAS and are indications for CEA. The complication rate of the surgeon must also be taken into account when weighing the risk and benefits of carotid intervention for the individual patient.

320

Intraoperative Anesthetic Considerations and Management

Carotid revascularization can be performed under general anesthesia or under local anesthesia. The primary advantage of local anesthesia is the ability to continuously monitor neurologic function in an awake patient, which may more reliably detect cerebral ischemia than the neuromonitoring methods used under general anesthesia. Because the need for intraoperative intervention in an awake patient may be detected more promptly and reliably, it can minimize the risks of intervention such as embolic risk of shunt placement. Local anesthetic techniques may also avoid hemodynamic extremes and cardiorespiratory morbidity associated with general anesthesia. General anesthesia, on the other hand, has the benefits of increased patient comfort, decreased patient anxiety, and airway control. It also avoids the need for emergent intraoperative conversion because of complications such as seizure and airway compromise.

Patient outcomes after general versus local anesthesia have been the subject of extensive study. The largest and most well-known study is the General Anaesthesia versus Local Anaesthesia for carotid surgery (GALA) trial, which randomized more than 3500 patients undergoing CEA at 95 medical centers in 24 countries to either general anesthesia or local anesthesia. In this investigation, there were no differences in major adverse events between the two groups with respect to death, stroke, MI, length of stay (LOS), and quality of life. Patients undergoing general anesthesia were more at risk for hemodynamic instability and perioperative cognitive dysfunction; subsequent analysis, however, demonstrated that intraoperative shunting was the main risk factor variable associated with perioperative cognitive dysfunction. A recent large meta-analysis demonstrated that anesthetic technique had no effect on death, stroke, MI, postoperative cardiopulmonary complications, hospital LOS, or patient satisfaction after CEA. The available literature does not support the use of one anesthetic technique over another for carotid surgery, and survey of practice patterns suggests variability in perioperative practice for carotid surgery. The decision for general versus local anesthesia should consider both patient and surgeon preferences, as well as unique patient characteristics, that might favor one technique over another. Regardless of technique, the goals of the anesthetic are the same: maintain hemodynamic norms and ensure smooth, rapid recovery from anesthesia to allow for early neurologic assessment.

Local Anesthesia Technique for Carotid Endarterectomy

Local anesthesia is performed with a nerve block, usually in conjunction with IV sedation to minimize patient discomfort and anxiety. It is important to limit sedation so as to maintain the ability to monitor the neurologic status. Local anesthetic options include cervical epidural or superficial cervical plexus block with or without deep cervical plexus block. Superficial cervical plexus block has been found to be as effective as a deep or combined block, while avoiding the complications of a deep cervical plexus block such as subarachnoid injection, phrenic nerve blockade, Horner syndrome, and increased risk of conversion to general anesthesia.

The ability to rapidly convert to a general anesthetic must be ensured before undertaking CEA under local anesthesia. Indications for conversion to general anesthesia include patient intolerance or request, accidental subarachnoid injection with brainstem anesthesia, seizure (related to intravascular injection of local anesthetic), airway compromise (from surgery or oversedation), or other hemodynamic or surgical complication. Patient selection is key for the success of local anesthesia. The patient cannot be claustrophobic (drapes are immediately adjacent to and across the patient's face) and must be able to lie flat and still for the duration (arthritis, chronic obstructive pulmonary disease [COPD], heart failure [HF], and other comorbidities may make this difficult for patients). Consideration must be given to the fact that intraoperative conversion may require airway management after sterile draping and surgical incision. As such, it may be prudent to consider having advanced airway equipment readily available, such as video laryngoscopy, to minimize disruption or difficulty during an emergent intubation. Despite these concerns, the rate of conversion to general anesthesia has been reported to be relatively low, occurring in only 4% of patients in the GALA trial.

General Anesthetic Technique for Carotid Endarterectomy

A major goal during the induction and maintenance of a general anesthetic is to avoid hemodynamic extremes such as the lows (during induction with agents with vasodilatory effects) and the highs (during periods of intense sympathetic stimulation, such as intubation and surgical incision). To this end, a variety of anesthetic agents can and have been used. Typically a balanced anesthetic technique is used. Induction of general anesthesia should involve the slow titration of a short-acting hypnotic agent, titrated to effect. The addition of a short-acting opioid may blunt the hemodynamic response to endotracheal intubation. In general, endotracheal intubation is preferred because of limited access to the airway during the procedure and the greater ability to manipulate ventilation. Normocapnia should be maintained during the procedure to avoid both a decrease in cerebral blood flow associated with hyperventilation and vasoconstriction, as well as potential intracerebral "steal" during permissive hypercapnia. Invasive arterial blood pressure monitoring should be considered because of the potential for sudden hemodynamic changes as a result of anesthesia or surgical manipulation. General anesthesia can be maintained effectively with either volatile or IV agents. Anesthetics must be titrated to minimize interference with any intraoperative monitoring techniques such as electroencephalography (EEG).

Additional Intraoperative Monitoring

Stroke during carotid intervention may result from inadequate cerebral perfusion because of hypotension, thrombosis, embolism, or carotid clamping in the setting of insufficient collateral flow from the circle of Willis. Cerebral ischemia can be mitigated if the insult is detected in timely fashion and appropriate interventions are made. An intact neurologic examination in an awake patient remains the gold standard for neurologic monitoring and provides a rationale for carotid intervention under local anesthesia. In this setting, a baseline neurologic assessment is performed before administration of sedative medication. Thereafter the sedation is titrated to achieve both patient comfort and cooperation with serial neurologic evaluations during the procedure, especially during carotid manipulation and clamping. A change in neurologic function may require interventions to restore cerebral perfusion such as shunt placement or permissive systemic hypertension to augment collateral flow via the circle of Willis.

When a general anesthetic technique is chosen, a variety of neuromonitoring techniques are available to monitor for cerebral ischemia during carotid intervention such as EEG, carotid stump pressure, somatosensory evoked potentials, transcranial Doppler, and cerebral oximetry. Intraoperative EEG is a commonly used neuromonitoring modality. Unprocessed EEG is preferred over processed EEG (e.g., bispectral index) because bispectral index monitoring has not been reliably shown to predict cerebral ischemia in this patient population. Significant alterations during carotid intervention in the EEG tracings such as complete signal loss, a 50% decrease in background activity, or an increase in delta wave activity may indicate intraoperative ischemia and the need for intervention. The clinical studies supporting the utility of routine EEG monitoring during carotid intervention are limited and not conclusive. Because both IV and volatile anesthetic agents may affect the EEG tracings, close communication between the anesthesia and neuromonitoring teams remains essential to minimize this anesthetic interference and to maximize both the sensitivity and specificity of EEG to detect cerebral ischemia during the carotid procedure.

Although EEG is the most commonly used monitor, other options are available to detect cerebral ischemia. Although an intraoperative carotid stump pressure less than 50 mm Hg may predict for stroke after carotid intervention, it has limited utility as the sole method for detecting intraoperative cerebral ischemia and the need for interventions such as shunting. Transcranial Doppler (TCD) measures blood velocity in the middle cerebral artery for detection of significant intraoperative microemboli. This alert may prompt the surgical team to avoid further carotid manipulation that could lead to stroke. Although TCD can detect cerebral ischemia, it is not always accurate. Cerebral oximetry is another monitoring modality that uses near-infrared spectroscopy to detect cerebral oxygen saturation; however, data to support its use for carotid surgery are mixed.

Given the current neuromonitoring choices for detection of stroke during carotid intervention under general anesthesia, it is clear that no technique is perfect. The primary role for neuromonitoring during CEA under general anesthesia is to guide decision for selective shunting. In the setting of routine shunting for CEA, there is less of a role for these modalities, given that the shunt maintains cerebral perfusion despite the clamped segment of the carotid artery. Ultimately, the choice of neuro-monitoring technique—and whether to routinely use neuromonitoring at all—is left to the discretion and expertise of the operative team.

Anesthesia for Carotid Artery Stenting

Carotid artery stenting is a minimally invasive procedure that can usually be performed under local anesthesia or monitored anesthesia care (MAC). Sedation is carefully titrated to allow for continuous neurologic examination throughout the procedure. If a general anesthetic technique is used, short-acting agents are typically used to allow for a rapid emergence and neurologic evaluation. Because peripheral endovascular access is obtained rather than direct surgical manipulation of the head and neck, a laryngeal mask airway may be chosen rather than endotracheal intubation to attenuate the hemodynamic lability encountered on induction and emergence of general anesthesia. As with any endovascular technique, it may become necessary to convert to open repair. As such, monitoring and vascular access should be planned accordingly.

Perioperative Challenges

Both CEA and CAS may be associated with hemodynamic lability of both heart rate and blood pressure because of altered baseline carotid baroreceptor sensitivity as well as intraoperative manipulation of the carotid baroreceptors. Carotid baroreceptor manipulation, either directly or via endovascular manipulation, may result in a profound parasympathetic response with bradycardia and hypotension. Conversely, periods of significant stimulation (such as endotracheal intubation or surgical dissection) may lead to increased sympathetic outflow with resultant hypertension and tachycardia, which may not be well tolerated by patients with concomitant CAD. Hemodynamic lability may continue into the postoperative period because of continued altered baroreceptor function or uncontrolled pain.

Carotid cross-clamping may precipitate ipsilateral cerebral ischemia from decreased carotid blood flow and inadequate collateral flow via the circle of Willis. Blood pressure should be maintained in a normal to slightly higher-than-baseline range before cross-clamping to optimize cerebral blood flow. Carotid unclamping may be complicated by impaired autoregulation and disrupted baroreceptor function, resulting in increased cerebral blood flow.

Cerebral hyperperfusion syndrome is a rare but clinically important complication, which results from impaired cerebral autoregulation after relief of high-grade stenosis. The clinical presentation may progress from severe headache to seizure to, at worst presentation, intracerebral hemorrhage. Thus it is important to monitor the patient closely for complaint of headache in the postoperative period. Management is supportive with strict control of blood pressure to minimize the risk of intracerebral hemorrhage.

Postoperative hematoma after CEA is usually a result of diffuse oozing after heparin administration and concurrent antiplatelet therapy. Although a relatively uncommon occurrence, with a reported incidence of 0.5% to 3%, it can result in life-threatening airway compromise. Injury to the recurrent or superior laryngeal nerve may result in paralysis of the ipsilateral vocal cord.

Carotid artery angioplasty and stenting may present unique concerns such as stent kinking, stent thrombosis, carotid dissection, or atheroembolism. Technical issues with the stent may often be amenable to observation or additional stent placement, and acute thrombosis typically necessitates immediate conversion to open CEA. The incidence of clinically important embolization has significantly decreased with the use of embolic protection devices. In the event of significant distal embolization, management options include catheter-directed thrombolysis, aspiration thrombectomy, and aggressive anticoagulation.

Abdominal Aortic Disease

The aorta is the major arterial conduit from the heart to the systemic circulation and provides vascular inflow to all of the major abdominal and pelvic organs as it traverses the abdomen. The abdominal aorta is a retroperitoneal structure that begins at the diaphragmatic hiatus and ends at the level of the fourth lumbar vertebra, where it bifurcates into the common iliac arteries. The aorta tapers gradually from the thorax to the abdomen such that its normal diameter at the level of the renal arteries is approximately 2.0 cm. An aneurysm is typically defined as a greater than 50% dilation of the expected normal arterial diameter. Aortic aneurysm occurs most commonly in the abdominal aorta. Aneurysms of the thoracic and thoracoabdominal aorta occur far less commonly.

Abdominal aortic aneurysms (AAAs) are classified by location as infrarenal (originating below the level of the renal arteries), juxtarenal (originating at the level of the renal arteries), or suprarenal (originating above the renal arteries). This distinction is important because it dictates the complexity of the surgical repair as well as the potential for hemodynamic derangements, particularly with open intervention and the accompanying aortic cross-clamp. Whereas the majority of AAAs are infrarenal, approximately 5% to 15% involve the suprarenal aorta.

It has recently been recognized that the process of aneurysm formation is a distinct degenerative progression from atherosclerotic disease, with features such as vessel wall infiltration by macrophages, destruction of elastin and collagen, loss of smooth muscle cells, and neovascularization. Although inflammation and macrophage infiltration are common to both atherosclerotic and aneurysmal disease, atherosclerosis is primarily noted within the intima and media, but aneurysmal disease typically affects the media and adventitia. Although the overwhelming majority of AAAs are caused by degenerative disease, less common etiologies include infection, inflammatory diseases, trauma, and congenital conditions.

Considerations for Intervention

The single greatest risk factor for aneurysm rupture is size. Current evidence-based guidelines suggest repair when aneurysm diameter exceeds 5.0 to 5.5 cm. Rapid aneurysm growth, defined as greater than 10 mm per year, is also an indication for intervention. Urgent repair is recommended in the setting of symptomatic nonruptured AAA, regardless of size. In the setting of excessive perioperative risk, medical rather than surgical management may be considered in patients with multiple significant comorbidities.

Historically, open repair has been the definitive treatment for AAA. Open AAA repair is associated with significant perioperative morbidity and mortality. Although clinical outcomes have steadily improved because of ongoing refinements in perioperative management, including advances in anesthetic and surgical techniques, current estimates of perioperative mortality rates for elective open AAA repair range from 1 to 5%, with perioperative mortality rates for emergent repair reported to be as high as 30%. Perioperative morbidity may result from all major organ systems, including cardiovascular complications, renal failure, respiratory failure, mesenteric ischemia, bleeding, and infection.

With ongoing improvements in endovascular technology and proceduralist skill, endovascular aortic repair (EVAR) has become the mainstay of treatment for AAA. Even complex AAAs involving abdominal viscera may be candidates for endovascular repair using advanced techniques such as fenestrated stent grafts or snorkel techniques. Multiple high-quality randomized controlled trials comparing endovascular with open abdominal aortic repair have demonstrated a significant difference in 30-day mortality rates and major morbidity for patients who undergo EVAR. This perioperative survival advantage has not been sustained in intermediate- to long-term follow up. Furthermore, follow-up studies suggest a significantly higher rate of reintervention in patients who undergo EVAR, although the majority were also endovascular-based procedures associated with low mortality. In the current era, open AAA repair tends to be reserved for patients who are not candidates for EVAR, but the decision for open versus endovascular repair for the individual patient depends on multiple factors such as aortic anatomy, urgency, patient preference, and surgical expertise.

Intraoperative Anesthetic Considerations and Management

Open Abdominal Aortic Aneurysm Repair

General anesthesia is the most commonly used technique for open AAA repair. Surgical exposure is obtained by either a midline transabdominal or lateral retroperitoneal incision. Given the extensive incision and frequency of concomitant COPD, epidural analgesia should be considered in this setting to facilitate high-quality pain control, to limit the side effects of parenteral narcotics, and to preserve respiratory function. A recent meta-analysis has suggested that this strategy can decrease major complications in AAA repair such as postoperative mechanical ventilation, MI, gastrointestinal morbidity, and renal injury.

Although general anesthesia can be induced by a variety of agents, particular consideration is given to maintaining the patient's baseline hemodynamics in order to maintain adequate end-organ perfusion (typically within 20% of baseline values), while minimizing sympathetic stimulation to noxious events such as endotracheal intubation and placement of invasive monitors. Moderate doses of narcotics and/or IV lidocaine upon anesthetic induction may prove useful in this regard. Volatile and/or IV anesthesia may be used for maintenance of general anesthesia. Although recent evidence suggests a cardioprotective effect of volatile agents in cardiac surgery, this benefit is less clear in AAA repair.

Invasive blood pressure monitoring is mandatory for tight control of blood pressure during periods of hemodynamic instability and rapid blood loss. Consideration should be given to placement of an arterial catheter before the induction of general anesthesia to guide titration of induction agents to ensure steady hemodynamics during this labile period. Reliable large-bore IV access is required and should also be present before surgical incision. Adequate blood product availability and assisted means for expeditious transfusion should be available as needed. Cell-saving techniques may decrease the amount of autologous blood needed and mitigate the risks of transfusion. Central venous access should be obtained to facilitate monitoring of overall volume status and to ensure rapid and reliable administration of vasoactive drugs. Invasive monitoring of cardiac output (CO), either by pulmonary artery catheter or TEE, is reasonable, especially in high-risk patients and those undergoing complicated surgical repairs requiring high or prolonged aortic cross-clamp times.

Endovascular Abdominal Aortic Aneurysm Repair

Endovascular aortic repair can be successfully performed under local anesthesia, neuraxial anesthesia, or general anesthesia. Very limited evidence exists on the best choice of anesthesia for a standard EVAR, and even less for complex endovascular repair. No randomized controlled trials have been performed that compare anesthetic techniques for EVAR. The data that exist are limited to retrospective analyses that must be interpreted cautiously because of the inherent risk for selection biases. A recent meta-analysis of the existing data found no difference in 30-day mortality or major morbidity rates among techniques. Locoregional anesthesia was associated with shorter procedural times, hospital LOS, and lower likelihood of ICU admission. Both the Society for Vascular Surgery as well as the European Society for Vascular Surgery practice guidelines suggest the use of locoregional techniques; however, wide variability exists in practice patterns.

Surgical access is obtained via surgical cutdown or percutaneous access of the femoral vessels. Locoregional anesthesia may be provided by neuraxial anesthesia (single-shot spinal, continuous spinal, or epidural catheter), regional blocks (ilioinguinal and hypogastric nerve blocks or bilateral transversus abdominis plane blocks), or surgical skin infiltration. As delivery devices improve, the need for surgical cutdown has decreased significantly, increasing the likelihood of success with local infiltration. Locoregional anesthesia has several potential intraoperative benefits for EVAR. Avoiding the myocardial depressant effects of general anesthetic agents and the potentially stimulating periods of induction and emergence may afford better intraoperative hemodynamic stability. Pulmonary outcomes may be improved by avoiding mechanical ventilation and maintaining baseline respiratory mechanics. An awake, conversant patient may also serve as an early monitor for complications such as anaphylactic reactions to iodinated contrast agents (e.g., pruritus or dyspnea) or arterial rupture (e.g., sudden retroperitoneal pain) that may not be immediately evident in an unconscious patient. Locoregional anesthesia may require supplementation with titrated sedation. Small doses of short-acting agents should be titrated carefully to provide adequate cooperation, sedation, analgesia, and anxiolysis. Care must be taken to avoid oversedation, airway obstruction, and hypoxemia. The ability to convert rapidly and safely to a general anesthetic remains important in the case of either surgical or anesthetic misadventure.

General anesthesia eliminates concerns regarding patient comfort, anxiety, and the ability to lie immobile and flat for a prolonged duration. It also obviates emergent conversion to general anesthesia, although the reported conversion rate from locoregional to general anesthesia (usually precipitated by surgical complication) is less than 1%. Additional advantages of general anesthesia include dampened bowel peristalsis and precise control of respiration, which may enhance the quality of intraoperative imaging to facilitate accurate stent deployment.

Both surgical factors and patient preference should be considered when choosing an anesthetic technique. Anatomically complex lesions requiring advanced endovascular techniques may be lengthy operations and can be associated with significant blood loss despite the minimally invasive nature. As such, complex endovascular repairs may be better suited for general anesthesia. Certain patient populations may also be unsuitable candidates for locoregional anesthesia, including patients with significant anxiety, medical comorbidities that preclude their ability to lie flat, and patients with whom communication is limited (e.g., baseline cognitive dysfunction or language barrier).

There is typically less hemodynamic instability during EVAR than an open aortic intervention because the need for aortic cross-clamping is avoided, although periods of ballooning and stent deployment are analogous to the placement of an endoclamp and may result in transient lability. Thus, from this perspective, the requirement for invasive arterial blood pressure monitoring is less imperative for EVAR. The ability to place an arterial catheter rapidly in an emergency situation is limited in EVAR, however, because both arms are usually tucked to allow intraoperative fluoroscopy, and both groins are usually surgically accessed for the repair. Given these constraints, elective direct arterial blood pressure monitoring is often selected as a precaution in case of arterial rupture and conversion to open repair. Continuous arterial pressure monitoring may also allow for more precise hemodynamic manipulation during critical periods such as stent positioning and deployment, although there are no studies to suggest benefit compared with noninvasive blood pressure monitoring.

Although EVAR has a lower risk of bleeding and transfusion compared with open aortic intervention, large-bore peripheral IV access is still preferred because of the small, but real, risk of conversion to an open approach. Central venous access is typically not required unless a significant need for vasoactive medication is anticipated or reliable large-bore peripheral access cannot be established.

Perioperative Challenges

Hemodynamic Management of Aortic Clamping and Unclamping

Hemodynamic management during open AAA repair is challenging and requires constant communication with the surgical team (Box 13.3). Hemodynamic perturbations during open AAA repair are influenced by factors such as aortic clamping (AXC), rapid blood loss, significant fluid shifts, and acute cardiac dysfunction. The application of an AXC initiates an array of physiologic derangements governed primarily by the level at which the clamp is applied (Fig. 13.3). Increases in mean arterial pressure (MAP) and systemic vascular resistance (SVR) caused by impeded arterial flow are the most consistent responses to AXC, with an increase in arterial pressure of 10% or more with infrarenal aortic cross-clamping. The potential for substantially greater increases exists if the aorta is clamped at a higher level such as above the celiac axis where flow to the abdominal viscera is also interrupted.

The hemodynamic effects of an AXC below the level of the celiac axis allows for shifting of blood flow to the splanchnic circulation, which in turn augments its venous capacitance (Fig. 13.4). The typical result of this volume redistribution is little change in venous return and CO unless major swings in splanchnic venous tone occur. When the clamp is placed above the celiac artery, the splanchnic circulation cannot serve as a reservoir. Rather, venous capacitance below the clamp decreases, expelling blood from the splanchnic system to the central circulation, with resultant increases in filling pressures and venous return. The redistribution of blood volume in this setting is also affected by blood loss, fluid loading, anesthetic depth, and administered vasopressors.

Baseline myocardial contractility reserve may also affect the response to AXC during AAA repair. The increases in preload and afterload acutely increase myocardial work and

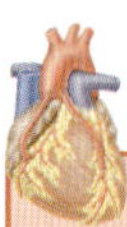

BOX 13.3 *Considerations and Management Strategies for Aortic Cross-Clamping*

- Maintain blood pressure on the low side of tolerable range in the minutes preceding aortic cross-clamp, anticipating an increase in afterload with the placement of aortic cross-clamp. This can be accomplished with increasing anesthetic depth or with the use of vasodilating agents (e.g., nitroprusside, nicardipine, local anesthetic bolus via epidural catheter).
- The higher the placement of the cross-clamp, the more significant the increase in afterload.
- Minimize fluid loading before aortic cross-clamp placement to avoid overloading the heart.
- Monitor closely for evidence of cardiac ischemia or failure with ECG, PAC, or TEE and support accordingly.
- Maintain blood pressure on the high side of tolerable range during the period of aortic cross-clamping to maximize perfusion distal to the clamp via collateral circulation.

ECG, Electrocardiography; *PAC,* pulmonary artery catheter; *TEE,* transesophageal echocardiography.

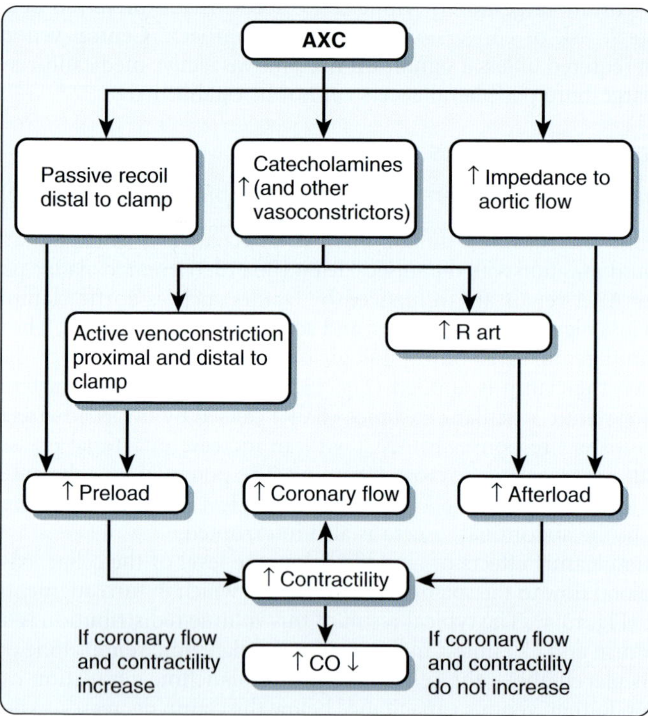

Fig. 13.3 Physiologic changes with aortic cross-clamp placement. Typical hemodynamic response to aortic cross-clamp placement. The level of cross-clamp placement, changes in circulating blood volume, depth of anesthesia or anesthetic agents used, and other physiologic factors may have varying effects. *AXC,* Aortic cross-clamping; *CO,* cardiac output; *R art,* increased arterial resistance. (Modified from Gelman S. The pathophysiology of aortic cross-clamping and unclamping. *Anesthesiology.* 1995;82:1026–1060.)

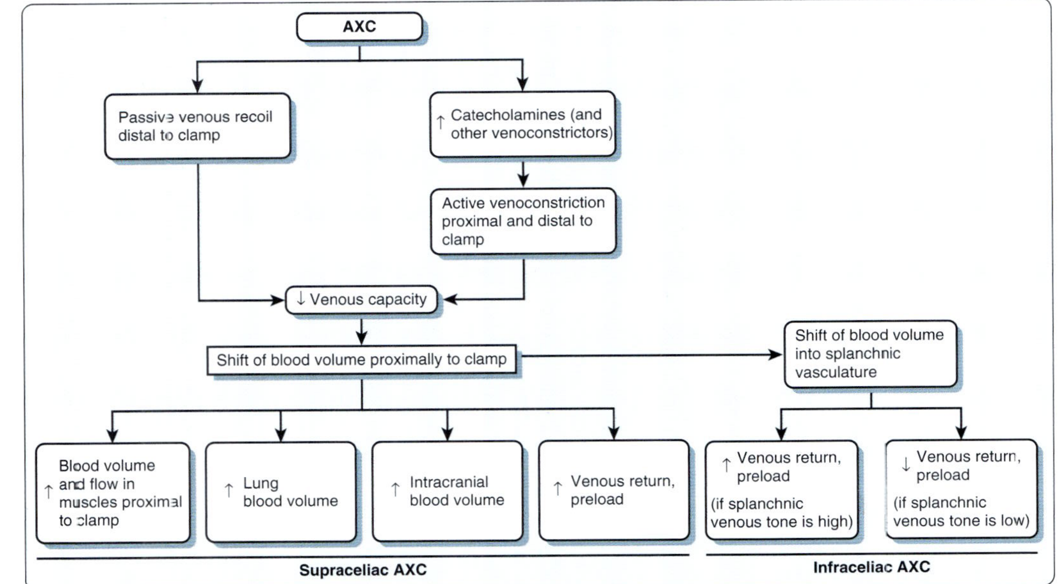

Fig. 13.4 Changes in blood volume distribution during aortic cross-clamping (AXC). The shifting of blood volume with AXC is dependent on the level of cross-clamp placement (supraceliac vs. infraceliac), release of catecholamines and administration of vasoactive medications, and overall blood volume. (Modified from Gelman S. The pathophysiology of aortic cross-clamping and unclamping. *Anesthesiology*. 1995;82:1026–1060.)

oxygen demand, particularly with supraceliac clamping. The physiologic response to this increased demand is to increase myocardial perfusion via coronary vasodilation. Thus patients without significant CAD and preserved ventricular function may tolerate these increases in preload and afterload with minimal effect on CO. TEE has demonstrated regional wall motion abnormalities in 33% of patients during suprarenal clamping and in 92% of patients during supraceliac clamping. In the setting of concomitant CAD in which the coronary vasculature is already maximally vasodilated or has preexisting left ventricular (LV) dysfunction, the acute increase in myocardial oxygen demand during AXC may precipitate myocardial ischemia or overt HF.

Hemodynamic management during AXC primarily focuses on decreasing afterload and LV wall stress with arteriolar dilators and normalizing preload with venous dilators. Typically, short-acting vasoactive agents (e.g., sodium nitroprusside, nitroglycerin, nicardipine, and/or clevidipine) are titrated to achieve these hemodynamic goals in a fashion that adapts rapidly to a changing clinical scenario. Because myocardial ischemia and HF may present acutely during this critical period, agents to improve myocardial oxygen supply as well as inotropic agents should be available to support ventricular function as necessary. Close communication between the surgical and anesthetic teams is paramount so that pathophysiologic derangements can be anticipated and appropriately managed.

The release of an aortic cross-clamp also requires close attention and preparation (Box 13.4). There are several episodes of aortic clamp release during open aortic repair (Fig. 13.5). After completion of the proximal aortic anastomosis, the initial superior aortic clamp is then applied lower on the new aortic graft to minimize ischemic time to the visceral organs. The typically brief initial clamp time for the proximal aortic anastomosis results in minor hemodynamic disruption from reperfusion of the celiac and renal vascular territories. In contrast, after completion of the entire AAA repair, release of the distal AXC is frequently associated with dramatic hypotension. The mechanism for hypotension is multifactorial (Fig. 13.6). Distal aortic unclamping results in an immediate and profound (≤70%–80%) decrease in systemic vascular resistance. This distal vasodilation as a result of tissue hypoxia and release of vasoactive mediators promotes sequestration of blood distal to the AXC, resulting in a relative central hypovolemia. These vasoactive and inflammatory mediators such as lactic acid, oxygen free radicals, prostaglandins, endotoxins, and cytokines promote vasodilation and myocardial depression upon release of the AXC. This hypotensive response can

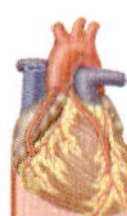

BOX 13.4   *Considerations and Management Strategies for Aortic Cross-Clamp Release*

- Maintain blood pressure on the high side of tolerable range in the minutes preceding aortic cross-clamp release to attenuate the sudden and profound vasoplegia that occurs upon release.
- Volume load during the period of aortic cross-clamping, anticipating a relative hypovolemia upon cross-clamp release related to vasoplegia and sequestration of blood in areas distal to the cross-clamp following release.
- Minimize surgical cross-clamp time and move clamp distal as each anastomosis or reimplantation is complete to minimize ischemic time to vital organs.
- Consider administering vasopressor or inotropic agents (or both) with cross-clamp release.
- Remove cross-clamp slowly to attenuate hypotensive response. Reapply cross-clamp and further medically optimize if patient does not tolerate attempt at cross-clamp release (e.g., additional fluid or administration of a vasopressor or inotrope).

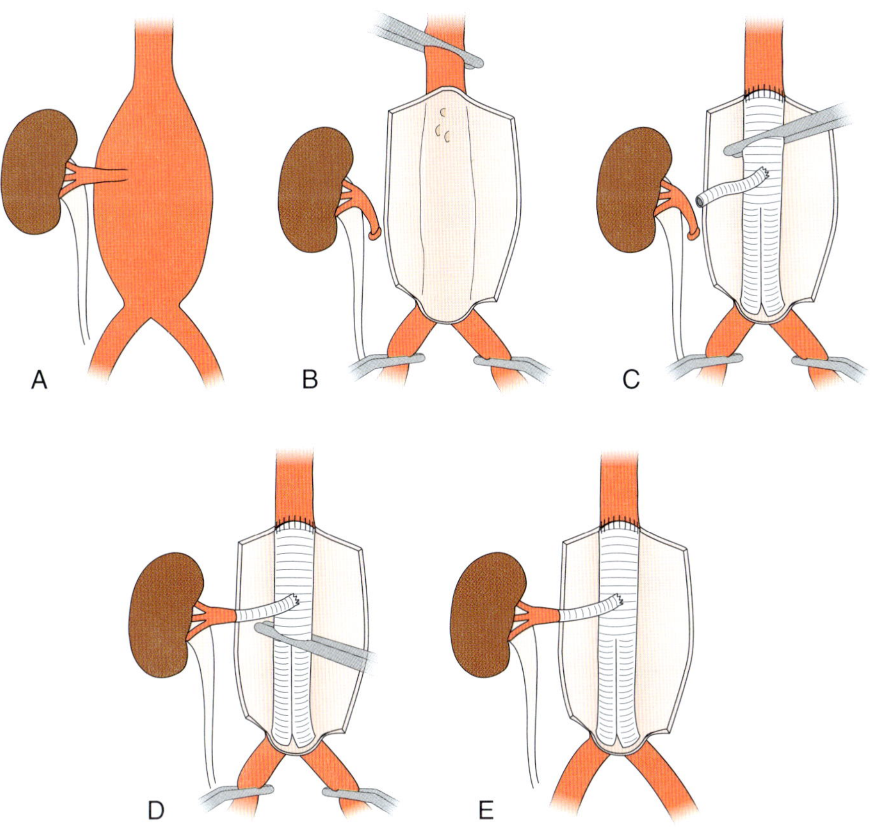

Fig. 13.5 Mobilization of aortic cross-clamp during open abdominal aortic aneurysm repair. To minimize unnecessary ischemic time on visceral organs, the aortic cross-clamp is moved sequentially lower on the graft as each anastomosis is completed. Each cross-clamp release will result in metabolic washout to the previously ischemic organs, although the subsequent quick replacement of the cross-clamp lower on the graft will mitigate some of the hemodynamic alterations. (A) Native aneurysm with right renal artery. (B) The aortal and iliac arteries are clamped. The aneurysm sack is opened, and the right renal artery is dissected. (C) Aortobifemoral graft with a separate arterial graft is sewn in. The aortic clamp is moved from the native aorta to the proximal graft. (D) The right renal artery is anastomosed, with perfusion to the right kidney achieve by moving the aortic cross-clamp distal. (E) Reperfusion of the legs: all arterial clamps are removed. (Modified from Woo EY, Damrauer SM. Abdominal aortic aneurysms: open surgical treatment. In: Cronenwett JL, Johnston KW, eds. *Rutherford's Vascular Surgery*. 8th ed. Philadelphia: Elsevier; 2014:2024–2045.)

be mitigated by surgical techniques such as minimizing ischemic time and gradual AXC release.

Adequate volume loading should be performed during the period of AXC in anticipation of the profound vasodilation and relative hypovolemia that accompany clamp removal. Vasodilatory agents during the AXC period may prove useful in this regard. In anticipation of AXC release, vasodilatory agents should be discontinued, and vasopressor agents should be immediately available. A slow release of the AXC or opening of iliac artery clamps one at a time may allow for a more gradual metabolic washout with less profound hemodynamic derangements. In case of profound hypotension, the AXC may be reapplied. As with AXC placement, clear communication between the surgical and anesthesia teams is necessary during this critical time.

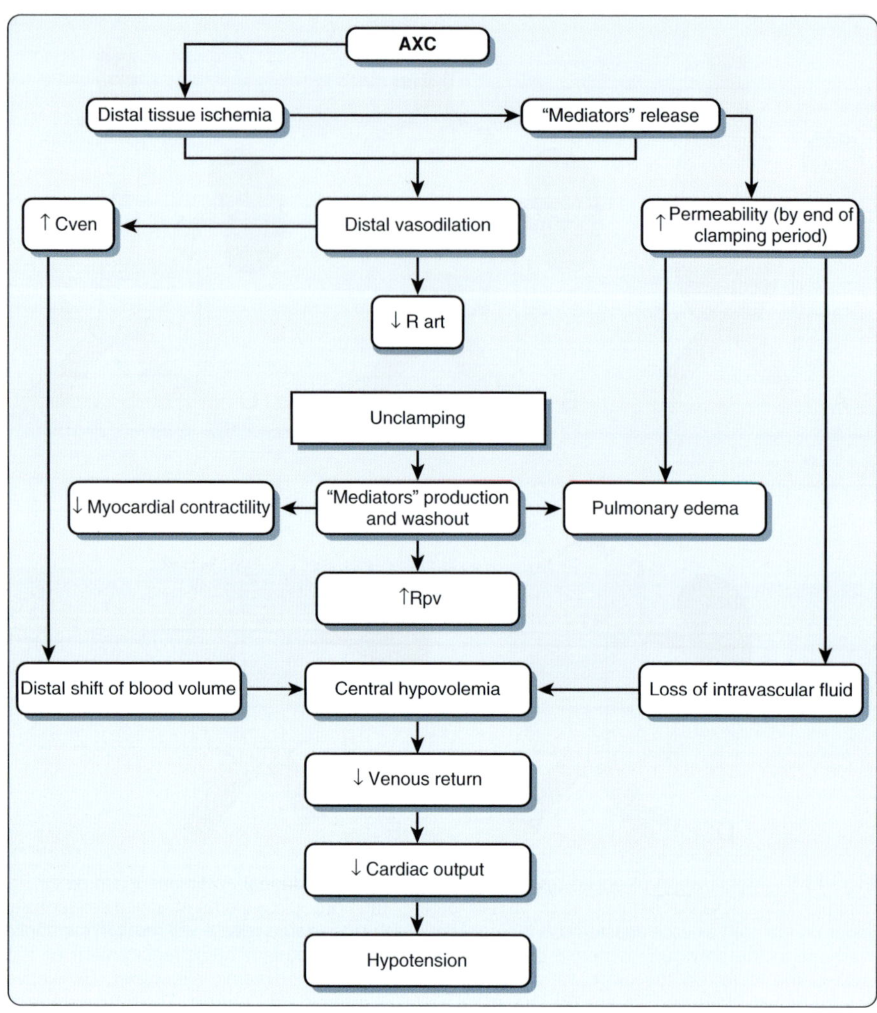

Fig. 13.6 Physiologic changes with aortic cross-clamp release. Typical hemodynamic response to aortic cross-clamp release. *AXC,* Aortic cross-clamping; *Cven,* venous capacitance; *R art,* arterial resistance; *Rpv,* pulmonary vascular resistance. (Modified from Gelman S. The pathophysiology of aortic cross-clamping and unclamping. *Anesthesiology.* 1995;82:1026–1060.)

In general, EVAR is associated with less extreme hemodynamic perturbations owing to the lack of the AXC compared with open AAA repair. Even though endovascular aortic occlusion during stent deployment may result in transient increases in MAP and afterload similar to those seen with external AXC application, their relative brevity rarely necessitates hemodynamic intervention. Brief deliberate hypotension may be used at the time of deployment to position the stent precisely and minimize the risk of distal migration. This can be accomplished by a variety of short-acting vasodilatory agents titrated to effect.

Renal Protection and Function

Postoperative renal dysfunction is a major source of morbidity in AAA repair. During open repair, AXC at all levels reduces renal blood flow. Even infrarenal AXC may decrease renal blood flow by 40%, accompanied by an increase in renal vascular resistance, with decreases in renal cortical blood flow and glomerular filtration rate. These renal effects are mediated by the renin–angiotensin and sympathetic nervous systems. Renal atheroemboli from AXC may also have a deleterious effect on renal function.

Multiple trials since the 1980s have explored whether agents such as mannitol, furosemide, dopamine, fenoldopam, and *N*-acetylcysteine are nephroprotective during AAA repair. Although these interventions are still frequently used, there is inadequate evidence to support this practice. Intraoperative maneuvers such as minimizing AXC time and maintaining adequate hemodynamics are the most prudent measures to limit renal injury during open AAA repair.

Renal dysfunction after EVAR is typically a result of iodinated contrast agents, although atheroemboli and graft impingement of the renal artery ostia may also contribute. In this setting, perioperative maneuvers that minimize the risk of contrast-induced nephropathy include limitation of contrast volume, adequate resuscitation with isotonic fluid, and systemic sodium bicarbonate.

Respiratory Challenges

Pulmonary complications are also common after AAA repair. Mechanical ventilation is commonly continued into the immediate postoperative period for open AAA repair, particularly for more complicated procedures. Frequent ongoing resuscitation needs for the first 24 to 48 postoperative hours after repair may make it prudent to "rest" the patient until hemodynamic stability is achieved, particularly in patients with underlying pulmonary compromise such as COPD. Although the majority of patients are liberated from mechanical ventilation thereafter, pulmonary infection still remains a common postoperative complication occurring in 17% of patients. In contrast, most patients undergoing EVAR either do not require mechanical ventilation or undergo tracheal extubation in the OR at the end of the procedure. Consequently, pulmonary complications after EVAR are less common with a reported incidence of 3% to 7%. Perioperative interventions such as adequate analgesia, aggressive pulmonary toilet, and early ventilator liberation may all help to minimize pulmonary complications after AAA repair.

Unique Complications of Endovascular Intervention

Patients undergoing EVAR are at increased risk for subsequent intervention to manage unique complications. Endoleak is defined as a failure to exclude the aneurysm from the circulation after device deployment because of a persistent flow of blood into the aneurysm sac. Endoleaks are important because they pressurize the aneurysm sac for a continued risk of expansion and rupture. Five types of endoleak exist, categorized by location and route of blood flow into the space between the graft and the native aneurysm (Fig. 13.7). Meticulous intraoperative imaging will typically identify the presence of an endoleak requiring immediate intervention. Management options include the placement of additional stents, embolization of feeding vessels, or conversion to open repair.

Endovascular graft kinking has been associated with an increased risk for endoleak, stent migration, stent thrombosis, and acute limb ischemia. Graft kinking is more common after endovascular compared with open AAA repair. Surgical options in this setting include additional stent placement, thrombectomy, and open surgical repair. Because stent complications such as separation and migration typically occur beyond the perioperative period, follow-up remains essential after EVAR.

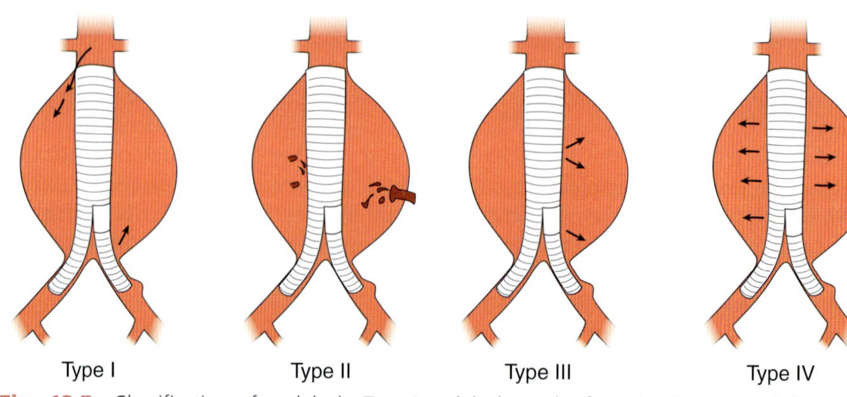

Fig. 13.7 Classification of endoleak. Type I endoleak results from inadequate seal from the proximal or distal end of the endograft. Type II endoleak is caused by inflow from a visceral vessel. Type III endoleak occurs as a result of a defect in the graft, a disconnection of modular graft components, or an inadequate seal. Type IV endoleak occurs as a result of porosity of the graft fabric. Type V endoleak, also known as endotension, is an elevation in aneurysm sac pressure without a demonstrable source of endoleak. (Modified from Fairman RM, Wang GJ. Abdominal aortic aneurysms: endovascular treatment. In: Cronenwett JL, Johnston KW, eds. *Rutherford's Vascular Surgery*. 8th ed. Philadelphia: Elsevier; 2014:2046–2061.)

ABDOMINAL AORTIC DISSECTION

Aortic dissection is an aortic syndrome characterized by a tear in the intima that may subsequently be propagated by pulsatile blood flow with development of a false lumen between the dissected layers of the arterial wall. Aortic dissections are classified both temporally and anatomically. Classically, dissections are labeled acute when clinical symptoms have lasted for 14 days or less and chronic if symptom duration exceeds 2 weeks. Recent work, however, suggests four distinct time periods: hyperacute (symptom onset <24 hours), acute (2–7 days), subacute (8–30 days), and chronic (>30 days), with a mortality rate that continues to increase significantly even into what is traditionally considered the chronic phase. The majority of late deaths are from rupture of the false lumen because its long-term patency sets the stage for aneurysmal dilation and rupture.

Anatomically, two classification systems are used to describe aortic dissections. DeBakey first identified variations in aortic dissection based on both the origin of the initial tear as well as the extent of aortic dissection. The Stanford classification system simplifies the schema by entry site only, with Stanford type A dissection originating in the ascending aorta and Stanford type B dissection originating in the descending aorta. In this chapter, discussion of aortic dissection will be limited to abdominal aortic dissections. For an in-depth discussion of thoracic and thoracoabdominal aortic dissection, please refer to the seventh edition of *Kaplan's Cardiac Anesthesia*, pp. 843–882.

Acute type B dissections are responsible for approximately one-third of all aortic dissections. Isolated dissection of the abdominal aorta is rare; most commonly, the intimal tear originates within a few centimeters of the left subclavian artery. The clinical presentation of isolated abdominal aortic dissection may vary depending on end-organ compromise; abdominal pain, visceral ischemia, acute renal failure, and limb ischemia have all been reported. Anesthetic considerations in this patient population are similar to those undergoing AAA repair and both open and endovascular surgical techniques have been used.

AORTOILIAC OCCLUSIVE DISEASE

Aortoiliac occlusive disease is a manifestation of PAD that ultimately results in partial or total vascular occlusion. Atherosclerosis is the most common cause of both PAD and aortoiliac occlusive disease; thus the risk factors are similar and include smoking, age, family history, diabetes, hypertension, and hyperlipidemia, as well as more recently identified risk factors such as hyperhomocysteinemia.

Aortoiliac occlusive disease typically begins in the distal aortic segment and the origin of the common iliac arteries and progresses indolently over time. An extensive collateral circulation, primarily from the lumbar and hypogastric arteries, frequently reconstitutes the infrainguinal vessels in disease limited to the aortoiliac segment. Thus although isolated aortoiliac disease may lead to claudication symptoms (manifested by intermittent thigh, hip, or buttock pain or impotence from inadequate flow through the internal pudendal artery), it rarely leads to critical limb ischemia. Indications for intervention include disabling or progressive claudication, ischemic rest pain, and tissue loss. The extent to which claudication is disabling is a somewhat subjective decision made jointly by the surgeon and patient based on symptomatology and limitations on quality of life. Current guidelines recommend either endovascular or surgical intervention for patients who have significant functional disability that is vocational or lifestyle limiting, who are unresponsive to medical or exercise therapy, and who have a reasonable likelihood of symptomatic improvement.

The Trans-Atlantic Inter-Society Consensus (TASC) classifies aortoiliac occlusive disease by location and severity of disease (Fig. 13.8). Historically, open surgical reconstruction has been the gold standard, including both aortoiliac or femoral bypass or endarterectomy procedures. Extraanatomic bypass procedures such as axillofemoral bypass are typically reserved for high-risk patients with aortoiliac occlusive disease, but they are less durable, with reported patency rates below 80%. Because extraanatomic bypass, by definition, does not involve the aortic segment, the hemodynamic lability of aortic cross-clamping is avoided. Increasingly, an endovascular-first approach is used for even the most complex aortoocclusive disease. No contemporary randomized controlled trials exist to definitively establish the superiority of open surgical versus endovascular repair. The choice of revascularization should consider individual patient comorbidities, the anatomic complexity of the lesion, and the overall vascular center's competence and experience.

Open surgical repairs are typically performed under general anesthesia because of the length of the operation, risk for hemodynamic lability (particularly for direct bypasses), and the need for extensive resuscitation. Endovascular procedures are typically performed under locoregional anesthesia. Considerations are similar to open AAA repair, whether open or endovascular. An arterial catheter and large-bore IV access are typically warranted because of patient comorbidities, risk for hemorrhage, and risk of hemodynamic changes (albeit less severe) with peripheral vascular clamping.

LOWER EXTREMITY ARTERIAL DISEASE

Lower extremity ischemia has a spectrum of clinical presentation, ranging from exertional muscle pain to gangrene and tissue loss. The clinical manifestations of lower extremity arterial disease (LEAD) depend on the location and severity of arterial occlusion as well as the extent of collateral vessels. Risk factors for LEAD include advanced age, tobacco abuse, hypertension, hyperlipidemia, and diabetes mellitus. Although LEAD may be asymptomatic in up to 50% of patients, it remains a sentinel

Type A lesions

- Unilateral or bilateral stenoses of CIA
- Unilateral or bilateral single short (≤3 cm) stenosis of EIA

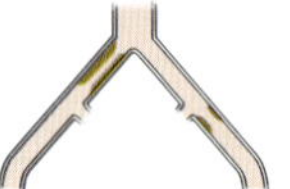

Type B lesions

- Short (≤3 cm) stenosis of infrarenal aorta
- Unilateral CIA occlusion
- Single or multiple stenosis totaling 3–10 cm involving the EIA not extending into the CFA
- Unilateral EIA occlusion not involving the origins of internal iliac or CFA

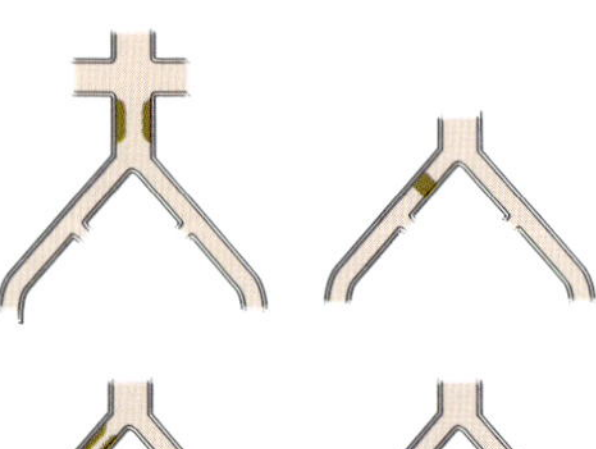

Type C lesions

- Bilateral CIA occlusions
- Bilateral EIA stenoses 3–10 cm long not extending into the CFA
- Unilateral EIA stenosis extending into the CFA
- Unilateral EIA occlusion that involves the origins of internal iliac and/or CFA
- Heavily calcified unilateral EIA occlusion with or without involvement of origins of internal iliac and/or CFA

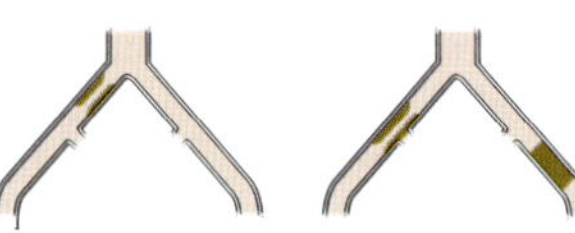

Type D lesions

- Intrarenal aortoiliac occlusion
- Diffuse disease involving the aorta and both iliac arteries requiring treatment
- Diffuse multiple stenoses involving the unilateral CIA, EIA, and CFA
- Unilateral occlusions of both CIA and EIA
- Bilateral occlusions of EIA
- Iliac stenoses in patients with AAA requiring treatment and not amenable to endograft placement or other lesions requiring open aortic or iliac surgery

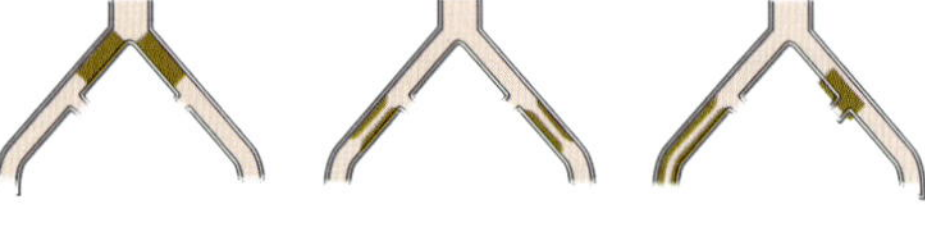

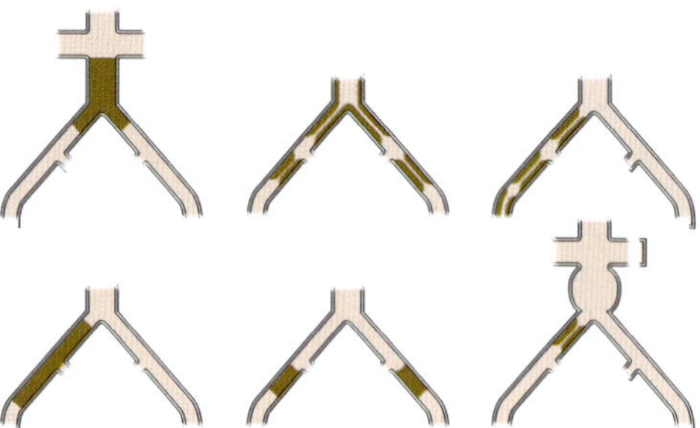

Fig. 13.8 Trans-Atlantic Inter-Society Consensus (TASC) II classifications of aortoiliac disease. Classification of aortoiliac disease based on location, laterality, and disease severity. *AAA,* Abdominal aortic aneurysm; *CFA,* common femoral artery; *CIA,* common iliac artery; *EIA,* external iliac artery. (Modified from Norgren L, Hiatt WR, Dormandy JA, et al. Inter-society consensus for the management of peripheral arterial disease [TASC II]. *J Vasc Surg.* 2007;45[suppl S]:S5–S67.)

marker for adverse cardiovascular outcomes because it is frequently associated with atherosclerotic CAD.

Intermittent claudication is the presenting feature of LEAD in up to 35% of patients. Intermittent claudication is defined as a reproducible discomfort in a defined muscle group that is induced by exercise and relieved with rest. In general, claudication in the buttock and hip typically results from aortoiliac occlusion, and claudication in the thigh or lower leg results from progressively distal arterial disease. The natural history of PAD is usually a slow, progressive decline in function. With aggressive medical management, lifestyle adjustment, and exercise therapy, the vast majority of patients do not progress to more advanced disease.

In a minority of patients, the disease will progress to critical limb ischemia when existing arterial blood flow is insufficient to meet the basic metabolic demands of resting tissue. The clinical presentation in this setting ranges from rest pain to tissue loss (nonhealing ulcers or gangrene). Risk factors that increase the risk for accelerated disease progression include age, diabetes, smoking, and hyperlipidemia. Unlike claudication, critical limb ischemia includes a high risk of limb loss because of a more aggressive LEAD with multisegmental involvement. Within 1 year, it is estimated that 25% of patients will progress to amputation, and 25% will die from CV mortality. Approximately 50% of patients with critical limb ischemia will also have advanced coronary and cerebrovascular artery disease, with a higher mortality risk from MI, stroke, or both. The management of critical limb ischemia involves aggressive risk factor reduction, wound care, and a low threshold for revascularization.

Considerations for Intervention

The majority of patients with intermittent claudication have a relatively indolent progression of their disease process. The decision for procedural intervention is a highly individualized decision and must weigh the perceived benefit of relief of symptomatology versus the risks of intervention. In general, intervention is considered for patients who have intolerable symptoms despite aggressive medical therapy and lifestyle interventions. Tolerability of symptoms may be highly variable between patients; a relatively active patient may find even minor symptoms life limiting, while more sedentary individuals may not be bothered by even more severe disease. In contrast to intermittent claudication, critical limb ischemia typically mandates intervention because of the high rate of limb loss without intervention.

After the decision has been made for surgical intervention, the selection of open versus endovascular intervention must then also be individualized based on procedural risk, medical comorbidity, overall life expectancy, and expected extent of clinical improvement. Open surgical bypass has a long history of success and durability, with long-term patency rates greater than 95%. Despite this track record, endovascular intervention has become the preferred approach for most patients with LEAD because of the low associated mortality and low morbidity rates. Endovascular procedures, however, have proven less durable in the long term than surgical bypass and require a higher incidence of reintervention.

Intraoperative Anesthetic Considerations and Management

Open Lower Extremity Arterial Bypass

Open lower extremity revascularization procedures are amenable to anesthetic techniques such as regional blocks, neuraxial anesthesia, and general anesthesia. Although studies have suggested that regional and neuraxial techniques enhance hemodynamic stability and decrease catecholamine responses, these differences likely occur primarily during induction and emergence from general anesthesia. Thus careful management of hemodynamics during these critical periods may be just as efficacious. Although regional and neuraxial anesthetic techniques may enhance lower extremity blood flow because of the concomitant sympathectomy, clinical trials have inconsistently demonstrated higher graft patency rates due to anesthetic technique. There is currently no compelling evidence to favor a particular anesthetic technique, given that the literature suggests at least equivalent outcomes. The final choice of anesthetic technique is left to the discretion of the provider, bearing in mind both patient risks and preferences.

A general anesthetic alleviates concerns of patient anxiety, discomfort, and cooperation. No trials have examined the use of one general anesthetic technique over another. The most important consideration when general anesthesia is used is careful attention to perioperative hemodynamics, particularly during periods of known lability such as induction, intubation, cross-clamp placement or release, and emergence from anesthesia. A variety of agents can be used to this end. It is prudent to have a variety of short-acting hemodynamic agents readily available to control changes in hemodynamics, including heart rate and blood pressure.

If a regional technique is used, neuraxial anesthesia is the most commonly used technique. Cutaneous innervation of the lower extremity is provided by the lumbar (primarily above the knee) and lumbosacral (primarily below the knee) plexi. The lumbar plexus is composed of the ventral rami from L1 to L4, with variable contribution from T12 (ultimately dividing into the femoral, lateral femoral cutaneous, and obturator nerves), and the lumbosacral plexus is composed of the ventral rami of L4 to S3 (ultimately forming the sciatic nerve, which branches to become the tibial and common peroneal nerves). In general, local anesthetics are carefully titrated to slowly bring the anesthetic level to approximately T10 to allow for adequate surgical anesthesia while minimizing hemodynamic compromise. Light sedation with short-acting agents may be considered as supplementation to neuraxial or peripheral anesthesia.

Although the hemodynamic and physiologic derangements of peripheral cross-clamping are typically less severe than with aortic cross-clamping, the risk for significant blood loss and hemodynamic lability observed in this patient population makes arterial blood pressure monitoring ideal. Adequate IV access and blood product availability should be assured. Central venous access is rarely warranted unless specific patient factors warrant placement or if peripheral access is problematic.

Endovascular Lower Extremity Peripheral Arterial Repair

In general, infrainguinal endovascular interventions are very amenable to MAC or local anesthesia. Arterial access can be obtained percutaneously or via small surgical cutdown, typically under local anesthetic block performed by the surgical team. A variety of short-acting agents have been successfully used for MAC. Most commonly, short-acting opioids (e.g., fentanyl or remifentanil), benzodiazepines, or low doses of sedative agents such as propofol or dexmedetomidine are used in this regard. In general, hemodynamic perturbations and blood loss during endovascular management are minimal. Invasive monitoring is rarely warranted. As always, the anesthesia team must be prepared for rapid conversion to a general anesthetic if complications occur with either the surgical or anesthetic management. Some patients may be poor candidates for MAC (e.g., cannot lie flat or cannot follow commands); in this case, general anesthesia may be a more prudent strategy.

Perioperative Challenges

Intraoperative challenges during infrainguinal vascular repair are usually secondary to hemodynamic changes related to peripheral vascular clamping and unclamping. In general, compared with AXC, peripheral vascular clamping is fairly well tolerated, with relatively mild changes in afterload, hemodynamics, and myocardial wall stress. Release of the peripheral cross-clamp, as with an AXC, may result in hypotension as a result of a decrease in SVR and release of inflammatory mediators. Adequate volume loading, the availability of vasopressor and inotropic support, and close communication with the surgical team can help prevent profound derangements in hemodynamics during this critical period.

SUGGESTED READING

Barnett HJ, Taylor DW, Eliasziw M, et al. Benefit of carotid endarterectomy in patients with symptomatic moderate or severe stenosis. North American Symptomatic Carotid Endarterectomy Trial Collaborators. *NEJM*. 1998;339:1415–1425.

Becquemin JP, Pillet JC, Lescalie F, et al. A randomized controlled trial of endovascular aneurysm repair versus open surgery for abdominal aortic aneurysms in low- to moderate-risk patients. *J Vasc Surg*. 2011;53:1167–1173.e1.

Conte MS, Pomposelli FB, Clair DG, et al. Society for Vascular Surgery practice guidelines for atherosclerotic occlusive disease of the lower extremities: management of asymptomatic disease and claudication. *J Vasc Surg*. 2015;61(3 suppl):2S–41S.

De Bruin JL, Baas AF, Buth J, et al. Long-term outcome of open or endovascular repair of abdominal aortic aneurysm. *NEJM*. 2010;362:1881–1889.

Endarterectomy for asymptomatic carotid artery stenosis. Executive Committee for the Asymptomatic Carotid Atherosclerosis Study. *JAMA*. 1995;273:1421–1428.

Fleisher LA, Fleischmann KE, Auerbach AD, et al. 2014 ACC/AHA guideline on perioperative cardiovascular evaluation and management of patients undergoing noncardiac surgery: a report of the American College of Cardiology/American Heart Association Task Force on practice guidelines. *J Am Coll Cardiol*. 2014;64:e77–e137.

Greenhalgh RM, Brown LC, Kwong GP, Powell JT, Thompson SG. Comparison of endovascular aneurysm repair with open repair in patients with abdominal aortic aneurysm (EVAR trial 1), 30-day operative mortality results: randomised controlled trial. *Lancet*. 2004;364:843–848.

Greenhalgh RM, Brown LC, Powell JT, et al. Endovascular versus open repair of abdominal aortic aneurysm. *NEJM*. 2010;362:1863–1871.

Halliday A, Mansfield A, Marro J, et al. Prevention of disabling and fatal strokes by successful carotid endarterectomy in patients without recent neurological symptoms: randomised controlled trial. *Lancet*. 2004;363:1491–1502.

Hobson RW 2nd, Weiss DG, Fields WS, et al. Efficacy of carotid endarterectomy for asymptomatic carotid stenosis. The Veterans Affairs Cooperative Study Group. *NEJM*. 1993;328:221–227.

Kent KC. Clinical practice. Abdominal aortic aneurysms. *NEJM*. 2014;371:2101–2108.

Lederle FA, Freischlag JA, Kyriakides TC, et al. Outcomes following endovascular vs open repair of abdominal aortic aneurysm: a randomized trial. *JAMA*. 2009;302:1535–1542.

Lederle FA, Freischlag JA, Kyriakides TC, et al. Long-term comparison of endovascular and open repair of abdominal aortic aneurysm. *NEJM*. 2012;367:1988–1997.

Levine GN, Bates ER, Bittl JA, et al. 2016 ACC/AHA guideline focused update on duration of dual antiplatelet therapy in patients with coronary artery disease: a report of the American College of Cardiology/American Heart Association Task Force on Clinical Practice Guidelines. *J Am Coll Cardiol*. 2016;68(10):1082–1115.

Lewis SC, Warlow CP, Bodenham AR, et al. General anaesthesia versus local anaesthesia for carotid surgery (GALA): a multicentre, randomised controlled trial. *Lancet*. 2008;372:2132–2142.

Liu ZJ, Fu WG, Guo ZY, et al. Updated systematic review and meta-analysis of randomized clinical trials comparing carotid artery stenting and carotid endarterectomy in the treatment of carotid stenosis. *Ann Vasc Surg*. 2012;26:576–590.

Norgren L, Hiatt WR, Dormandy JA, et al. Inter-society consensus for the management of peripheral arterial disease (TASC II). *J Vasc Surg*. 2007;45(suppl S):S5–S67.

Pandit JJ, Satya-Krishna R, Gration P. Superficial or deep cervical plexus block for carotid endarterectomy: a systematic review of complications. *Br J Anaesth*. 2007;99:159–169.

Prinssen M, Verhoeven EL, Buth J, et al. A randomized trial comparing conventional and endovascular repair of abdominal aortic aneurysms. *NEJM*. 2004;351:1607–1618.

Randomised trial of endarterectomy for recently symptomatic carotid stenosis: final results of the MRC European Carotid Surgery Trial (ECST). *Lancet*. 1998;351:1379–1387.

TASC Steering Committee. An update on methods for revascularization and expansion of the TASC lesion classification to include Below-the-Knee arteries: a supplement to the Inter-Society consensus for the management of peripheral arterial disease (TASC II). *Vasc Med*. 2015;20(5):465–478.

Zammert M, Gelman S. The pathophysiology of aortic cross-clamping. *Best Pract Res Clin Anaesthesiol*. 2016;30(3):257–269.

Chapter 14

The Cardiac Patient for Thoracic Noncardiac Surgery

Alexander Huang, MD, FRCPC • Peter D. Slinger, MD, FRCPC • Steven M. Neustein, MD • Edmond Cohen, MD

Key Points

1. Cardiac patients and those who have had previous cardiac surgery often present for intrathoracic diagnostic or therapeutic noncardiac procedures.
2. Patients with coronary artery disease, valvular heart disease, cardiomyopathies, or pulmonary hypertension may require surgery involving lung isolation and one-lung ventilation (OLV). OLV can carry a significant risk for hypoxia. A stepwise approach to management of hypoxia during OLV is important.
3. Patients with low cardiac output tend to desaturate quickly during OLV and often require inotropic support for thoracotomy or thoracoscopy.
4. Double-lumen endobronchial tubes and bronchial blockers are used for OLV during thoracic surgery. Bronchial blockers are useful options for lung isolation in patients with difficult airways or those who will remain intubated postoperatively. However, double-lumen tubes are used more often because they are stable during surgery and can be suctioned.
5. Transesophageal echocardiography is a useful tool in noncardiac thoracic surgery. It can be used to assess the relationship between mediastinal lesions and adjacent structures (heart, lungs, great vessels) or to diagnose and assist in management during hemodynamic instability.
6. It is very important for the anesthesiologist to review the chest imaging before any intrathoracic or airway procedure so that an appropriate airway management strategy can be planned.
7. Management of rigid bronchoscopy is fundamental to anesthesia for a lower airway lesion.
8. Patients with mediastinal masses require careful assessment and investigation to avoid cardiorespiratory collapse during the induction of anesthesia. This may require awake intubation, the availability of rigid bronchoscopy, or the use of cardiopulmonary bypass (CPB). Alternatively, a less invasive procedure should be considered for masses with considerable compression.

Patients with underlying cardiac disease and patients who have had previous cardiac surgery may subsequently present for intrathoracic diagnostic or therapeutic procedures for noncardiac problems. This chapter is not a comprehensive review of anesthesia for thoracic surgery; resources for this are available in the Suggested Reading. This chapter presents the essential perioperative management considerations for patients with cardiac diseases who require noncardiac thoracic surgery.

ANESTHETIC MANAGEMENT FOR PULMONARY RESECTION IN PATIENTS WITH CARDIAC DISEASE

Coronary Artery Disease

Because smoking is prevalent among patients presenting for thoracic surgery, these patients are also at risk for having cardiovascular disease, including coronary and peripheral vascular disease. In particular, patients with coronary disease need to be optimized medically before proceeding with surgery. These patients may have atherosclerosis and hypertension and may be taking β-blockers and statins, which should be continued through the perioperative period, including the day of surgery. Statin use has been shown to reduce perioperative cardiovascular risk in patients undergoing vascular surgery.

Patients with coronary disease may also be taking aspirin unless contraindicated. If a coronary stent has been placed, aspirin is generally required for lifetime use. Most coronary stents currently being placed are drug eluting and necessitate taking another antiplatelet drug such as clopidogrel, which also may need to be continued for 1 year. Typically, clopidogrel is stopped at least 5 days before surgery and preferably 7 days to allow for placement of neuraxial analgesia. Aspirin should be continued both preoperatively and postoperatively and especially needs to be continued if the stent has been recently placed. American College of Cardiology guidelines suggest that, if possible, surgery should be delayed for 1 year after a drug-eluting stent placement. This delay is not likely to be feasible in the presence of a possible lung cancer, which could spread during a prolonged delay. However, some studies have upheld the 6-week delay after bare-metal stents but suggested the risks after drug-eluting stents are minimal after 6 months (Fig. 14.1). The risk of the stent thrombosing perioperatively

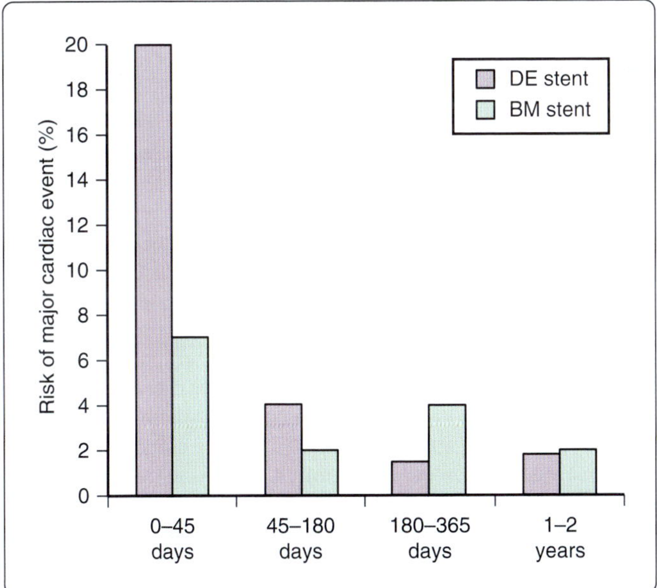

Fig. 14.1 Risk of major 30-day postoperative cardiac events after elective noncardiac surgery in more than 2000 patients after coronary artery stents. The risks after bare-metal (BM) stents become minimal after 6 weeks and after 6 months for drug-eluting (DE) stents. (Data from Wijeysundera ND, Wijeysundera HC, Wasowicz M, et al. Risk of elective major noncardiac surgery after coronary stent insertion. *Circulation*. 2012:126:1355.)

would generally outweigh the additional risk of bleeding with continuing aspirin therapy. A recent large prospective study of slightly more than 10,000 patients did show that continuing aspirin perioperatively increased bleeding risk without impacting cardiovascular risk. However, that study excluded patients with drug-eluting stents placed within 1 year.

Intraoperatively, avoiding excessive myocardial oxygen demand, which could cause myocardial ischemia, is important. Elevated heart rate can be controlled with β-blockade. The short-acting β-blocker esmolol may be useful to acutely control the tachycardia and hypertension that may result from sympathetic stimulation during laryngoscopy, intraoperative stimulation, and emergence from general anesthesia. The placement of a double-lumen tube (DLT) may be more difficult than placement of a single-lumen tube (SLT), and prolonged laryngoscopy is more likely to cause sympathetic stimulation. Nitroglycerin can also be useful to treat hypertension in these situations and can be used together with esmolol, especially if the heart rate is high and hypertension persists. Nitroglycerin can provide both venodilation and dilation of coronary arteries.

In addition to demand-related ischemia, adequate supply of oxygen to the myocardium must be maintained. A relatively low hemoglobin oxygen saturation, which may occur during one-lung ventilation (OLV), may not be tolerated in patients at risk for myocardial ischemia. The lowered oxygen blood content could contribute to the development of myocardial ischemia, which could also lead to arrhythmias. If the oxygen saturation level does drop, it may be necessary to reinstitute two-lung ventilation or add continuous positive airway pressure (CPAP) in such situations. In surgeries via thoracoscopy, it may only be possible to use a limited amount of CPAP without impairing surgical conditions.

The presence of anemia can impact both myocardial supply and demand. A lowered hemoglobin level reduces the oxygen blood content. In addition, anemia may lead to a compensatory tachycardia, increasing myocardial oxygen demand. Anemia, especially in the presence of tachycardia, will not be well tolerated, and these patients should be transfused accordingly. Patients who are treated with β-blockers intraoperatively may not tolerate anemia well.

Recovering from a thoracotomy incision would be accompanied by more pain than from a thoracoscopy. The pain causes sympathetic stimulation and increases myocardial demand. Effective postoperative pain control is especially important in such patients, and an epidural or paravertebral catheter is recommended if possible. Advanced planning is needed in the case of a patient taking clopidogrel, such that it is discontinued 1 week in advance, as per the guidelines of the American Society of Regional Anesthesia. Otherwise, the surgery will either need to be postponed or performed without the benefit of an epidural or paravertebral catheter, which might increase the perioperative pulmonary risk in patients with severe lung disease.

Patients with smoking history and significant coronary disease may have experienced prior myocardial infarction and have resulting cardiomyopathy. Such patients may have an internal cardioverter-defibrillator, which will require a perioperative management strategy. A high inspired oxygen concentration is needed to help tolerate OLV without hypoxemia, limiting the ability to use nitrous oxide (N_2O_2). Most commonly, potent inhaled agents are used, although the use of more than 1 minimum alveolar concentration (MAC) may interfere with hypoxic pulmonary vasoconstriction (HPV). Patients with a low left ventricular (LV) ejection fraction may not tolerate the myocardial depressant effects of higher doses of the potent inhaled agents. The concomitant intraoperative use of remifentanil can provide analgesia without vasodilation or myocardial depression and will facilitate a rapid emergence after surgery without prolonged respiratory depression. Its use may allow for a reduction in the amount

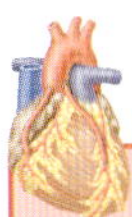

of potent inhaled agent. Although higher amounts of the potent inhaled agents can inhibit HPV, the use of sevoflurane has been shown to reduce the level of inflammatory mediators during thoracic surgery compared with propofol and remifentanil. It may be necessary to infuse a vasopressor concomitantly with the anesthetic agents to maintain an adequate perfusion pressure. If the cardiomyopathy is severe, it may be prudent to place a central venous catheter to provide central access for the administration of medications such as norepinephrine or phenylephrine. Strategies to manage patients with coronary artery disease are summarized in Box 14.1.

Valvular Heart Disease

Patients with coexisting valvular disease also need special consideration when presenting for thoracic surgery. Patients with aortic stenosis, in particular, need maintenance of cardiac preload, systemic vascular resistance (SVR), and myocardial contractility. Such patients may not tolerate higher amounts of potent inhaled agents because of vasodilation and myocardial depression. Patients with aortic stenosis are likely to have compensatory concentric LV hypertrophy and diastolic dysfunction. Patients undergoing thoracic surgery are prone to atrial arrhythmias, especially if there is a thoracotomy incision. Patients with aortic stenosis and ventricular hypertrophy are likely to poorly tolerate such arrhythmias because of an increased dependence on the atrial contraction for ventricular filling. The sympathetic block and vasodilation associated with epidural analgesia may also not be well tolerated. A dilute concentration of local anesthesia should be used, such as 0.1% bupivacaine, and the epidural should be activated gradually. In addition to maintaining adequate hydration and avoiding excessive myocardial depression and vasodilation, it may be necessary to also infuse a vasoconstrictor during the general anesthetic. The addition of intravenous (IV) remifentanil may be a beneficial adjunct to provide analgesia without myocardial depression or vasodilation.

In the case of a subvalvular outflow tract obstruction, the intraoperative management would differ from that with valvular aortic stenosis. A subvalvular outflow tract obstruction may occur with hypertrophic cardiomyopathy. If there is a significant pressure gradient, it is important to avoid increases in myocardial contractility; β-blockade may be useful in this situation. It is particularly important to maintain adequate preload and afterload to avoid outflow tract obstruction and systolic anterior motion of the mitral valve with its associated mitral regurgitation. As with aortic stenosis and associated ventricular hypertrophy, atrial arrhythmias are poorly tolerated. Patients with regurgitant valvular disease are likely to better tolerate the use of inhaled

14

potent agents because of the associated vasodilation that promotes forward flow with such disease present. It is important to also maintain adequate cardiac preload in these patients.

In the past, the placement of a pulmonary catheter would have been indicated in the presence of significant ventricular dysfunction or valvular disease for monitoring pulmonary artery pressures (PAPs) and measurement of cardiac outputs. Currently, the vast majority of thoracic operations are done without the use of this monitoring technique, which has not been shown to improve outcome. Pulmonary artery catheters (PACs) are also prone to being misused because of misinterpretation of data. The presence of severe pulmonary hypertension, however, is an indication for monitoring with a PAC to guide the administration of nitric oxide (NO) or other pulmonary vasodilators.

The use of the arterial tracing for evaluation of systolic pressure or pulse pressure variation is predictive of fluid responsiveness. A respiratory-related decrease of greater than 13% would suggest that the patient would be fluid responsive. A change of 9% to 13% has been shown to reflect an intermediate range of predictability, a gray zone in which the patient may be fluid responsive. If the systolic pressure or pulse pressure variation is less than 9%, it is unlikely that the patient would be fluid responsive. There has been some question about the usefulness of central venous pressure (CVP) to predict fluid responsiveness during anesthesia. However, in the open-chest context of thoracotomy, CVP may be more useful than the dynamic preload monitors to predict fluid responsiveness. A general goal of fluid management for thoracic surgery is to avoid excessive fluid administration and possible pulmonary edema that is more likely to occur after larger lung resections, particularly right pneumonectomy. An accurate prediction of fluid responsiveness might avoid the use of unnecessary IV fluid challenges.

Cardiomyopathies

During OLV for thoracotomy or thoracoscopy, there will be an obligate 20% to 30% shunt through the nonventilated lung. If the cardiac output also is decreased, the fall in mixed venous oxygen saturation will lead to a fall in arterial oxygen saturation. Thus patients with cardiomyopathies may tolerate OLV poorly. They need monitoring of venous saturation and inotropes to support cardiac output. This is particularly a concern in patients having video-assisted thoracoscopic (VATS) cardiac sympathectomy procedures for refractory ventricular arrhythmias. These procedures are being done with increasing frequency for ventricular tachyarrhythmias refractory to medical or ablative therapies and for long QT syndrome. The approach is by left or bilateral VATS. Intraoperative considerations include reprogramming of implanted electronic antitachycardia devices, percutaneous defibrillator pads, and provisions to optimize cardiac output and oxygenation during OLV. These patients recover slowly from episodes of desaturation during OLV, so it is best to avoid desaturation with prophylactic measures discussed later in the section on management of OLV.

Pulmonary Hypertension

Patients with pulmonary hypertension (mean pulmonary artery [PA] pressure >25 mm Hg by catheterization or systolic PAP >50 mm Hg on echocardiography) may present for a variety of noncardiac thoracic surgical procedures, including pulmonary resections for malignant or benign lesions, esophageal surgery, or vascular surgery. Compared with patients with normal pulmonary pressures, patients with pulmonary hypertension are at increased risk of respiratory complications and the need for prolonged intubation after noncardiac surgery. Much has been written about anesthesia for patients with pulmonary hypertension. The classification of pulmonary hypertension is discussed in Chapter 7, and it includes primary and secondary causes of pulmonary hypertension, including pulmonary arterial hypertension, pulmonary venoocclusive disease, left heart disease, lung disease and chronic hypoxemia, pulmonary thromboembolic disease, and a variety of autoimmune, metabolic, and systemic disorders. Anesthesiologists often encounter two main types of pulmonary hypertension: pulmonary hypertension caused by left heart disease and pulmonary hypertension caused by lung disease (Box 14.2). Most of the anesthesia literature has focused on patients with underlying cardiac disease. However, patients who present for noncardiac surgery are more likely to have pulmonary hypertension secondary to lung disease and the anesthetic management is very different for these two types of pulmonary hypertension. This section focuses on patients with pulmonary hypertension caused by lung disease. Much of what has been learned about anesthesia for patients with this type of pulmonary hypertension has come from clinical experience with pulmonary endarterectomies and lung transplantation.

Although estimates vary widely depending on disease severity and the method of measurement, the prevalence of pulmonary hypertension in severe chronic lung disease ranges from 40% to 50%. As PAP rises, evidence of cor pulmonale develops as increased strain causes the right ventricle to hypertrophy and become dysfunctional. In the United States, cor pulmonale accounts for 10% to 30% of all heart failure admissions, of which 84% are secondary to chronic obstructive pulmonary disease. The risk of right ventricular (RV) ischemia is also increased. The right ventricle is normally perfused throughout the cardiac cycle. However, the increased RV transmural and intracavitary pressures associated with pulmonary hypertension may restrict perfusion of the right coronary artery during systole, especially as PAPs approach systemic levels. Avoiding hypotension is key to managing these patients.

The impact of pulmonary hypertension on RV dysfunction has several anesthetic implications. The hemodynamic goals are similar to other conditions in which cardiac output is relatively fixed. Care should be taken to avoid physiologic states that will increase pulmonary vascular resistance (PVR) such as hypoxemia, hypercarbia, acidosis, and hypothermia. Conditions that impair RV filling, such as tachycardia and arrhythmias, are not well tolerated. Ideally, under anesthesia, RV contractility and SVR are maintained or increased, and PVR is decreased. This would ensure forward flow and

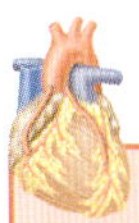

BOX 14.2 *Modified Classification of Pulmonary Hypertension for Anesthesia*

Left Heart Disease

- Systolic dysfunction
- Diastolic dysfunction
- Mitral valvular disease: stenosis, regurgitation
- Congenital cardiac disease

Lung Disease

- Pulmonary vascular disease
- Chronic lung diseases, hypoxemia, sleep apnea
- Thromboembolic pulmonary hypertension
- Miscellaneous: autoimmune, metabolic, and systemic disorders

minimize the risk of RV ischemia. In practice, these goals can be a challenge to achieve because anesthetics are commonly associated with a decrease in SVR (e.g., propofol and inhalational agents) and a variable effect on PVR.

Ketamine is a useful anesthetic agent in pulmonary hypertension caused by lung disease. Ketamine is well known for its sympathomimetic effects: ketamine increases cardiac contractility and SVR. However, its effect on PVR is controversial. Although concern is often raised over ketamine's potential to worsen pulmonary hypertension, animal and human clinical studies have suggested that in some contexts it may decrease PVR. Anecdotally, at the authors' (A.H., P.D.S.) institution, ketamine is commonly and safely used for anesthetic induction of patients with severe pulmonary hypertension. Inodilators such as dobutamine and milrinone may improve hemodynamics in patients with pulmonary hypertension secondary to left heart disease. However, they tend to cause tachycardia and decreased SVR, potentially leading to hemodynamic deterioration of patients with pulmonary hypertension caused by lung disease. To maintain a systemic blood pressure that is greater than the pulmonary artery pressure, vasopressors, such as phenylephrine or norepinephrine, are commonly used. Of the two, norepinephrine is preferable in pulmonary hypertension because it maintains cardiac index and decreases the ratio of PAP to systemic blood pressure (SBP). In contrast, phenylephrine causes the cardiac index to drop while the PAP:SBP ratio remains unchanged. Increasingly, vasopressin is also used to maintain systemic pressures. Vasopressin appears to significantly increase SBP without affecting PAP in patients with pulmonary hypertension (Fig. 14.2). In patients with severe pulmonary hypertension, selective inhaled pulmonary vasodilators, including NO (10–40 ppm) or nebulized prostaglandins (prostacyclin 50 ng/kg per minute) (Fig. 14.3), should be considered. A useful pharmacologic management strategy for the failing right ventricle in patients with pulmonary

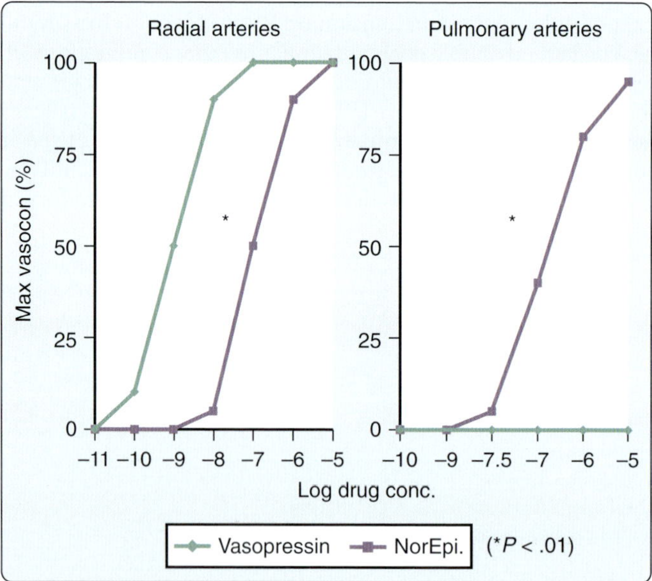

Fig. 14.2 In vitro maximal vasoconstriction dose-response curves of human radial *(left)* and pulmonary *(right)* arteries to vasopressin and norepinephrine (NorEpi.). All vasoconstrictors studied (including phenylephrine and metaraminol) showed similar dose-response patterns in both types of arteries except vasopressin, which showed no constriction of pulmonary arteries. (Data from Currigan DA, Hughes RJA, Wright CE, et al. Vasoconstrictor responses to vasopressor agents in human pulmonary and radial arteries. *Anesthesiology.* 2014;121:930–936.)

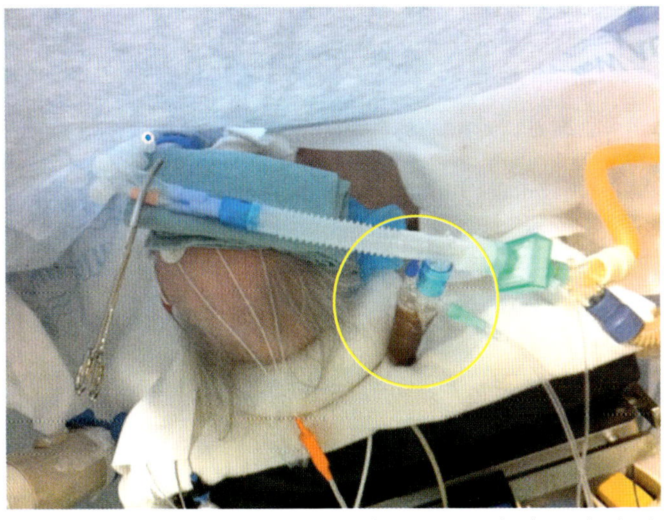

Fig. 14.3 Prostacyclin can be delivered continuously into a standard anesthetic circuit and the dose titrated as needed. In the image, prostacyclin is delivered by nebulization to the ventilated lung via a double-lumen tube during thoracic surgery and one-lung ventilation in a patient with pulmonary hypertension.

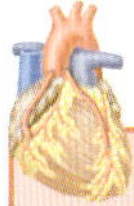

BOX 14.3	*Management Principles for Pulmonary Hypertension Secondary to Lung Disease*

1. Avoid hypotensive and vasodilating anesthetic agents whenever possible.
2. Ketamine does not exacerbate pulmonary hypertension.
3. Support mean systolic arterial pressure with vasopressors: norepinephrine, phenylephrine, vasopressin.
4. Use inhaled pulmonary vasodilators (nitric oxide, prostacyclin) in preference to IV vasodilators PRN.
5. Use thoracic epidural local anesthetics cautiously and with inotropes PRN.
6. Monitor cardiac output.

IV, Intravenous; *PRN,* as needed.

hypertension caused by lung disease is the combination of a potent IV vasoconstrictor and an inhaled pulmonary vasodilator (Box 14.3). Patients requiring inhaled NO can be weaned with oral sildenafil postoperatively.

The extremes of tidal volumes (high and low) can cause compression of the extraalveolar or interalveolar blood vessels, both of which contribute to an increased PVR. As a result, a ventilation strategy that avoids atelectasis as well as lung hyperinflation should be used.

Echocardiography is useful for diagnosis and management of patients with pulmonary hypertension. However, it should be appreciated that transthoracic echocardiographic assessments of RV systolic pressure may be ±10 mm Hg compared with catheterization measurements in more than 40% of patients, with a tendency toward underestimation. Transesophageal echocardiography (TEE) is commonly recommended for intraoperative monitoring of RV function in patients with pulmonary hypertension. Although echocardiography is extremely useful to differentiate between a normally functioning right ventricle and a dilated hypokinetic right ventricle (and this correlates with outcome in cardiac surgery), for minute-to-minute continuous objective monitoring of RV function, TEE is not yet the ideal monitor. This is because the right ventricle is a very complex nongeometric structure in three dimensions. At present, continuous monitoring of minor changes in regional RV function with standard two-dimensional TEE is, at best, difficult. Advances in echocardiography technology, particularly three-dimensional TEE, may make continuous objective monitoring of RV function possible in the future.

At present, the basis of intraoperative monitoring for patients with pulmonary hypertension having noncardiac thoracic surgery remains the PAC. However, it must be understood that PA data alone can be misleading in these patients. Rising PAPs are almost always a bad sign. Falling PAPs may be a good sign indicating pulmonary vasodilation or may be a very bad sign indicating impending RV decompensation. Thus PAP data must be followed in concert with cardiac output, mixed venous saturation, and CVP data.

Although there have been multiple case reports of the successful use of lumbar epidural analgesia and anesthesia in obstetric patients with pulmonary hypertension, there are very few reports of the use of thoracic epidural analgesia in pulmonary hypertension. Patients with pulmonary hypertension caused by lung disease seem to be extremely dependent on tonic cardiac sympathetic innervation for normal hemodynamic stability. In patients undergoing thoracotomy for lung resection, the use of a thoracic epidural impaired baseline RV contractility, but did not affect the compensatory increase in RV contractility brought on by an acute increase in RV afterload. Because of the increased risk of postoperative respiratory complications in these patients, the use of postoperative thoracic epidural analgesia is often desirable. However, it must be appreciated that these patients will often require a low-dose infusion of inotropes or vasopressors during thoracic epidural local analgesia. This may necessitate continued central venous catheterization and intensive care unit admission. Paravertebral analgesia has been associated with better postthoracotomy hemodynamic stability versus thoracic epidural analgesia in patients with normal cardiac function, but this has not been studied specifically in pulmonary hypertensive patients.

The patient populations discussed above (coronary artery disease, cardiomyopathies, and pulmonary hypertension) are those who would be considered to be at high risk for thoracic surgery by open thoracotomy, carrying an increased risk for cardiac, pulmonary, and overall complications. Traditionally, these patients may not have been considered appropriate surgical candidates as a result. However, new evidence has demonstrated the safety of VATS techniques in high-risk patients, with reduced complication rates compared with high-risk patients undergoing open thoracotomy and comparable complication rates to non–high-risk patients undergoing VATS.

LUNG ISOLATION FOR CARDIAC PATIENTS HAVING THORACIC PROCEDURES

Procedures in the thoracic cavity are greatly facilitated by the use of OLV. Procedures on the lung, esophagus, thoracic aortic, or resection of mediastinal masses frequently require a collapsed lung for a motionless surgical field and optimal surgical exposure.

The Robertshaw-type DLTs have been used in clinical practice for more than half a century and are considered the gold standard to achieve lung separation. A left 37-Fr DLT is most commonly used for women, and a 39-Fr DLT is used in the average man. The right-sided DLT is less commonly used. It has a donut-shaped bronchial cuff, allowing a right upper lobe ventilation slot to ride over the right upper lobe orifice. The Univent tube (Fuji Corp.) or independent endobronchial blockers (EBBs) were introduced to clinical practice as an alternative to the DLT. These blockers have a steering mechanism to direct them into the selected bronchus. With the Arndt blocker (Cook Medical), the fiberoptic bronchoscopy (FOB) is passed through the loop and guided into the desired mainstem bronchus. The Cohen Flexitip Endobronchial Blocker (Cook Medical) uses a flexible soft tip that can be deflected by the rotation of a wheel and the Uniblocker (Fuji Corp.) has a fixed curve like a hockey stick. The EZ-Blocker (Teleflex Medical Incorporated), recently introduced into clinical practice, is a 7.0-Fr catheter designed with two Y-shaped distal extensions that ride over the carina; each lung can be selectively deflated. Whether a DLT or EBB is used to provide lung separation, proper position should be confirmed by FOB.

The choice of the device to be used for lung isolation depends on individual experience, comfort, and patient safety. The practicing anesthesiologist should be familiar with the variety of available devices so as to select the best choice for each individual patient. Patients with significant cardiac disease and associated comorbidities who are scheduled for surgery requiring lung separation present a challenge to the anesthesiologist. These patients are highly sensitive to any hemodynamic instability and poorly tolerate any periods of hypoxemia. When selecting the best method of providing lung separation for cardiac patients undergoing surgery on the lung, there are several issues to take into consideration, detailed next.

Double-Lumen Tubes

Advantages

Whenever the nondiseased lung is potentially exposed to contamination by blood or pus from the diseased lung, the lungs must be isolated. When lung isolation is required, DLTs are preferable to EBBs because they provide a superior protective seal to prevent contamination of the unaffected lung. The use of EBBs is not recommended for these indications because the low pressure and high volume of the EBB cuff usually cannot provide a complete seal. Second, DLTs are preferred for bilateral procedures such as bilateral lung transplantation, bilateral sympathectomy, and bilateral lung wedge resection. When in place, they minimize the manipulation and resulting hemodynamic response. DLTs are more stable after being positioned and have less tendency to dislocate during surgical manipulation and patient positioning. This is important in patients with cardiac disease in whom any irritation of the tracheobronchial tree can induce tachycardia, hypertension, and ischemia. In addition, it is easier to suction thick secretions or blood clots through the lumen of the DLT. Aggressive pulmonary toilet is particularly crucial in cardiac patients. Finally, most anesthesiologists and surgeons are familiar with DLTs and are comfortable managing them.

Disadvantages

DIFFICULT INTUBATION

Double-lumen tubes are somewhat bulky and may be more difficult to insert and position compared to SLTs. It may be challenging to switch from a DLT to an SLT and vice versa if the patients require postoperative ventilatory support. The use of tube exchange catheters may trigger a cardiovascular response, which can be detrimental to patients with cardiac disease. Tracheal intubation causes a stress response, resulting in increased sympathetic activity that may result in hypertension, tachycardia, and arrhythmias. These changes in hemodynamics can be harmful to patients with hypertension and myocardial ischemia because of inadequate perfusion of the coronary arteries.

14

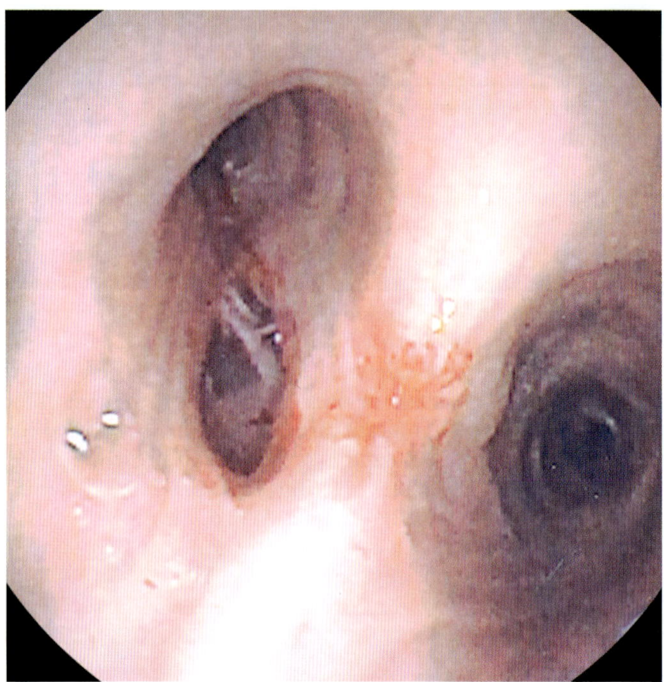

Fig. 14.4 Image taken through a fiberoptic bronchoscope of a laceration of the posterior membranous portion of the left mainstem bronchus just distal to the carina caused by a left-sided double-lumen tube.

AIRWAY INJURIES

Previous studies have found a higher incidence of postoperative sore throat; hoarseness; and in some cases, pharyngeal or bronchial tree laceration (Fig. 14.4) associated with DLT use. Use of an EBB is associated with decreased postoperative hoarseness and fewer days with a sore throat compared with a DLT. Moreover, the blocker technique was associated with a decreased incidence of vocal cord injuries. Any added injury to patients with cardiac disease, who are often on anticoagulant therapy for cardiac stents or arrhythmia, can add a significant increased risk of complications and prolong recovery.

Endobronchial Blockers for Lung Separation

Endobronchial blockers can be placed to achieve lung separation and may offer several advantages to patients with cardiac disease. The most significant advantage is the decrease in hemodynamic stress. Because the EBB is inserted through an SLT, it is less stimulating than the insertion and manipulation of a DLT. EBBs can be advantageous in patients with difficult airways or abnormal tracheobronchial trees. In addition, patients with tracheostomies or those who require a nasal intubation are often managed with EBBs. Finally, some patients arrive from the intensive care unit to the operating room (OR) with endotracheal tubes (ETTs) in place; insertion of an EBB would be the best option to avoid changing of the existing SLT.

350

Lung Separation in Thoracic Aortic Aneurysm Surgery

Because of the close anatomic relationship, a thoracic aortic aneurysm can potentially compress the airway at the level of the trachea or, more often, left mainstem bronchus (LMB). Patients who present with a descending thoracic aortic aneurysm and LMB compression who require lung isolation should be managed with a right-sided DLT (Fig. 14.5). Placement of a left-sided DLT is both difficult and dangerous in these patients, presenting the risk of airway trauma and rupture of the aneurysm. A DLT in a descending thoracic aortic aneurysm repair improves surgical exposure and makes it easier to remove blood and secretions. The use of EBBs for thoracic aneurysm repair should be limited to situations in which intubation or endobronchial placement of a DLT is difficult.

Lung Separation for Esophageal Surgery

In the United States, 17,000 new patients are diagnosed each year with esophageal cancer, and 15,000 die from the disease. The most common type of esophageal cancer is squamous cell carcinoma, usually in sicker patients with history of heavy smoking and alcohol abuse, who may be physically debilitated, with chronic obstructive pulmonary disease (COPD) and poor lung function. Adenocarcinoma is usually found in patients with gastroesophageal reflux disease.

There are three techniques of surgical approach for esophageal resection: (1) Ivor Lewis esophagectomy: abdominal incision followed by open right thoracotomy with an

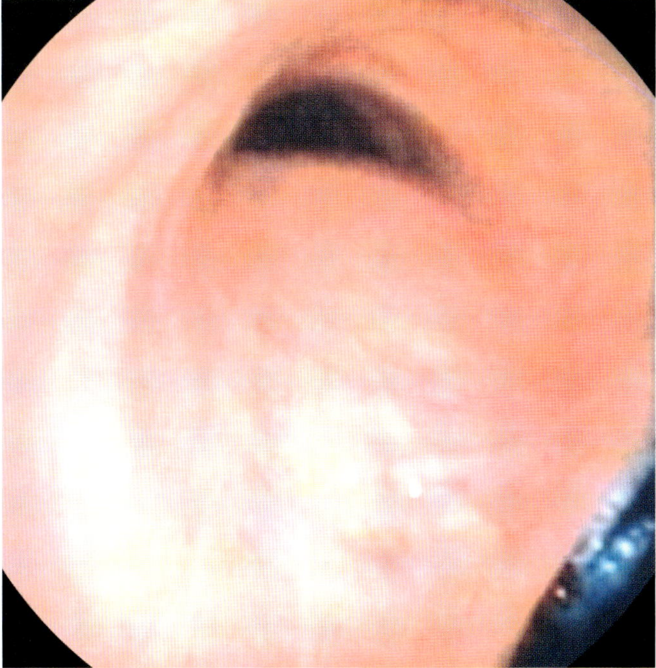

Fig. 14.5 Image taken through a fiberoptic bronchoscope of a posterior compression of the left mainstem bronchus caused by an aneurysm of the descending thoracic aorta.

anastomosis located in the upper chest; (2) transhiatal esophagectomy: the esophageal tumor is removed through an abdominal incision without thoracotomy in which the stomach is pulled posterior to the sternum to perform an anastomosis in the left neck; and (3) minimally invasive esophagectomy: both the abdominal and the thoracic procedures are performed through laparoscopy and thoracoscopy, respectively.

For procedures in which the surgeon has to perform dissections in the right hemithorax, OLV can be provided either by a DLT or by independent EBB. There are several reasons to prefer EBBs for these procedures. Aspiration is a major concern in these patients. Residual food may be present proximal to the obstruction or previous radiation therapy may compromise esophageal function. A rapid-sequence or awake intubation is recommended, and securing the airway with an SLT followed by placement of an EBB is the safest approach. These procedures can be lengthy and with significant amounts of fluid administration, which may cause airway edema. If the patient requires postoperative respiratory support, changing the DLT to an SLT carries the risk of losing control of the airway and should be performed with the help of tube exchange catheters and videolaryngoscopy. Regardless of which device is used, ultimately, the level of familiarity and comfort of the anesthesiologist and surgeon dictate the best management of the patient.

MANAGEMENT OF ONE-LUNG VENTILATION

During OLV, the anesthesiologist has the unique and often conflicting goals of trying to maximize atelectasis in the nonventilated lung to improve surgical access while trying to avoid atelectasis in the ventilated lung (usually the dependent lung) to optimize gas exchange. This can be particularly challenging in patients with underlying cardiac disease. The gas mixture in the nonventilated lung immediately before OLV has a significant effect on the speed of collapse of this lung. Because of its low blood-gas solubility, nitrogen (or an air-oxygen mixture) will delay collapse of this lung. This is a problem at the start of minimally invasive surgery when surgical visualization in the operative hemithorax is limited. It is important to thoroughly denitrogenate the operative lung by ventilating with oxygen immediately before it is allowed to collapse.

During the period of two-lung anesthesia before the start of OLV, atelectasis will develop in the dependent lung. It is useful to perform a recruitment maneuver of the dependent lung (similar to a Valsalva maneuver), holding the lung at an end-inspiratory pressure of 20 cm H_2O for 15 to 20 seconds immediately after the start of OLV to decrease this atelectasis. Recruitment is important to maintain PaO_2 levels during subsequent OLV.

Hypoxemia

A major concern that influences anesthetic management for thoracic surgery is the occurrence of hypoxemia during OLV. There is no universally acceptable value for the safest lower limit of oxygen saturation during OLV. An arterial oxygen saturation of 90% (PaO_2 ~60 mm Hg) is commonly seen as the lowest acceptable limit. However, the lowest acceptable saturation will be higher in patients with organs at risk of hypoxia because of limited regional blood flow (e.g., coronary or cerebrovascular disease) and in patients with limited oxygen transport (e.g., anemia or decreased cardiopulmonary reserve). It has been shown that during OLV, patients with COPD desaturate more quickly during isovolemic hemodilution than normal patients.

Previously, hypoxemia occurred frequently during OLV. Reports from 1950 to 1980 described an incidence of hypoxemia (arterial saturation <90%) of 20% to 25%.

Current reports describe an incidence of less than 5%. This improvement is most likely due to several factors: improved lung isolation techniques such as routine FOB to prevent lobar obstruction from DLTs, improved anesthetic agents that cause less inhibition of HPV, and better understanding of the pathophysiology of OLV. The pathophysiology of OLV involves the body's ability to redistribute pulmonary blood flow to the ventilated lung. The anesthesiologist's goal during OLV is to maximize PVR in the nonventilated lung while minimizing PVR in the ventilated lung. Key to understanding this physiology is the appreciation that PVR is correlated with lung volume in a hyperbolic fashion. PVR is lowest at functional residual capacity (FRC) and increases as lung volume rises or falls above or below FRC. The anesthesiologist's aim, to optimize pulmonary blood flow redistribution during OLV, is to maintain the ventilated lung as close as possible to its FRC while facilitating collapse of the nonventilated lung to increase its PVR.

Most thoracic surgery is performed in the lateral position. Patients having OLV in the lateral position have significantly better PaO_2 levels than patients during OLV in the supine position because of gravitational enhancement of blood flow to the dependent, ventilated lung. This applies both to patients with normal lung function and to those with COPD.

Hypoxic Pulmonary Vasoconstriction

Hypoxic pulmonary vasoconstriction can decrease the blood flow to the nonventilated lung by as much as 50%. The stimulus for HPV is primarily the alveolar oxygen tension (PAO_2), which stimulates precapillary vasoconstriction redistributing pulmonary blood flow away from hypoxemic lung regions via a pathway involving NO or cyclooxygenase synthesis inhibition. The mixed venous PO_2 (P_vO_2) is also a stimulus, although it is considerably weaker than PAO_2. HPV has a biphasic temporal response to alveolar hypoxia. The rapid-onset phase begins immediately and reaches a plateau by 20 to 30 minutes. The second (delayed) phase begins after 40 minutes and plateaus after several hours. The offset of HPV is also biphasic, and PVR may not return to baseline for several hours after a prolonged period of OLV. This may contribute to increased desaturation during the collapse of the second lung during bilateral thoracic procedures. HPV also has a preconditioning effect, and the response to a second hypoxic challenge will be greater than to the first challenge.

The surgical trauma to the lung can affect pulmonary blood flow redistribution. Surgery may oppose HPV by the release of vasoactive metabolites locally in the lung. Conversely, surgery can dramatically decrease blood flow to the nonventilated lung by deliberately or accidentally mechanically interfering with either the unilateral pulmonary arterial or venous blood flow. Ventilation increases blood flow through a hypoxic lung more than in a normoxic lung, which is generally not of clinical relevance but does complicate studies of HPV. HPV is decreased by vasodilators such as nitroglycerin and nitroprusside. In general, vasodilators can be expected to cause a deterioration in P_aO_2 during OLV. Thoracic epidural sympathetic blockade probably has little or no direct effect on HPV, which is a localized chemical response in the lung. However, thoracic epidural anesthesia can have an indirect effect on oxygenation during OLV if it is allowed to cause hypotension and a fall in cardiac output.

Choice of Anesthetic

All the volatile anesthetics inhibit HPV in a dose-dependent fashion. The older volatile agents were potent inhibitors of HPV, which may have contributed to the high incidence

14

of hypoxemia reported during OLV in the 1960s and 1970s; many of these studies used 2- to 3-MAC doses of halothane.

In doses of 1 MAC or less, the modern volatile anesthetics (isoflurane, sevoflurane, and desflurane) are weak and equipotent inhibitors of HPV. The inhibition of the HPV response by 1 MAC of a volatile agent such as isoflurane is approximately 20% of the total HPV response, and this could account for only a net 4% increase in total arteriovenous shunt during OLV, which is a difference too small to be detected in most clinical studies. In addition, volatile anesthetics cause less inhibition of HPV when delivered to the active site of vasoconstriction via the pulmonary arterial blood than via the alveolus. This pattern is similar to the HPV stimulus characteristics of oxygen. During established OLV, the volatile agent only reaches the hypoxic lung pulmonary capillaries via the mixed venous blood. No clinical benefit in oxygenation during OLV has been shown for total IV anesthesia above that seen with 1 MAC of the modern volatile anesthetics.

The use of nitrous oxide–oxygen (N_2O–O_2) mixtures is associated with a higher incidence of postthoracotomy radiographic atelectasis (51%) in the dependent lung than when air–oxygen mixtures are used (24%). N_2O also tends to increase PAPs in patients who have pulmonary hypertension, and N_2O inhibits HPV. For these reasons, N_2O is usually avoided during thoracic anesthesia.

Cardiac Output

The effects of alterations of cardiac output during OLV are complex. Increasing cardiac output tends to cause increased PAPs and passive dilation of the pulmonary vascular bed, which in turn opposes HPV and has been shown to be associated with increased arteriovenous shunt (Qs/Qt) during OLV. However, in patients with a relatively fixed oxygen consumption, as is seen during stable anesthesia, the effect of an increase in cardiac output is to increase the mixed venous oxygen saturation (S_vO_2). Thus increasing cardiac output during OLV tends to increase both shunt and S_vO_2, which have opposing effects on PaO_2. There is a ceiling effect to the amount that S_vO_2 can be increased. Increasing the cardiac output to supranormal levels by administering inotropes such as dopamine tends to have an overall negative effect on PaO_2. Conversely, allowing the cardiac output to fall will lead to falls in both shunt and S_vO_2 with a net effect of decreasing PaO_2. It is very important to maintain cardiac output in patients with limited cardiac reserve.

Ventilation Strategies During One-Lung Ventilation

The strategy used to manage the ventilated lung during OLV plays an important part in the distribution of pulmonary blood flow between the lungs. It has been the practice of many anesthesiologists to use the same large tidal volume (e.g., 10 mL/kg ideal body weight) during OLV as during two-lung ventilation. This strategy decreases hypoxemia, probably by recurrently recruiting atelectatic regions in the dependent lung, and may result in higher PaO_2 values during OLV when compared with smaller tidal volumes. However, there is a trend to use smaller tidal volumes with positive end-expiratory pressure (PEEP) during OLV for several reasons. First, the incidence of hypoxemia during OLV is much lower than 20 to 30 years ago. Second, there is a risk of causing acute injury to the ventilated lung with prolonged use of large tidal volumes. And third, a ventilation pattern that allows cyclic atelectasis and recruitment of lung parenchyma seems to be injurious. The ventilation technique needs to be individualized depending on the patient's underlying lung mechanics.

Respiratory Acid-Base Status

The efficacy of HPV in a hypoxic lung region is increased in the presence of respiratory acidosis and is inhibited by respiratory alkalosis. However, there is no net benefit to gas exchange during OLV from hypoventilation because the respiratory acidosis preferentially increases the pulmonary vascular tone of the well-oxygenated lung, and this opposes any clinically useful pulmonary blood flow redistribution. Overall, the effects of hyperventilation usually tend to decrease pulmonary vascular pressures.

Positive End-Expiratory Pressure

Resistance to blood flow through the lung is related to lung volume in a biphasic pattern and is lowest when the lung is at its FRC. Keeping the ventilated lung as close as possible to its normal FRC using modest amounts of PEEP favorably encourages pulmonary blood flow to this lung. Several intraoperative factors that are known to alter FRC tend to cause the FRC of the ventilated lung to fall below its normal level; these include lateral position, paralysis, and opening the nondependent hemithorax, which allows the weight of the mediastinum to compress the dependent lung. Attempts to measure FRC in human patients during OLV have been complicated by the presence of a persistent end-expiratory airflow in COPD patients. Many patients do not actually reach their end-expiratory equilibrium FRC lung volume as they try to exhale a relatively large tidal volume through one lumen of a DLT. These patients develop dynamic hyperinflation and an occult positive end-expiratory pressure (auto-PEEP).

Auto-PEEP

Auto-PEEP (also called intrinsic PEEP) is most prone to occur in patients with decreased lung elastic recoil such as older adults and those with emphysema. Auto-PEEP increases as the inspiratory/expiratory (I:E) ratio increases (i.e., as the time of expiration decreases). This auto-PEEP, which averages 4 to 6 cm H_2O in most series of lung cancer patients studied, opposes the previously mentioned factors, which tend to diminish dependent-lung FRC during OLV. The effects of applying external PEEP through the ventilator circuit to the lung in the presence of auto-PEEP are complex. Patients with a very low auto-PEEP (<2 cm H_2O) will experience a greater increase in total PEEP from a moderate (5 cm H_2O) external PEEP than those with a high level of auto PEEP (>10 cm H_2O). Whether the application of PEEP during OLV will improve a patient's gas exchange depends on the individual's lung mechanics. If the application of PEEP tends to shift the expiratory equilibration position on the compliance curve towards the lower inflection point (LIP) of the curve (i.e., toward the FRC), then external PEEP is of benefit (Fig. 14.6). However, if the application of PEEP raises the equilibration point such that it is further from the LIP, then gas exchange deteriorates.

Auto-PEEP is difficult to detect and measure using currently available anesthetic ventilators. To detect auto-PEEP, the respiratory circuit must be held closed at the end of a normal expiration until an equilibrium appears in the airway pressure. Most current intensive care ventilators can be used to accurately measure auto-PEEP, but most anesthesia ventilators cannot.

Tidal Volume

There will be an optimal combination of tidal volume, respiratory rate, I:E ratio, and pressure- or volume-control ventilation for each individual patient undergoing OLV.

14

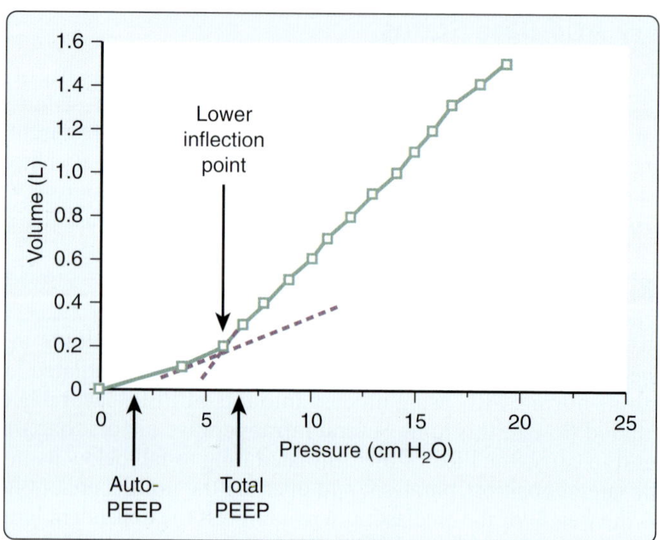

Fig. 14.6 Inspiratory static compliance curve of a young patient with normal pulmonary function during one-lung ventilation (OLV) (in this case for removal of a mediastinal tumor). The lower inflection point of the curve (functional residual capacity) was at 6 cm H_2O. The patient had 2 cm H_2O occult positive end-expiratory pressure (auto-PEEP) during OLV. Adding 5 cm H_2O PEEP to the ventilator raised the total PEEP to 7 cm H_2O and improved PaO_2. Young patients and patients with increased lung elastic recoil (e.g., because of restrictive lung diseases) have an increase in PaO_2 from PEEP during OLV. (Data from Slinger P, Kruger M, McRae K, Winton T. Relation of the static compliance curve and positive end-expiratory pressure to oxygenation during one-lung ventilation. *Anesthesiology.* 2001;95:1096.)

However, to try to assess each of these parameters while still providing anesthesia with the available anesthetic ventilators is not practical, and the clinician must initially rely on a simplified strategy (Table 14.1). The results of alterations in tidal volume are unpredictable. This may be due in part to the interaction of tidal volume with auto-PEEP. The use of 5 to 6 mL/kg ideal body weight tidal volumes plus 5 cm H_2O PEEP initially for most patients (except those with COPD) seems a logical starting point during OLV. Tidal volume should be managed so that peak airway pressures do not exceed 35 cm H_2O. This will correspond to a plateau airway pressure of approximately 25 cm H_2O. Peak airway pressures exceeding 40 cm H_2O may contribute to hyperinflation injury of the ventilated lung during OLV. Turning the patient to the lateral position will increase respiratory dead space and the arterial to end-tidal CO_2 tension gradient ($Pa_{ET}CO_2$). This usually requires a 20% increase in minute ventilation to maintain the same $PaCO_2$. Individual variations in $Pa_{ET}CO_2$ gradient become much larger and $P_{ET}CO_2$ is less reliable as a monitor of $PaCO_2$ during OLV. This effect is possibly because there are differences in the excretion of CO_2 between the dependent and nondependent lungs.

Volume-Controlled Versus Pressure-Controlled Ventilation

Traditionally, volume-controlled ventilation has been used in the OR for all types of surgery. The recent availability of anesthesia ventilators with pressure-control modes has made it possible to study and use this form of ventilation during thoracic surgery. Pressure-controlled ventilation has not been shown to improve oxygenation versus

Table 14.1 Suggested Ventilation Parameters for One-Lung Ventilation

Parameter	Suggested	Guidelines/ Exceptions
Tidal volume	5–6 mL/kg	Maintain: Peak airway pressure <35 cm H_2O Plateau airway pressure <25 cm H_2O
Positive end-expiratory pressure	5 cm H_2O	Patients with COPD: no added PEEP
Respiratory rate	12 breaths/min	Tolerate mild hypercapnia $PaCO_2$ (<60 mm Hg); $P_{a\text{-}ET}CO_2$ will usually increase 1–3 mm Hg during OLV
Mode	Volume or pressure controlled	Pressure control for patients at risk of lung injury (e.g., bullae, pneumonectomy, after lung transplantation)
F_IO_2	Initially 1.0	Decrease as tolerated with air to maintain acceptable SpO_2

COPD, Chronic obstructive pulmonary disease; *OLV,* one-lung ventilation; F_IO_2, fraction of inspired oxygen; $P_{a\text{-}ET}CO_2$, arterial to end-tidal CO_2 tension gradient; *PEEP,* positive end-expiratory pressure; SpO_2, functional oxygen saturation.

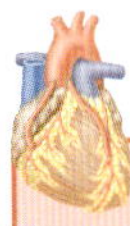

BOX 14.4 *Factors That Correlate With an Increased Risk of Desaturation During One-Lung Ventilation*

1. High percentage of ventilation or perfusion to the operative lung on preoperative V/Q scan
2. Poor PaO_2 during two-lung ventilation, particularly in the lateral position intraoperatively.
3. Right-sided thoracotomy.
4. Normal preoperative spirometry (FEV_1 or FVC) or restrictive lung disease.
5. Supine position during one-lung ventilation

FEV₁, Forced expiratory volume in 1 second; *FVC,* forced vital capacity; *V/Q,* ventilation/perfusion.

---

volume-controlled ventilation for most patients, although the peak airway pressures are lower. The decrease in peak pressure with pressure-controlled ventilation may be largely in the anesthetic circuit and not at the distal airway. Pressure-controlled ventilation will avoid sudden increases in peak airway pressures that may result from surgical manipulation in the chest. This will be of benefit in patients at increased risk for lung injury from high volumes or pressures such as after lung transplantation or during a pneumonectomy. Because of the rapid changes of lung compliance that occur during pulmonary surgery, when pressure-controlled ventilation is used, the delivered tidal volume needs to be closely monitored as this may change suddenly.

Prediction of Hypoxemia During One-Lung Ventilation

The problem of hypoxemia during OLV has prompted much research in thoracic anesthesia. Hypoxemia during OLV is predictable (Box 14.4), preventable, and treatable in the vast majority of cases.

Preoperative Ventilation/Perfusion Scan

The shunt and P_aO_2 during intraoperative OLV are highly correlated with the fractional perfusion of the ventilated lung as determined by a preoperative ventilation/perfusion (V/Q) scan. Patients with long-standing unilateral disease on the operative side develop a unilateral decrease of ventilation and perfusion and tolerate OLV very well. Similarly, patients who intraoperatively have a higher proportion of gas exchange in the dependent lung during OLV tend to have better oxygenation during OLV.

Side of Operation

Patients having right-sided thoracotomies tend to have a larger shunt and lower PaO_2 during OLV because the right lung is larger and normally receives 10% more blood flow than the left. The overall mean PaO_2 difference between left and right thoracotomies during stable OLV is approximately 100 mm Hg.

Two-Lung Oxygenation

Patients who have better PaO_2 levels during two-lung ventilation in the lateral position tend to have better oxygenation during OLV. These patients may have better abilities to match ventilation and perfusion (individual variability of HPV response), or they may have less atelectasis in the dependent lung. This is a particularly relevant consideration in trauma patients who may require a thoracotomy but have a contusion of the dependent lung.

Preoperative Spirometry

Studies consistently show that when the previous factors are controlled, patients with better spirometric lung function preoperatively are more likely to desaturate and have lower PaO_2 values during OLV. Clinically, this is evident because patients with emphysematous lung volume reduction generally tolerate OLV very well. The explanation is not clear but may be related to maintenance of a more favorable FRC in patients with obstructive airways disease during OLV with an open hemithorax because of the development of auto-PEEP.

Treatment of Hypoxemia During One-Lung Ventilation

During OLV, there is a decrease in arterial oxygenation that usually reaches its nadir 20 to 30 minutes after the initiation of OLV. The O_2 saturation then stabilizes or rises slightly as HPV increases over the next 2 hours. The majority of patients who desaturate do so quickly and within the first 10 minutes of OLV. Hypoxemia during OLV responds readily to treatment in the vast majority of cases. Potential therapies are outlined in Box 14.5 and are as follows:

1. Resume two-lung ventilation. Reinflate the nonventilated lung and deflate the bronchial cuff of the DLT or the bronchial blocker. This will necessitate interruption of surgery but is necessary in case of severe or precipitous desaturation. After an adequate level of oxygenation is obtained, the diagnosis of the cause of desaturation can be made and prophylactic measures instituted before another trial of OLV is attempted.
2. Increase fraction of inspired oxygen (F_IO_2). Ensure that the delivered F_IO_2 is 1.0. This is an option in essentially all patients except those who have received bleomycin or similar therapies that potentiate pulmonary oxygen toxicity.

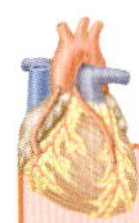

BOX 14.5   *Therapies for Desaturation During One-Lung Ventilation*

A. Severe or precipitous desaturation: Resume two-lung ventilation (if possible).
B. Gradual desaturation:
1. Ensure that delivered F_1O_2 is 1.0.
2. Check position of double-lumen tube or blocker with FOB.
3. Ensure that cardiac output is optimal; decrease volatile anesthetics to <1 MAC.
4. Apply a recruitment maneuver to the ventilated lung (this will transiently make the hypoxemia worse).
5. Apply PEEP 5 cm H_2O to the ventilated lung (except in patients with emphysematous pathology).
6. Apply CPAP 1–2 cm H_2O to the nonventilated lung (apply a recruitment maneuver to this lung immediately before CPAP).
7. Intermittent reinflation of the nonventilated lung.
8. Partial ventilation techniques of the nonventilated lung:
   a. Lung oxygen insufflation
   b. Lobar insufflation
   c. Lobar collapse (using a bronchial blocker)
9. Mechanical restriction of the blood flow to the nonventilated lung.

CPAP, Continuous positive airway pressure; *F_1O_2,* fraction of inspired oxygen; *FOB,* fiberoptic bronchoscopy; *MAC,* minimum alveolar concentration; *PEEP,* positive end-expiratory pressure.

3. Recheck the position of the DLT or bronchial blocker with FOB. Ensure that there is no lobar obstruction in the ventilated lung.
4. Check the patient's hemodynamics to ensure that there has been no decrease in cardiac output. It is very common for the surgeon to accidentally compress the inferior vena cava during pulmonary resections, and the fall in blood pressure and cardiac output that this causes leads to rapid desaturation during OLV. Treat the fall in cardiac output as indicated (e.g., inotropes or vasopressors if caused by thoracic epidural sympathetic blockade). Stop administration of vasodilators and decrease MAC of volatile anesthetics to less than 1 MAC.
5. Perform a recruitment maneuver of the ventilated lung. To eliminate any atelectasis, inflate the lung to 20 cm H_2O or more for 15 to 20 seconds. This may cause transient hypotension and will also cause a transient further fall in the PaO_2 as the blood flow is temporarily redistributed to the nonventilated lung.
6. Apply PEEP to the ventilated lung. It is necessary to perform a recruitment maneuver before applying PEEP to get the maximal benefit. PEEP will raise the end-expiratory volume of the ventilated lung toward the FRC in patients with normal lung mechanics and in those with increased elastic recoil because of restrictive disease. It is not possible to predict the optimal PEEP for individual patients, but a level of 5 cm H_2O is a useful starting point. PEEP will increase the end-expiratory lung volume of patients with significant levels of auto-PEEP (e.g., patients with emphysema). Unlike CPAP, application of PEEP does not require reinflation of the nonventilated lung and interruption of surgery. PEEP has been shown to be as effective for increasing PaO_2 levels during OLV in patients with normal lung function as CPAP to the nonventilated lung (Fig. 14.7). For patients with normal pulmonary function, it is logical to routinely apply a recruitment maneuver and PEEP from the start of OLV.

14

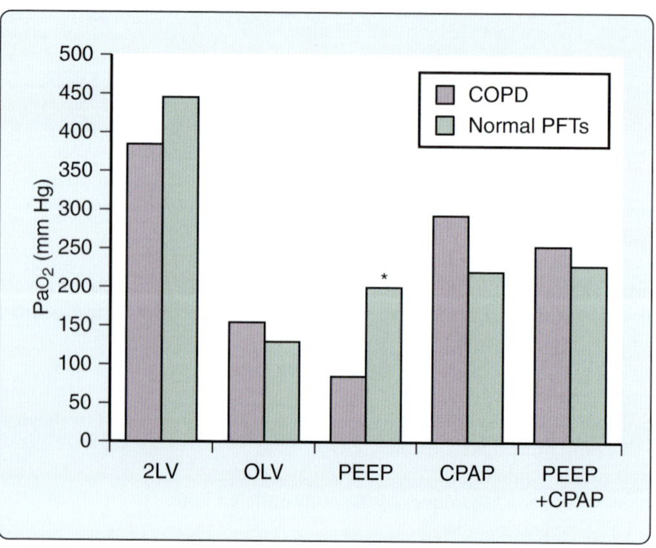

Fig. 14.7 Comparison of the effects of positive end-expiratory pressure (PEEP) to the ventilated lung and continuous positive airway pressure (CPAP) to the nonventilated lung on mean PaO_2 levels during one-lung ventilation (OLV). *COPD,* chronic obstructive pulmonary disease: a group of lung cancer surgery patients; normal *PFTs,* pulmonary function tests: a group of esophageal surgery patients with normal preoperative PFTs; *2LV,* two-lung ventilation. $*P < .05$ vs. OLV. (Data from Fujiwara M, Abe K, Mashimo T. The effect of positive end-expiratory pressure and continuous positive airway pressure on the oxygenation and shunt fraction during one-lung ventilation with propofol anesthesia. *J Clin Anesth.* 2001;13:473; and Capan LM, Turndorf H, Patel C, et al. Optimization of arterial oxygenation during one-lung anesthesia. *Anesth Analg.* 1980;59:847.)

7. CPAP with oxygen to the nonventilated lung is the next line of therapy after application of PEEP. There is an important caveat to be observed when CPAP is applied to the nonventilated lung, and that is that CPAP must be applied to an inflated (recruited) lung to be completely effective. The opening pressure of atelectatic lung regions is greater than 20 cm H_2O, and these units will not be recruited by simple application of CPAP levels of 5 to 10 cm H_2O. Even a period as short as 5 minutes of collapse before CPAP application can have deleterious effects on oxygenation during OLV. When CPAP is applied to a fully inflated lung, levels of CPAP as low as 1 to 2 cm H_2O can be used. Because the normal transpulmonary pressure of the lung at FRC is approximately 5 cm H_2O, levels of 5 to 10 cm H_2O CPAP applied to a fully recruited lung result in a large-volume lung that impedes surgery, particularly during minimally invasive procedures.

Continuous positive airway pressure levels less than 10 cm H_2O do not interfere with hemodynamics. The beneficial effects of low levels of CPAP are primarily caused by oxygen uptake from the nonventilated lung and not caused by blood flow diversion to the ventilated lung. CPAP is most effective when oxygen (F_iO_2 1.0) is applied to the nonventilated lung. Lower F_iO_2 levels of CPAP are of clinical benefit and can be used along with decreased F_iO_2 to the ventilated lung in patients at risk of oxygen toxicity.

Numerous anesthetic systems to apply CPAP to the nonventilated lung have been described. Essentially all that is required is a CPAP (or PEEP) valve and an oxygen source. Ideally, the circuit should permit variation of the CPAP level and include a reservoir bag to allow easy reinflation of the nonventilated lung and a manometer to measure the actual CPAP supplied. Such circuits are commercially available or can be readily constructed from standard anesthetic equipment. CPAP can be applied with either a DLT or through the suction channel of a bronchial blocker.

Continuous positive airway pressure, even when properly administered, is not completely reliable to improve oxygenation during OLV. When the bronchus of the operative lung is obstructed or open to atmosphere (as in a bronchopleural fistula or during endobronchial surgery), CPAP will not improve oxygenation. Also, in certain situations, particularly during thoracoscopic surgery, access to the operative hemithorax is limited and CPAP can significantly interfere with surgery.

Pharmacologic Manipulations

Eliminating known potent vasodilators, such as nitroglycerin, halothane, and large doses of other volatile anesthetics, will improve oxygenation during OLV. Selective administration of NO alone to the ventilated lung has not been shown to be of benefit in humans. The combination of inhaled NO (20 ppm) and an IV infusion of almitrine, which enhances HPV, has been shown to restore P_aO_2 values during OLV in humans to essentially the same levels as during two-lung ventilation. However, this may have been due primarily to the augmentation of HPV by almitrine. It is unlikely that almitrine, which was previously available in North America as a respiratory stimulant, will be reintroduced to this market because of side effects such as hepatic enzyme changes and lactic acidosis. However, the combination of NO and other pulmonary vasoconstrictors such as phenylephrine has been shown to improve oxygenation in ventilated intensive care unit patients with acute respiratory distress syndrome, and this may have applications in OLV.

Intermittent Reinflation of the Nonventilated Lung

Hypoxic pulmonary vasoconstriction becomes more effective during repeated hypoxic exposure. Often after reinflation, the oxygen saturation will be more acceptable during a second period of lung collapse. Reexpansion can be performed by regular reexpansion of the operative lung via an attached CPAP circuit.

Partial Ventilation Methods

Several alternative methods of OLV, all involving partial ventilation of the nonventilated lung, have been described and improve oxygenation during OLV. These techniques are useful in patients who are particularly at risk of desaturation, such as those who have had previous pulmonary resections of the contralateral lung. These alternatives include:

1. Intermittent positive airway pressure to the nonventilated lung. This can be performed by a variety of methods. Attaching a standard bacteriostatic filter to the nonventilated lumen of the DLT with a 2 L oxygen inflow attached to the CO_2 port of the filter allows for intermittent insufflation. Manual occlusion of the filter for 2 seconds gives an insufflation of approximately 66 mL of oxygen to the nonventilated lung. This could be repeated at 10-second intervals with minimal interference with surgical exposure.
2. Selective insufflation of oxygen to recruit lung segments on the side of surgery but remote from the site of surgery (Fig. 14.8). A useful technique in minimally invasive surgery is intermittent insufflation of oxygen using a fiberoptic bronchoscope. A 5 L oxygen flow is attached to the suction port of a fiberoptic bronchoscope,

14

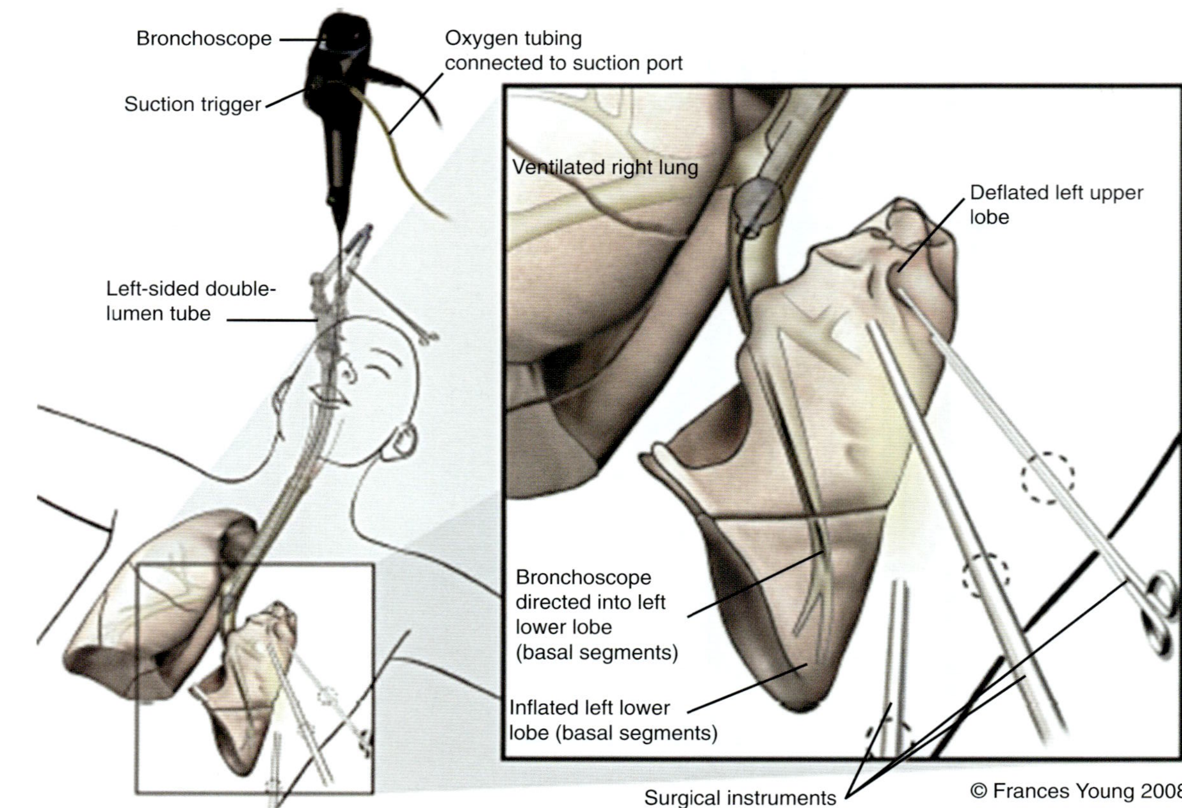

Fig. 14.8 Intermittent oxygen insufflation during thoracoscopic surgery to segments of the nonventilated lung on the side of surgery using a fiberoptic bronchoscope. (From Slinger P. Principles and Practice of Anesthesia for Thoracic Surgery. New York: Springer; 2011.)

which is passed under direct vision into a segment of the lung remote from the site of surgery, which is then reinflated by triggering the suction on the fiberoptic bronchoscope. The surgeon aids this technique by observing the lung inflation with the thoracoscope to avoid overdistention of the recruited segment(s).
3. Selective lobar collapse of only the operative lobe in the open hemithorax. This is accomplished by placement of a blocker in the appropriate lobar bronchus of the ipsilateral operative lung.
4. Mechanical restriction of pulmonary blood flow.

It is possible for the surgeon to directly compress or clamp the blood flow to the nonventilated lung. This can be done temporarily in emergency desaturation situations or definitively in cases of pneumonectomy or lung transplantation. Another technique of mechanical limitation of blood flow to the nonventilated lung is the inflation of a PAC balloon in the main pulmonary artery (PA) of the operative lung. The PAC can be positioned at induction with fluoroscopic or TEE guidance and inflated as needed intraoperatively. This has been shown to be a useful technique for resection of large pulmonary arteriovenous fistulae.

Hypoxemia Prophylaxis

The majority of the treatments outlined as therapies for hypoxemia can be used prophylactically to prevent hypoxemia in patients who are at high risk of desaturation during OLV. The advantage of prophylactic therapy of hypoxemia, in addition to the obvious patient safety benefit, is that maneuvers involving CPAP or alternative ventilation patterns of the operative lung can be instituted at the onset of OLV in a controlled fashion and will not require interruption of surgery and emergent reinflation of the nonventilated lung at a time that may be extremely disadvantageous.

Bilateral Pulmonary Surgery

Because of mechanical trauma to the operative lung, the gas exchange in this lung will always be temporarily impaired after OLV. Also, HPV offset may be delayed after reinflation of the first lung collapsed. Desaturation during bilateral lung procedures is particularly a problem during the second period of OLV (i.e., during OLV of the lung that has already had surgery). Thus for bilateral procedures, it is advisable to operate first on the lung that has better gas exchange and less propensity to desaturate during OLV. For the majority of patients, this means operating on the right lung first.

TRANSESOPHAGEAL ECHOCARDIOGRAPHY FOR NONCARDIAC THORACIC SURGERY

Transesophageal echocardiography is recommended as a category I indication for noncardiac surgery in the circumstances of life-threatening unexplained hypoxemia or hypotension. It is also recommended when patients have known or suspected cardiovascular pathology that may impact outcomes. In clinical practice, intraoperative TEE is used in a wide variety of procedures in noncardiac thoracic surgery, including to assess cardiac or great vessel compression from intrathoracic masses, hemodynamic instability, to assess changes in RV and LV preload and contractility, and in thoracic trauma. The basics and clinical applications of TEE to cardiac and vascular surgery are discussed elsewhere in this text. This section concentrates on TEE for intrathoracic noncardiac surgery but will not discuss lung transplantation or pulmonary endarterectomy.

Transesophageal echocardiography can be useful to assess the existence or extent of cardiac involvement from benign or malignant tumors of the lung or mediastinum (Figs. 14.9 to 14.11). It is often difficult for the surgeon to assess this during thoracotomy or sternotomy. TEE can also be useful to assess the extent of compression of the SVC, which can occur with lung tumors of the right upper lobe.

Transesophageal echocardiography can also be useful to assess hemodynamic instability in patients having noncardiac thoracic surgery. Pericardial tamponade, pulmonary embolism, hypovolemia, and left or right heart failure may be diagnosed by TEE when other clinical signs or monitors are misleading (Fig.14.12).

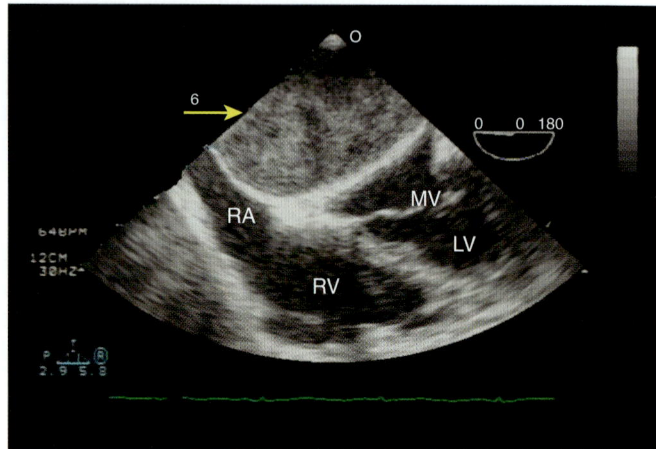

Fig. 14.9 Initial intraoperative midesophageal four-chamber transesophageal echocardiographic (TEE) view at 0 degrees of the heart a patient with a posterior mediastinal tumor that was compressing the left atrium, showing near complete compression of the left atrium by the tumor *(yellow arrow)* posteriorly and also compression of the right atrium (RA). Although the left atrium was severely compressed by the tumor (a mediastinal schwannoma), there is no clear evidence that the tumor extends through the wall of the atrium. *LV,* Left ventricle; *MV,* mitral valve; *RV,* right ventricle.

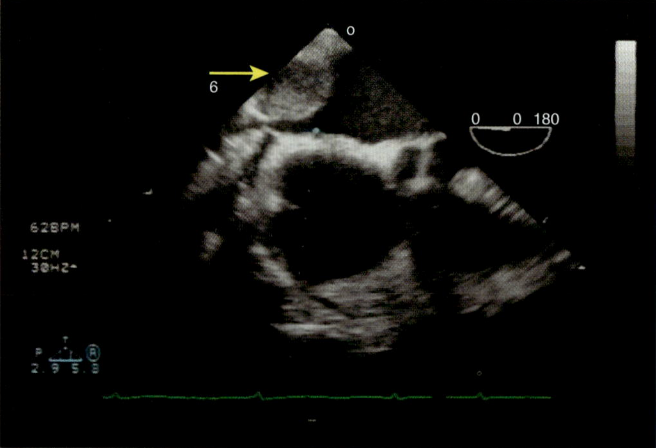

Fig. 14.10 Modified four-chamber transesophageal echocardiographic (TEE) view at 0 degrees after surgical resection of the posterior mediastinal tumor. TEE shows that one lobe of the tumor *(yellow arrow)* remains adherent to the posterior left atrial wall. This was not initially evident to the surgeon.

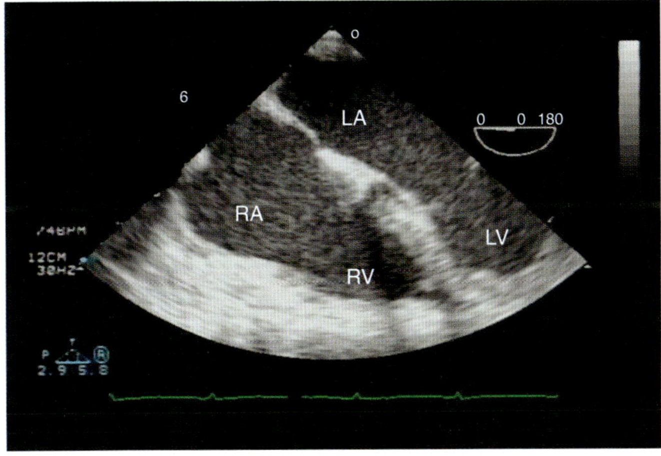

Fig. 14.11 Mid-esophageal four-chamber transesophageal echocardiographic view after excision of the remaining portion of the mediastinal tumor. *LA,* Left atrium; *LV,* left ventricle; *RA,* right atrium; *RV,* right ventricle.

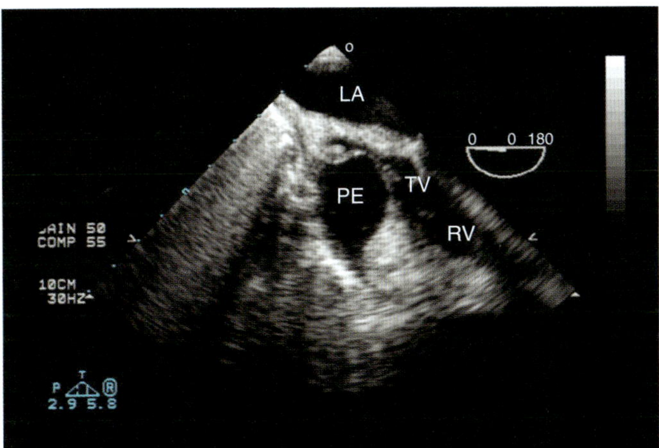

Fig. 14.12 Intraoperative midesophageal four-chamber transesophageal echocardiographic (TEE) view of a patient with bilateral pleural effusions thought to be secondary to metastatic breast cancer, performed for the diagnosis of severe refractory hypotension after induction of anesthesia. There is a loculated pericardial effusion (PE), which is nearly completely obliterating the right atrium and causing a cardiac tamponade. Based on the TEE diagnosis, it was possible to add a video-assisted thoracoscopic pericardial window to the originally planned surgery. *LA,* Left atrium; *RV,* right ventricle; *TV,* tricuspid valve.

AIRWAY SURGERY

Anesthetic Management for Diagnostic or Therapeutic Airway Procedures

Patients with underlying cardiac disease may present for a variety of surgical procedures involving the airways. Flexible FOB is a diagnostic and therapeutic procedure of great value in the clinical practice of thoracic surgery and anesthesia. In many centers, it is common practice to perform flexible FOB before airway or other thoracic surgeries, to reconfirm the diagnosis (if a tumor compresses the airway), or to determine the invasion and obstruction of the distal airway. There are multiple techniques for flexible FOB. Options include awake versus general anesthesia and oral versus nasal approaches. Options for local anesthesia include topical anesthesia via a nebulizer, handheld aerosol, or soaked pledgets; nerve blocks (laryngeal or glossopharyngeal nerves) or direct administration of local anesthetic through the bronchoscope ("spray as you go" technique), with or without sedation or opioid or antisialagogues. Options during general anesthesia include spontaneous versus positive-pressure ventilation with or without muscle relaxation. Airway management during general anesthesia can be with an ETT or a supraglottic airway (SGA). A swivel bronchoscopy connector with a self-sealing valve is used to facilitate the ventilation and manipulation of the bronchoscope at the same time inhalation or IV agents (or both) can be used for anesthesia. Patients who have copious secretions in the preoperative period should receive anticholinergic medication to ensure a dry field, which provides optimal visualization with the flexible bronchoscope.

The advantages of an SGA technique include that it allows visualization of the vocal cords and subglottic structures and there is a lower airway resistance versus an ETT when the bronchoscope is inserted (Fig. 14.13). This is particularly useful in a patient with a difficult airway when maintaining spontaneous respiration may be the safest method or anesthetic management. Self-expanding flexo-metallic tracheal and bronchial stents can be placed with fiberoptic or rigid bronchoscopy. However, silastic airway stents require rigid bronchoscopy for placement.

Rigid bronchoscopy has traditionally been considered the technique of choice for the preoperative diagnostic assessment of an airway obstruction involving the trachea and in the therapy of massive hemoptysis and foreign bodies in the airway. The role of interventional bronchoscopy with laser, bronchial dilation, or stent insertion is well established for the treatment of malignant and benign central airway and endobronchial lesions. Rigid bronchoscopy is the procedure of choice for operative procedures such as dilation of tracheal stenosis.

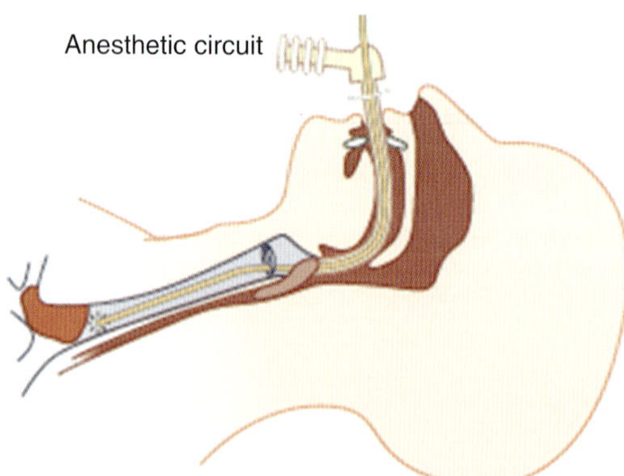

Fig. 14.13 Diagram of fiberoptic bronchoscopy performed via a laryngeal mask airway (LMA) during general anesthesia in a spontaneously breathing patient with a carinal tumor, in this case for diagnosis and Nd:YAG laser tumor excision. The LMA permits visualization of the vocal cords and subglottic structures with the bronchoscope, which is not possible when fiberoptic bronchoscope is performed via an endotracheal tube. (From Slinger PD, Cambs JH. Anesthesia for thoracic surgery. In: Miller RD, Eriksson Li, eds. *Miller's anesthesia.* 8th ed. Philadelphia: Elsevier; 2015.)

Patients undergoing rigid bronchoscopy should have a complete preoperative evaluation including radiologic studies. Chest radiographs and chest computed tomography (CT) scans should be reviewed in the preoperative evaluation. If time permits, it is recommended that patients with severe stridor receive pharmacologic interventions for temporary stabilization of the condition. Treatments may include inspired cool saline mist, nebulized racemic epinephrine, and the use of systemic steroids.

There are four basic methods of ventilation management for rigid bronchoscopy:

1. Spontaneous ventilation. The addition of topical anesthesia or nerve blocks to the airway decreases the tendency to breath-hold and cough when volatile anesthetics are used.
2. Apneic oxygenation (with or without insufflation of oxygen). This requires thorough preoxygenation, and the anesthesiologist will have to interrupt surgery to ventilate the patient before desaturation occurs. This should allow the surgeon working intervals of 3 minutes or longer depending on the underlying condition of the patient.
3. Positive-pressure ventilation via a ventilating bronchoscope. This allows the use of a standard anesthetic circuit but may cause significant air leaks if there is a discrepancy between the size of a smaller bronchoscope and a larger airway.
4. Jet ventilation. This can be performed with a handheld injector such as the Sanders injector or with a high-frequency ventilator. These techniques are most useful with IV anesthesia because they entrain gas from either the room air or an attached anesthetic circuit and the dose of any volatile agent delivered will be very uncertain.

The use of anticholinergic agents (e.g., glycopyrrolate 0.2 mg IV) before manipulation of the airway will decrease secretions during the bronchoscopic examination. For a patient undergoing rigid bronchoscopy, the surgeon must be at the bedside for the induction of anesthesia and be prepared to establish airway control with the rigid bronchoscope. Anesthesia in children for rigid bronchoscopy is most commonly with spontaneous ventilation (method 1) and a volatile anesthetic. In adults, IV anesthesia and the use of muscle relaxants are more common, with ventilation by a combination of methods 3 and 4.

For cases in which the use of muscle relaxants is not contraindicated, a short-acting agent (succinylcholine) can be used initially to facilitate intubation with either a small SLT or rigid bronchoscope. Nondepolarizing relaxants may be needed for prolonged procedures such as stent placement or tumor resection. Mouthguards should be used to protect the upper and lower teeth and gums from the pressure of the bronchoscope. Remifentanil and propofol infusions can be administered if an IV regimen is the planned anesthetic. This is a useful technique if the surgeon needs repeated access (for suction or instrumentation) to the open airway because it maintains the level of anesthesia and avoids contaminating the OR with anesthetic vapors.

In cases in which a neodymium-doped yttrium aluminum garnet (Nd:YAG) laser is used, the inspired fraction of oxygen should be maintained in the lowest acceptable range (i.e., <30% if possible) according to patient oxygen saturation to avoid the potential for fire in the airway. Because any common material (including porcelain and metal) can be perforated by the Nd:YAG laser, it is best to avoid any potentially combustible substance in the airway when the Nd:YAG laser is used. Because of its high energy and short wavelength, the Nd:YAG laser has several advantages for distal airway surgery over the CO_2 laser that is used in upper airway surgery. The Nd:YAG laser penetrates tissue more deeply, so it causes more coagulation in vascular tumors, and it can be refracted and passed in fibers through a flexible or rigid bronchoscope.

However, there is a higher potential for accidental reflected laser strikes, and there is more delayed airway edema.

Rigid bronchoscopes have different sizes, commonly from 3.5- to 9-mm diameters, with a ventilating side port to facilitate ventilation when the bronchoscope is placed into the airway. If excessive leak of tidal volume occurs around the bronchoscope with positive-pressure ventilation, it may be necessary to place throat packs to facilitate ventilation. Continuous communication with the surgeon or pulmonologist is necessary in case desaturation occurs. If desaturation does occur, it must be corrected by stopping surgery and allowing the anesthesiologist to ventilate and oxygenate the patient, either via the rigid bronchoscope or by removing the bronchoscope and ventilating with a mask, SGA, or ETT.

Pulse oximetry is vital during rigid bronchoscopy because there is a high risk of desaturation. There is no simple way to monitor end-tidal CO_2 or volatile anesthetics because the airway remains essentially open to atmosphere. For patients with underlying cardiac disease, an arterial line is usually placed for rigid bronchoscopy to facilitate rapid hemodynamic control. For prolonged procedures, it is useful to perform repeated arterial blood gas analysis to confirm the adequacy of ventilation. An alternative is to interrupt surgery and ventilate the patient with a standard circuit and a mask or ETT to assess the end-tidal CO_2.

Unlike during FOB via an ETT, with rigid bronchoscopy, the airway is never completely secure, and there is always the potential for aspiration in patients at increased risk, such as those with a full stomach, hiatus hernia, or morbid obesity. It is always best to defer rigid bronchoscopy to decrease the aspiration risk if possible in these patients. When there is no benefit to be gained by deferring or the airway risk is acute (e.g., aspiration of an obstructing foreign body), there is no simple solution, and each case must be managed on an individual basis depending on the context and competing risks.

Other rigid bronchoscopic procedures that require anesthesia include dilation for benign airway stenosis, core-out of malignant lesions in the trachea, laser ablation of endobronchial and carinal tumors, and therapeutic bronchoscopic interventions before surgical resection of lung cancer. Additionally, interventional bronchoscopy is often used for the management of airway complications after lung transplantation. Rigid bronchoscopy can be performed in combination with extracorporeal membranous oxygenation (ECMO) or CPB in high-risk patients.

Complications of rigid bronchoscopy include airway perforation, mucosal damage, hemorrhage, postmanipulation airway edema, and potential airway loss at the end of the procedure. In some situations, it may be necessary to keep the patient intubated with a small (e.g., 6.0 mm internal diameter) SLT after a rigid bronchoscopy if an edematous airway is suspected or the patient is not able to be extubated. These patients may require the use of steroids, nebulized racemic epinephrine, or helium and oxygen mixtures to treat stridor in the postoperative period.

Anesthesia for Tracheal Resection

Tracheal resection and reconstruction is indicated in patients who have a tracheal obstruction as a result of a tracheal tumor, previous tracheal trauma (most commonly postintubation stenosis), congenital anomalies, vascular lesions, and tracheomalacia. For patients who have operable tumors, approximately 80% undergo segmental resection with primary anastomosis, 10% undergo segmental resection with prosthetic reconstruction, and the remaining 10% undergo placement of a T-tube stent.

Diagnostic studies are reviewed as part of the preoperative evaluation. The CT scan is a useful diagnostic tool to evaluate the degree, level, and length of the lesion.

Bronchoscopy is one of the definitive diagnostic tests for tracheal obstruction. Bronchoscopy for a patient with tracheal stenosis should be carried out in the OR, where the surgical and anesthesia teams are present and ready to intervene if loss of airway occurs. An advantage of rigid bronchoscopy over flexible bronchoscopy is that it can bypass the obstruction and provide a ventilation pathway if complete obstruction occurs. During surgery, all patients should have an invasive arterial catheter placed to facilitate measurement of arterial blood gases, as well as measure arterial blood pressure. CVP catheters are only used if the patient requires CPB.

A variety of methods for providing adequate oxygenation and elimination of CO_2 have been used during tracheal resection. The alternatives include (1) standard orotracheal intubation, (2) insertion of a sterile SLT into the opened trachea or bronchus distal to the area of resection, (3) high-frequency jet ventilation (HFJV) through the stenotic area, (4) high-frequency positive-pressure ventilation (HFPPV), and (5) the use of CPB or ECMO.

Induction of anesthesia in patients with a compromised airway requires good communication between the surgical team and the anesthesiologist. The surgeon should always be in the OR during induction and available to manage a surgical airway if this becomes necessary. A rigid bronchoscope must be immediately available. The patient should be thoroughly preoxygenated with 100% O_2 before induction. The airways of patients with congenital or acquired tracheal stenosis are unlikely to collapse during induction of anesthesia. However, intratracheal masses may lead to airway obstruction with induction of anesthesia and should be managed similarly to anterior mediastinal masses (see later). One airway management technique is to begin the case with rigid bronchoscopy and tracheal dilation and then to pass an SLT through the stenosis. This tube is withdrawn into the proximal trachea after the distal trachea is opened, and a second sterile SLT is placed into the distal trachea by the surgeon. Ventilation is via a sterile anesthetic circuit passed across the drapes into the surgical field. With a low tracheal lesion, a right thoracotomy provides the optimal surgical exposure. A sterile SLT is used to provide ventilation to the lung distal to the resection. After the posterior anastomosis is completed, the endobronchial tube is removed, and the original SLT is advanced past the site of resection. This technique can also be used for carinal resections.

Another technique for airway management during tracheal resection includes HFJV through a small-bore ETT or catheter. With this technique, a small-bore uncuffed catheter is placed through the stenotic area, and ventilation is accomplished by intermittently exposing the lung to a high flow of fresh gas through the catheter. Other techniques that have been used for oxygenation during distal airway resections include HFPPV, helium–oxygen mixtures, and CPB.

After the tracheal resection is completed, most patients are kept in a position of neck flexion to reduce tension on the suture line. Replacement of the SLT by an SGA for emergence facilitates bronchoscopy if required. A thick chin-sternum suture ("Grillo-stitch") may be placed for several days to maintain neck flexion, or a cervical splint may be used. A T-tube with upper limb 0.5 to 1 cm above the vocal cords may be inserted at the end of surgery in cases when glottic edema is a concern or for patients requiring ventilatory support. If a tracheostomy is performed, it will be done distal to the anastomosis. Early extubation is highly desirable. If a patient requires reintubation, it should be performed with a flexible fiberoptic bronchoscope by advancing an SLT under direct vision over the bronchoscope and then placing it in the patient's trachea. The patient is kept in a head-up position to diminish swelling. Steroids may be useful in these cases to decrease airway edema.

One of the complications in the postoperative period is tetraplegia, with hyperflexion of the neck having been implicated as a potential cause. In these cases, it is necessary

14

to cut the chin stitch. An infusion of propofol and remifentanil, with FOB guidance and full patient cooperation, can aid extubation.

Pulmonary Hemorrhage

Massive hemoptysis is defined as expectoration of more than 200 mL of blood in 24 to 48 hours. The most common causes are carcinoma, bronchiectasis, and trauma (blunt, penetrating, or secondary to a PAC). Death can occur quickly from asphyxia. Management requires four sequential steps: lung isolation, resuscitation, diagnosis, and definitive treatment. The anesthesiologist is often called to deal with these cases outside of the OR. There is no consensus on the best method of lung isolation for these cases. The initial method for lung isolation will depend on the availability of appropriate equipment and an assessment of the patient's airway. All three basic methods of lung isolation have been used: DLTs, SLTs, and bronchial blockers. FOB is usually not helpful to position endobronchial tubes or blockers in the presence of torrential pulmonary hemorrhage, and lung isolation must be guided by clinical signs (primarily auscultation). DLTs will achieve rapid and secure lung isolation. Even if a left-sided tube enters the right mainstem bronchus, only the right upper lobe will be obstructed. However, suctioning large amounts of blood or clots is difficult through the narrow lumens of a DLT. An option is initial placement of an SLT for oxygenation and suctioning and then replacement with a DLT either by laryngoscopy or with an appropriate tube exchanger. An uncut single-lumen ETT can be advanced directly into the right mainstem bronchus or rotated 90 degrees counterclockwise for advancement into the left mainstem bronchus. A bronchial blocker will normally pass easily into the right mainstem bronchus and is useful for right-sided hemorrhage (90% of PAC-induced hemorrhages are right sided). Except for cases with blunt or penetrating trauma, after lung isolation and resuscitation have been achieved, diagnosis and definitive therapy of massive hemoptysis are now most commonly performed in interventional radiology (Fig. 14.14).

Pulmonary Artery Catheter–Induced Hemorrhage

Hemoptysis in a patient with a PAC must be assumed to be caused by perforation of a pulmonary vessel by the PAC until proven otherwise. The mortality rate may exceed 50%. This complication seems to be occurring less than previously, possibly related to stricter indications for the use of PACs and more appropriate management of PACs with less reliance on wedge measurements. Therapy for PAC-induced hemorrhage should follow an organized protocol, with some variation depending on the severity of the hemorrhage (Box 14.6).

During Weaning From Cardiopulmonary Bypass

Weaning from CPB is one of the times when PAC-induced hemorrhage is most likely to occur. Management of the PAC during CPB by withdrawal from a potential wedge depth and observing the PAP waveform to avoid wedging during CPB may decrease the risk of this complication. When hemoptysis does occur in this situation, the anesthesiologist should resist the temptation to rapidly reverse the anticoagulation to quickly discontinue CPB because this can lead to fatal asphyxiation from hemorrhage. Resumption of full CPB ensures oxygenation while the tracheobronchial tree is suctioned and then visualized with FOB. The use of a PA vent may be required to decrease the pulmonary blood flow sufficiently to define the bleeding site (usually the right lower lobe). The pleural cavity should be opened to assess the lung parenchymal damage.

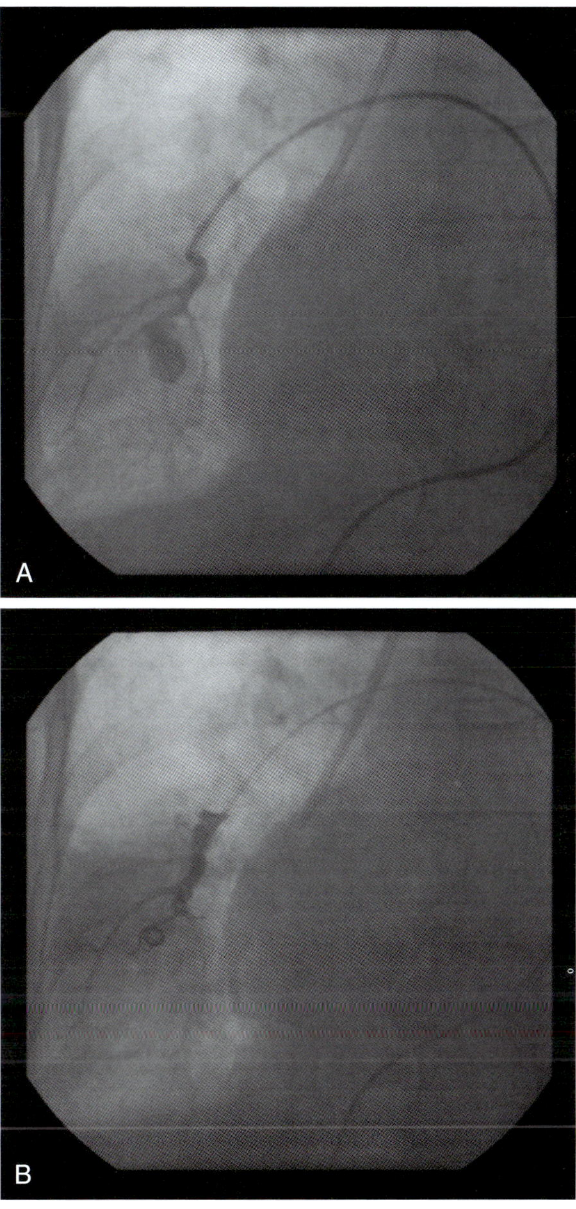

Fig. 14.14 (A) Radiographic dye injection showing a false aneurysm of the pulmonary artery of the right lower lobe following massive hemoptysis induced by pulmonary artery catheter rupture. (B) A coil has been placed by interventional radiology in the false aneurysm of the right lower pulmonary artery in the same patient. Dye injection shows that the aneurysm has embolized with no further leakage.

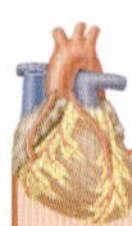

> **BOX 14.6** **Management of the Patient With a PA Catheter–Induced Pulmonary Hemorrhage**
>
> 1. Initially position the patient with the bleeding lung dependent.
> 2. Perform endotracheal intubation, oxygenation, airway toilet.
> 3. Isolate lung with endobronchial double- or single-lumen tube or bronchial blocker.
> 4. Withdraw the PA catheter several centimeters, leaving it in the main PA; do not inflate the balloon (except with fluoroscopic guidance).
> 5. Position the patient with the isolated bleeding lung nondependent; provide PEEP to the bleeding lung if possible.
> 6. Transport to medical imaging for diagnosis and embolization if feasible.
>
> *PA,* Pulmonary artery; *PEEP,* positive end-expiratory pressure.

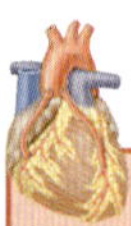

> **BOX 14.7** **Management of Tracheo-innominate Artery Fistula Hemorrhage**
>
> 1. Overinflate the tracheostomy cuff to tamponade the hemorrhage. If this fails:
>   - Replace the tracheostomy tube with an oral endotracheal tube. Position the cuff with fiberoptic bronchoscopy guidance just above the carina.
> 3. Provide digital compression of the innominate artery against the posterior sternum using a finger passed through the tracheostomy stoma. If this fails:
>   - Slowly withdraw the endotracheal tube and overinflate the cuff to tamponade.
> 5. Proceed with definitive therapy: sternotomy and ligation of the innominate artery.

Conservative management with lung isolation, avoiding lung resection, is optimal therapy if possible. In patients with persistent hemorrhage who are not candidates for lung resection, temporary lobar PA occlusion with a vascular loop during and after weaning from CPB may be an option and subsequent transport to a location for interventional radiology.

Posttracheostomy Hemorrhage

Hemorrhage in the immediate postoperative period after a tracheostomy is usually from local vessels in the incision such as the anterior jugular or inferior thyroid veins. Massive hemorrhage 1 to 6 weeks postoperatively is most commonly caused by trachea-innominate artery fistula. A small sentinel bleed occurs in most patients before a massive bleed. The management protocol for trachea-innominate artery fistula is outlined in Box 14.7.

Mediastinal Masses

Patients with mediastinal masses, particularly masses in the anterior or superior mediastinum, present unique problems for anesthesiologists. Patients may require anesthesia for biopsy of these masses by mediastinoscopy or VATS, or they may require definitive resection via sternotomy or thoracotomy. Tumors of the mediastinum include thymoma, teratoma, lymphoma, cystic hygroma, bronchogenic cyst, and thyroid tumors. Mediastinal masses may cause obstruction of major airways, main pulmonary arteries, atria, or the superior vena cava. During induction of general anesthesia in patients with an anterior or superior mediastinal mass, airway obstruction is the most common and feared complication. It is important to note that the point of tracheobronchial compression usually occurs distal to an ETT, and it is not possible to forcibly pass an ETT through the airway after it has collapsed. A history of supine dyspnea or cough should alert the clinician to the possibility of airway obstruction upon induction of anesthesia. Life-threatening complications may occur in the absence of symptoms in children. The other major complication is cardiovascular collapse secondary to compression of the heart or major vessels. Symptoms of supine presyncope suggest vascular compression.

Anesthetic deaths have mainly been reported in children. These deaths may be the result of the more compressible cartilaginous structure of the airway in children or because of the difficulty in obtaining a history of positional symptoms in children. The most important diagnostic test in a patient with a mediastinal mass is the CT scan of the trachea and chest. Children with tracheobronchial compression greater than 50% on CT scan cannot be given general anesthesia safely. Flow-volume loops, specifically the exacerbation of a variable intrathoracic obstructive pattern (expiratory plateau) when supine, are unreliable for predicting which patients will have intraoperative airway collapse. Preoperative transthoracic echocardiography is indicated for patients with vascular compression symptoms.

General anesthesia exacerbates extrinsic intrathoracic airway compression in three ways. First, reduced lung volume occurs during general anesthesia, and tracheobronchial diameters decrease according to lung volume. Second, bronchial smooth muscle relaxes during general anesthesia, allowing greater compressibility of large airways. Third, paralysis eliminates the caudal movement of the diaphragm seen during spontaneous ventilation. This eliminates the normal transpleural pressure gradient that dilates the airways during inspiration and minimizes the effects of extrinsic intrathoracic airway compression.

Management of patients with mediastinal masses is guided by their symptoms and the CT scan. Patients with uncertain distal airways should have diagnostic procedures performed under local or regional anesthesia whenever possible. Patients with uncertain airways requiring general anesthesia need a step-by-step induction of anesthesia with continuous monitoring of gas exchange and hemodynamics. This "NPIC" (*noli pontes ignii consumere*, or "don't burn your bridges") anesthetic induction can be an inhalation induction with a volatile anesthetic, such as sevoflurane or IV titration of propofol with or without ketamine, maintaining spontaneous ventilation until either the airway is definitively secured or the procedure is completed. Awake intubation of the trachea before induction is a possibility in some adult patients if the CT scan shows an area of noncompressed distal trachea to which the ETT can be advanced before induction. If muscle relaxants are required, ventilation should first be gradually taken over manually to ensure that positive-pressure ventilation is possible, and only then can a short-acting muscle relaxant be administered (Box 14.8).

Development of airway or vascular compression upon anesthetic induction requires that the patient be awakened as rapidly as possible and then other options for the procedure be explored. Intraoperative life-threatening airway compression usually has responded to one of two therapies: either repositioning of the patient (it must be determined before induction if there is a position that causes less compression and fewer symptoms) or rigid bronchoscopy and ventilation distal to the obstruction (this means that an experienced bronchoscopist and equipment must always be immediately available in the OR for these cases). The rigid bronchoscope, even if passed into only one mainstem bronchus, can be used for oxygenation during resuscitation (see Rigid Bronchoscopy earlier). After adequate oxygenation has been

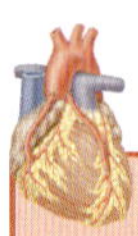

> **BOX 14.8** *Management for All Patients With a Mediastinal Mass and an Uncertain Airway for General Anesthesia*
>
> 1. Determine optimal positioning of patient preoperatively.
> 2. Secure the airway beyond stenosis (with the patient awake if feasible).
> 3. Use a rigid bronchoscope and have a surgeon available at induction.
> 4. Maintain spontaneous ventilation if possible (NPIC).
> 5. Monitor for airway compromise postoperatively.
>
> *NPIC, Noli pontes ignii consumere* ("don't burn your bridges").

restored, the rigid bronchoscope can be used to position an airway exchange catheter over which an ETT is passed after the bronchoscope is withdrawn. An alternative technique to secure the airway with rigid bronchoscopy is to first mount an ETT over a small rigid bronchoscope (e.g., 6 mm) and then perform rigid bronchoscopy using the bronchoscope to deliver the ETT distal to the obstruction.

Institution of femoral–femoral CPB before induction of anesthesia is a possibility for some adult patients who are unsafe for NPIC general anesthesia (Fig. 14.15). However, the concept of CPB "standby" during attempted induction of anesthesia is fraught with danger because there is not enough time after a sudden airway collapse to establish CPB before hypoxic cerebral injury occurs. The salient points in managing a patient with an anterior or superior mediastinal mass include:

1. In virtually all adults with a mediastinal mass, diagnostic procedures and imaging can be performed, if necessary, without subjecting the patient to the risks of general anesthesia.
2. An extrathoracic source of tissue for diagnostic biopsy (pleural effusion or extrathoracic lymph node) should be sought as an initial measure in every patient.
3. Regardless of the proposed diagnostic or therapeutic procedure, the flat (supine) position is never mandatory.

With improved awareness of the risk of acute intraoperative airway obstruction in these patients, life-threatening events are now less likely to occur in the OR. In children, these events now tend to occur preoperatively if the patient is forced to assume a supine position for imaging. In adults, acute airway obstruction is now more likely to occur postoperatively in the recovery room. Vigilance must be maintained throughout the entire perioperative period.

VASCULAR ANOMALIES WITH AIRWAY COMPRESSION

A spectrum of congenital vascular abnormalities can cause tracheal, bronchial, or esophageal compression. These include double aortic arch, right aortic arch with anomalous origin of the left subclavian artery, left aortic arch with anomalous right subclavian, and Kommerell diverticulum. Kommerell diverticulum is an aneurysm at the origin of an anomalous subclavian artery that represents an embryologic remnant of the interrupted fourth aortic arch between the carotid and subclavian arteries. In combination with the ligamentum arteriosum or a patent ductus, it may cause a complete vascular ring compressing the trachea. Symptoms involve varying degrees

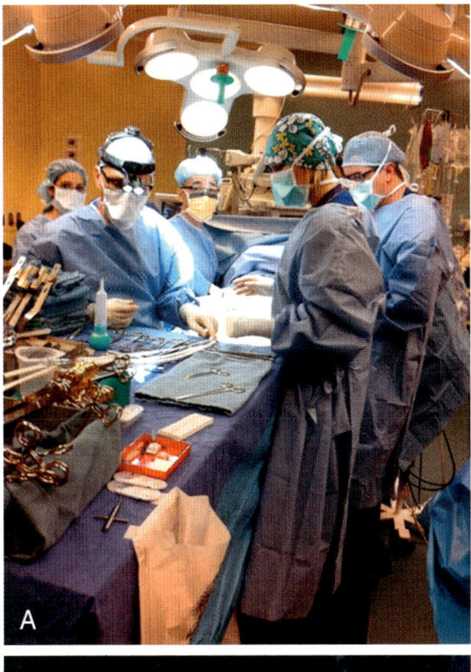

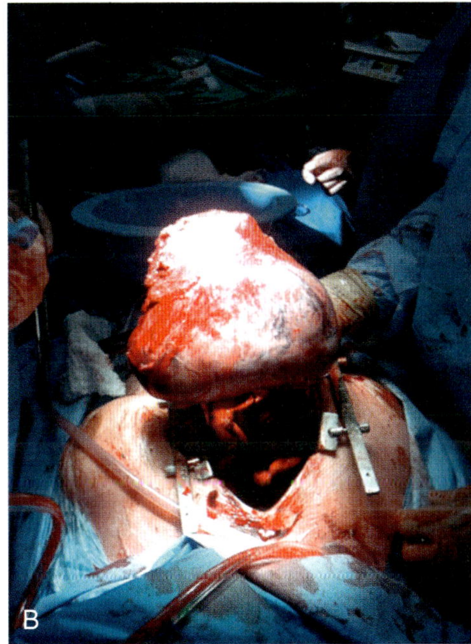

Fig. 14.15 (A) A patient with a large anterior mediastinal mass is placed on femoral-femoral arteriovenous cardiopulmonary bypass (CPB) before induction of anesthesia. The perspective is from the foot of the operating room table. The patient was reclined to 45 degrees for cannulation. The patient's head and upper body are concealed behind the surgical drapes. (B) A large anterior mediastinal sarcoma is removed from the same patient by sternotomy after induction of anesthesia with spontaneous ventilation while on CPB. The perspective is from the head of the operating room table over the surgical drapes.

of esophageal or airway obstruction and may present at any age. There is a tendency for airway symptoms to predominate in children and esophageal symptoms in adults. Respiratory symptoms and simple bronchoscopy can lead to a misdiagnosis of congenital tracheal stenosis. The diagnosis is confirmed by CT scan (Figs. 14.16 to 14.18), magnetic resonance imaging, and barium swallow. Surgical correction should follow diagnosis because of the tendency for rupture or dissection of these abnormal vessels. Depending on the anatomy, surgical correction may range from thoracoscopic ligation of the ligamentum arteriosum to sternotomy, with vascular and airway reconstruction potentially requiring hypothermic cardiac arrest.

As with all other lower airway abnormalities, airway management requires a flexible plan and full understanding of the anatomy by the anesthesiologist based on the preoperative imaging. After induction of anesthesia, a complete FOB via a SGA is usually performed to guide further airway management. Lung isolation when needed may then require placement of a DLT or SLT with bronchial blocker. A rigid bronchoscope should be available in the OR during induction and emergence from anesthesia in case of distal airway collapse. Consideration should be given to the use of corticosteroids to potentially decrease airway edema postoperatively.

There is the potential for postoperative tracheomalacia in patients who have had severe airway compression. Extubation should be approached in a cautious, controlled fashion with the patient alert and sitting, and after a leak test of the ETT, recognizing that the ETT cuff leak test is not infallible. Another option to consider is extubation during general anesthesia, with spontaneous ventilation and observation of the airway via a fiberoptic bronchoscope through an SGA during emergence.

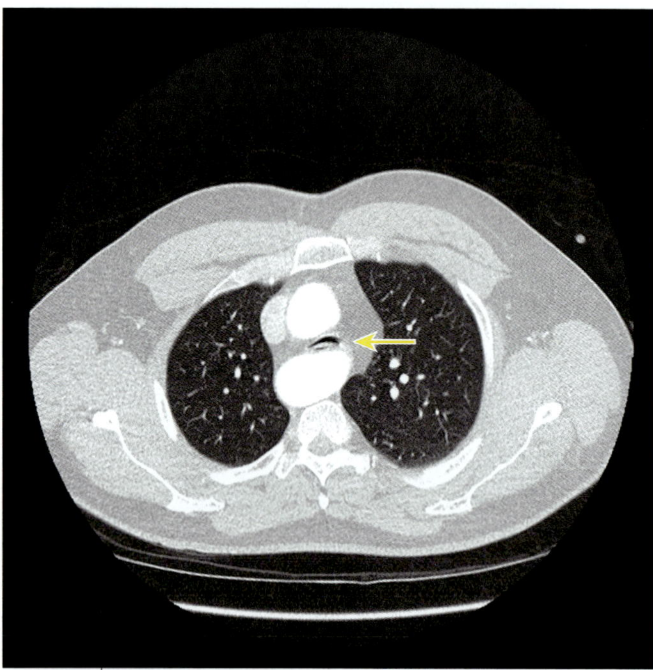

Fig. 14.16 Chest computed tomography scan of an adult with a Kommerell diverticulum showing mid-distal tracheal compression *(arrow)*. The anteroposterior tracheal diameter was 3 mm at its narrowest point.

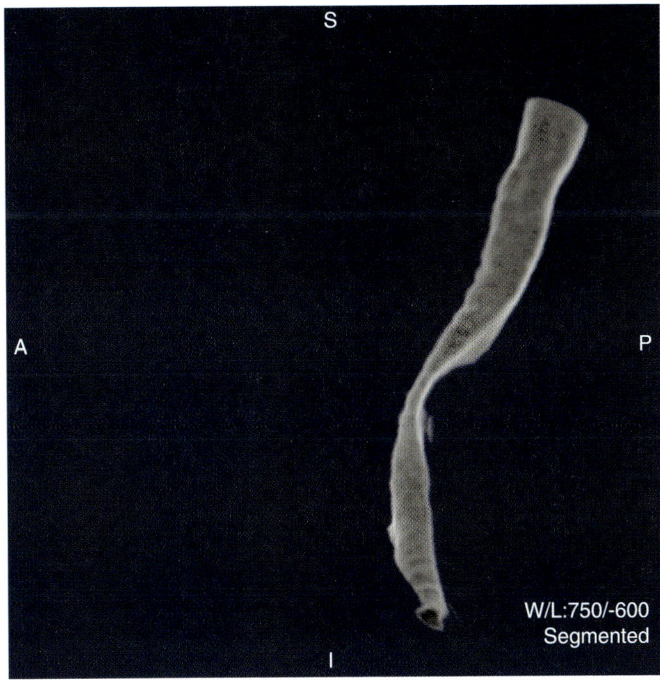

Fig. 14.17 Left lateral computed tomography reconstruction of the trachea in the same patient showing the posterior compression of the mid-distal trachea.

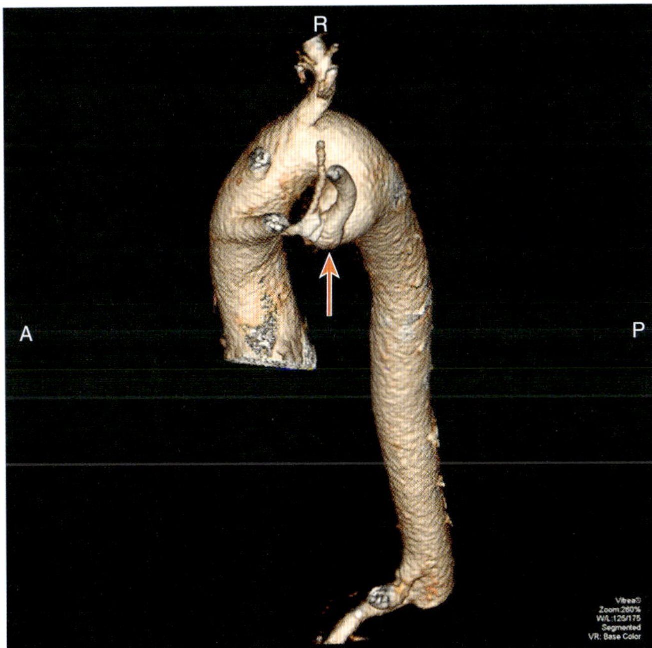

Fig. 14.18 Three-dimensional computed tomography angiogram from the left lateral perspective of the same patient. The patient has a right-sided aortic arch. The trachea is compressed by the ring formed by the aberrant take-off of the left subclavian artery and the Kommerell diverticulum, which forms the origin of the left common carotid *(arrow)*.

SUGGESTED READING

Bechard P, Letourneau L, Lacasse Y, et al. Perioperative cardiorespiratory complications in adults with mediastinal mass: incidence and risk factors. *Anesthesiology*. 2004;100:826.

Blank RS, Colquhoun DA, Durieux ME, et al. Management of one-lung ventilation: impact of tidal volume on complications after thoracic surgery. *Anesthesiology*. 2016;124:1286.

Clayton-Smith A, Bennett K, Alston RP, et al. A comparison of the efficacy and adverse effects of double-lumen endobronchial tubes and bronchial blockers in thoracic surgery: a systematic review and meta-analysis of randomized controlled trials. *J Cardiothorac Vasc Anesth*. 2015;29:955.

Donahoe LL, de Valence M, Atenafu EG, et al. High risk for thoracotomy but not thoracoscopic lobectomy. *Ann Thorac Surg*. 1730;103:2017.

Fleisher LA, Fleischmann KE, Auerbach AD, et al. ACC/AHA guidelines on perioperative cardiovascular evaluation and management of patients undergoing noncardiac surgery: executive summary: a report of the American College of Cardiology/American Heart Association Task Force on Practice Guidelines. *J Am Coll Cardiol*. 2014;64:2373.

Hosseinian L. Pulmonary hypertension and noncardiac surgery: implications for the anesthesiologist. *J Cardoiothorac Vasc Anesth*. 2014;28:1064.

Kozian A, Schilling T, Schutze H. Ventilatory protective strategies during thoracic surgery. *Anesthesiology*. 2011;114:1009.

Lumb AB, Slinger P. Hypoxic pulmonary vasoconstriction: physiology and anesthetic implications. *Anesthesiology*. 2015;122:932.

Mahmood F, Christie A, Maytal R. Transesophageal echocardiography for noncardiac surgery. *Sem Cardiothorac Vasc Anesth*. 2008;12:265.

Maxwell BG, Jackson E. Role of ketamine in the management of pulmonary hypertension and right ventricular failure. *J Cardiothorac Vasc Anesth*. 2012;26:e24.

Slinger P, ed. *Principles and Practice of Anesthesia for Thoracic Surgery*. New York: Springer; 2011.

Pritts CD, Pearl RG. Anesthesia for patients with pulmonary hypertension. *Curr Opin Anaesthesiol*. 2010;23:411.

Russell WJ, James MF. The effects on arterial haemoglobin oxygen saturation and on shunt of increasing cardiac output with dopamine or dobutamine during one-lung ventilation. *Anaesth Intens Care*. 2004;32:644.

Schwarzkopf K, Klein U, Schreiber T, et al. Oxygenation during one-lung ventilation: the effects of inhaled nitric oxide and increasing levels of inspired fraction of oxygen. *Anesth Analg*. 2001;92:842.

Slinger P, Campos J. Anesthesia for Thoracic Surgery. In: Miller RD, eds. *Miller's Anesthesia*. 8th ed. New York: Elsevier; 2014.

Slinger P, Karsli C. Management of the patient with a large anterior mediastinal mass: recurring myths. *Curr Opinion Anaesthesiol*. 2007;20:1.

Subramaniam K, Yared JP. Management of pulmonary hypertension in the operating room. *Semin Cardiothorac Vasc Anesth*. 2007;11:119.

Wijeysundera ND, Wijeysundera HC, Wasowicz M, et al. Risk of elective major non-cardiac surgery after coronary stent insertion. *Circulation*. 2012;126:1355.

Wink J, de Wilde RBP, Wouters PF, et al. Thoracic epidural anesthesia reduces right ventricular systolic function w\with maintained ventricular-pulmonary coupling: clinical perspective. *Circulation*. 2016;134:1163.

Chapter 15

Anesthesia for Cardioversion and Electrophysiologic Procedures

Marshall K. Lee, MD • Neal S. Gerstein, MD, FASE •
Peter M. Schulman, MD • Peter M. Jessel, MD, FHRS

Key Points

1. Tachyarrhythmias result from one of three mechanisms (reentry, automaticity, and triggered activity), with reentry being the mechanism most commonly treated in the electrophysiology (EP) laboratory.
2. Anesthetic agents influence cardiac conduction and arrhythmogenesis and can adversely affect EP procedures.
3. Opioids may have an antiarrhythmic effect in the setting of myocardial ischemia.
4. While the arrhythmic properties of volatile anesthetics are controversial, overall they have an antifibrillatory effect.
5. Two new, more minimally invasive cardiac implantable electrical devices include the subcutaneous implantable cardioverter-defibrillator and leadless pacemaker.
6. General anesthesia is becoming increasingly preferred for atrial fibrillation ablation because of the longer procedure time and predictable thoracic excursion with mechanical ventilation.
7. Atrial fibrillation is responsible for more than 35% of ischemic strokes, with the left atrial appendage being the most common place for thrombus formation.
8. Complications of procedures performed in the EP laboratory are secondary to vascular access, thromboembolism, arrhythmias, pericardial effusions, air embolism, pulmonary vein stenosis, atrioesophageal fistula formation, and phrenic nerve injury.

Cardiac arrhythmias cause significant morbidity and mortality. In the United States, cardiac arrhythmias account for nearly 400,000 deaths annually. Since the implantation of the first cardiac pacemaker in 1958, clinical electrophysiology (EP) has become increasingly complex and now includes a variety of sophisticated therapeutic and diagnostic procedures. Although sedation for many EP cases has historically been performed by a nurse under the direction of the proceduralist, because of a number of factors (complexity of many of these cases, long procedural times, potential significant hemodynamic instability, and significant patient comorbidities often present), an anesthesia provider is now frequently integral to providing safe and effective EP care. Understanding the basic principles of how these procedures are performed, the mechanisms of cardiac arrhythmias, and the impact that anesthetic agents have on the cardiac conduction system is paramount for anesthesia providers working in this environment.

Table 15.1 Commonly Used Abbreviations in Clinical Electrophysiology

AF	Atrial fibrillation	ICD	Implantable cardioverter-defibrillator
AFL	Atrial flutter		
AT	Atrial tachycardia	ICE	Intracardiac echocardiogram
AVNRT	Atrioventricular nodal reentrant tachycardia	LAA	Left atrial appendage
		NavX	Navigation system (St. Jude Medical)
AVRT	Atrioventricular reciprocating tachycardia		
		PDNA	Proceduralist-directed nurse-administered
CARTO	Navigation system produced by Biosense Webster		
		PSVT	Paroxysmal supraventricular tachycardia
CIED	Cardiovascular implantable electronic device		
		PVC	Premature ventricular contraction
CS	Coronary sinus		
EC	Electrical cardioversion	PVI	Pulmonary vein isolation
EP	Electrophysiology	SVT	Supraventricular tachycardia
EGM	Electrogram (generally intracardiac)	TdP	Torsades de pointes
		VF	Ventricular fibrillation
hRA	High right atrium	VT	Ventricular tachycardia

This chapter provides an overview of clinical EP for anesthesia providers. It discusses the effects of the most commonly used anesthetic agents in the EP laboratory on cardiac conduction. It reviews the salient details and anesthetic considerations of each of the main EP procedures as well as the associated complications that might arise during the periprocedural period. See Table 15.1 for commonly used abbreviations in clinical EP.

OVERVIEW OF ELECTROPHYSIOLOGY PROCEDURES

Electrophysiology Laboratory

Initially, the main purpose of the EP laboratory was for diagnostic studies. However, its focus has evolved to include many therapeutic procedures such as catheter ablation and cardiac rhythm device implantation and extraction. The EP laboratory is divided into the control room, which is shielded from radiation by a glass partition and doorway, and the area where the procedure is performed, which contains the patient table and imaging equipment. While the procedure is being performed, a technician (and sometimes a second electrophysiologist) in the control room monitors the patient's cardiac rhythm and performs various pacing maneuvers. A large amount of equipment is required (e.g., single or biplane fluoroscopy, mapping patches, electrocardiogram [ECG] leads, catheters, boom with multiple screens), limiting access to the patient during the procedure and thus complicating anesthetic care. Some laboratories also contain a magnetic catheter navigation system (e.g., Stereotaxis Inc.), which occupies even more space and introduces the logistical considerations (i.e., magnetic resonance imaging [MRI]-compatible monitors and anesthesia machine) and potential dangers of a ferromagnetic field. Because fluoroscopy is constantly used in the EP laboratory, necessary radiation safety precautions (e.g., lead aprons or shields, eye protection) must be followed. Radiation dosimeters should be worn by personnel who routinely work in this environment.

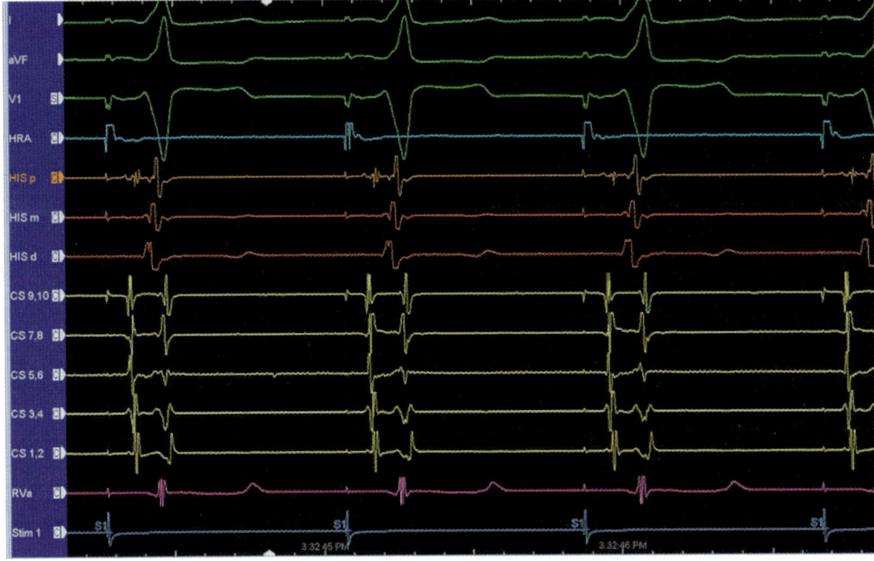

Fig. 15.1 Intracardiac electrograms obtained during a standard electrophysiology study in a patient with ventricular preexcitation. This screen shot shows the intracardiac and surface electrocardiogram (ECG) recordings obtained while a high right atrial catheter was used to pace the atrium. Displayed are three surface ECG leads (I, aVF, V1), and the following intracardiac recordings: high right atrial (HRA), three His (proximal, mid, distal), five coronary sinus (CS), and a right ventricular apex (RVa). The bottom-most tracing is a stimulation channel (Stim 1), which confirms pacing is being performed. The pacing artifact seen on the surface ECG may not necessarily be seen on the anesthesia team's monitor, and review of the stimulation channel on the screen can confirm that pacing is occurring. In this patient, the short PR interval and delta wave visible on the surface ECG leads are characteristic of ventricular preexcitation.

Catheter Placement and Generation of Intracardiac Electrograms

Right heart catheter placement is most often performed via the femoral vein; however, the internal jugular, subclavian, or brachial vein can be used. Multiple intravenous (IV) sheaths are placed so that catheters can be advanced into the heart to record intracardiac signals (electrograms). In contradistinction to the surface ECG, which provides summed vectors of the heart's electrical activity, the intracardiac electrogram records a discrete local signal from a small area of the myocardium. These diagnostic catheters, some with multiple electrode pairs, are used to determine information such as signal voltage, complexity, and local activation (timing compared with a reference). The exact type and location of the catheters placed depend on the procedure being performed and physician preference.

To perform a basic EP study, several electrograms are typically obtained by placing catheters into the high right atrium (hRA), coronary sinus (CS), His bundle, and RV apex (RVa) (Fig. 15.1). A variable number of surface ECGs leads are also displayed. To better visualize the signals, they are displayed at a sweep speed of 100 mm/s compared with 25 mm/s for a standard ECG. Real-time signals are viewed on one screen, and an additional screen is available for measurements and static review.

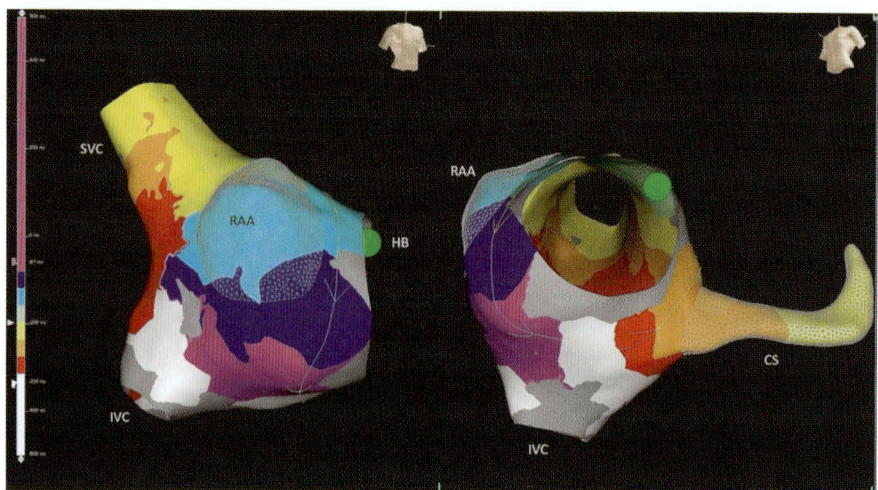

Fig. 15.2 An activation map showing typical atrial flutter with counterclockwise rotation *(arrows)*. The color bar (located on the left edge of the image) provides a reference for timing and color correlation. Earliest activation sites are noted by white followed by red, with purple indicating the last activated site compared to the reference time. A macroreentrant circuit is continuous; thus early and late are arbitrarily defined, but the so-called "early meets late" pattern supports the mechanism as reentry rather than a focal tachycardia. The right atrium is seen in both the right anterior oblique view (image on left) and left anterior oblique caudal view (image on right). *CS,* Coronary sinus; *HB,* His bundle; *IVC,* inferior vena cava; *RAA,* right atrial appendage; *SVC,* superior vena cava.

Catheter Mapping System

Mapping systems are used to collect and display information gathered from intracardiac recordings. A three-dimensional (3D) shell of the chamber(s) of interest is generated along with pertinent timing and voltage information. These systems reduce radiation exposure compared with fluoroscopy alone by integrating preprocedural images obtained from computed tomography (CT) or magnetic resonance (MR) or use intraprocedural ultrasound to improve anatomic relationships. During an arrhythmia, an activation map is produced by measuring the timing of different cardiac events and then using color coding or an animation to display the wavefront proceeding across the 3D map (Fig. 15.2). The map helps the electrophysiologist determine the area that should be targeted for ablation by pinpointing the source of a focal tachycardia or the area of slow conduction in the case of a macroreentrant tachycardia. Voltage mapping is used in addition to or in lieu of activation mapping if an arrhythmia is noninducible and provides important information about the scar substrate responsible for reentrant rhythms.

Mechanisms of Cardiac Arrhythmias

Arrhythmias are classified as slow (bradyarrhythmia) or fast (tachyarrhythmia) based on whether the heart rate is less than 60 beats/min or greater than 100 beats/min, respectively.

Bradyarrhythmias

A bradyarrhythmia results from failure of impulse formation or conduction. The most commonly treated bradyarrhythmia in the EP laboratory is sinus node (SN)

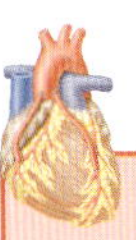

> **BOX 15.1** *Tachyarrhythmia Mechanisms*
>
> - Reentry (mechanism most commonly addressed in electrophysiology procedures)
> - Automaticity
> - Triggered

dysfunction, which occurs when impulse formation is impaired within the SN. Conduction system disease is most often from advanced age or underlying cardiovascular disease and results in three main forms of atrioventricular (AV) block—first, second, or third degree.

First-degree AV block is actually a misnomer because in this condition conduction through the AV node is simply slowed, which results in a prolonged PR interval on the ECG and requires no treatment. Second-degree AV block is subdivided into types I and II; these conditions partially impair but do not entirely block impulses from conducting to the ventricles. On the ECG, type I is diagnosed by progressive PR prolongation until a dropped ventricular beat occurs. In contrast, type II is characterized by intermittent nonconducted P-waves without progressive PR prolongation. Type II is important to identify because it indicates infranodal conduction disease, can progress to third-degree heart block, and might warrant pacemaker implantation. In third-degree heart block, there is complete AV dissociation, which requires a junctional or ventricular escape rhythm to maintain perfusion.

Tachyarrhythmias

Tachyarrhythmias are caused by one of three mechanisms (Box 15.1). In the EP laboratory, the most commonly treated mechanism is reentry. A reentrant tachycardia is defined by its continuous circular path in which the wavefront of excitability returns to the site of initiation. Requirements of reentry include two adjacent pathways with differing EP properties that connect proximally and distally to form a single circuit with a nonexcitable central area. Unidirectional block is required and occurs when differences in refractory periods allow an impulse to initially conduct down one pathway but not the other. Because of slow conduction, by the time the wavefront reaches the end of the first pathway, the second pathway is no longer refractory and accepts the impulse. The impulse then continues until it returns to its origin and thus completes one cycle of tachycardia. There is often an area of slow conduction that facilitates reentry and may be targeted for ablation (e.g., the cavotricuspid isthmus in typical atrial flutter [AFL]).

The remaining two mechanisms, automaticity and triggered activity, are abnormalities in impulse formation rather than conduction. Automaticity is spontaneous impulse formation and is normal behavior when occurring in specialized conduction tissue. Failure of automaticity may result in a bradyarrhythmia such as sinus bradycardia. Alternatively, increased automaticity in diseased or ischemic atrial or ventricular myocardial cells may result in a sustained tachyarrhythmia or induce premature beats that initiate reentry. Triggered activity requires a preceding impulse and is caused by oscillations in the cellular membrane potential called afterdepolarizations. Afterdepolarizations are further characterized as early or delayed depending on when they occur during the action potential. Clinical examples of early and delayed afterdepolarizations include torsades de pointes in long-QT syndrome and digoxin toxicity, respectively. Table 15.2 summarizes key characteristics of the different tachyarrhythmias treated in the EP laboratory.

Table 15.2	Tachyarrhythmias Treated in the Electrophysiology Laboratory		
Arrhythmia	**Mechanism**	**Ablation Target**	**Sedation Level Needed**
AV nodal reentry	Reentry	Slow pathway	Moderate
AV reciprocating tachycardia	Reentry	Accessory pathway	Moderate
Atrial tachycardia	Reentry, triggered activity, automaticity	Origin of focal tachycardia	Moderate
Atrial flutter	Reentry	Area of slow conduction	Moderate
Atrial fibrillation	Multiple mechanisms coexist	Pulmonary vein isolation initially	Moderate to general anesthesia
PVCs	Automaticity, reentry, triggered activity	PVC focus (outflow tract most common)	Moderate
VT with a structurally normal heart	Automaticity, reentry, triggered activity	VT focus	Moderate
VT with structural heart disease	Reentry caused by fibrosis	Critical isthmus or extensive substrate modification	General anesthesia

AV, Atrioventricular; *PVC,* premature ventricular contraction; *VT,* ventricular tachycardia.

ANESTHETIC AGENTS AND CARDIAC CONDUCTION

Many anesthetic agents influence cardiac conduction and arrhythmogenesis and thus have the propensity to adversely impact the efficacy of the diagnostic and therapeutic procedures performed in the EP laboratory. The most commonly used sedative and anesthetic agents along with a description of their varying effects on the cardiac conduction system are provided next. A summary of this information is also contained in Table 15.3.

Propofol

Propofol (2,6-di-isopropylphenol) is perhaps the most commonly used anesthetic agent because of its efficacy, potency, rapid titratability, and short duration of action. Because propofol induces a profound level of sedation or even general anesthesia, it is postulated to indirectly modify atrial electrical activity and AV conduction. It also inhibits vagal tone in a dose-dependent manner. Because it decreases P-wave dispersion (i.e., the difference between the widest trand narrowest P-wave duration), it might be partially responsible for the conversion of atrial fibrillation (AF) to sinus rhythm.

The magnitude and significance of propofol's aforementioned indirect effects on cardiac conduction are controversial. However, its proarrhythmic and antiarrhythmic effects are thought to be dose dependent. Typically, low doses have minimal effects on cardiac conduction; the impact of larger doses might be more significant. Propofol does not directly affect sinoatrial (SA) node activity or atrial electrical conduction.

Table 15.3 Summary of Anesthetic Agent Effects on Cardiac Conduction and Electrical Properties

Agent	Antiarrhythmic Properties	Proarrhythmic Properties	Acceptable for Use in Cardioversion	Effect on P-R Interval	Effect on QTc Interval	Benefits	Adverse Effects
Propofol	May terminate SVT May convert AF May terminate VT	Bradycardia Lengthens SA node interval Slows AVN conduction/prolongs AVN effective refractory period Slows atrial rate Case reports of TdP	Yes	May shorten	Varying reports: Primarily prolongs May shorten	Rapid onset and recovery	Vasodilation Dose-dependent decrease in blood pressure Possible P-wave dispersion
Etomidate	None	None	Yes	NR	NR	Minimal cardiac depressive effects	Adrenocortical suppression
Midazolam	NR	NR	Yes	NR	None	Amnesia Minimal HD effects	Mild venous dilation but no significant impact on contractility
Dexmedetomidine	Bradycardic effect has been used in SVT, VT, AFL, junctional ectopic tachycardia	SA node interval lengthening in some reports Slows AVN conduction or blockade	Yes	Prolongs	Prolongs	Rapid onset/clearance	Use with caution in heart block, bradycardia, and heart transplant Caution when coadministered with β-blockade
Sevoflurane	Antifibrillatory	Atrial ectopy in pediatric reports Slowing of AVN conduction time	Yes	NR	Prolongs	Not noxious to airways	Dose-dependent vasodilation
Desflurane	Antifibrillatory	Slowing of AVN conduction time	Yes	NR	Prolongs	Lowest blood:gas solubility of the three listed volatile agents	Dose-dependent vasodilation

Continued

Table 15.3 Summary of Anesthetic Agent Effects on Cardiac Conduction and Electrical Properties—cont'd

Agent	Antiarrhythmic Properties	Proarrhythmic Properties	Acceptable for Use in Cardioversion	Effect on P-R Interval	Effect on QTc Interval	Benefits	Adverse Effects
Isoflurane	Antifibrillatory	Slowing of AVN conduction time APERP prolongation in preexcitation syndromes	Yes	NR	Prolongs	Inexpensive	Dose-dependent vasodilation
Fentanyl	Antifibrillatory; elongates the sinus node recovery time	Bradycardia	Yes	NR	None	Inexpensive	No amnestic effect Ventilation depressant May affect accuracy of atrial mapping during EP procedures
Morphine	Decreases the occurrence of reperfusion-induced arrhythmias Antifibrillatory	Bradycardia	Yes	NR	None	Inexpensive	Vasodilation secondary to histamine release
Remifentanil	NR	Bradycardia Slows SA node function Slows AVN conduction and prolongs AVN ERP	Yes	NR	None; may attenuate QTc prolongation in hypertensive patients	Ultrarapid onset and recovery	No amnesia Ventilation depressant Hypotension Bradycardia Caution with β-blockade

AF, Atrial fibrillation; *AFL,* atrial flutter; *APERP,* accessory pathway effective refractory period in pre-excitation syndromes; *AVN,* atrioventricular node; *EP,* electrophysiology; *ERP,* effective refractory period; *HD,* hemodynamic; *NR,* none reported; *SA,* sinoatrial; *SVT,* supraventricular tachycardia; *TdP,* torsades de pointes; *VT,* ventricular tachycardia.

Despite its potential to indirectly affect conduction, the impact is likely modest at best, and available data (albeit limited) support the use of propofol for these procedures.

Antiarrhythmic Qualities

Propofol can inhibit cardiac conduction and has been demonstrated to convert supraventricular and ventricular tachycardias. The mechanism for its conduction effects is not fully elucidated but likely involves a combination of cardiomyocyte ion channels (inward and outward ion currents (I_{Na}, I_{Ca}, I_{KR}, I_{KS}), the autonomic nervous system, and cardiac cell gap junctions (intercellular channels that electrically and metabolically connect cardiomyocytes). Propofol shortens the cardiac action potential duration and suppresses both sympathetic and parasympathetic tone. The aggregate of these effects leads to both the antiarrhythmic and proarrhythmic properties of propofol.

Propofol has been shown to shorten the PR interval associated with Wolff-Parkinson-White syndrome, as well as shorten the QT interval, and prevent episodes of ventricular tachycardia (VT). Propofol also inhibits arrhythmias associated with ischemia-reperfusion injuries after episodes of myocardial ischemia.

Proarrhythmic Qualities

In a dose-dependent manner, propofol has been demonstrated to impede various components of the cardiac conduction system, including lengthening of the SA interval, inhibition of atrioventricular node (AVN) activity, slowing of atrial rates, and prolongation of the stimulus-to-His bundle interval length. Importantly, there are reports of clinically significant bradycardia associated with high-dose propofol including polymorphic VT and Brugada type 1 ECG pattern (upward concave ST elevation in leads V_1–V_3).

Etomidate

Etomidate, a carboxylated imidazole compound that acts as a γ-aminobutyric acid type A ($GABA_A$) receptor agonist, is primarily used as an anesthetic induction agent. There is no evidence that etomidate possesses significant antiarrhythmogenic or proarrhythmogenic effects, and it specifically does not impact the duration of repolarization of cardiac conduction tissue.

Opioids

Opioids are primarily vagotonic; thus they can cause bradycardia and a concomitant decrease in cardiac metabolic demand. In animal studies, opioids have been shown to attenuate the excitatory influence of the sympathetic nervous system. In the setting of myocardial ischemia, they might have an antiarrhythmic effect. Opioids have had no effect on VT inducibility. The most frequently used opioids include fentanyl, morphine, hydromorphone, and remifentanil.

Fentanyl

Fentanyl, a synthetic μ-opioid receptor agonist, enhances vagal tone and has been reported to be associated with sinus tachycardia, hypertension, hypotension, arrhythmias, vasodilation, bradycardia, and bigeminy. Fentanyl indirectly raises the ventricular fibrillation (VF) threshold because of its sympatholytic effects, not by activation of vagal efferent pathways. Compared with morphine, fentanyl produces more profound bradycardia.

In pediatric patients, fentanyl has been shown to significantly elongate the SN recovery time, but not SA conduction time. Fentanyl's effect on SA function parallels

15

that of propranolol by affecting automaticity but not SA conduction times. The clinical implication of this effect is that during EP procedures in certain patients, enhanced vagal tone may facilitate the generation of paroxysmal supraventricular tachycardia (PSVT) through its effect on refractoriness of the slow and fast AV nodal conduction pathways. Moreover, autonomic nervous system imbalances during an EP study may attenuate PSVT heart rates compared with spontaneous PSVT, and these fentanyl-induced changes in autonomic nervous system function may ultimately affect the accuracy of an EP study.

Morphine

Morphine, a μ-opioid receptor agonist, increases parasympathetic and reduces sympathetic activity. It has minimal direct cardiac conduction effects. Primarily vagally mediated, it has been reported to be associated with tachycardia, AF, hypertension, hypotension, and bradycardia. Morphine has been thought to raise the VF threshold because of its effect on altering autonomic tone.

In animal models, morphine reduces ischemia-induced membrane depolarization, attenuates myocardial ischemia-related decreases in action potential amplitude, decreases the occurrence of conduction block related to myocardial ischemia, and decreases the occurrence of reperfusion-induced arrhythmias.

Remifentanil

Remifentanil is a selective μ-opioid receptor agonist. Metabolism involves rapid hydrolysis by nonspecific tissue and plasma esterases, which leads to a very rapid onset and short duration of action that provide intense analgesia without prolonged respiratory depression.

Remifentanil has been associated with bradyarrhythmias and asystole both in children and adults. Bradycardia and hypotension have been reported and are likely caused by a centrally mediated increase in vagal nerve activity. EP studies demonstrate that remifentanil is associated with a dose-dependent slowing of SA and AV node function, causing a prolongation of SN recovery time, SA conduction time, and Wenckebach cycle length. Hence, remifentanil should be used cautiously in patients at risk for bradyarrhythmias.

Benzodiazepines

Benzodiazepines bind to stereospecific benzodiazepine receptors on central nervous system (CNS) GABA$_A$ receptors, leading to increased neuronal membrane permeability to chloride ions. GABA$_A$ receptor agonism by benzodiazepines results in sedative, hypnotic, anxiolytic, antiepileptic, and muscle relaxant properties. The vast majority of patients undergoing EP procedures receive a benzodiazepine for sedation and anxiolysis.

Of the available agents, midazolam is the most frequently used because of its IV formulation, rapid onset (3–5 minutes when administered intravenously), and predictable pharmacokinetics, including an effective duration between 2 and 6 hours. Midazolam transiently depresses baroreceptor-mediated heart rate responses. Whether benzodiazepines prolong the QTc interval is controversial.

Dexmedetomidine

Dexmedetomidine has a complex mechanism of action involving both presynaptic and postsynaptic receptor activation. Activation of presynaptic α$_2$-receptors in the CNS is responsible for its sympatholytic effects. Dexmedetomidine causes bradycardia

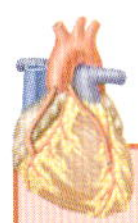

> ### BOX 15.2 *Dexmedetomidine Effects*
>
> - Presynaptic α_2-receptor: sympatholysis, bradycardia, hypotension
> - Peripheral α_{2b}-receptors: hypertension

and hypotension because of inhibition of norepinephrine release from presynaptic neurons. However, hypertension caused by activation of peripheral α_{2b}-adrenergic receptors may occur with rapid IV administration or with high-dose infusion rates (Box 15.2).

Antiarrhythmic Qualities

Dexmedetomidine causes central activation of α_2-receptors involving the dorsal motor nucleus of the vagus nerve, the nucleus ambiguous, and the nucleus of the tractus solitarius, which are all involved in modifying vagal tone. The subsequent impact leads to a decrease in cardiomyocyte cyclic adenosine monophosphate and a reduction in L-type calcium ion currents, resulting in prolonged repolarization and refractory periods.

These aforementioned mechanisms explain the bradycardic effects of dexmedetomidine, which has been used specifically for its antiarrhythmic properties in the context of SVT, AFL, VT, and junctional ectopic tachycardia. Although some concern exists about dexmedetomidine's potential to suppress tachyarrhythmias, this agent may still be used in the EP laboratory because unlike some of the other aforementioned agents, dexmedetomidine has minimal respiratory depressant effects. Furthermore, dexmedetomidine has less risk of delirium in older adults compared with the benzodiazepines.

Proarrhythmic Qualities

In children, dexmedetomidine has been shown to prolong the QTc, increase SN cycle length, and increase SN recovery time. AVN block has been reported, with a prolonged Wenckebach cycle length and PR interval. Hence, dexmedetomidine should be used cautiously or avoided in those at risk for heart block, significant bradycardia, heart transplant patients, and those with known preexisting cardiac conduction defects.

Volatile Anesthetics

Potent volatile anesthetic agents include isoflurane, desflurane, and sevoflurane. The arrhythmic properties of the volatile anesthetics are controversial. The effects of volatile anesthetics on ventricular arrhythmias vary in different experimental models and according to the mechanism of the arrhythmia. Overall, the potent volatile anesthetics have an antifibrillatory effect, especially in the context of acute ischemia.

All volatile anesthetics lead to a prolongation of cardiomyocyte repolarization time, including slowing of AVN conduction time and prolongation of the QTc. Pediatric and adult clinical studies have demonstrated this effect for desflurane, sevoflurane, and isoflurane. In the context of pediatric dental surgery, supraventricular ectopy associated with sevoflurane has been reported. Sevoflurane has also been reported to prolong accessory pathway effective refractory periods in preexcitation syndromes. This has led to difficulty in inducing SVT despite the use of pacing and isoproterenol.

Isoflurane has also been reported to cause prolongation of accessory pathway effective refractory periods in preexcitation syndromes. Nonetheless, isoflurane, desflurane, and sevoflurane have an overall low arrhythmogenicity potential, and the small doses administered during ablative procedures likely have minimal effects on EP studies.

Although no longer administered or available in most developed countries, halothane is still used in many nondeveloped nations. Halothane is notably associated with arrhythmias, particularly its ability to lower the epinephrine dose needed to provoke significant ventricular arrhythmias. Especially in children, halothane is notably more arrhythmogenic than isoflurane, desflurane, or sevoflurane.

CARDIOVERSION

Electrical cardioversion (EC) is performed to restore sinus rhythm in patients with a tachyarrhythmia. EC entails using a defibrillator to administer a shock to the heart that is synchronized to the R wave of the ECG. The defibrillator's capacitor is charged to a selected voltage, and then energy is delivered to the myocardium through electrodes (i.e., pads) applied to the patient's chest in an anterolateral or anteroposterior position. The amount of energy actually provided is contingent on the voltage selected and the patient's transthoracic impedance (which varies based on patient size and other factors). Although defibrillators can use either a monophasic or biphasic waveform, the biphasic waveform is now used almost exclusively because it is more efficacious at lower energy levels. Although the precise mechanism is debated, by simultaneously depolarizing a critical mass of myocardium and prolonging the refractory period, clinicians can terminate supraventricular and ventricular tachyarrhythmias caused by reentry (i.e., AF, AFL, atrioventricular nodal reentrant tachycardia [AVNRT], VT). EC may only transiently terminate arrhythmias caused by enhanced automaticity or triggered activity and has a relative contraindication in the case of tachyarrhythmias caused by digoxin toxicity, which has been attributed to both of these mechanisms.

Complications of EC include inadvertent shock delivery on the T-wave precipitating VF, transient myocardial depression, arrhythmia recurrence, and thromboembolism (e.g., stroke) (Box 15.3). Because of a high risk of thromboembolism, patients with AF or AFL of more than 48 hours' duration should be therapeutically anticoagulated for a minimum of 3 weeks before scheduled EC and for a minimum of 4 weeks afterward. Patients with AF/AFL of more than 48 hours' duration requiring EC before a 3-week course of anticoagulation can be completed should receive a screening transesophageal echocardiogram (TEE) immediately before EC to rule out left heart thrombus with the left atrial appendage (LAA) being the most common location. EC should not be carried out until therapeutic anticoagulation has been achieved or left heart thrombus ruled out.

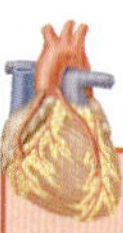

BOX 15.3   *Potential Complications of Cardioversion*

- Ventricular fibrillation (i.e., R-on-T)
- Myocardial depression (transient)
- Arrhythmia recurrence
- Thromboembolism

Anesthetic Considerations

Although EC is a brief and relatively simple procedure, it is highly stimulating and uncomfortable, and its anesthetic management may be confounded by several factors. Even though only a brief period of deep sedation or general anesthesia (GA) is required, hemodynamic and respiratory stability can be challenging to maintain because of adverse effects of the anesthetic agents and comorbid disease that is sometimes present (e.g., structural heart disease, heart failure, obstructive sleep apnea). Moreover, EC is a procedure often performed in a location remote from the operating room or EP laboratory, where unique logistical challenges exist.

As delineated by the American Society of Anesthesiologists (ASA), minimum monitoring standards for such cases include pulse oximetry, blood pressure, electrocardiography, and capnography. Even when GA is not planned, emergency equipment such as a functioning bag-mask device capable of delivering 100% oxygen, an airway kit with oral airway, laryngoscope, endotracheal tubes, and suction apparatus must be immediately available. The ideal anesthetic for EC would result in rapid loss of consciousness and arousal with minimal adverse hemodynamic and respiratory effects. Unfortunately, no such agent currently exists, and the optimal anesthetic regimen remains controversial. Another controversy surrounds whether an anesthesia provider should always administer the sedation for this procedure or if proceduralist-directed nurse-administered (PDNA) sedation is appropriate.

The pharmacologic effects of propofol cannot be reliably predicted by simple dosing formulas, and progression from moderate to deep sedation and then to GA depends on a litany of factors including patient age, cardiovascular status, speed of injection, and the concomitant administration of other medications. For these reasons, the Centers for Medicare and Medicaid Services prohibits PDNA deep sedation (e.g., propofol), and specifically stipulates that it must be administered by a licensed independent practitioner who is privileged to administer GA. Furthermore, the individual must not also be performing the procedure.

Various anesthesia provider–administered anesthetic regimens for EC have also been investigated. Multiple drugs have been studied for their use in EC, including sodium thiopental, methohexital, etomidate, propofol, and midazolam. Although any of these agents may be used effectively and safely, midazolam has been typically deemed inferior because of its association with significantly longer induction, awakening, and recovery times. In comparisons between midazolam and propofol, oxygen desaturations were higher in the midazolam groups compared with age-matched counterparts in the propofol groups. Propofol has also been reported to be a better option for older patients because it is associated with shorter recovery times, fewer side effects, and increased comfort. Recently, a trial compared the use of fentanyl and propofol versus fentanyl and etomidate. There was no difference in the number of shocks needed to restore sinus rhythm or the number of unsuccessful cardioversion attempts. Patients in the etomidate group had a shorter time to loss of consciousness and to administration of the first shock, and patients in the propofol group had a more pronounced decline in systolic blood pressure. The need for positive-pressure ventilation was not statistically different between groups. It was concluded that although both propofol + fentanyl and etomidate + fentanyl regimens provided excellent conditions for EC, etomidate was associated with a quicker induction and better hemodynamic stability. The same trial concluded that when sedating patients for EC using these regimens, the presence of an anesthesiologist is necessary to recognize and manage potential airway obstruction or apnea.

Although EC is straightforward and quick to perform, the anesthetic management of this procedure is complicated by several factors. A typical sedation regimen for EC can include benzodiazepines, opioids, propofol, or dexmedetomidine. At present, there is insufficient evidence to support any one specific approach. Although benzodiazepines are relatively easy to use, can be titrated to effect, and provide hemodynamic stability, in many cases, these drugs may not be the best choice. Compared with benzodiazepines, propofol and etomidate have a more rapid onset and offset, and the capability of more reliably and effectively achieving a deep plane of sedation. Other advantages of these agents include their ability to blunt or even abolish laryngeal reflexes and to minimize the chance of recall. Regardless of the drug or approach used, postanesthetic care is always required. During this time, particular attention should be paid to arrhythmia recurrence and signs of thromboembolism. Same-day discharge home after elective EC is often reasonable.

CARDIAC IMPLANTABLE ELECTRONIC DEVICES

More than 500,000 pacemakers and implantable cardioverter-defibrillators (ICDs) are implanted in the United States every year. Initially developed to manage symptomatic bradyarrhythmias and sustained ventricular tachyarrhythmias, the indications for these cardiac implantable electronic devices (CIEDs) have evolved considerably and now also include patients with heart failure who might benefit from cardiac resynchronization therapy (CRT), which is otherwise known as biventricular pacing.

Conventional CIED systems consist of a pulse generator and one to three leads. The pulse generator is typically implanted below the clavicle in a subcutaneous pectoral pocket, and the leads are inserted directly into the heart (i.e., right atrium [RA], right ventricle [RV], or coronary sinus [CS]) through the superior vena cava (SVC). An atrial lead is indicated for SN dysfunction as well as atrial monitoring. An RV lead is used to circumvent AV block; monitor RV rhythms; and in the case of an ICD, deliver antitachycardia therapy (i.e., antitachycardia pacing [ATP] and shocks). Patients in the United States with SN disease, but without AV block at the time of implant, almost always receive an RV lead in addition to an RA lead because of the concern that AV block might occur later. Finally, a CS lead is used to pace the left ventricle for CRT. Epicardial lead placement (affixing a lead to the outside of the heart) requires invasive surgery and is thus only performed when transvenous placement is not possible or contraindicated (e.g., mechanical tricuspid valve or congenital cardiac anomalies). Of note, in addition to delivering antitachycardia therapy, all modern transvenous ICDs perform all of the functions of a PM (i.e., can be used to manage bradyarrhythmias as well as tachyarrhythmias).

Recent technologic advances have resulted in the US Food and Drug Administration (FDA) approving two new, more minimally invasive CIEDs: a subcutaneous ICD (S-ICD) and leadless pacemaker. The S-ICD has two main components, a pulse generator and subcutaneously tunneled single-coil electrode that allows the device to sense malignant cardiac rhythms and deliver a shock when indicated. Implanting an electrode under the skin in lieu of a lead in the heart reduces the potential for both acute and long-term complications. However, this device has several important drawbacks: its high-voltage output is nonprogrammable, it cannot perform ATP, and its antibradycardia pacing capabilities are extremely limited (Box 15.4).

The leadless pacemaker can currently only provide single-chamber RV pacing. However, it is implanted percutaneously and is about one-tenth the size of a traditional PM. Two versions of this device have been developed, and the Micra (Medtronic, Dublin, Ireland) is now widely available in the United States.

A third minimally invasive nontherapeutic CIED is the implantable loop recorder, a subcutaneous single-lead ECG monitoring device used for diagnostic purposes only. The current generation is small enough to be implanted with local anesthetic only.

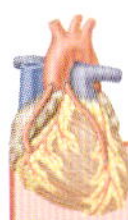

> **BOX 15.4** *Subcutaneous Implantable Cardioverter-Defibrillator Limitations*
>
> - High-voltage output is nonprogrammable
> - Lack of ATP
> - Limited antibradycardia pacing

Anesthetic Considerations

Although CIED insertion is relatively safe, serious complications do occur and in the acute setting include bleeding, vascular injury, pneumothorax, hemothorax, and cardiac tamponade.

Cardiac implantable electronic device implantation is frequently performed with local anesthetic and moderate sedation because a deeper level of sedation is rarely needed. Moreover, limited retrospective data suggest that sedation instead of GA for these cases is associated with shorter procedure and recovery times, reduced analgesic requirements, and lower costs. Commonly used agents include benzodiazepines, narcotics, and propofol.

When moderate sedation is planned, it is not clear whether PDNA sedation is appropriate or whether an anesthesia provider should always be required, because to date, no prospective randomized trial specifically comparing these two approaches for ICD or CRT implants has been performed. However, it is important to understand that there is always a risk of inadvertent progression from moderate to deep sedation, especially when propofol is used, because the pharmacology of propofol cannot be predicted by simple dosing formulas alone.

Also, despite its purported advantages, moderate sedation is not always suitable for these cases. For example, during ICD implantation, deep sedation is mandatory whenever defibrillation threshold testing is performed (because VF is induced and then terminated by delivering a shock). Deep sedation or GA may also be prudent for patients receiving a CRT device because these cases sometimes require many hours of procedural time. Finally, many ICD and CRT patients have structural heart disease, poor left ventricular function, obstructive sleep apnea, and other comorbidities, placing them at higher risk for sedation-related and periprocedural complications.

For these reasons, when at least moderate sedation is planned or necessary, it may be prudent to have an anesthesia provider administer sedation for these cases.

CATHETER ABLATIONS

Paroxysmal Supraventricular Tachycardia

Paroxysmal supraventricular tachycardia describes sudden onset and offset arrhythmias that include AVNRT, atrioventricular reciprocating tachycardia (AVRT), and atrial tachycardia (AT). An EP study and ablation are performed when symptomatic PSVT fails to respond to medical therapy or if the patient prefers curative ablation over chronic medical management.

Diagnostic catheters are placed into the right heart, as described previously. Pacing is performed from the ventricle and atrium to evaluate conduction properties and induce the arrhythmia. When induced, the patient may be left in SVT for long periods of time for further pacing maneuvers or mapping. Isoproterenol is commonly used to promote arrhythmia induction if initial attempts fail. If the patient does not tolerate PSVT hemodynamically, which is uncommon, pacing performed from the control room can terminate PSVT. Ablation is most commonly performed in the RA, but if a left-sided accessory pathway or left atrial focus is identified, left atrial access is obtained. There is often a 30-minute waiting period after ablation to assess for recurrence via EP testing.

Atrioventricular Nodal Reentrant Tachycardia

Atrioventricular nodal reentrant tachycardia is a small reentrant circuit involving the fast and slow pathways of the AV node. As with most reentrant circuits, the slow pathway is targeted, and ablation is performed between the tricuspid valve and coronary sinus using an approach guided by anatomy and intracardiac electrograms in sinus rhythm. Catheter stability during ablation of the slow pathway is important because movement can result in heart block caused by proximity to the AV node. Maneuvers to limit airway obstruction and apnea may be requested to reduce movement. Some electrophysiologists may use a cryoablation catheter, rather than radiofrequency energy, because of improved stability after it adheres to the myocardium. Injury to the AV node is often reversible, but cryoablation has been shown to have a higher arrhythmia recurrence rate. The ideal endpoint is complete elimination of the slow pathway, but modification of the slow pathway with only a single atrial "echo beat" (an impulse that goes down the slow pathway and up the fast pathway resulting in a retrograde P wave but failing to continue as AVNRT) is acceptable and is not associated with an increased risk of recurrence.

Atrioventricular Reciprocating Tachycardia

Atrioventricular reciprocating tachycardia is classified as an SVT but is mediated by an accessory pathway that traverses both the atrium and the ventricle; therefore the circuit of the tachycardia uses both the atrium and ventricle. Ventricular preexcitation evident on resting surface ECG (i.e., Wolf-Parkinson-White syndrome) indicates the presence of an accessory pathway; however, some pathways are concealed (i.e., retrograde conduction only) and are only revealed upon EP study. AVRT more commonly results in a narrow-complex tachycardia because conduction occurs antegrade down the AV node and back to the atrium via the accessory pathway. Alternatively, if the wavefront occurs in the reverse direction, a wide-complex tachycardia is observed because conduction is antegrade down the accessory pathway insertion into the ventricle and back up to the AV node. The most common accessory pathway location is the left lateral mitral annulus, although many sites are possible along the mitral and tricuspid valves. A transseptal approach or a retrograde aortic approach via the femoral artery may be used for left-sided access. Ablation is ideally performed at the midportion of the accessory pathway because the atrial and ventricular insertions may be up to a few centimeters away because of the oblique course along the annulus. Elimination of both antegrade and retrograde pathway conduction is the optimal endpoint.

Atrial Tachycardia

Focal AT may be caused by an automatic or triggered focus as well as micro-reentry. Focal AT will display centrifugal activation emanating from a single point like the ripples from a stone dropped in a pond. AT can occur from any atrial tissue but tends to occur more frequently in specific locations such as the crista terminalis, coronary sinus, pulmonary veins, SVC, mitral and tricuspid valves, and atrial septum. AT is less common than the other PSVTs referred for ablation but increases with age and is associated with underlying cardiac disease. Occasionally, AT is challenging to induce and sustain. Therefore the sedation level may need to be minimized for the procedure. Particular to AT, a sustained arrhythmia is helpful to map the focus. The endpoint for an AT ablation relies on lack of inducibility compared with AVRNT and AVRT in which the conduction properties of the substrate ablated can be used to determine success.

Atrial Flutter

Atrial flutter is a macroreentrant arrhythmia. When it perpetuates in a counterclockwise direction around the atrial side of the tricuspid valve, which can be identified by the 12-lead ECG, it is called "typical" AFL. Typical AFL is cavotricuspid isthmus dependent, which means that the region extending along the floor of the RA from the tricuspid valve to the inferior vena cava is the zone of slow conduction that facilitates this rhythm. It is unnecessary for the patient to be in AFL for ablation because an anatomic approach is generally taken with RF energy delivered along the cavotricuspid isthmus. Because of the risk of stroke when converting AFL to sinus, many of these patients will have continued therapeutic anticoagulation; thus the bleeding risk may be increased. However, the risk for tamponade remains low given the thickness of the isthmus.

Multipolar catheters are placed around the tricuspid valve and isthmus to evaluate the endpoint of ablation. Pacing across the cavotricuspid isthmus should show bidirectional block (i.e., conduction fails to cross the line of ablation from either direction). Termination of AFL is not a reliable endpoint because most patients will continue to have isthmus conduction. Bidirectional block is usually observed for 30 minutes to ensure electrical reconnection does not occur. AF frequently accompanies AFL, and if AF occurs and does not spontaneously terminate, a cardioversion is performed. Atypical AFL is defined as all noncavotricuspid isthmus–dependent macroreentrant atrial arrhythmias. Atypical AFLs are often associated with prior ablation, cardiac surgery, congenital heart disease, or other structural heart disease. An anatomic approach is usually not possible, and cardiac mapping during sustained atypical AFL will be performed to locate and ablate the circuit.

Atrial Fibrillation and Left Atrial Ablations

The cornerstone of AF ablation is isolating all pulmonary veins, which are known triggers and substrate for potentiating AF. Pulmonary vein isolation is performed with an anatomic approach, either with point-by-point RF ablation widely encircling the antrum of the pulmonary veins or with a balloon-based catheter. Before the procedure, cardiac CT, TEE, or both is used to exclude left atrial thrombus and evaluate for anomalous pulmonary vein anatomy. Left atrial access requires a transseptal puncture that is usually performed under fluoroscopic and intracardiac ultrasound guidance. Patient stability is important, and many centers prefer performing AF or left AFL ablation using GA given the longer duration of these procedures.

When using point-by-point RF ablation catheters, GA is associated with an improved long-term outcome of freedom from AF, but with a higher incidence of esophageal injury compared with sedation. Many centers insert a probe to evaluate esophageal temperature and an EP mapping catheter to localize the esophagus on the 3D map.

It is often easier to place the mapping catheter via the nasopharynx with patient cooperation while awake. Patients are frequently on therapeutic anticoagulation, and the risk of nasopharyngeal bleeding is significant. Radiofrequency ablation uses an irrigated catheter tip, and the patient will receive up to an additional liter or more of fluid; thus a Foley may be needed for these cases. Furosemide may be requested at the conclusion of these procedures to prevent a heart failure exacerbation. Arterial catheter monitoring provides early warning of hypotension caused by tamponade and may be performed by anesthesiology at the radial artery or at the femoral artery by the electrophysiologist.

After transseptal puncture, anticoagulation is achieved with a heparin bolus. The goal is an activated clotting time (ACT) of greater than 300 to 350 seconds, although many centers prefer to achieve a therapeutic ACT after venous access but before transseptal puncture. If any hemodynamic changes occur that cannot be readily explained by the effects of anesthesia, the electrophysiologist should be notified given the potential for tamponade. The patient should not be paralyzed during ablation, particularly for balloon-based ablation technologies, because there is increased risk for phrenic nerve injury. During laser or cryoballoon ablation of the right-sided pulmonary veins, a catheter is used to pace the right phrenic nerve, and diaphragmatic capture is palpated. Additionally, a diaphragmatic potential can confirm capture and provide early warning of phrenic nerve injury if a modified surface lead I is positioned across the diaphragm on lead setup.

The endpoint for paroxysmal AF ablation is pulmonary vein isolation (electrical disconnection of the vein from the atrium), which is confirmed by placing a multipolar catheter into each pulmonary vein. If the patient has persistent AF, additional ablation may be performed, but there is a gap in knowledge regarding the next best approach. This may include lines of ablation across the left atrial roof, mitral annulus, posterior left atrium, ablation of complex fractionated atrial electrograms, or nonpulmonary vein triggers induced by high-dose isoproterenol. Many patients will need to be cardioverted toward the end of the procedure if they remain in AF. There are variable approaches to hemostasis after left atrial ablation. Use of large venous sheaths in the EP laboratory has resulted in increasing use of a "z-stitch," which obviates the need for protamine reversal and avoids longer waiting periods for hemostasis to be achieved via manual pressure.

Ventricular Tachycardia and Premature Ventricular Contraction Ablation

The approach to VT ablation can be separated by the presence or absence of underlying structural heart disease. For patients with macroreentrant VT caused by scar, such as ischemic or nonischemic cardiomyopathy, the goal is to ablate the critical isthmus responsible for the VT or ablate sufficient substrate to reduce the risk of future VT. This is typically a long procedure (>4 hours) and is often associated with hemodynamic instability. On occasion, patients are in VT electrical storm with numerous prior defibrillator shocks despite medical therapy. Patients with poor cardiac output may require percutaneous hemodynamic support with a mechanical circulatory support device. If VT is tolerated, the patient will likely be left in this rhythm to facilitate mapping. An area within or near endocardial scar in the left ventricle is most commonly targeted, although some patients may have an epicardial source that can be ablated via percutaneous subxiphoid epicardial access. Epicardial procedures are associated with increased postprocedural pain, and there is also an increased risk of pericarditis.

Irrigated radiofrequency catheters are generally used for VT ablation, and volume overload from the additional fluid is possible. Arterial access is recommended given the risk of tamponade and hemodynamic instability during VT. Heparin will be given to maintain an ACT longer than 300 seconds when catheters are in the systemic circulation.

Alternatively, premature ventricular contractions (PVCs) and idiopathic VT (no underlying structural heart disease) generally arise from an isolated focus that requires precise mapping but with fewer ablation attempts. The most common locations for idiopathic VT are the right or left ventricular outflow tracts, with the majority localized to the right. Ablation is performed where the earliest activation time during VT or PVCs occurs or where the best pacemap is obtained. Pacemapping is a technique that compares the pacing morphology on the surface ECG produced by the mapping or ablation catheter, with the clinical PVC or VT morphology saved as a template. The site that is a perfect match should be the origin of the arrhythmia. The endpoint for ablation is lack of inducible PVCs or VT despite aggressive pacing with or without isoproterenol.

Anesthetic Considerations

PDNA and GA have both been successfully used for ablation procedures. Generally, minimal sedation offers hemodynamic stability; however, some patients may not be able to tolerate lying supine or immobile for a significant period of time. Additionally, GA may be mandated because of certain procedure characteristics (e.g., length of time, transseptal puncture, use of TEE, extensive radiofrequency ablation).

Most SVT and AFL ablations are relatively short in duration (~2 hours) and may be performed under local anesthesia with monitored anesthetic care. Minimal use of sedation may also be beneficial because deep sedation or GA potentially can suppress arrhythmia inducibility. A typical setup from the anesthetic perspective for these ablations includes standard ASA monitors and one to two peripheral IV catheters depending on ease of access to the patient's extremities. Tubing extension for IV catheters and end-tidal CO_2 ($ETCO_2$) monitoring are helpful. Sedation can be achieved with benzodiazepines and opioids or with continuous infusions of propofol or dexmedetomidine. If radiofrequency ablation is used, a deeper plane of sedation may be required because of the pain associated with the heat transferred.

Atrial fibrillation ablations and other left-sided atrial ablations are lengthier procedures (3–6 hours) that often require patient immobility in key portions of the procedure. GA is becoming increasingly preferred. Typically, there is a higher incidence of procedure success with shorter procedure times when using GA because of patient immobility and predictable thoracic excursions using mechanical ventilation, both of which lead to improved catheter stability and mapping accuracy. Jet ventilation and high-frequency oscillatory ventilation have been proposed to offer further catheter stability.

In addition to standard ASA monitors, these procedures may also require an invasive arterial catheter for frequent laboratory draws and to ensure rapid identification of hemodynamic instability, an esophageal stethoscope for temperature monitoring in cryofrequency or radiofrequency ablations, and a nasogastric or orogastric tube to help indicate the position of the esophagus. In addition, these procedures often require monitoring of the phrenic nerve and observation of diaphragmatic contraction, which precludes long-term paralysis. Finally, total IV anesthesia is required with jet ventilation (Box 15.5).

Ventricular tachycardia ablations also are associated with long procedure times (>4 hours) and with hemodynamic instability stemming from the underlying

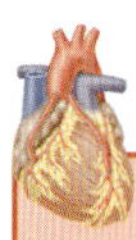

> **BOX 15.5** *Mechanical Ventilation for Atrial Fibrillation Ablation Procedures*
>
> - Associated with better catheter stability and mapping accuracy
> - Jet ventilation and high-frequency oscillatory ventilation have also been proposed
> - Jet ventilation mandates total intravenous anesthesia

arrhythmia. For these reasons, these patients are placed under GA with invasive blood pressure monitoring. Conversely, patients undergoing PVC ablation and focal VT with a structurally normal heart are kept moderately sedated because anesthetic agents may suppress the induction of the ventricular arrhythmia.

Ultimately, the anesthetic technique preferred is institutionally or proceduralist dependent. Clear communication with the EP team to identify patient and procedural concerns is prudent to optimize safe and effective anesthetic care.

LEFT ATRIAL APPENDAGE CLOSURE

Atrial fibrillation is a frequently encountered tachyarrhythmia associated with an increased risk of a cerebrovascular event. In fact, AF likely is responsible for greater than 35% of ischemic strokes and is associated with larger, more debilitating strokes presumed to be related to larger embolic clots than those seen in carotid stenosis. The LAA is thought to be the most common place for thrombus formation, leading to these embolic strokes in nonvalvular AF. The standard prevention and treatment for stroke associated with AF have been utilizing anticoagulants, most notably warfarin or the novel oral anticoagulants, including rivaroxaban, apixaban, and dabigatran. However, patients may have risk factors that preclude the use of anticoagulants, and patients on warfarin often have subtherapeutic INRs. For these reasons, there have been a variety of devices created to isolate and close the LAA in hopes of reducing thrombus formation and thereby reducing stroke risk. The most commonly used LAA closure devices are discussed next.

Endovascularly Delivered Closure

The endovascularly driven LAA closure procedure is similar to AF ablation because left atrial access is a key step. Periprocedural imaging is essential to evaluate the LAA dimensions and direct precise device positioning. Most centers use TEE for this purpose; other centers with more experience may opt for intracardiac echocardiography or even fluoroscopy alone. After TEE examination, femoral venous access is obtained through a large introducer sheath. If intracardiac echocardiography is used, an additional venous access point is established. At this point, a bicaval view of the RA on TEE can aid the proceduralist in identifying a location for transseptal puncture, which is usually inferoposterior to the fossa ovalis. IV heparin is typically delivered before or immediately after left atrial access occurs, with a goal ACT of longer than 250 seconds. A sheath is introduced transseptally, and subsequent imaging is used to introduce the closure device into the appropriate anatomic position within the LAA before deployment. After deployment, the catheters and introducer sheaths are removed, and manual compression, stitches, or percutaneous closure devices are used. The procedure length can range from 1 to 3 hours depending on imaging and difficulty with device orientation. The two most frequently used devices are the Watchman and the Amplatzer.

Watchman

The Watchman device (Boston Scientific), approved by the FDA in 2015, is composed of a self-expanding nickel-titanium frame and a permeable polyethylene terephthalate membrane. This device has been well studied in multiple prospective, randomized clinical trials. As compared to anticoagulation with warfarin or antiplatelet therapy, the Watchman is an efficacious mechanism for LAA occlusion with an acceptable risk (~2.5%) of pericardial effusion.

Amplatzer

The Amplatzer (St. Jude Medical) is a percutaneous occlusion device made of nickel-titanium alloy mesh of varying diameters. When used for LAA occlusion, it demonstrates a favorable risk reduction in stroke and bleeding rates compared with anticoagulation. It has a reported complication rate of about 5%, which is mainly related to periprocedural stroke and cardiac tamponade. It is currently undergoing an investigational device exemption trial seeking FDA approval. In this trial, patients will be randomized to receive either the Amplatzer or the FDA-approved Watchman device, with the primary outcomes being procedural complications, incidence of ischemic stroke or systemic embolism, and successful occlusion of the LAA by TEE.

Percutaneous Closure

Lariat

The Lariat Suture Delivery Device (SentreHEART International) also permits LAA closure percutaneously. The procedure itself is preferably done under GA given that patients undergo perioperative TEE to rule out intracardiac thrombi and monitor procedure progress. As with most EP procedures, femoral venous access is obtained. In this procedure, the pericardium is also accessed with a Tuohy epidural needle. After subxiphoid pericardial access, transseptal puncture is performed and anticoagulation initiated upon accessing the left atrium. An angiogram helps identify the LAA, which is then wired so that a balloon-tipped catheter can be positioned into the ostium. A second wire is then introduced epicardially, which makes contact with the endocardial LAA wire magnetically. The LARIAT loop is then deployed followed by endocardial balloon inflation to aid in the deployment. Radiographic and echocardiographic imaging confirm successful device deployment, at which point the endocardial wire and balloon are disengaged from the LAA. The LARIAT is then tightened, and a pericardial drain is placed before removal of any additional hardware. The appendage eventually necroses as a result of mechanical strangulation, which results in electrical isolation, but painful pericarditis can be a consequence.

Anesthetic Considerations

Left atrial appendage closures should invariably be treated like left atrial ablation procedures. GA is often preferred, especially if TEE imaging is required. However, experienced institutions not employing TEE may perform closures using moderate to deep sedation. As with left atrial procedures, an invasive arterial catheter can be useful for frequent laboratory testing (e.g., ACT monitoring) and rapid identification of hemodynamic compromise.

COMPLICATIONS

The overall incidence of complications is about 3%, with the highest complication rates occurring in ablation procedures for AF and VT with structural heart disease.

The types of periprocedural complications are numerous, and not all are associated with each type of procedure performed. Generally, complications can occur during one of five procedure intervals: vascular access; transseptal access; catheter manipulation; ablative energy delivery; or side effects from anesthesia, sedation, or medications.

Vascular Complications

Vascular access complications comprise the majority of complications seen with EP procedures and are reported to occur in 2% to 8% of procedures. They include hematomas, lacerations, retroperitoneal hematomas, pseudoaneurysms, and arteriovenous fistula formations. The rate of vascular complications has not decreased significantly over the years, which can likely be attributed to using multiple sheaths (often three or more) that are often large (up to 16 Fr [5.33 mm] in diameter). Other risk factors for vascular access complications include older age, obesity, and peripheral vascular disease. Typically, these complications are identified during access closure or postoperatively, but at times may become evident in the intraoperative period (e.g., hypotension, anemia).

The management of vascular injuries depends on the location and degree of insult. Most can be managed conservatively with manual or mechanical compression. However, certain vascular injuries require surgical repair. Prevention of these complications lies in the use of ultrasonography during the initial access and ensuring hemostasis after sheath removal.

Thromboembolism

Thromboembolic complications can be as high as 3%, especially in regard to ablation for AF. Although AF and AFL inherently represent risks for cardioembolic events, catheter ablation procedures likely further increase this risk by activating the coagulation cascade with placement of catheters, disruption of endothelium, EC, arrhythmia ablation, and atrial stunning.

The premise of thromboembolism management resides in the prevention of a thromboembolic event. Intraoperative prevention strategies include the use of TEE and intracardiac echocardiography as well as the administration of IV heparin.

Iatrogenic Cardiac Arrhythmias

Catheter manipulation within the cardiac chamber can induce iatrogenic cardiac arrhythmias, including high-grade AV nodal blockade to VF. These arrhythmias are most often short-lived and innocuous; however, care must be taken to recognize more significant arrhythmias and act accordingly. EP patients should have defibrillation pads placed before the procedure to allow for transcutaneous pacing or defibrillation if warranted.

Pericardial Effusion

Pericardial effusion is more common in catheter ablation procedures and can occur during catheter manipulation, radiofrequency or cryoballoon ablation, or transseptal puncture in a systemically anticoagulated patient. The overall incidence remains low at 0.2% of all EP procedures but increases to 2% when considering only radiofrequency ablations.

Small pericardial effusions can be asymptomatic, but because of the acute nature of pericardial fluid accumulation in the EP laboratory, even small effusions can result in tamponade physiology and require pericardiocentesis. The diagnosis can be made by transthoracic echocardiography, TEE, intracardiac ultrasound, or the absence of lateral heart border movement on fluoroscopy. After confirmation, anticoagulation should be reversed and a pericardiocentesis with drain placement completed. If bleeding is brisk or persists, cardiac surgery consultation should be considered for possible open surgical repair of a tear.

During lead extraction procedures, vascular injuries typically occur in the SVC, and a high number of these will also result in tamponade given the communication with the pericardium. Fortunately, there is a new compressible balloon designed to occlude the SVC, which provides hemostasis while the tear is surgically repaired. To use this balloon, a long wire is placed from the femoral vein into the right internal jugular vein before the percutaneous extraction. Contrast is then used to inflate the balloon under fluoroscopy to visualize its proper location and stability if an SVC injury occurs. Experts recommend occluding the SVC even before attempting peri-cardiocentesis in these cases.

Air Embolism

Air embolism may occur on the right, left, or both sides of the cardiac system. Systemic air embolism is more frequently encountered with the introduction of a transseptal catheter or in patients who have a patent foramen ovale or other cardiac septal defects. Systemic air embolism commonly presents as heart block or acute inferior ischemia, given the anterior location of the right coronary ostium. Detection of air emboli may be possible with echocardiography, and arterial air emboli may be seen on neurovascular imaging. Management is largely supportive because restoration of flow will help with the resolution of the embolism. Increasing the fraction of inspired oxygen will also aid with resorption.

Pulmonary Vein Stenosis

Pulmonary vein stenosis was historically a common complication of catheter-based ablations of arrhythmogenic foci on the pulmonary vein. With time, electrophysiologists have focused their ablation farther outside the pulmonary vein ostia at the antrum and reduced the incidence of this complication. The pathogenesis of pulmonary vein stenosis is unclear but may be from intimal proliferation and fibrosis or thrombus formation.

The presentation of pulmonary vein stenosis generally occurs several months after ablation and can range from asymptomatic to severe dyspnea, hemoptysis, and recurrent respiratory infections. Today intracardiac electrocardiography is used intraoperatively to prevent ablation within the pulmonary veins and diagnosis in the postprocedural period can be made by CT or MRI. Treatment for severe pulmonary vein stenosis is balloon angioplasty or stent placement (or both).

Atrioesophageal Fistula

Atrioesophageal fistula, a rare complication of AF and other left-sided ablations, carries with it a high mortality rate. The posterior wall of the left atrium and the esophagus are located within several millimeters of each other, and direct thermal injury is postulated to be the cause of fistula formation. Multiple modalities are used to prevent this devastating complication, including intracardiac echocardiography, esophageal temperature monitoring, and electroanatomic mapping systems. These techniques attempt to visualize catheter placement, avoid excessive thermal energy to the posterior atrial wall, and provide continuous esophageal temperature measurements.

The presentation of an atrioesophageal fistula typically occurs 2 to 4 weeks after an ablation procedure. Symptoms can include fever, chest pain, dysphagia, and hematemesis and can even progress to a severe neurologic or cardiac event secondary to air embolism or septic shock. If suspected, a diagnosis can be made by CT or MRI, and endoscopy should be avoided. Treatment entails esophageal stenting or operative repair of the fistula; however, the mortality rate remains high.

Phrenic Nerve Injury

Phrenic nerve injury can occur during radiofrequency ablation procedures but is much more common with balloon-based ablation. Right phrenic nerve injury is more frequent and is associated with ablations near the right pulmonary veins or the SVC. Given its anatomic location, the left phrenic nerve is associated with ablation of the LAA.

Affected patients may be asymptomatic or present with cough, dyspnea, and hiccups. The diagnosis is typically confirmed by unilateral hemidiaphragm elevation on imaging. In the majority of cases, phrenic nerve function recovers within 1 year. Electrophysiologists try to avoid this complication by identifying high-risk areas with pacemapping phrenic nerve capture. Before balloon-based ablation, many centers prepare a modified ECG lead I across the right diaphragm and measure a compound motor action potential (CMAP), which provides early warning for phrenic nerve injury while pacing the diaphragm. If the CMAP amplitude decreases by 30% compared to baseline, ablation should be terminated.

Death

Death is an infrequent complication of EP procedures. The overall 30-day mortality rate after an EP procedure is approximately 0.6%; however, the majority of these deaths have been attributed to worsening of the patient's underlying condition rather than to the procedure itself. Procedural complications most often associated with death include cardiac tamponade, atrioesophageal fistula, and ischemic brain injury.

CONCLUSION

Clinical EP is experiencing a period of growth in both volume and complexity. Little prospective evidence is available to guide the best anesthetic plan or which EP procedures require management by an anesthesiologist. However, given the increasing involvement of anesthesiologists, it seems prudent for anesthesia providers to become familiar with the breadth of EP procedures.

SUGGESTED READING

Anderson R, et al. Anesthetic considerations for electrophysiologic procedures. *Anesthesiol Clin.* 2013;31(2):479–489.

Ashley EMC. Anaesthesia for electrophysiology procedures in the cardiac catheter laboratory. *Continuing Education Anaesthesia, Critical Care, and Pain.* 2012;12(5):230–236.

Bohnen M, et al. Incidence and predictors of major complications from contemporary catheter ablation to treat cardiac arrhythmias. *Heart Rhythm.* 2011;8(11):1661–1666.

Calkins H, et al. HRS/EHRA/ECAS Expert consensus statement on catheter and surgical ablation of atrial fibrillation. *J Interv Card Electrophysiol.* 2012;33(2):171–257.

Di Biase L, et al. Ablation of stable VTs versus substrate ablation in ischemic cardiomyopathy: the VISTA randomized multicenter trial. *J Am Coll Cardiol.* 2015;66(25):2872–2882.

Di Biase L, et al. General anesthesia reduces the prevalence of pulmonary vein reconnection during repeat ablation when compared with conscious sedation: results from a randomized study. *Heart Rhythm.* 2011;8(3):368–372.

Issa AF, et al. Electrophysiologic testing. In: *Clinical Arrhythmology and Electrophysiology.* Philadelphia.: Saunders; 2009:27–56.

Zipes DP. Mechanisms of clinical arrhythmias. *J Cardiovasc Electrophysiol.* 2003;14(8):902–912.

Chapter 16

Cardiac Patients Requiring Emergent Noncardiac Surgery

Lev Deriy, MD • Neal S. Gerstein, MD, FASE •
Pramod Panikkath, MD • Harish Ram, MD, FASE, FACC •
Brian Starr, MD

Key Points

1. Cardiac patients presenting for emergency noncardiac surgery have higher risk for perioperative morbidity and mortality. Emergency surgeries are associated with two to five times the risk of major adverse cardiac events compared with elective procedures. Preoperative evaluation and patient optimization are limited by the nature of emergency surgery.
2. The main anesthetic goals in patients with cardiac disease undergoing emergency noncardiac surgery are prevention, detection, and treatment of myocardial ischemia by optimization of myocardial oxygen (O_2) supply and demand.
3. The older trauma patients have higher rates of established cardiac disease than younger patients; hence, they are more susceptible to the effects and vicissitudes of trauma. A second significant population that may be encountered in the trauma arena are adults with uncorrected or corrected congenital heart disease.
4. The central pathophysiology involved in most trauma involves hemorrhage and resultant hypovolemia. Uncontrolled hemorrhage progresses to hypovolemic shock, which results in a constellation of physiologic and organ-related perturbations.
5. Neurosurgical emergencies that require emergent surgery and care by an anesthesiologist are mostly caused by head or spinal cord trauma, rupture of cerebral aneurysms or arteriovenous malformations, hematomas, acute hydrocephalus, and intracranial tumors with possible brain herniation.
6. Patients with severe traumatic brain injury or spinal cord injury (SCI) also tend to have other injuries. In addition, if these patients also have significant cardiac disease, management is complex and requires a multidisciplinary approach.
7. Vascular surgical procedures are associated with a two- to fourfold higher risk of adverse cardiac events (myocardial infarction, cardiac death) compared with other types of noncardiac operations. Coronary artery disease (CAD) shares similar risk factors with noncoronary vascular disease, with atherosclerosis the most common pathologic process affecting coronary arteries, cerebral arteries, the aorta, and peripheral arteries. Consequently, as many as 50% of patients with atherosclerotic disease in one vascular distribution have concomitant disease in at least one other location.
8. The vascular procedure with the highest associated mortality rate is open surgical repair of abdominal aortic aneurysmal rupture (rAAA), followed by elective thoracoabdominal aortic replacement, lower extremity arterial bypass, and carotid endarterectomy. In addition, patients requiring lower extremity amputation frequently have diffuse and severe CAD.

9. rAAA is a surgical emergency that requires rapid diagnosis, efficient preoperative evaluation, and prompt transfer to the operating room for open or endovascular repair. The mortality rate of patients with rAAA who reach the hospital has not changed significantly over the past few decades and still approaches 50% compared with 6% for elective repair.

10. Emergency abdominal surgeries, commonly encountered in practice, include, but are not limited to, cholecystectomy, appendectomy, acute intestinal obstruction from a variety of causes, and acute abdomen caused by perforated bowel and intraabdominal sepsis.

11. The unique risks associated with emergency abdominal surgeries include abdominal distention causing cardiovascular and respiratory issues, risk of aspiration of gastric contents, rapid fluid shifts, electrolyte and acid-base changes, and increased risk of associated sepsis.

12. The most common types of surgical orthopedic emergencies are spine injury with spinal cord compromise, open fractures, septic joints, and acute compartment syndrome. These orthopedic emergencies range in acuity from needing immediate operative management versus waiting up to 24 hours. When time is available regarding the cardiac patient, as much of the preoperative history, physical examination including airway examination, laboratory analysis, and other studies (electrocardiography, chest radiography, echocardiography) should be obtained.

13. The majority of truly emergent otolaryngologic surgeries involve processes that immediately threaten the patient's airway and include emergency tracheostomy, emergencies of airway compromise (Ludwig angina, postoperative hematoma, acute epiglottitis, angioedema), and neck dissections for neck abscesses. Emergency otolaryngologic surgery ranges in acuity from the need for operative management in minutes to seconds (emergency tracheostomy, postoperative hematoma compressing the airway) to potentially several hours (posttonsillectomy hemorrhage, malignant otitis externa [MOE]). When possible, especially regarding cardiac patients, as much preoperative information should be gathered as possible.

14. Ophthalmologic emergencies occur relatively infrequently on the spectrum of emergency surgery; however, these patients often require prompt operative intervention to preserve vision in the affected eye. Patients requiring emergency eye surgery have most often sustained trauma to the eye (ruptured globe) or have been affected by an ongoing or suddenly acute disease process (acute glaucoma, retinal detachment, infection).

Cardiac patients undergoing emergency surgery are at increased risk of perioperative cardiovascular events compared with those undergoing elective surgery. A decision has already been made to proceed with surgery as soon as possible, thereby limiting preoperative evaluation, risk stratification, and optimization. The 2014 American College of Cardiology/American Heart Association (ACC/AHA) guidelines clearly mention that patients must proceed to the operating room (OR) if surgery is deemed emergent (defined as a situation that is limb or life threatening if surgery is not performed promptly, typically within 6 hours) mandating the perioperative team to anticipate and be prepared to manage adverse cardiovascular events in case they arise. Emergency surgeries are associated with two to five times the risk of major adverse cardiac events (MACEs), including myocardial ischemia, heart failure, cardiac arrest, conduction abnormalities, and death, compared with elective procedures.

ANESTHESIA FOR CARDIAC PATIENTS UNDERGOING EMERGENT ABDOMINAL SURGERY

This section focuses on anesthetic implications in cardiac patients undergoing emergency abdominal surgeries that are commonly encountered in practice, which include but are not limited to cholecystectomy, appendectomy, acute intestinal obstruction from a variety of causes, and acute abdomen caused by perforated bowel or intraabdominal sepsis. The general principles included in this section are also applicable to urogynecologic emergencies such as acute ovarian or testicular torsion or urosepsis that typically present as an acute abdomen. Vascular emergencies such as abdominal aortic aneurysm rupture (rAAA), acute mesenteric arterial occlusion, and abdominal trauma are covered elsewhere in this chapter. Although transplant of abdominal organs such as the liver, kidney, pancreas and intestine are technically emergent surgeries, they differ in that patients often have undergone extensive workup to determine their candidacy for transplant. Transplant surgery in cardiac patients is discussed elsewhere in this text.

Emergency abdominal surgeries are associated with certain unique risks, including:

- An advanced age population with multiple comorbidities. Aging and chronic illness deplete physiologic reserve, and superimposed acute illness potentially shifts them to a state of critical illness.
- Risk of aspiration of gastric contents
- Rapid fluid shifts. An acute abdomen is a state of absolute hypovolemia in both extracellular and intracellular compartments, with an increase in the release of stress hormones such as vasopressin (antidiuretic hormone) and activation of the renin–angiotensin–aldosterone axis that conserve salt and water. To maintain circulating volume, there are increases in myocardial work and cardiac output (CO) driven by catecholamines and widespread capillary leak.
- Electrolyte and acid-base changes
- Increased risk of associated sepsis
- Abdominal distention causing cardiovascular and respiratory issues

Preoperative Concerns

The AHA/ACC guidelines recommending proceeding with surgery also recommend assessing clinical risk factors, collecting information about preexisting cardiac illness, and incorporating them to help determine the surgical strategy and to optimize perioperative monitoring and management. In reality, most of the time, the cardiac status of these emergent patients is unknown or possibly manifested intraoperatively with unstable hemodynamics (which may be an indicator of an underlying cardiac condition). In such instances, evaluation and management must go hand in hand, preferably in the hands of an anesthesia provider capable of performing and interpreting point-of-care procedures such as bedside echocardiography or pulmonary artery catheter (PAC) data.

A prudent approach includes aggressive perioperative medical management of the unstable cardiac condition with a goal to shift cardiac interventional therapies, if deemed required, to the immediate postoperative period. In such instances, the conflicting risks and benefits of emergent surgery versus the unstable cardiac condition could put immense pressure on the entire perioperative team with implications on outcomes. A multidisciplinary approach is best if implemented at the time of initial evaluation and must involve all persons available, including the patient, family, surgical team, cardiology and primary care team, if possible.

In most emergency situations, it is often possible to obtain available clinical information and perform a rapid history and physical examination. Additionally, available laboratory and diagnostic data should be reviewed. Routine blood work, if already not sent, should be drawn at the time of intravenous (IV) catheter placement.

Table 16.1   Emergency Reversal of Anticoagulation Agents

Agent	Notes
Antiplatelet agents (e.g., clopidogrel, prasugrel, ticagrelor, eptifibatide)	Platelet transfusion may be required for reversal
Warfarin or coumadin	1. PCC + vitamin K (preferable, especially in a cardiac patient who is volume loaded) or 2. FFP + vitamin K
Unfractionated heparin	Protamine
LMWH: enoxaparin	Protamine[a]
Direct thrombin inhibitors	Novel agent idarucizumab specifically for dabigatran reversal No specific reversal agent available for bivalirudin, lepirudin, desirudin, or argatroban
Direct factor Xa inhibitors (e.g., apixaban, edoxaban, rivaroxaban)	PCC[b]

[a]Per American College of Chest Physicians recommendation to be administered to a bleeding patient if LMWH has been given for less than 8 hours. Only incompletely reverses LMWH and ineffective in case of fondaparinux.

[b]High-dose four-factor PCC is possibly effective but remains an off-label use because there is no Food and Drug Administration–approved reversal agent yet available.

FFP, Fresh-frozen plasma; *LMWH,* low-molecular-weight heparin; *PCC,* prothrombin complex concentrate.

Coagulation studies and blood type and crossmatch should be included. If required, anticoagulation reversal should be initiated (Table 16.1).

Monitoring needs will depend on the patient's cardiac disease and clinical state. Invasive monitoring, if required, may include an arterial catheter or central catheter. Placement of an introducer sheath allows for both volume resuscitation as well as potential PAC placement if indicated. If clinically indicated, invasive monitoring may be placed preoperatively and is usually well tolerated by most conscious patients under adequate local anesthesia and ultrasound guidance. Handheld ultrasound or bedside echocardiography permits easy and prompt recognition of significant cardiac lesions, and such information provides the operating team an opportunity to incorporate measures to optimize perioperative outcomes. It has been shown that use of such devices can recognize major cardiac abnormalities, especially the presence of unrecognized left ventricular (LV) systolic dysfunction or valvular heart disease.

A significant number of patients presenting for emergency abdominal surgery present with systemic inflammatory response syndrome, sepsis, or septic shock. Early antibiotic administration and goal-directed resuscitation must be initiated when indicated. Significant intracellular and interstitial fluid depletion may exist despite the appearance of normal cardiovascular measurements (blood pressure, CO, stroke volume). Patients typically require administration of resuscitation fluids to maintain blood pressure and circulating volume during emergency abdominal surgery, but must be performed judiciously in a cardiac patient to prevent pulmonary edema or acute ventricular dysfunction. Also, electrolyte and acid–base abnormalities should be corrected. Occasionally, after relieving obstruction (in cases of urosepsis, obstructive jaundice, or intestinal obstruction), there is a potential for patients to become overtly septic or prone to arrhythmia.

Antiaspiration prophylaxis in the form of nonparticulate antacid and, if time permits, an H_2 blocker or proton pump inhibitor, must be administered to reduce risk of aspiration. Metoclopramide, because of its prokinetic properties, is best avoided in emergency abdominal surgery.

Intraoperative Concerns

Overall, there is no specific anesthetic technique recommended. General anesthesia (GA) is typically indicated because of the emergent nature of the case, with an open abdomen and likelihood of hemodynamic instability with attendant need for ongoing resuscitation. Anticipation of increased sensitivity to anesthetic agents and hemodynamic perturbations is essential. Decreased doses and gently titrated anesthetic agents with close monitoring of the hemodynamics are required.

After initiating emergency fluid resuscitation as needed and placement of appropriate monitors, a modified rapid-sequence induction often balances the risk-to-benefit equation of competing goals of preventing aspiration versus cardiovascular stability. Agents that minimally depress the cardiovascular system (judicious propofol, etomidate, or ketamine for induction and high-dose rocuronium for intubation) are recommended to achieve this goal.

Patients undergoing emergency abdominal surgeries are prone to volume shifts, and use of the arterial tracing for evaluation of systolic pressure or pulse pressure variation is predictive of fluid responsiveness. A goal-directed fluid therapy approach may assist in appropriate fluid resuscitation. A respiratory-related change of more than 13% suggests that the patient would be fluid responsive. A change of 9% to 13% has been shown to reflect an intermediate range of predictability, a gray zone, in which the patient may be fluid responsive. If the systolic pressure or pulse pressure variation is less than 9%, it is unlikely that the patient would be fluid responsive.

In patients with coronary artery disease (CAD), it is important to avoid excessive myocardial oxygen demand (MVO_2), which could elicit or exacerbate myocardial ischemia. Elevated heart rate (HR) can be controlled with a short-acting β-blocker, such as esmolol, especially to blunt the sympathetic response during laryngoscopy, surgical stimulation, and emergence from GA. Nitroglycerin can also be useful to treat hypertension, especially if the HR is low and hypertension persists. Nitroglycerin can provide both venodilation and dilation of coronary arteries. In addition to demand-related ischemia, adequate supply of oxygen to the myocardium must be maintained in the form of correction of anemia, hypovolemia, and prevention of desaturation. Vasopressor or inotropic infusion might be necessary with the anesthetic agents to maintain an adequate perfusion pressure or if cardiomyopathy is severe. A central venous catheter (CVC) can be placed to provide central access for the administration of a vasopressor or inotrope. Patients with cardiomyopathies may not tolerate rapid fluid shifts during emergency abdominal surgeries and therefore may need monitoring of mixed venous oxygen saturation or CO to direct vasoactive agent therapy. Because of third spacing, frequent monitoring and replacement of electrolytes is necessary. Severe hyperglycemia should be controlled with IV insulin, and hypothermia must be prevented.

Patients with coexisting valvular heart disease need special consideration, particularly patients with aortic stenosis who require maintenance of cardiac preload, systemic vascular resistance (SVR), and myocardial contractility. Rapid correction of arrhythmias is necessary because patients with aortic stenosis and associated LV hypertrophy are likely to poorly tolerate such arrhythmias. Although the usage of PACs is declining, the presence of severe pulmonary hypertension (PH) or severe LV or right ventricular (RV) dysfunction may be an indication for monitoring with a PAC to guide the administration of nitric oxide or other pulmonary vasodilators.

Transesophageal echocardiography (TEE) is used for real-time evaluation of cardiac function and restrictive fluid management during surgery. Perioperative hemodynamic management with TEE may be useful for gastrointestinal tract surgeries in patients with severe cardiac disease. See Chapter 10 for an approach to using TEE for fluid resuscitation.

Despite maximal medical management, if a patient continues to be unstable during emergency abdominal surgery, mechanical support for the ventricle (e.g., intraaortic balloon pump [IABP] or percutaneous ventricular assist device [VAD]) or venoarterial extracorporeal membrane oxygenator (ECMO) can be initiated intraoperatively to facilitate successful completion of surgery and hemodynamic stabilization. This requires resources, early planning, and communication with various teams. Additionally, there is the added time constraint, especially after a sudden collapse, to establish mechanical support or initiation of extracorporeal circulation before hypoxic cerebral injury occurs.

Postoperative Period

An elevated level of postoperative care is necessary in cardiac patients who have undergone emergency abdominal surgery, and intensive care unit (ICU) admission should be considered for these patients for prompt recognition and management of complications. In the immediate postoperative period, there is usually relative hypovolemia from third spacing with associated increased myocardial work. During this phase, resuscitation fluids should be administered cautiously guided by invasive hemodynamic monitoring and circulatory support in the form of vasopressor/inotrope, to prevent precipitation of heart failure. Over the ensuing postoperative days, a state of equilibrium develops when active sequestration stops, followed by a phase of diuresis during which the patient mobilizes fluid and recovers. These fluid shifts are associated with intracellular movement of ions. Hypophosphatemia, hypomagnesemia, and, in particular, hypokalemia are usually evident, requiring regular serum chemistry monitoring. During the equilibrium phase, administration of IV fluid is balanced on whether the current aim is to augment intravascular volume to ensure adequate organ perfusion or to prevent further tissue edema. During the diuretic phase, the main goals are to allow the patient to return to baseline body weight and to aggressively replete electrolytes. Due to the risk of postoperative sepsis, respiratory, and cardiac events being the most common causes of death after discharge from the ICU, patients should be continued to be watched carefully on the floor.

EMERGENT TRAUMA SURGERY IN CARDIAC PATIENTS

In the United States, the number of patients aged 65 years and older is expected to rise from 46 million currently, to 82 million by 2040, and exceeding 98 million individuals by 2060 (which will constitute nearly one-quarter of the U.S. population). Trauma victims are typically represented by a younger demographic. However, older trauma patients have higher rates of established cardiac disease compared with younger patients; hence, older patients are more susceptible to the effects and vicissitudes of trauma. A second high-risk population that may be encountered in the trauma arena are adults with uncorrected or corrected congenital heart disease (CHD). By 2015, more than 80% of all children with CHD had survived to adulthood and after trauma may present to a hospital without prior experience with CHD. Adult trauma victims with CHD are similar to the older adult trauma patient in that they present unique clinical and care challenges.

The central pathophysiology involved in most trauma involves hemorrhage and resultant hypovolemia. Hemorrhage may be distant from structures most germane to cardiac patients (great vessels, heart, lungs) or may be caused by their direct injury. Uncontrolled hemorrhage progresses to hypovolemic shock, which results in a constellation of physiologic and end-organ–related perturbations. Hypovolemic shock is associated with metabolic acidosis, which leads to regulatory cell enzyme dysfunction, resulting in cellular swelling, phospholipid membrane disruption, and ultimately cell death. Many of the normal compensatory mechanisms that counter the aforementioned shock cascade are impaired in cardiac patients. In the following section, caring for stereotypical older trauma patients with cardiac disease, as well as younger trauma patients with corrected CHD, will be addressed.

Recognition of Preexisting Cardiac Disease in Trauma Patients

Trauma victims frequently arrive to the receiving hospital emergency department (ED) unconscious, intubated, or unable to provide a history. History from emergency medical workers or family may reveal the details of the trauma patient's cardiac history. However, this often may not be readily available. For a trauma patient brought emergently to the OR when a brief history is unattainable, various signs may indicate the presence of prior or current cardiac disease.

A cursory physical examination revealing a midline sternotomy scar is likely associated with prior cardiac surgery. In an older patient, evidence of a prior sternotomy should alert the physician to either prior coronary bypass grafting surgery and history of CAD or potentially prior valve surgery. Clinicians should consider the presence of congenital correction in a younger trauma patient with a sternotomy scar. Other evidence of cardiac disease includes the presence of an implanted cardiac electronic device (i.e., implanted pacemaker or defibrillator) or the battery pack and driveline of a VAD.

Additionally, rapidly identified physical examination clues of current cardiac disease may include clubbing of digits indicating uncorrected cyanotic heart disease, a heave on chest palpation indicating an enlarged cardiac chamber, an audible or palpable thrill demonstrative of severe valvular abnormality, or the auscultation of the click associated with mechanical prosthetic valves. The electrocardiogram (ECG) may reveal pacer spikes in a pacer-dependent patient.

Consideration should also be given to the potential concomitant use of outpatient anticoagulation and antiplatelet medications in trauma patients with possible prosthetic heart valves, CAD, or other implanted devices (e.g., VADs). Plans should be made for immediate coagulation testing and possible massive blood product administration in this context.

Finally, in older trauma patients without obvious signs or symptoms of cardiac disease, the clinician should presume that at least mild diastolic dysfunction exists, and consideration should be made for rational fluid management and resuscitation with appropriate monitoring.

Preparation for Trauma Patients With Cardiac Disease

Trauma patients with cardiac disease require careful planning and preparation. This planning should include a review, time permitting, of the patient's prior medical and surgical history, a review of the current trauma presentation (including mechanism, issues with transport, field or ED resuscitative efforts), preoperative imaging, and

Table 16.2　Preparatory Items for Emergent Trauma Surgery in the Cardiac Patient

Induction Drug Issues	Venous Access Issues	Monitoring Issues
Propofol: myocardial depressant and vasodilator	Peripheral IV catheter: based on Hagen-Poiseuille law: short- or large-bore IV will have highest flow rate	Invasive arterial blood pressure: mandatory in significant trauma or significant coexisting cardiac disease
Etomidate: minimal cardiac effects, but concern for postoperative adrenal suppression	Central IV catheter: better suited than peripheral IV if vasoactive drug administration needed; requires increased time and access to neck, chest, or groin, which may not be feasible depending on trauma location	CVP: may be helpful in guiding resuscitative efforts, although there is robust literature demonstrating no correlation between CVP and volume status
Ketamine: usually minimal cardiovascular effects	Intraosseous line: less familiarity for some clinicians; less commonly used; limited flow rate	TEE: may be helpful in guiding resuscitation as well as monitoring or diagnosing preexisting or new cardiac issues; requires expertise; may be contraindicated in penetrating abdominal or chest trauma
Midazolam: minimal cardiac effects but may be significantly sympatholytic if combined with fentanyl or other induction agents		Pulse-pressure wave analysis (i.e., FloTrac): provides real-time cardiac output from invasive arterial catheter; requires specialized equipment; may be invalid in certain surgical procedures, arrhythmias, or with certain vasoactive drug use

CVP, Central venous pressure; *IV,* intravenous; *TEE,* transesophageal echocardiography.

any recent studies (cardiac catheterization, echocardiography, device interrogation). When time is limited and patients present directly to the OR, as much history as possible should be obtained before induction, as well as a limited physical examination focusing on signs of heart failure, previous cardiac surgery, and the presence of existing implanted devices (pacemakers, defibrillators, VADs, medication pumps).

During this preparatory period, consideration should be given to induction agents, circulatory access, and monitoring needs (Table 16.2).

Vasoactive Drugs for Emergent Trauma Preparation

In addition to the preparation of appropriate induction drugs and anesthetic maintenance agents, clinicians should also prepare basic cardiac vasoactive drugs for the purposes of optimizing intraoperative hemodynamics. In a time-limited emergency scenario, preparation of three basic vasoactive drugs (nitroglycerin, epinephrine, norepinephrine) enables the rapid management of most hemodynamic issues for the majority of cardiac patients. Nitroglycerin (starting dosage of 0.5–1.0 µg/kg per minute) provides varying degrees of venous, coronary, and arterial dilation; epinephrine (starting dose of 0.01–0.05 µg/kg per minute) provides arterial vasoconstriction and inotropic support, and norepinephrine (starting dose of 0.01–0.05 µg/kg per minute) provides primarily arterial vasoconstriction with a small degree of inotropic support.

Trauma Care in Older Patients With Established Cardiac Disease

Overview of Aging Effects on Cardiac Function

Numerous cardiac structural and functional changes accompany aging (Table 16.3). In addition to age-related cardiac changes, cardiac-related medications, such as antihypertensive drugs, may also affect the care of older trauma patients. β-Blockers and calcium channel blockers have both negative chronotropic and inotropic effects, which attenuate the normal trauma-induced adrenergic response. Hence, intrinsic compensatory responses to injury may be blunted, and there may be diagnostic challenges because of the lack of an expected HR increase in response to hypovolemia. In addition, there may be issues in the inadequate physiologic response with relation to implanted cardiac devices, which include VADs and implanted electronic devices (defibrillators, pacemakers).

Determination of the severity and degree of hypovolemia in cardiac trauma in older adults may be difficult because of the aforementioned reasons. It is well established that the expected baroreceptor reflex findings of tachycardia and hypotension may be minimal or absent in older adults. Therefore older patients may be significantly hypovolemic but not demonstrate tachycardia or hypotension until extremes of blood loss have occurred.

Table 16.3	Age-Related Structural and Functional Cardiac Changes
Changes	**Impact on Cardiac Function**
Expected	
Myocyte number decreases; replaced with noncontractile matrix	Diminished ventricular compliance; increase in diastolic dysfunction
Sinoatrial node and conduction fiber dysfunction	Conduction defects, increased risk for brady- and tachyarrhythmias
Decrease in aortic and pulmonary artery compliance	Contributor to diastolic dysfunction
Decrease in cardiac adrenergic receptors	Diminished effects of exogenous catecholamines
Pathologic	
Atherosclerosis or coronary artery disease	Myocardial oxygen supply–demand mismatch leading to possible myocardial ischemia
Valvular disease (mitral regurgitation and aortic regurgitation less common than aortic stenosis)	Increased risk for development of acute heart failure, especially with aortic stenosis
Right heart dysfunction secondary to left heart or pulmonary disease	Increased risk of right heart failure, especially with trauma-associated hypoxia or acidosis

Management of Trauma Patients With Cardiac Disease

Management of trauma patients with concomitant CAD poses multiple challenges. The hemodynamic goals in this context are similar to those in nontrauma patients with CAD: to optimize the ratio of myocardial oxygen supply to demand. Trauma and the loss of oxygen-carrying hemoglobin, a high sympathetic tone situation, and hypotension may all contribute to exacerbating existing coronary disease or unmasking occult disease. Table 16.4 displays the factors governing oxygen supply and demand. Of note, HR is the most important determinant of oxygen demand. Therefore appropriate attention to the rapid reinstitution of hemodynamic stability and oxygen-carrying capacity is paramount to limit the impact on patients with CAD.

Patients with valvular disease additionally may not tolerate the high sympathetic tone seen with hypotension. In particular, those with stenotic lesions (i.e., aortic or mitral stenosis) do not tolerate significant tachycardia without leading to impaired ventricular filling, further exacerbated by the hypovolemic state. Appropriate resuscitation and hemodynamic control are essential. Intraoperative monitoring with TEE can serve as both a diagnostic modality for patients with unknown valvular disease and as a monitor to guide resuscitation in such patients.

Procoagulant Agent Use During Trauma: Impact on Patients With Coronary Artery Disease

The use of antifibrinolytics (aminocaproic acid, tranexamic acid) in major trauma is becoming increasingly frequent. Moreover, other procoagulants (e.g., prothrombin complex concentrates, recombinant factor VIIa) are also used on occasion in the context of trauma-related coagulopathy. Clearly, there is an indication for the use of these agents when hemorrhage or coagulopathy is overwhelming and hindering an adequate resuscitation. However, in patients with flow limitation in their native coronary arteries, stented arteries, or grafted arteries, these agents may lead to intraarterial thrombosis and precipitate significant myocardial ischemia. Careful consideration should be given to the use of procoagulant agents in these patients. Any patient with a recently implanted coronary stent or graft (or any vascular stent or graft) should be considered at risk for stent or graft occlusion and these procoagulant agents should be administered with extreme caution and only when they are deemed lifesaving. Similar considerations should apply to patients with cardiac prostheses such as mechanical prosthetic valves or LV assist devices.

16

Table 16.4 Myocardial Ischemia: Factors Governing Oxygen Supply and Demand	
Oxygen Supply	**Oxygen Demand**
Heart rate[a]	Heart rate[a]
O_2 content	Contractility
Hgb, SAT%, PaO_2	Wall tension
Coronary blood flow	Afterload
CPP = DP − LVEDP[a]	Preload (LVEDP)[a]
CVR	

[a]Affects supply and demand.

CPP, Coronary perfusion pressure; *CVR,* coronary vascular resistance; *DP,* diastolic blood pressure; *Hgb,* hemoglobin; *LVEDP,* left ventricular end-diastolic pressure; *PaO₂,* partial pressure of oxygen, *SAT%,* percent oxygen saturation.

Trauma Care in Adults With Congenital Heart Disease

There are a wide variety of corrected CHD defects that may exist into adulthood and therefore may potentially present in trauma patients, including defects ranging from simple atrial and ventricular septal defects to complex repairs of single ventricles or truncus arteriosus. As of 2017, there were approximately 1.4 million adults with corrected CHD. CHD that is considered complex and of higher risk includes prior Fontan procedures, severe pulmonary arterial hypertension, cyanotic CHD, complex CHD with malignant arrhythmias, and any pregnant patient with CHD (Table 16.5). Although there are recommendations that adults with CHD be cared for in specialized centers, there is always the potential that a trauma victim may be brought to any given hospital at any given time.

Preoperative Preparation for Adult Trauma Patients With Congenital Heart Disease

Three groups of CHD patients who may present as trauma victims may be generalized: those with uncorrected CHD, those who have received palliative surgery, and those with corrected CHD. Even with the same structural cardiac lesion, each of these three CHD patients may differ greatly from each other from an anatomy or physiology standpoint. For example, multiple variants of tetralogy of Fallot exist with a range of pulmonary stenosis, leading to a spectrum of "pink" to severely cyanotic patients. Hence, any and all preoperative history and physical examination findings should be obtained to help guide planning and intraoperative management.

Ideally, the following four parameters should be determined preoperatively, time permitting:

Table 16.5	Basic Anesthesia-Related Hemodynamic Issues Associated With Congenital Heart Disease			
Congenital Heart Disease Type	**Common or Major Coexisting Problems**	**Intraoperative Issues**	**Key Hemodynamic Issues**	**Intraoperative Variables to Avoid**
Fontan population	Supraventricular arrhythmias Heart failure Pulmonary AVF Liver cirrhosis	Positive pressure induced hemodynamic instability caused by passive lung perfusion	Impaired systolic function Preload dependence Impaired chronotropy	Tachycardia Bradycardia Hypovolemia Positive-pressure ventilation
Cyanotic heart disease with shunt repairs (intracardiac, vascular, complex): all are usually left to right		Shunt reversal or cyanosis possible if PVR↑, SVR↓, RVOTO	Maintain SVR Minimize PVR	Acidosis Hypercarbia Hypoxia Hypothermia Systemic hypotension

AVF, Arteriovenous fistula; *PVR,* pulmonary vascular resistance; *RVOTO,* right ventricular outflow tract obstruction; *SVR,* systemic vascular resistance.

1. The patient's anatomic disease and the clinical status: What exactly is the anatomic or structural and physiologic nature of the CHD? That is, what shunts exist, and what is the nature of the blood flow in these shunts? Is the patient fully compensated, or is there coexistent heart failure? It should be noted that heart failure is the leading cause of death in the adult CHD population, and the presence of compensated heart failure should be strongly considered in adults with complex CHD. Are there coexisting arrhythmias or conduction disturbances? Malignant arrhythmias are the second leading cause of morbidity and mortality in the CHD population, with supraventricular tachyarrhythmias being most common. Is there residual PH, and is it fixed or reversible? Last, a large number of patients with CHD receive chronic antiplatelet and anticoagulation therapy, which should be factored into the preoperative planning.
2. The patient's prior cardiac interventions: What has the patient's CHD course been? What surgeries or interventions have been undertaken to date? Is the patient palliated or considered corrected?
3. The patient's additional comorbidities: What are other comorbidities (renal, hepatic, hematologic, neurologic, infectious, endocrine) associated with the patient's CHD?
4. The currently planned traumatic surgery: What is the planned procedure in relation to cardiac anatomy? (For example, emergent exploratory laparotomy has fewer potential anatomic implications than emergency thoracotomy.)

Intraoperative Care of Trauma Patients With Congenital Heart Disease

In many regards, the anesthetic considerations for the intraoperative management of the trauma patient with CHD are analogous to considerations in older cardiac patients. First, consideration should be given to the need for GA. Regional anesthesia lends itself to potentially fewer hemodynamic fluctuations along with obviating the need for mechanical ventilation. It is important to note that local anesthetic–induced methemoglobinemia (e.g., use of prilocaine) may be fatal in the context of cyanotic CHD. Nonetheless, most abdominal, chest, or neurotrauma demands GA. Although GA using a balanced technique is common in nonemergent surgery in the CHD population, it is similarly recommended in trauma patients. The most important principle is an understanding of the resultant anesthesia-induced hemodynamic changes in the context of the given CHD. The effects of anesthesia, volume status, and sympathetic state on CHD will depend on whether the CHD issue relates to intracardiac shunting, pressure overload, or volume overload of the systemic or pulmonary ventricle. See Chapter 8 for further discussion on specific CHD pathologies.

Similar to older trauma patients requiring GA, invasive blood pressure monitoring is mandatory, and adjunctive monitors should be considered (e.g., TEE, central venous pressure [CVP] monitoring). In preparation of venous lines and hemodynamic drips, attention to removing air bubbles is essential because CHD patients may have residual cardiac shunting.

EMERGENT NEUROLOGIC SURGERY IN PATIENTS WITH CARDIAC DISEASE

Introduction

Neurosurgical emergencies that require immediate surgery and care by an anesthesiologist are mostly caused by head or spinal cord trauma, rupture of cerebral aneurysms

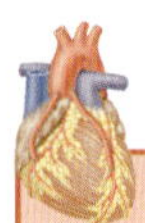

> **BOX 16.1** *Preanesthesia Assessment of Head-Injured Patients*
>
> - Airway (cervical spine)
> - Breathing: ventilation and oxygenation
> - Circulatory status
> - Associated injuries
> - Neurologic status (Glasgow Coma Scale)
> - Preexisting chronic illness
> - Circumstances of the injury
>   - Time of injury
>   - Duration of unconsciousness
>   - Associated alcohol or drug use
>
> Modified from Cottrell JE, Young, WL. *Cottrell and Young's Neuroanesthesia.* 5th ed. Philadelphia: Elsevier; 2010.

or arteriovenous malformations, hematomas, acute hydrocephalus, and intracranial tumors with possible brain herniation. Intracranial hematomas may arise epidurally, subdurally, or intracerebrally and can expand rapidly or slowly. Emergencies affecting the spinal cord include tumors or hematomas causing compression of the spinal cord, which can cause acute spinal cord injuries (SCI).

Patients with severe traumatic brain injury (TBI) or SCI also tend to have other injuries. In addition, if these patients also have significant cardiac disease, management is complex and requires a multidisciplinary approach. Surgery and anesthesia can also subject the injured brain to other secondary injuries as a result of hypotension or hypertension, hypoxemia, hypocarbia or hypercarbia, hypoglycemia or hyperglycemia, fever, or increased intracranial pressure (ICP) that can cause further adverse outcomes.

Preoperative Evaluation

Preanesthesia evaluation should be as complete as possible but is frequently limited by the emergency of the clinical situation. The preanesthetic considerations for patients with cardiac disease involve assessing cardiac and overall health risk, identifying factors that may cause significant perioperative issues, working with cardiology to help optimize cardiac issues if time permits, assessing the risk for a perioperative cardiac event, and developing an anesthetic plan to avoid cardiovascular complications. Patients with coexisting cardiac disease who require urgent or emergent surgical procedures are at increased risk for cardiovascular complications, regardless of the severity of the disease and baseline risk (Box 16.1).

The preanesthetic assessment includes:

- Airway assessment and management plan (Fig. 16.1)
- Severity and chronicity of the cardiac lesion
- Effects of the surgical procedure and anesthetic technique on the preexisting condition and cardiac function
- Plan regarding the use of invasive monitoring and risks and benefits of planned invasive monitors

416

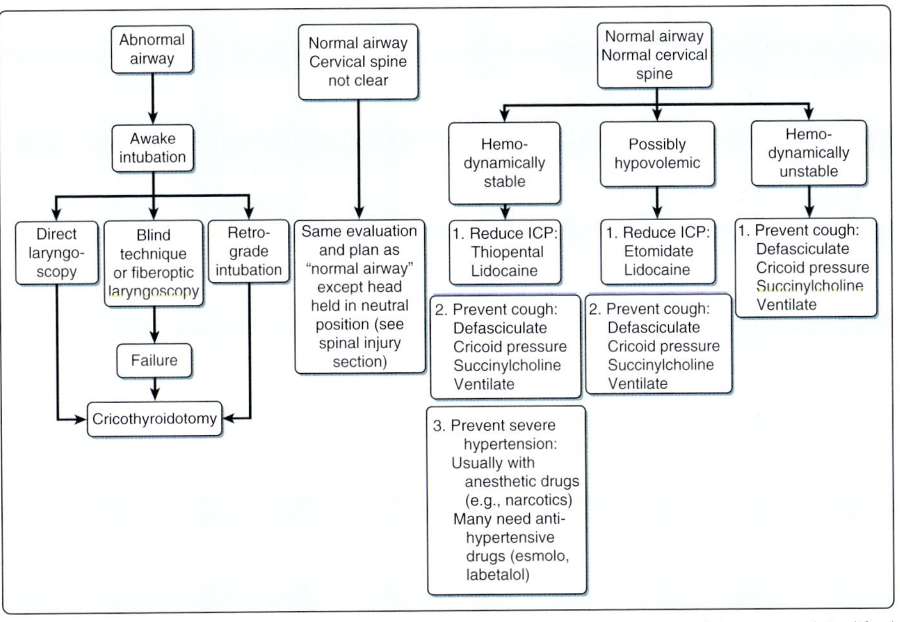

Fig. 16.1 Airway management in a patient with a head injury. *ICP,* Intracranial pressure. (Modified from Cottrell JE, Young, WL. *Cottrell and Young's Neuroanesthesia.* 5th ed. Philadelphia, PA: Elsevier; 2010.)

- Plan regarding the selection and use of vasoactive agents
- Use of surface echocardiography for quick assessment of cardiac status and use of TEE based on hemodynamics

When these patients are brought to the OR emergently, there is usually minimal time for a complete preoperative assessment. In these situations, obtaining any significant cardiac history can be extremely difficult, either because of a lack of reliable source of history or the patient being unable to communicate because of mental status changes. The anesthesiologist may have to depend on physical signs and symptoms to look for signs of heart disease or dysfunction. The presence of chest scars may indicate possible prior heart surgery. Physical examination of the chest and listening to the heart sounds may also provide valuable clues to the presence of heart disease. Signs and symptoms of CHF should be carefully assessed. They include rales, wheezing, hepatomegaly, jugular venous distention, ascites, and edema. Physical deconditioning may also be present in patients with significant preexisting cardiac disease. Close monitoring of vital signs as the patient is brought in to the operating suite is vitally important.

Patients who have had a recent myocardial infarction (MI) within the past 4 weeks and require emergent surgery are at extremely high risk for a perioperative cardiac event. For emergent surgery, the goals should be to prevent, detect, and treat ischemia. Consultation should be obtained from a cardiologist if needed and feasible for risk stratification and further management.

Patients with recent cardiac percutaneous coronary intervention (PCI) are also at increased risk if noncardiac surgery is performed within 6 weeks of stenting. This is closely associated with the cessation of antiplatelet therapy in the setting of a surgery-induced prothrombotic state. In patients requiring emergent surgery, the risk of surgical bleeding by continuing antiplatelet drugs has to be balanced against the risk of adverse cardiac events. This can be particularly problematic in patients requiring emergent neurologic surgery because bleeding into the brain can be devastating. Patients in this scenario usually require platelet transfusions in the perioperative period.

Rapid neurologic assessment is performed using the Glasgow Coma Scale (GCS) to stratify the severity of the TBI. A key priority in the management of patients with neurosurgical emergencies is a rapid and accurate diagnosis with computed tomography (CT) to evaluate an expanding lesion that requires immediate surgical intervention. Lesions such as epidural hematomas, subdural hematomas, intracerebral hematomas, and contusions should be evacuated as soon as possible.

Goals in the Anesthetic Management of Neurologic Emergencies in Patients With Head Injury

The primary goal in neurologic emergencies is the prevention of secondary neurologic injury. In the past few decades, the understanding of the causes and the early treatment of secondary brain injury have led to a decrease in the mortality rate of patients with acute neurologic injury. The outcomes of acute neurologic injury are determined by the presence or absence of secondary brain injury. The main contributors to secondary injuries include hypoxia, hypotension, hypercapnia, intracranial hypertension, and brainstem herniation. These factors can also significantly impact the cardiac status of patients with significant cardiac disease (Table 16.6). The duration of systemic hypotension, hypoxia, and pyrexia have all been found to be strongly associated with death. High-dose steroids do not reduce ICP in head trauma and have not been shown to affect outcome. They are not routinely used in the management of these patients. Steroids may be useful in reducing edema in patients with a brain tumor, however.

Some of the key points to be considered while managing these patients include (Box 16.2):

- Maintain cerebral perfusion pressure and treat increased ICP.
- Avoid secondary injuries such as hypotension, hypoxia, hypercarbia and hypocarbia, hypoglycemia and hyperglycemia, and coagulation abnormalities.
- Provide adequate anesthesia and analgesia.

Table 16.6 Impact of Hypoxia and Hypotension on Outcome After Severe Head Injury (Glasgow Coma Scale Score <8)

		Outcome (% of Patients)		
Secondary Insults	Number of Patients	Good or Moderate	Severe or Vegetative	Dead
Total number of cases	699	43	21	37
Neither insult	456	51	22	27
Hypoxia (Pao$_2$ <60 mm Hg)	78	45	22	33
Hypotension (systemic blood pressure <90 mm Hg)	113	26	14	60
Both	52	6	19	75

Modified from Cottrell JE, Young, WL. *Cottrell and Young's Neuroanesthesia.* 5th ed. Philadelphia: Elsevier; 2010.

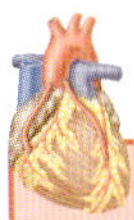

> **BOX 16.2**   *Major Goals in the Acute Care of the Brain-Injured Patient*
>
> A. Prevention of hypoxemia: maintain PaO_2 >60 mm Hg or SaO_2 >90%:
>   1. Increase inspired oxygen tension.
>   2. Treat pulmonary pathologic condition.
>   3. Consider positive end-expiratory pressure ($\leq$10 cm H_2O).
> B. Maintenance of blood pressure:
>   1. Prevent hypotension—maintain systolic blood pressure >90 mm Hg:
>   a. Avoid glucose-containing solutions.
>   b. Maintain intravascular volume status; aim for euvolemia.
>   2. Treat hypertension:
>   a. Sympathetic nervous system overactivity
>   b. Increased intracranial pressure
>   c. Light anesthesia
> C. Reduction in intracranial pressure:
>   1. Head position
>   2. Brief periods of hyperventilation
>   3. Hyperosmolar therapy
>   4. Sedation
>   5. Hypothermia
>   6. Surgical procedures: drainage of cerebrospinal fluid and evacuation of hematoma
>
> Modified from Cottrell JE, Young, WL. *Cottrell and Young's Neuroanesthesia.* 5th ed. Philadelphia: Elsevier; 2010.

Prevention of Hypoxia

Aggressive attempts at the treatment of hypoxia are essential in head injury patients because hypoxemia is associated with the development of secondary brain injury, worsening neurologic outcomes, and increased mortality rate, and these are worse when associated with systemic hypotension (Table 16.6). The goal should be to maintain an oxygen saturation of 90% or higher or a PaO_2 greater than 60 mm Hg. Many patients with significant brain injury require intubation to maintain these goals. There is concern that positive end-expiratory pressure (PEEP) may cause an increase in ICP in patients with neurologic injury because it may decrease cerebral venous outflow and thus increase cerebral venous volume.

Blood Pressure Management

HYPOTENSION

Any episode of hypotension, defined as systolic blood pressure less than 90 mm Hg, has been correlated with higher morbidity and mortality rates in patients with neurologic injury. These episodes of hypotension can also be significantly detrimental to patients with cardiac disease. The common causes of hemodynamic instability in patients with neurologic injury are hypovolemia caused by blood loss and diuresis caused by mannitol use.

The injured brain does not tolerate hypotension well, and adequate resuscitation is required to restore intravascular volume. Hypotension may become severely exacerbated when the brain is decompressed. Patients with ischemic heart disease and aortic stenosis also poorly tolerate hypotension.

Table 16.7	Concomitant Rates of Atherosclerotic Disease in Major Vascular Beds[a]		
	Cerebrovascular Disease (%)	Abdominal Aortic Disease (%)	Peripheral Artery Disease (%)
Coronary artery disease	8–40	30–40	4–40
Cerebrovascular disease	—	9–13	17–50
Abdominal aortic disease	—	—	7–12

[a]Significant overlap exists in risk factors for coronary, cerebrovascular, aortic, and peripheral arterial disease. As many as 50% of patients with atherosclerotic disease in one vascular bed will have concomitant disease present in at least one other vascular distribution.

Data from Beck AW, Goodney PP, Nolan BW, et al. Predicting 1-year mortality after elective abdominal aortic aneurysm repair. *J Vasc Surg.* 2009;49:838-843; Nathan DP, Brinster CJ, Woo EY, et al. Predictors of early and late mortality following open extent IV thoracoabdominal aortic aneurysm repair in a large contemporary single-center experience. *J Vasc Surg.* 2011;53:299-306; and Fransen GA, Desgranges P, Laheij RJ, et al. Frequency, predictive factors, and consequences of stent-graft kind following endovascular AAA repair. *J Endovasc Ther.* 2003;10:913-918.

HYPERTENSION

In some situations, after trauma when there is an isolated neurologic injury, stress-induced activation of the sympathetic nervous system may lead to a release of catecholamines generating systemic hypertension. Because neuroautoregulation is usually impaired after head injury, hypertension can cause hyperemia and lead to increases in ICP. Before pharmacologically treating hypertension, causes such as increased ICP and light anesthesia should be addressed. Patients with neurologic injury may also need to be treated with β-blockade to reduce tachycardia, ST and T-wave changes, and myocardial necrosis that may be associated with severe neurologic injury. This is particularly important in patients with preexisting cardiovascular disease (Table 16.7).

Blood Glucose Control

Stress-induced hyperglycemia is common in neurologically injured patients, and this has been associated with increased morbidity and mortality rates after head trauma and cardiac arrest. Multiple mechanisms (mitochondrial damage, intracellular acidosis, endothelial damage, and inflammation) have been described for the hyperglycemia-related increased neurologic damage, but the exact cause is still unclear. The exact level about which injury occurs is not known but appears to be less than 200 mg/dL. On the other hand, tight glycemic control is also detrimental because of the high incidence of hypoglycemia and thus worsening of outcome. Solutions that contain glucose should not be administered to patients with neurologic injury. Part of the difficult management comes from determining the safe level of blood glucose.

Hyperthermia

A core temperature greater than 38°C is strongly associated with worse neurologic outcomes and increased mortality rates in patients with neurologic injury. It can also lead to detrimental effects in patients with cardiac disease because it can increase oxygen consumption and lead to demand ischemia. Infusion of warm IV fluids, in the setting of hypovolemia, should be performed cautiously, with the risk of hyperthermia in mind.

The different modalities to decrease temperature in patients with acute neurologic injuries include antipyretic drugs, external devices such as cooling blankets, and internal cooling such as infusion of cold saline and endo-cooling devices.

Intracranial Hypertension

Reducing ICP is a major goal in the acute management of patients with brain injury. It can be achieved with changes in head position, hyperventilation, hyperosmolar fluids or diuretics, barbiturates, and sometimes surgical intervention.

Head-up position or reverse Trendelenburg (up to 30 degrees) position with the neck being neutral promotes cerebral venous drainage and can potentially decrease ICP, assuming the venous pathways are still patent. Tight endotracheal tube ties around the neck should be avoided because they can potentially restrict venous drainage and increase the ICP.

Hypocapnia from hyperventilation is a useful therapeutic tool in the management of increased ICP. Although this can lower ICP, it has to be used with caution because it can also increase cerebral ischemia.

Hyperosmolar therapy using mannitol decreases brain water content and ICP mainly by increasing the plasma osmolality and hence creating an osmotic gradient across the blood-brain barrier. Transient hypotension may occur after rapid administration of mannitol, which may be problematic in patients with significant cardiac disease. After the transient blood pressure drop, mannitol then increases blood volume and cardiac index. These hemodynamic changes should be closely watched because they can be poorly tolerated in patients with significant cardiac disease.

Diuretics, such as furosemide, can lower ICP when used in larger doses, up to 1 mg/kg, or in smaller doses when combined with mannitol. Using furosemide may be advantageous in patients with a coexisting cardiac disease because it does not increase blood volume. Still, it has to be used with caution because it can acutely decrease blood pressure, which can be detrimental to patients with significant cardiovascular disease.

Barbiturates and other sedatives can also be used to reduce cerebral metabolism and ICP. Barbiturates work well in the acute control of ICP, but as a class of drugs, barbiturates are myocardial depressants, which may restrict their use in patients with preexisting cardiac disease. Propofol, also a myocardial depressant, can also be used with care in similar situations. Other options include midazolam with or without opioids.

Goals in Anesthetic Management of Patients With Spinal Cord Emergencies

Similar to patients with head injury, one of the primary goals in the management of SCI is the prevention of secondary cord injury. A key way to do this is to immobilize the spine, and subsequent treatment has involved anatomic realignment and stabilization with or without surgery.

Secondary neurologic injury is further prevented by maintaining spinal cord perfusion and correcting hypoxia. Autoregulation can be impaired for several hours after injury. Hence, vasopressors, mainly norepinephrine, should be used to maintain mean arterial pressures (MAPs) of at least 65 mm Hg to improve spinal cord perfusion pressure. This may also be required in patients with CAD to maintain cardiac perfusion. Hypertension is also not helpful because it can cause hemorrhage and increase spinal cord edema.

Hyperglycemia should also be avoided after SCI. Blood glucose levels above 177 mg/dL have been associated with worsening neurologic outcomes. Glucose-containing solutions should be avoided in the first 24 hours, and hyperglycemia should be carefully treated.

Large doses of steroids, especially methylprednisolone, have been reported to improve outcomes in patients with spinal injuries in some studies but not confirmed in others. Currently, the administration of steroids remains an institutional or physician preference.

Anesthetic Management of Patients With Cerebral Aneurysm Surgery

Cerebral aneurysm surgery may be emergent in situations when patients present with a subarachnoid hemorrhage. Preoperative evaluation includes assessment of the patient's neurologic condition and grading of the subarachnoid hemorrhage, assessment of the intracranial pathology with review of CT scans and angiograms, monitoring of ICPs, and evaluation of other systemic issues, including cardiac issues.

Careful management of blood pressure during anesthesia induction is particularly important in these patients. Aneurysm rupture or rebleeding during induction of anesthesia may be precipitated by sudden increases in blood pressure during intubation and is associated with a high mortality rate. The risk of ischemia from a reduction in cerebral perfusion pressure has to be balanced with the benefit of reduced chance of aneurysmal rupture, taking into consideration the clinical Hunt-Hess grade. Patients with lower grades usually have normal ICP, but patients with higher grades tend to have higher ICPs, and these patients tolerate hypotension poorly. This has also to be balanced against the risk of myocardial ischemia in patients with CAD or critical aortic stenosis. The use of high dose narcotics during induction is common to prevent the rise in blood pressure with intubation. Although succinylcholine has been reported to cause an increase in ICP, it has been successfully used in many aneurysm patients with no known sequelae. Many anesthesiologists tend to use nondepolarizing agents. In patients with a full stomach, the risk of aspiration must be balanced against the risk of aneurysm rupture.

In addition to standard GA monitors, monitoring should also include an arterial catheter, preferably placed before induction. Careful blood pressure management is needed during head pinning because this can also increase the blood pressure and potentially cause aneurysm rupture. A central venous catheter (CVC) is usually placed to manage the large fluid shifts and potential need for resuscitation. Placement of a CVC in the internal jugular vein should be discussed with the neurosurgeon because of the potential for venous obstruction to cerebral venous outflow. Placement of a PAC in patients with significant cardiac disease should also be considered. Other less frequently used monitors include jugular bulb oxygen saturation and transcranial Doppler.

The main goals during maintenance of anesthesia are to provide a "relaxed" brain, maintenance of cerebral perfusion, reduction in transmural pressure during final clipping of an aneurysm if necessary, and to allow early neurologic assessment if possible at the end of surgery. Sometimes the neurosurgeon requests cardiac standstill to facilitate clipping of a large aneurysm, and this can be achieved with a bolus of adenosine. This has to be done with extreme caution and is frequently contraindicated in patients with significant cardiac disease. Some large aneurysms may also require circulatory arrest with cardiopulmonary bypass.

Electrophysiology monitoring with electroencephalography, somatosensory and motor evoked potentials (SSEPs and MEPs) are sometimes used as additional monitoring tools. They may allow an intraoperative detection of cerebral ischemia.

The incidence of intraoperative rupture varies with the size and location of the aneurysm. Management of rupture during surgery depends on the ability to maintain blood pressure. If the leak is small, sometimes the surgeon is able to gain control with suction and permanent clipping. At other times, temporary clipping is needed to gain control. Communication between the surgeon and anesthesiologist regarding optimal management of emergence and postoperative management is essential (e.g., early extubation to assess neurologic status versus airway protection for patients who come in for emergent surgery).

Anesthetic Management of Patients With Emergencies in Interventional Neuroradiology

Interventional neuroradiology is the discipline that uses endovascular methods to treat vascular conditions of the central nervous system (CNS). Common goals in the anesthetic management of patients in interventional neuroradiology include maintaining immobility during the procedure, rapid recovery to assess neurologic function, managing anticoagulation, treating and managing unexpected procedure-related complications, and medical management of transportation. Although some of the procedures done in interventional neuroradiology tend to be of an elective nature, two common emergencies are intracranial aneurysm ablation and thrombolysis or thrombectomy of acute stroke.

Intracranial Aneurysm Ablation

The two basic approaches are occlusion of the proximal parent artery and obliteration of the aneurysmal sac. Patients with aneurysmal subarachnoid hemorrhage often have increased ICP or decreased compliance, usually caused by the subarachnoid hemorrhage, hydrocephalus, or parenchymal injury.

The management of these cases involves being prepared for aneurysmal rupture and a new acute subarachnoid hemorrhage at all times. This can happen from spontaneous rupture of a leaky sac, injury from vascular manipulation, or arterial occlusion. The morbidity and mortality rates are high for an intraprocedural rupture. If a rupture does occur, anticoagulation must be quickly reversed, and cerebral perfusion pressure must be maintained at adequate levels. Most patients develop a Cushing response, with hypertension and bradycardia. Emergency placement of an external ventricular drain by the surgeon must be considered, and emergency imaging should be obtained to assess extent of damage and to plan further management.

Thrombolysis and Thrombectomy of Acute Thromboembolic Stroke

In an acute thromboembolic stroke, attempts are made to recanalize the occluded vessel by highly selective intraarterial thrombolytic therapy using agents that are delivered in high concentration through a microcatheter that is navigated close to the clot. Neurologic deficits may be reversed if treatment is completed within several hours of onset of ischemia in the carotid territory and somewhat longer if ischemia is in the vertebrobasilar territory. Another new method is to remove the thromboembolic material from the vessels using retrieval devices.

Both tissue plasminogen activator administration and retrieval with a device have the risk of promoting hemorrhage. Anesthetic challenges involved in the acute care of these patients are that they are generally older, and commonly little is known

16

about their comorbidities. These types of cases can be done under GA or sedation. The options have to be carefully considered, weighing the ability to monitor neurologic status and the risk of patient agitation and movement. Most of these patients also have vasculopathy and systemic hypertension. This can complicate the management because frequently there is the need to maintain MAPs at higher levels because of inadequate collateral circulation, and balancing the risk of vessel rupture or clot propagation.

Special Considerations in Anesthetic Management

Patients With Ischemic Heart Disease

When patients with ischemic heart disease present for emergency neurologic surgery, in addition to the above-mentioned goals, close attention must be given to prevention, detection, and treatment of myocardial ischemia.

HEART RATE

Low to normal HR should be maintained while maintaining blood pressure. Tachycardia compromises oxygen supply and demand. Tachycardia shortens the duration of diastole, the primary interval for coronary artery blood flow. The relationship between HR and diastolic time is not linear. Oxygen consumption in the myocardium more than doubles when the HR doubles. Treatment of tachycardia has to be prompt, initially by deepening the anesthetic or adding an opioid. A β-blocker, such as esmolol, may be added when these measures are not effective.

BLOOD PRESSURE

Every attempt should be made to maintain the blood pressure within 20% of the baseline, but with an increased ICP and the associated reflex hypertension, this may be untenable. Diastolic blood pressure should be maintained because of the role it plays in coronary perfusion. Prompt treatment of hypotension is needed to prevent ischemia, but this should be done with caution because hypertension may precipitate demand ischemia by increasing ventricular wall stress. Treatment of hypertension can be done by deepening the anesthetic or adding an opioid. Sometimes the addition of a vasodilating agent may be required. For hypertensive patients who develop persistent myocardial ischemia, an IV infusion of nitroglycerin, starting at 0.1 to 4 µg/kg per minute, may need to be titrated to control the blood pressure. Nitroglycerin causes dilatation of the coronary arteries and decreases the LV preload because of venodilation.

FLUID STATUS

Fluid status should be managed carefully to avoid volume overload or overt heart failure, especially in patients with diastolic heart disease. CVP can sometimes be used as a surrogate but has multiple limitations as a volume status surrogate. Patients can also be hypotensive because of being vasoplegic due to prior administration of angiotensin-converting enzyme (ACE) inhibitors or from being in septic shock. These patients may require vasopressin boluses or infusion (usually at 0.04 U/min).

ARTERIAL OXYGEN CONTENT

Hemoglobin levels must be adequate (> 8 gm/dL), to attempt to maximize the amount of oxygen in coronary arterial blood. Patients with known ischemic heart disease may need to be transfused to keep their hemoglobin levels closer to 10 g/dL for optimal oxygen delivery.

TEMPERATURE

Hyperthermia is associated with worsening neurologic injury. Although hypothermia is sometimes used for neuroprotection, it is associated with shivering, which can increase myocardial oxygen demand and can lead to ischemia.

The above factors have to be closely considered throughout the entire perioperative period because myocardial ischemia can continue to occur in the recovery room or the ICU.

Patients With Valvular Heart Disease

AORTIC STENOSIS

Severe aortic stenosis leads to obstruction of LV outflow, LV pressure overload, and concentric hypertrophy over time. Hemodynamic management includes carefully monitoring the following key factors.

Cardiac Rhythm

Patients with aortic stenosis have a large fraction of diastolic filling from the left atrial contraction or the "atrial kick." Hence, maintenance of normal sinus rhythm is of significant importance in these patients. Development of arrhythmias in these patients can lead to hypotension caused by reduced LV filling and reduced stroke volume. Attempts to restore sinus rhythm must be made, and in patients with hemodynamic instability, cardioversion may be required.

Heart Rate

Attempts must be made to maintain HR in the normal range. Tachycardia can lead to reduced LV filling or can even lead to ischemia caused by existing concentric hypertrophy. Bradycardia can lead to decreased CO.

Systemic Vascular Resistance

For patients with significant aortic stenosis, sudden drops in SVR can lead to decreased myocardial perfusion. SVR should be maintained within 20% of baseline or MAPs around 70 mm Hg or more.

MITRAL STENOSIS

Severe mitral stenosis leads to reduced LV filling caused by left atrial outflow obstruction. The increased left atrial pressure also leads to increased pulmonary artery pressures and pulmonary capillary wedge pressures. Patients with long-standing mitral stenosis also have PH. Hemodynamic management includes consideration of the following factors.

Heart Rate

Avoidance of tachycardia is important in these patients. Tachycardia that leads to inadequate LV filling is problematic because of the left atrial outflow obstruction that is present in these patients.

Volume Status

Volume must be adequate to maintain CO. Careful titration of fluid boluses is required because aggressive fluid administration can lead to pulmonary congestion.

Cardiac Rhythm

A large number of patients with mitral stenosis have chronic atrial fibrillation because of the presence of left atrial dilatation. There is less dependence on the atrial contraction ("atrial kick") for LV filling compared with patients with aortic stenosis. It is still important to control the ventricular rate in these patients.

Systemic Vascular Resistance

Patients with significant mitral stenosis have impaired compensatory responses to hypotension because the stroke volume cannot be significantly increased, which makes coronary perfusion dependent on SVR. As in the case of aortic stenosis, SVR should be maintained within 20% of baseline or MAPs around 70 mm Hg or more.

Contractility

Avoidance of drugs that can decrease cardiac contractility is important, such as high doses of propofol. RV function is often impaired in these patients, and avoiding further decrease in RV function is important.

AORTIC REGURGITATION

Chronic aortic regurgitation leads to eccentric dilation of the left ventricle. Ventricular contractility is usually preserved until the late stages of the disease when dilated cardiomyopathy occurs, leading to decreased CO. Key points in the hemodynamic management of patients with aortic regurgitation include the following.

Heart Rate

In contrast to patients with stenotic lesions, aortic regurgitation hemodynamics are improved with a slightly faster HR of around 80 to 95 beats/min. The faster HR decreases the duration of diastole, and regurgitant volume is decreased.

Cardiac Rhythm

Supraventricular tachyarrhythmias do not cause as much of a problem in patients with aortic regurgitation as they do with patients with aortic stenosis. Sinus rhythm is still the preferred rhythm when possible.

Volume Status

Patients with aortic regurgitation do better when volume status is maintained, and sometimes a restrictive fluid strategy is used to prevent volume overload and potential CHF exacerbation. This has to be balanced in the setting of neurosurgical trauma when trauma also involves other sites and active resuscitation is ongoing.

Systemic Vascular Resistance

Sudden, significant increases in SVR should be avoided. An increase in SVR leads to an increase in the regurgitant volume and decreases the forward flow. Hypertension can usually be managed by deepening the anesthetic or adding opioid agents.

MITRAL REGURGITATION

Longstanding mitral regurgitation (MR) leads to volume overload of the left atrium, which can lead to arrhythmias. With severe MR, there is an also elevated pulmonary arterial pressure. Secondary or functional MR occurs as a result of ischemia in patients with CAD. Hemodynamic goals in patients with MR include the following.

Heart Rate

For patients with MR, maintaining a normal to slightly faster HR of about 80 to 95 beats/min helps to reduce the regurgitant volume. Attempts must be made to avoid bradycardia. This approach has to be used cautiously in patients with CAD.

Cardiac Rhythm

Normal sinus rhythm is preferred in MR, but many patients with chronic MR have atrial fibrillation. Arrhythmias are better tolerated in patients with regurgitant lesions than patients with aortic stenosis. Patients with secondary MR associated with hypertrophic cardiomyopathy depend on atrial contraction for LV filling, and loss of the atrial kick can lead to hypotension in these patients.

Volume Status

A restrictive volume status can be helpful in patients with primary MR with evidence of volume overload. Aggressive fluid administration can lead to pulmonary congestion. Patients with secondary MR associated with hypertrophic cardiomyopathy need to have increased preload. Hypovolemia exacerbates the hypertrophic obstructive cardiomyopathy and the associated MR in these patients.

Systemic Vascular Resistance

Increased SVR leads to an increased regurgitant fraction and decreases the forward flow. In patients with primary MR, low-normal blood pressures are helpful to increase forward flow. Management of blood pressure for patients with ischemic MR is even more challenging because higher blood pressure helps with maintaining coronary perfusion, but higher blood pressure can reduce the forward flow of blood in the circulation because of increased regurgitant fraction.

The above goals have to be carefully balanced with factors important in the neurologic management of patients coming in for neurologic emergencies requiring surgery.

CARDIAC PATIENTS REQUIRING EMERGENCY VASCULAR SURGERY

General Considerations

Introduction

Vascular surgical procedures are associated with a two- to fourfold higher risk of adverse cardiac events (MI, cardiac death) compared with other types of noncardiac operations. Patients presenting for emergency vascular surgery have an even higher risk for perioperative morbidity and mortality. Many of these patients are at risk of having coexisting CAD. In fact, CAD is more common among patients undergoing vascular surgical procedures (with a prevalence ranging from 37% to 78%) than in other noncardiac surgical patients. The vascular procedure with the highest associated mortality rate is open surgical repair of rAAA followed by elective thoracoabdominal aortic replacement, lower extremity arterial bypass, and carotid endarterectomy. In addition, patients requiring lower extremity amputation frequently have diffuse and severe CAD.

Atherosclerosis is the most common pathologic process affecting coronary arteries, cerebral arteries, aorta, and peripheral arteries. Progressive narrowing of the intravascular lumen leads to downstream ischemia caused by oxygen supply and demand mismatch. Depending on the location of the atherosclerotic lesion, it may lead to MI, stroke, aneurysm rupture, or acute limb ischemia. CAD shares similar risk factors with noncoronary vascular disease. Consequently, as many as 50% of patients with atherosclerotic disease in one vascular distribution will have concomitant disease in at least one other location (Table 16.7). The risk factors for the development of atherosclerotic disease can be divided into nonmodifiable (age, male gender, ethnicity, and family history) and modifiable (smoking, hypertension, diabetes, dyslipidemia, obesity, diet, and physical activity).

Anesthetic Goals in Patients With Cardiac Disease

The main anesthetic goals in patients with cardiac disease undergoing emergency noncardiac surgery are prevention, detection, and treatment of myocardial ischemia by optimization of myocardial oxygen (O_2) supply and demand (Fig. 16.2). Prevention of

427

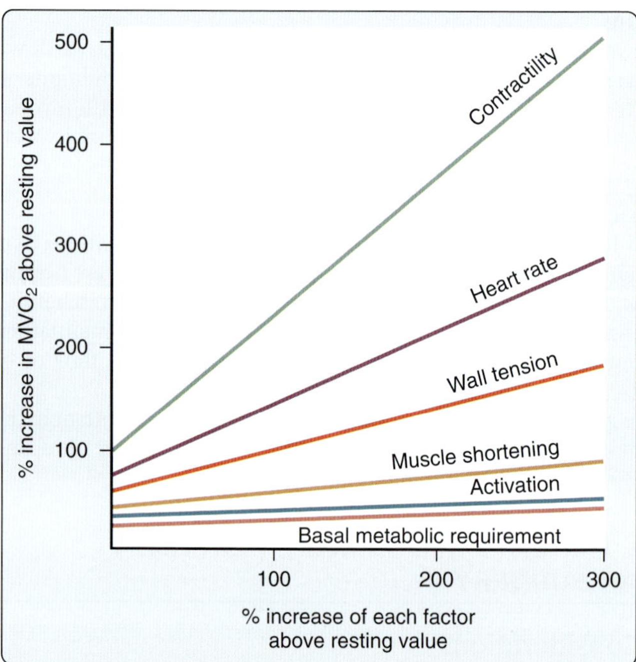

Fig. 16.2 Relative importance of variables that determine myocardial oxygen consumption (MVO₂). Each line roughly approximates the effect of manipulating one variable without changing the others. Most interventions cause changes in several of the variables at the same time. The importance of contractility, which is difficult to monitor in practice, is apparent. (Modified from Kaplan JA. *Kaplan's Cardiac Anesthesia.* 7th ed. Philadelphia: Elsevier; 2017.)

ischemia can be optimized via the following hemodynamic and physiologic parameters: HR, coronary perfusion pressure (CPP), arterial oxygen content, and body temperature. HR goals are typically 50 to 80 beats/min as higher HR compromises myocardial O_2 supply by limiting coronary perfusion time during diastole and linearly increases myocardial O_2 demand. CPP, defined as the difference between diastolic blood pressure and left ventricular end-diastolic pressure (LVED) (CPP = ADP − LVEDP), is optimized in two ways. Blood pressure is typically maintained within 20% of the baseline to increase O_2 supply while avoiding arterial hypertension and volume overload (wall stress) to decrease LVEDP and subsequent O_2 demand. Arterial O_2 content is maximized via optimizing arterial O_2 saturation and maintaining adequate hemoglobin levels (≥8 g/dL). Avoiding hypothermia and shivering is important because they may lead to increased myocardial oxygen demand ischemia.

Monitoring for ischemia is often accomplished via ECG. Myocardial ischemia is typically manifest by ST-segment changes, most commonly new horizontal or downsloping ST-segment depressions. Monitoring of leads II and V_5 allows detection of up to 80% of intraoperative myocardial ischemia. Other useful monitors in cardiac patients include intraarterial catheters; invasive blood pressure monitoring is mandatory for tight control of blood pressure during periods of hemodynamic instability and rapid blood loss. It can be useful in guiding the administration of vasoactive drugs and to facilitate frequent blood sampling. The intraarterial catheter should be placed before the induction of GA to guide titration of induction agents to ensure hemodynamic stability during this labile period.

Central venous catheters and PACs allow the monitoring of a variety of cardiac pressures. Although intraoperative changes in pulmonary artery pressure, specifically wedge pressure, and CVP are poor predictors of myocardial ischemia compared with ECG or TEE monitoring, they can be helpful in the management of patients with pulmonary arterial hypertension and RV failure. Central venous access should be obtained to facilitate high-volume resuscitation and to ensure rapid and reliable administration of vasoactive drugs.

Echocardiography is an excellent modality for the detection of ischemia. The echocardiographic manifestations of myocardial ischemia occur earlier and are more sensitive than the ECG. Segmental wall thickening of less than 30% suggests ischemia and can manifest within seconds of the onset of ischemia. Acute ischemia is diagnosed by a change in regional myocardial wall motion from baseline by two grades (i.e., normal to severe hypokinesis) in two or more segments. Complications of ischemia such as acute diastolic dysfunction, MR, and papillary muscle rupture can also aid in the diagnosis.

Treatment of intraoperative ischemia (Table 16.8) is based on the optimization of myocardial oxygen supply/demand ratio. In relation to tachycardia or hypertension, pain or inadequate anesthesia should be treated immediately by deepening of anesthetic or administering a dose of opioid. If tachycardia persists despite an adequate level of anesthesia, then short-acting β-blockers (esmolol) can be titrated as boluses or administered as an infusion. Tachycardia accompanied by hypertension can be treated with IV vasodilators such as nitroglycerin and nicardipine. Hypotension can be corrected by administering an α_1-receptor agonist (e.g., phenylephrine) or a direct or indirect sympathomimetic with β- and α-agonist effects (e.g., ephedrine) as appropriate. If hypotension persists, a continuous infusion of vasopressor (e.g., norepinephrine), inotrope (e.g., epinephrine), or both may be necessary.

Arterial O_2 saturation can be optimized with appropriate ventilation management. Transfusion of red blood cells may be necessary, particularly if there is evidence of ongoing bleeding, hypovolemia, or cardiac or other organ ischemia. Warming devices for IV fluids and blood products should be used to prevent hypothermia. Additionally, blankets and forced-air devices should be used for active warming.

Surgery for Ruptured Abdominal Aortic Aneurysm

Introduction

Ruptured abdominal aortic aneurysm is a surgical emergency that requires a rapid diagnosis, efficient preoperative evaluation, and prompt transfer to the OR for open or endovascular repair. The mortality rate of patients with rAAA who reach the hospital has not changed significantly over the past few decades and still approaches 50% compared with 6% for elective repair. Intraabdominal rupture (rupture in the free peritoneal cavity) is less common (25% of all rAAAs) but usually results in immediate exsanguination versus retroperitoneal rupture in which the expanding hematoma and surrounding tissue provide a tamponade effect.

Epidemiology

Ruptured abdominal aortic aneurysm is the 13th most common cause of death in the United States, with a prevalence of 5.9% in men between 50 and 79 years old. The incidence of abdominal aortic aneurysm (AAA) rupture ranges between 5.6 and 17.5 per 100,000 person-years, with the most significant predictor of rupture being large AAA size at presentation (the 1-year rupture risk of a 7 cm AAA is 30%). The average reported growth rate is 0.2 to 0.3 cm/year.

Table 16.8   **Acute Treatments for Suspected Intraoperative Myocardial Ischemia[a]**

Associated Hemodynamic Finding	Therapy	Dosage
Hypertension, tachycardia[b]	Deepen anesthesia IV β-blockade	 Esmolol, 20–100 mg ± 50–200 µg/kg/min PRN Metoprolol, 0.5–2.5 mg Labetalol, 2.5–10 mg
	IV nitroglycerin	Nitroglycerin, 10–500 µg/min[c]
Normotension, tachycardia[b]	Ensure adequate anesthesia, change anesthetic regimen	
	IV β-blockade	β-Blockade, as above
Hypertension, normal heart rate	Deepen anesthesia IV nitroglycerin or nicardipine	 Nicardipine, 1–5 mg ± 1–10 µg/kg/min Nitroglycerin, 10–500 µg/min[c]
Hypotension, tachycardia[b]	IV α-agonist	Phenylephrine, 25–100 µg Norepinephrine, 2–4 µg
	Alter anesthetic regimen (e.g., lighten)	
	IV β-blockade when normotensive	β-Blockade, as above
Hypotension, bradycardia	Lighten anesthesia IV ephedrine IV epinephrine IV atropine IV nitroglycerin when normotensive	 Ephedrine, 5–10 mg Epinephrine, 4–8 µg Atropine, 0.3–0.6 mg Nitroglycerin, 10–500 µg/min[c]
Hypotension, normal heart rate	IV α-agonist/ephedrine IV epinephrine Alter anesthesia (e.g., lighten) IV nitroglycerin when normotensive	α-Agonist, as above Epinephrine, 4–8 µg Nitroglycerin, 10–500 µg/min[c]
No abnormality	IV nitroglycerin IV nicardipine	Nitroglycerin, 10–500 µg/min[c] Nicardipine, 1–5 mg ±1–10 µg/kg/min

[a]Ensure the accuracy of oxygenation, ventilation, and intravascular volume status and consider surgical factors, such as manipulation of the heart with coronary grafts.

[b]Tachyarrhythmias (e.g., paroxysmal atrial tachycardia, atrial fibrillation) should be treated directly with synchronized cardioversion or specific pharmacologic agents.

[c]Bolus doses (25–50 µg) and a high infusion rate may be required initially.

IV, Intravenous; *PRN,* as needed.

Definitions

- AAA: greater than 50% dilation of the expected normal abdominal aortic diameter or aortic diameter greater than 3.0 cm
- Symptomatic unruptured AAA: AAA that has become painful but without breach of the aortic wall
- Ruptured AAA: bleeding outside the adventitia of a dilated aortic wall

Classification

* Infrarenal: originating below the level of the renal arteries (most common)
* Juxtarenal: originating at the level of the renal arteries
* Suprarenal: originating above the renal arteries

Clinical Presentation

Patients may have a variable presentation ranging from hemodynamically stable with abdominal or back pain with the presence of a pulsatile abdominal mass on physical examination to the extreme of shock or cardiovascular collapse from exsanguination.

Surgical Approach

The choice between open versus an endovascular aortic reconstruction (EVAR) primarily depends on the hemodynamic stability of the patient and the anatomic suitability of the aneurysm for EVAR. Hemodynamically unstable patients should be immediately transferred to the OR for open repair. There is a short-term survival benefit but no long-term survival benefit with EVAR compared with open repair. By avoiding aortic cross-clamping and abdominal incision, EVAR showed reductions in procedure time, blood loss, and ICU and hospital stays. Approximately 50% of patients with rAAAs have suitable anatomy for endovascular repair, which includes adequate proximal and distal landing zones and appropriately sized groin access vessels. Thus, if cardiovascular status permits, patients should be transferred to radiology for CT angiography to confirm the diagnosis and to assess the aneurysm morphology and possible suitability for EVAR. Alternatively, a transfemoral aortic occlusion balloon placed under local anesthesia can temporarily stabilize the patient and allow time to assess suitability for EVAR using angiography.

Anesthetic Management

PREOPERATIVE EVALUATION

As previously stated, preoperative evaluation and patient optimization are limited by the nature of emergency surgery. To minimize the "door to aortic cross-clamp" (AXC) time, a rapid targeted preoperative assessment should be performed. This includes obtaining pertinent patient history, including functional status, allergies, fasting status, relevant past medical (including cardiac) and surgical history, problems with prior anesthetics, and medications (including antiplatelet or anticoagulant agents). In addition, blood laboratory tests and relevant imaging studies should be reviewed, sufficient IV access (at least two large-bore peripheral IVs) and invasive arterial blood pressure monitoring should be established, and an order for blood type and crossmatch should be sent. The blood bank should be notified and massive transfusion protocol initiated.

PREPARATION

Equipment for insertion and monitoring of the intraarterial catheter, CVC, PAC, and TEE should be ready. Vasoactive drugs, including vasoconstrictors (norepinephrine, phenylephrine, vasopressin), vasodilators (nitroglycerin, nicardipine), inotropes (epinephrine, milrinone), and short-acting β-blockers (esmolol) should be set up and programmed via infusion pumps. Rapid-infusion systems, fluid warmers, and blood salvage equipment should be prepared in anticipation of significant blood loss. Body-warming devices (e.g., forced-air warmers) also should be prepared.

CHOICE OF ANESTHETIC TECHNIQUE: GENERAL ANESTHESIA VERSUS SEDATION PLUS LOCAL

Open emergency aortic reconstructions usually require GA. However, sedation with local anesthetic infiltration is a reasonable choice for EVAR. GA has some potential benefits for EVAR, including more favorable conditions for stent deployment (apnea, easily inducible hypotension, and patient immobility) and the ability to use TEE and quickly convert to open repair if EVAR fails; however, it also carries a risk of significant hemodynamic instability on induction. Sedation, on the other hand, avoids hemodynamic instability related to induction; maintains spontaneous ventilation, which preserves venous return; and improves postoperative analgesia. If sedation is used for EVAR, the anesthesia provider should be ready to convert to GA if necessary.

INDUCTION AND MAINTENANCE

There is a high risk for profound cardiovascular instability during the induction of GA because of the effects of anesthetic drugs, positive-pressure ventilation reducing venous return, reduction in sympathetic tone, and the loss of abdominal muscle tone maintaining tamponade, exacerbating intraabdominal bleeding. Therefore the surgical field should be prepped and draped before induction with the surgeon present in the OR ready to perform immediate incision and apply AXC. Alternatively, an aortic occlusion balloon placed in the proximal aorta under local anesthesia can restore the circulation and provide temporal stabilization to allow a controlled anesthetic induction.

There is no evidence that certain induction agents or a specific anesthetic technique improves outcomes. Consequently, GA can be induced by a variety of agents, with the primary goal to maintain hemodynamic stability and avoid significant hypotension to maintain adequate end-organ perfusion while minimizing sympathetic stimulation during laryngoscopy and endotracheal intubation. A modified rapid-sequence induction is typically performed with carefully titrated doses of an induction agent and opiates followed by a neuromuscular blocking agent. Ketamine and etomidate may provide more hemodynamically stable conditions in hemodynamically compromised patients, but both of these agents are not without side effects, including the cardiodepressant effect of ketamine in catecholamine-depleted patients and the adrenal suppressant effect from etomidate. Volatile or IV anesthesia may be used for maintenance of GA. Although recent evidence suggests a cardioprotective effect of volatile agents in cardiac surgery, this benefit is less clear in the context of AAA repair.

Hemodynamic and Fluid Management

Normotensive hemodynamic resuscitation with careful titration of fluids and vasoactive medications is currently recommended. The alternative strategy, controlled permissive hypotension, is a standard of care in some centers, with target systolic blood pressure kept to 50 to 100 mm Hg to minimize bleeding before AXC is applied, but it should be balanced against the risk of end-organ hypoperfusion and dysfunction. Hypertension should be aggressively treated with pain medications, β-blockers, and vasodilators. Excessive fluid resuscitation should be avoided before AXC application because of the risk of dilutional coagulopathy, clot disruption, and hematoma expansion.

Hemodynamic Challenges During Aortic Clamping and Unclamping

The physiologic changes (Figs. 16.3 and 16.4) of AXC placement depend on the level of AXC application (suprarenal vs. infrarenal; supraceliac vs. infraceliac). The increases in MAP and SVR are substantially greater with suprarenal versus infrarenal AXC. The increases in venous return and CO are substantially greater with AXC above the celiac artery versus below when the splanchnic circulation serves as a reservoir, alleviating

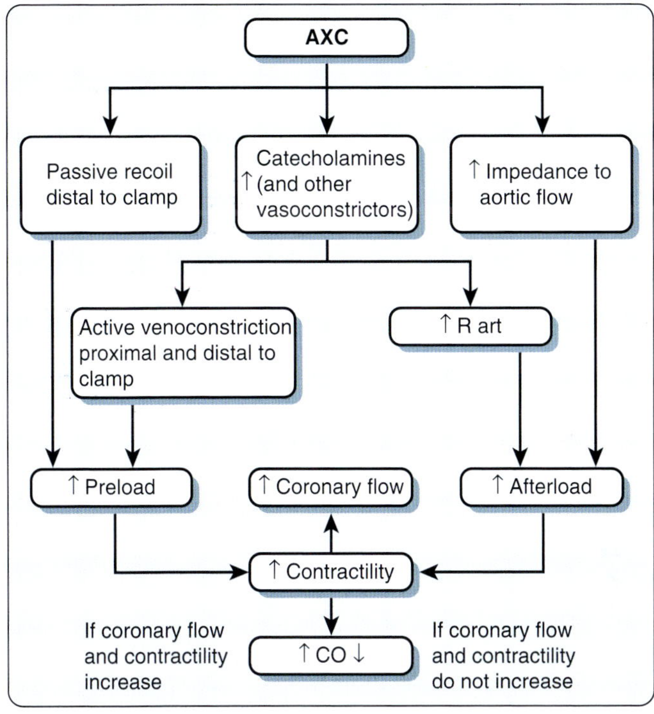

Fig. 16.3 Physiologic changes with aortic cross-clamp placement. Typical hemodynamic response to aortic cross-clamp placement. *AXC,* Aortic cross-clamping; *CO,* cardiac output; *R art,* increased arterial resistance. (Modified from Kaplan JA. *Kaplan's Cardiac Anesthesia.* 7th ed. Philadelphia: Elsevier; 2017.)

increases in venous return. The increases in preload and afterload acutely increase myocardial work and oxygen demand, and in the setting of concomitant CAD and LV dysfunction, they may precipitate myocardial ischemia.

The hemodynamic management of AXC placement includes decreasing afterload and LV wall stress with arteriolar dilators (e.g., sodium nitroprusside, nicardipine, clevidipine) and increasing venous capacitance with preload reduction via venous dilators (e.g., nitroglycerin). Close communication between the surgical and anesthetic teams is critical for timing of AXC placement and vasoactive drug administration.

Aortic cross-clamp removal (Fig. 16.5) is associated with a profound decrease in SVR. Distal vasodilation caused by tissue hypoxia and release of vasoactive mediators promotes sequestration of blood distal to the AXC, resulting in a relative central hypovolemia. Vasoactive and inflammatory mediators (e.g., lactic acid, oxygen free radicals, prostaglandins, endotoxins, and cytokines) promote vasodilation and myocardial depression. Hemodynamic management includes discontinuation of any vasodilator agents as well as initiation of vasopressor or inotropic therapy. A slow release of the AXC may allow for a more gradual metabolic washout with less profound hemodynamic derangements. In case of profound hypotension, the AXC may be reapplied. Again, clear communication between the surgical and anesthesia teams is paramount.

BLOOD AND COAGULATION MANAGEMENT (FIG. 16.6)

Significant blood loss is anticipated during open emergency rAAA repair or failed EVAR secondary to aortic rupture, disruption of retroperitoneal vessels during

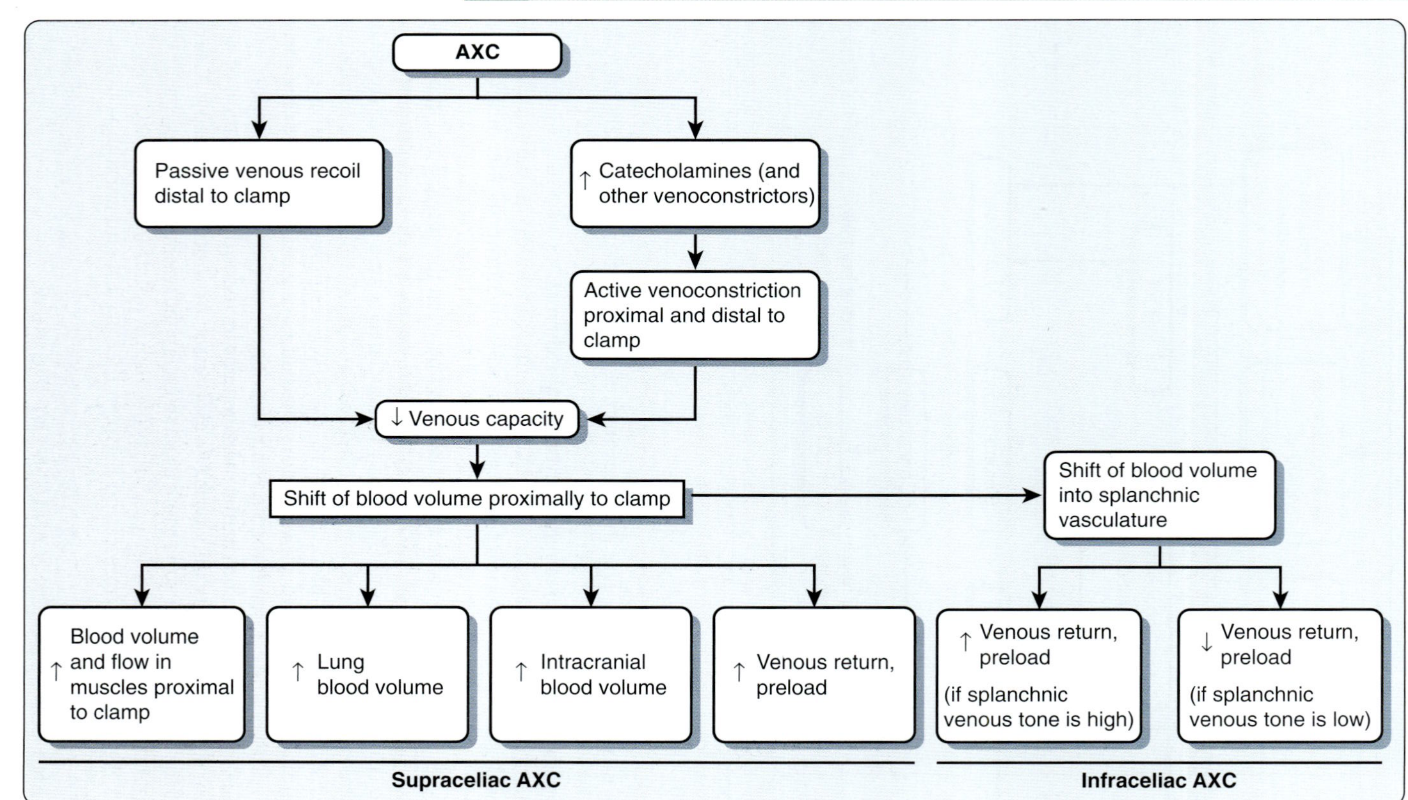

Fig. 16.4 Changes in blood volume distribution during aortic cross-clamping (AXC). The shifting of blood volume with aortic cross-clamping is dependent on the level of cross-clamp placement (supraceliac vs. infraceliac), release of catecholamines and administration of vasoactive medications, and overall blood volume. (Modified from Kaplan JA. *Kaplan's Cardiac Anesthesia.* 7th ed. Philadelphia: Elsevier; 2017.)

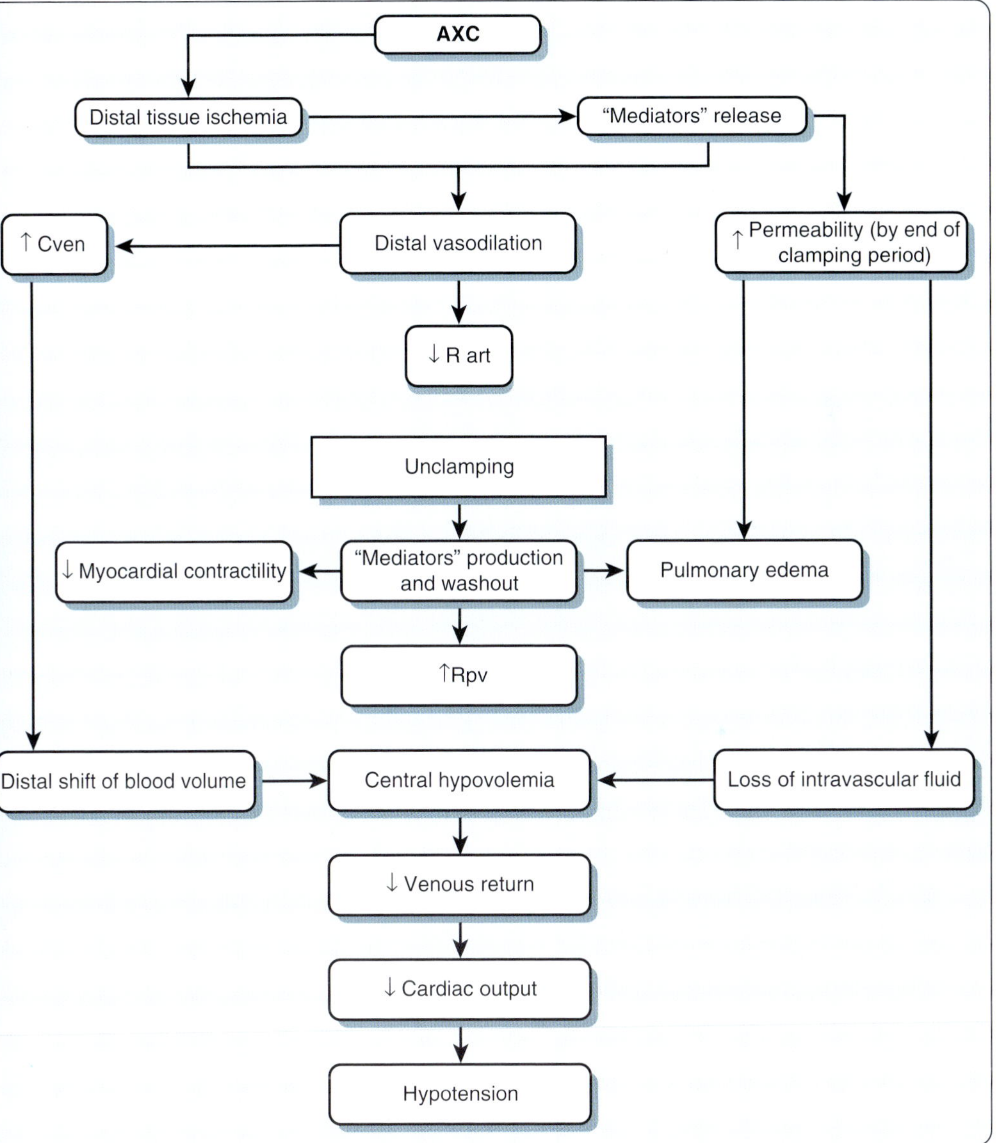

Fig. 16.5 Physiologic changes with aortic cross-clamp release. *AXC,* Aortic cross-clamping; *Cven,* venous capacitance; *R art,* arterial resistance; *Rpv,* pulmonary vascular resistance. (Modified from Kaplan JA. *Kaplan's Cardiac Anesthesia.* 7th ed. Philadelphia: Elsevier; 2017.)

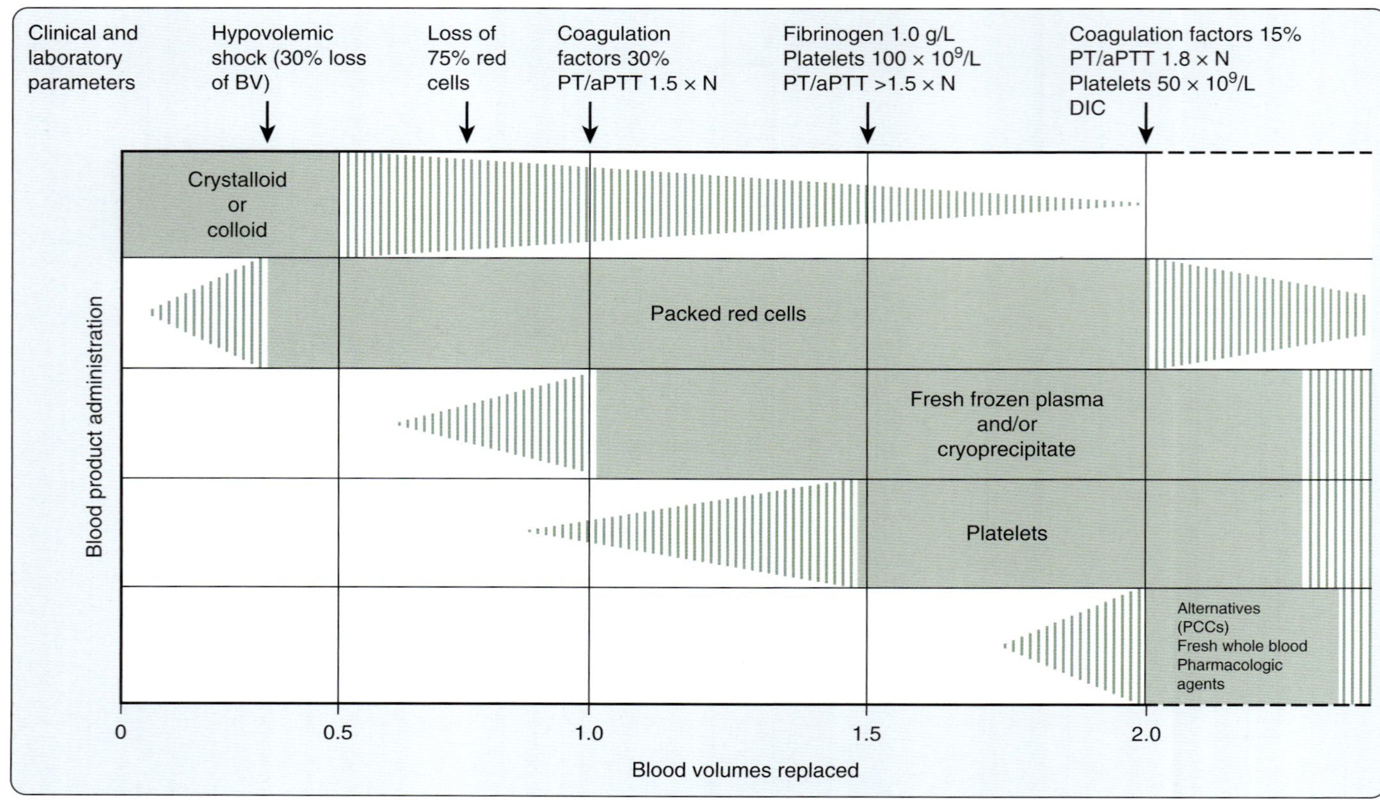

Fig. 16.6 Transfusion therapy for massive hemorrhage transfusion. *aPTT,* Activated partial thromboplastin time; *BV,* blood volume; *DIC,* disseminated intravascular coagulation; *FFP,* fresh-frozen plasma; *N,* normal; *PCC,* prothrombin complex concentrate; *PRBC,* packed red blood cell; *PT,* prothrombin time. (Modified from Kaplan JA. *Kaplan's Cardiac Anesthesia.* 7th ed. Philadelphia: Elsevier; 2017.)

dissection, and coagulopathy. Patients requiring massive transfusion in the perioperative period may become coagulopathic because of loss, hemodilution, consumption of coagulation factors, insufficient component replacement, and fibrinolysis induced by the AXC. Additionally, hypothermia can cause platelet dysfunction by its effect on platelet activation and adhesion and may contribute to reductions in clotting factor functional activity. Development of acidosis may act synergistically with hypothermia to further worsen coagulopathy through its impact on pH-sensitive enzyme complexes involved in the clotting cascade. The blood bank should be informed about potential high demand for a variety of blood products (packed red blood cells [PRBCs], fresh-frozen plasma [FFP], platelets, and cryoprecipitate). Massive transfusion protocol or its equivalent should be initiated with transfusion ratio of PRBCs, FFP, and platelets of 1:1:1. Point-of-care coagulation monitoring (thromboelastography, rotational thromboelastometry) can be used to provide targeted transfusion of deficient coagulation components. Replacement therapy (e.g., prothrombin complex concentrates, fibrinogen concentrates, factor VIIa) should be considered if coagulopathy persists despite transfusion of FFP and cryoprecipitate. Cell salvage techniques should be used to decrease need for allogeneic blood.

TEMPERATURE MANAGEMENT

Hypothermia is common in the perioperative period because of open abdomen, patient exposure, blood loss, and the large IV volumes transfused. Adverse consequences of perioperative hypothermia are impairment of coagulation, platelet, and immune functions as well as significant increase of O_2 consumption caused by shivering, which can precipitate myocardial ischemia in patients with limited coronary reserve. Every attempt should be made to achieve normothermia, including the use of forced-air warming blankets, warming all fluids and blood products, and increasing ambient temperature. Forced-air warming blankets should never be applied to the lower extremities to avoid heat injury during cross-clamping.

RENAL PROTECTION AND FUNCTION

Postoperative renal dysfunction is a major source of morbidity in rAAA repair, with incidence of renal failure reported as 16% to 26% after rAAA repair. Contributing factors include preexisting renal impairment, perioperative hypovolemia, hypotension, anemia, and AXC. Even infrarenal AXC may decrease renal blood flow by 40%, accompanied by an increase in renal vascular resistance with decreases in renal cortical blood flow and glomerular filtration rate. Renal atheroemboli from AXC may also have a deleterious effect on renal function.

There is inadequate evidence to support agents such as mannitol, furosemide, dopamine, fenoldopam, and N-acetyl-L-cysteine for nephroprotection during rAAA repair. Intraoperative maneuvers such as minimizing AXC time and maintaining adequate hemodynamics are the most prudent measures to limit renal injury during open rAAA repair.

Renal dysfunction after EVAR is typically a result of iodinated contrast agents, although atheroemboli and graft impingement of the renal artery ostia may also contribute. In this setting, perioperative maneuvers that minimize the risk of contrast-induced nephropathy include limitation of contrast volume, rehydration with isotonic fluid, and administration of systemic sodium bicarbonate.

SPINAL CORD PROTECTION

Spinal cord ischemia is a relatively rare but devastating complication of rAAA repair. Previous aortic surgery, length of coverage, sacrifice of new collateral vessels, AXC duration and location, and perioperative hemodynamic stability are all likely contributors. Spinal rescue in this setting includes permissive systemic hypertension with or without concurrent cerebrospinal fluid (CSF) drainage.

Postoperative Care

After open aortic reconstruction, most patients are transferred to the ICU intubated and sedated for further supportive care. Despite perioperative advances, there is still a significant perioperative rate of major adverse events after rAAA repair, including death, stroke, MI, renal failure, respiratory failure, paralysis, and death. Myocardial injury remains a common and serious complication after AAA repair, with higher rates reported in patients with preexisting cardiac disease.

Emergent Peripheral Vascular Surgery

Introduction

Acute peripheral arterial occlusion causing limb ischemia is a surgical emergency. Without urgent revascularization, it may result in limb necrosis and subsequent amputation. It is associated with a high morbidity rate and a greater than 25% 30-day mortality rate. Up to 40% of these patients have concomitant CAD. Patients usually present with pain, coldness, and numbness of the affected extremity, with diminished or absent peripheral pulse. Acute ischemia, if not promptly addressed, can lead to irreversible tissue injury within 4 to 6 hours.

Etiology

The most common causes of acute peripheral arterial occlusion are thrombosis in situ and embolism. The primary source of emboli to the lower extremity is cardiac in settings of atrial fibrillation or MI. The most common sites of embolic occlusion are the femoral artery bifurcation, iliac artery bifurcation, and popliteal artery. Thrombotic occlusions are more common than emboli and usually occur in the setting of severe and long-standing atherosclerosis.

Surgical Management

Initial management usually requires immediate systemic anticoagulation with IV heparin to prevent propagation of thrombus. Surgical approach depends on the etiology of acute occlusion. Acute embolism can be managed with embolectomy under local anesthesia with sedation. However, if the cause is an acute thrombosis in situ of a severely diseased atherosclerotic artery, immediate surgical revascularization under GA and invasive monitoring may be required. In addition, catheter-based thrombolysis can be used as a primary therapy or as adjuvant to surgery. If there are signs of compartment syndrome, fasciotomy or even amputation may be necessary.

Anesthetic Management

Emergent nature of the acute peripheral occlusion precludes a detailed preoperative evaluation and patient optimization. Brief targeted assessment should be performed. Pertinent patient information should be obtained addressing the functional status, allergies, fasting status, relevant past medical (including cardiac) and surgical history, airway examination, problems with prior anesthetics, and medications. The patient's laboratory data and imaging should be reviewed, adequate IV access obtained, and invasive monitoring and blood products ordered in case surgical revascularization is planned. The frequent use of heparin anticoagulation and thrombolytics precludes the use of regional and neuraxial anesthesia. The type of anesthesia usually depends on the surgery performed, the patient's overall health status, and underlying comorbidities. Sedation with local anesthetic infiltration is usually sufficient for embolectomy. GA with adequate peripheral or central IV access and invasive blood pressure monitoring is usually necessary for extensive surgical revascularization or fasciotomies.

CARDIAC PATIENTS REQUIRING EMERGENCY ORTHOPEDIC SURGERY

Introduction

Emergency orthopedic surgical procedures, including spine injury with cord compromise (SCI), open fractures, septic joint and acute compartment syndrome, occur daily in many OR suites around the world. A wide spectrum exists on which these surgeries fall, with some requiring surgery within 24 hours (open fractures) and others requiring surgery within hours or even minutes (spine stabilization surgery for SCI, compartment syndrome). These surgeries can occur in patients of all ages, and when these surgeries occur in cardiac-diseased patients (CAD, arrhythmia, valvulopathy, congestive heart failure), special attention and vigilance are important because all aspects of the perioperative course can be affected.

Epidemiology

Roughly 12,000 patients per year sustain a spinal cord injury. Estimates from data in 2010 suggested nearly 265,000 people live with SCIs in the United States, with males outnumbering females four to one. Motor vehicle accidents, falls, firearm injuries, and sports injuries comprise the majority of SCIs. Other causes include vascular disorders, tumors, infection, and iatrogenic injury (e.g., spinal or epidural needle injury). Open fractures can occur virtually anywhere on the body via a wide range of mechanisms. Open fractures require prompt attention because of the risk of infection and typically require, at a minimum, surgical irrigation and debridement within 24 hours of injury. Septic joints, also known as septic arthritis, occur in 20,000 patients per year (7.8 cases per 100,000 people). Infection of operative hardware from prosthetic joints now is a very common cause of septic arthritis. Acute compartment syndrome occurs when tissue pressure within a muscle compartment exceeds the perfusion pressure, leading to muscle and nerve ischemia. This most often occurs after a fracture but can result from the surgery itself. In patients with compartment syndrome, up to 69% had a fracture, and half of them were tibial fractures. Associated vascular injury increases the frequency of compartment syndrome drastically. Other causes of compartment syndrome include intensive muscle use (e.g., status post seizure), everyday exercise, burns, postischemic swelling, rhabdomyolysis, and deep vein thrombosis.

Pathophysiology

Spinal cord injury can lead to varying levels of motor and sensory deficits. With cervical or high thoracic spine injuries, respiratory compromise can occur (diaphragm innervated by C3–C5), and severe bradycardia can occur from loss of sympathetic tone to the cardiac accelerator fibers (T1–T4). Neurogenic shock may acutely occur, which leads to hypotension, bradycardia, and peripheral vasodilation—a dangerous combination for cardiac patients. This combination of vital signs can lead to worsening spinal cord perfusion and cardiac ischemia. Spinal cord perfusion

16

pressure is defined as MAP minus CSF pressure (SCCP = MAP − CSF pressure). Acute treatment is therefore aimed at raising MAP via inotropes, chronotropes, and vasoconstrictors.

Open fractures, as mentioned earlier, almost always require operative intervention because of the high risk of infection. Studies have shown that the timing should occur within 24 hours of injury for irrigation and debridement or operative repair. Open fractures, especially of the pelvis, can damage other nearby structures, including the bladder, rectum, pelvic vasculature, nerve supply, and arteries. A comprehensive examination and evaluation including radiologic studies can aid in the diagnosis of secondary injury and operative planning.

Septic arthritis occurs when there is a direct invasion of the joint space by microorganisms (bacteria, viruses, mycobacteria, and fungi). Bacteria remain the most significant pathogen because of their rapidly destructive nature. As noted earlier, a prosthetic joint infection can occur and has an estimated frequency of 2% to 10%. Organisms invade the joint via direct inoculation of the joint or via the bloodstream. A variety of microorganisms have been isolated from infected joints and can lead to destruction of the joint, chronic pain, and decreased range of motion. Sepsis ultimately can occur, which can be life threatening. Surgical intervention may range from minor irrigation and debridement to requiring complete explantation of affected hardware.

Compartment syndrome results from increased intracompartmental pressure leading to decreased perfusion, muscle and nerve ischemia, and potential loss of the limb. In general, compartment pressures exceeding 30 mm Hg require surgical intervention (i.e., fasciotomies). If left untreated for 6 to 10 hours, muscle infarction, nerve injury, and tissue necrosis occur.

Hip or femoral neck fractures are extremely common and prevalent in the older adult population. These patients often have many comorbidities such as CAD, aortic stenosis, severe hypertension, diabetes, stroke, and dementia. Although the morbidity and mortality rates are high, these surgeries often do not require truly emergent correction, so they are not discussed in this chapter.

Anesthetic Management of Cardiac Patients Requiring Emergency Orthopedic Surgery

Preoperative Evaluation

The aforementioned orthopedic emergencies range in acuity from needing immediate operative management versus waiting up to 24 hours. When time is available regarding the cardiac patient, as much of the preoperative history; physical examination, including airway examination; laboratory analysis; and other studies (ECG, chest radiography, echocardiography) should be obtained. For cardiac patients who have sustained SCIs requiring emergency repair, several insults to hemodynamics should be anticipated (bradycardia, hypotension). For patients with CAD, stenotic valve lesions, and depressed ejection fraction, these disturbances may not be tolerated well. When using neuromonitoring of spinal cord function (SSEPs, MEPs), partial or full total intravenous anesthesia (TIVA) may need to be planned. Invasive vascular access likely will be required (arterial catheter for blood pressure, CVC for vasoactive medications). Regarding open fractures, more preoperative time may be available because these patients usually require surgery within 24 hours of injury. Depending on which bone is broken (e.g., finger vs. femur), the type of anesthetic can be planned (regional vs. general), as well as the need for invasive vascular access or not. Surgery for compartment syndrome often requires immediate OR intervention for fasciotomies, so every effort should be made to obtain as much perioperative history as possible to assist with planning the anesthetic.

Anesthetic Technique

For the types of orthopedic surgical emergencies discussed earlier, MAC anesthesia is rarely adequate. An example in which MAC can be used is an open finger fracture in which MAC plus a digit block could suffice. Peripheral nerve blocks (PNBs) are used successfully thousands of times per day in elective orthopedic surgery; however, their use in orthopedic trauma is controversial. Many orthopedic surgeons believe the use of PNBs (e.g., popliteal/saphenous block for open tibia fracture or supraclavicular block for open elbow fracture) can make postoperative neurologic examinations for nerve function difficult or impossible. PNBs can conceal a postoperative compartment syndrome and potentially delay diagnosis. PNBs can be used for septic joints on a case-by-case basis, typically if systemic bacteremia is not present. However, PNBs may be less stressful physiologically to cardiac patients and should remain a potential option for emergency bone and joint surgery.

Spinal or epidural anesthesia can potentially be used for lower extremity joint or bone surgery, but these blocks can negatively affect patient hemodynamics, especially in cardiac patients. Spinal anesthesia can decrease SVR, dropping preload, reduce afterload, and decrease blood pressure, all of which can be detrimental to patients with CAD, stenotic valve lesions, or depressed LV function. Patient volume status also may be unclear (nothing by mouth [NPO] status, the degree of hemorrhage in the field), making neuraxial blocks an unlikely anesthetic choice in orthopedic emergencies.

Overwhelmingly, GA is the anesthetic of choice for many of the mentioned orthopedic emergencies. Most cardiac patients undergoing emergency GA will need endotracheal intubation, large-bore IV or central venous access, and invasive blood pressure monitoring. Vasoactive medications should be readily available as well as blood products and factors to potentially reverse coagulopathies. Occasionally, intraoperative TEE can be valuable in guiding fluid and medication administration. Regarding spine surgery, GA in the prone position is likely, presenting its own hemodynamic and anesthetic challenges (see later).

Induction and Maintenance of Anesthesia

Induction of anesthesia in any patient carries risk. Induction of anesthesia in cardiac patients requiring emergency surgery carries even higher risk. Induction and maintenance of anesthesia medications can depress cardiac function, decrease blood pressure, and decrease sympathetic tone. Instrumentation of the airway can lead to tachycardia and hypertension, also potentially detrimental for the cardiac patient. For patients with severe CAD, a moderate opioid-based induction may be more cardiostable; however, opioids may severely decrease sympathetic tone, which trauma or infected patients may be relying on for maintaining normal hemodynamics. For these reasons, a preoperative arterial catheter for blood pressure monitoring should be placed. Maintenance of anesthesia may occur with inhaled anesthetics or via TIVA. (TIVA is often required for neuromonitoring of patients with SCIs.) Blood products and vasoactive medications again should be immediately available and ready for administration (ideally via a CVC).

Emergence From Anesthesia

Occasionally, cardiac patients undergoing emergency orthopedic surgery (especially very long spine procedures or those who sustained a cardiac event intraoperatively) may require postoperative intubation and ICU care. For patients able to be extubated, emergence from anesthesia should occur as hemodynamically "smooth" as possible, avoiding large swings in HR and blood pressure that could precipitate ischemia or heart failure. Medications such as β-blockers and vasopressors should remain on hand to treat fluctuations in blood pressure, and invasive blood pressure management should continue during recovery from anesthesia.

Unique Considerations for Cardiac Patients and Orthopedic Surgery

Prone Positioning

Prone positioning for spine surgery presents several challenges. The risk of pressure point injury, nerve and plexus injury, neck injury, and cardiovascular or respiratory physiologic derangement must be at the forefront of the anesthesia provider's mind. Pressure point and nerve injury tend to occur in the extremes of body mass index. Great effort should be made to pad the knees, elbows, hips, genitalia, and eyes to prevent injury. The arms should be kept extended less than 90 degrees or should be tucked and padded at the patient's side. Absolutely all pressure should be kept off the eyes at all times (see Postoperative Vision Loss later). Perhaps of most importance in cardiac patients is how to pad the abdomen. Excess pressure over the abdomen can cause the viscera to force the diaphragm cephalad enough to impair ventilation. If this intraabdominal pressure exceeds venous pressure, then venous return of blood from the lower extremities and pelvis can be reduced or obstructed, leading to an increased risk of thrombosis. This venous congestion also transmits venous distention to the perivertebral and intraspinal surgical field, causing increased blood loss. Venous return to the heart ultimately can be decreased, leading to severe hypotension and decreased CO, putting the cardiac patient at increased risk of ischemia. Proper table, frame selection, and careful positioning can greatly reduce these complications.

Autonomic Dysreflexia

Autonomic dysreflexia (AD) occurs in patients with SCIs typically of T6 or higher and is characterized by acute hypertension and bradycardia. Typically, a noxious stimulus below the level of the cord lesion triggers AD (e.g., surgery, bladder catheter manipulation) (Fig. 16.7). AD results from unopposed sympathetic efferent outflow (extreme vasoconstriction; cool, pale skin; and severe hypertension) as a result of noxious stimuli below the spinal cord lesion, leading to reflex activation of parasympathetic outflow (bradycardia, cutaneous flushing) above the spinal cord lesion. Unopposed vasoconstriction persists because of blocked inhibitory responses at the spinal cord lesion. AD typically occurs 1 to 6 months after injury, but it can occur acutely after SCI. Regarding cardiac patients, severe hypertension is a major concern. It can lead to worsening myocardial ischemia, congestive heart failure, and occasionally cerebral hemorrhage. Prevention of AD can be accomplished with a deep regional block (spinal or PNB for lower extremity surgery; epidural block may be less effective due to sacral nerve sparing) or deep inhalation anesthesia. Treatment involves cessation of the noxious stimulus, deepening the anesthetic, and using antihypertensives. For cardiac patients and any patient in whom the index of suspicion is high for AD occurring, invasive arterial blood pressure management should be used with immediate treatment plans in place.

Venous Air Embolism

Venous air embolism (VAE) can occur in any surgery in which a pressure gradient occurs favoring air entrainment rather than bleeding, typically when the surgical site lies above the level of the heart. The prevalence of VAE is highest in posterior fossa neurosurgical patients, but also can occur during spine surgery, shoulder surgery

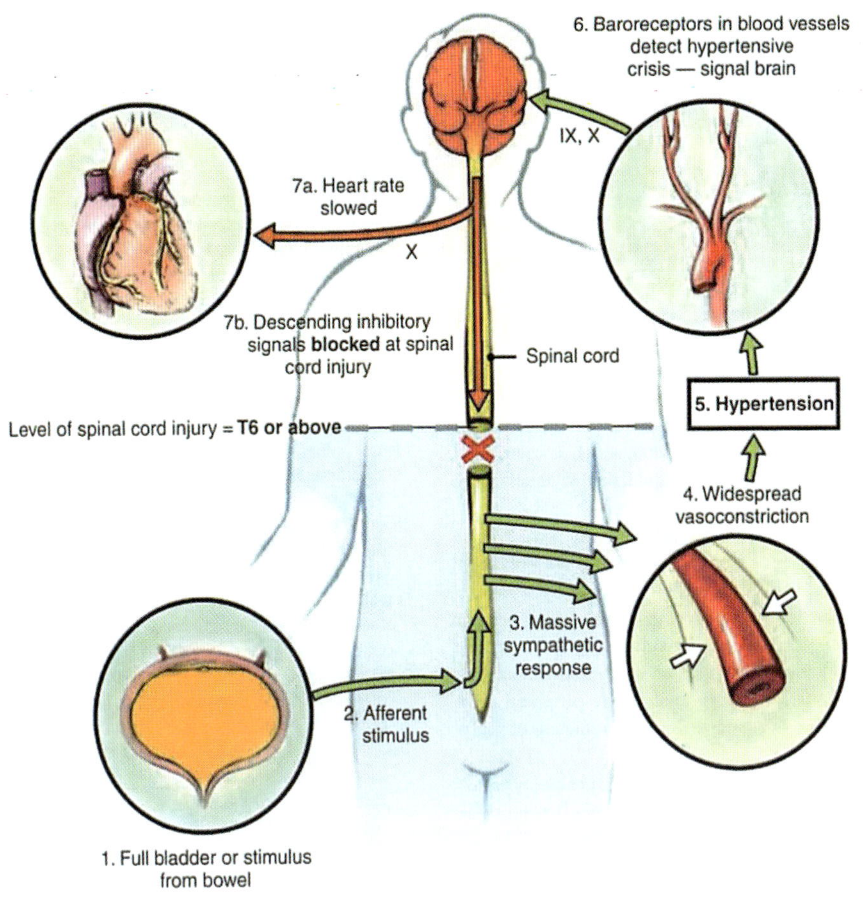

Fig. 16.7 Autonomic dysreflexia. (Modified from Murray MJ, Rose SH, Wedel DJ, et al. *Faust Anesthesiology Review.* 4th ed. Philadelphia: Elsevier; 2013.)

involving beach chair positioning, or hip or femur surgery. The consequences of VAE depend on the rate of air entry, with massive VAE causing an air lock in the right ventricle and cardiovascular collapse. More commonly, VAE occurs more slowly, leading to increased pulmonary vascular pressure, RV strain and failure, increased CVP, and systemic hypotension. Paradoxical air embolus is the passing of air via an intracardiac defect, leading to coronary artery obstruction (ischemia) or stroke. The diagnosis of VAE occurs best with TEE and precordial Doppler, but other modalities can also be used (Fig. 16.8).

Treatment of patients with VAE involves halting the entry of venous air (flooding the field with saline, bringing the surgical field below the level of the heart if possible, aspiration of air from the right atrium if a CVC has been placed), and circulatory support (fluids, vasoactive medications). The cardiac patient may tolerate a VAE poorly because of decreased cardiac reserve, potential lower ejection fraction, or from valvulopathy (especially stenotic lesions). If the index of suspicion for VAE occurring is high in a cardiac patient, then invasive arterial monitoring, central venous access (ideally with the tip in the right atrium for potential VAE aspiration), and potentially

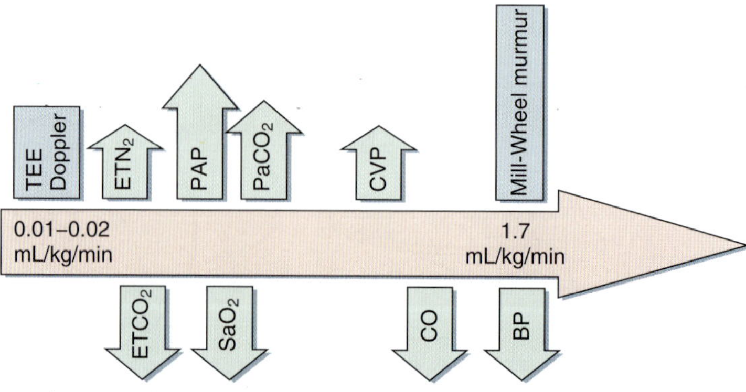

Fig. 16.8 Changes in detection parameters for venous air embolism with increasing volumes of air. *BP,* Blood pressure; *CO,* cardiac output; *CVP,* central venous pressure; *PaCO₂,* partial pressure of carbon dioxide; *PAP,* pulmonary artery pressure; *SaO₂,* arterial oxygen saturation; *TEE,* transesophageal echocardiography. (Modified from Murray MJ, Rose SH, Wedel DJ, et al. *Faust Anesthesiology Review.* 4th ed. Philadelphia: Elsevier; 2013.)

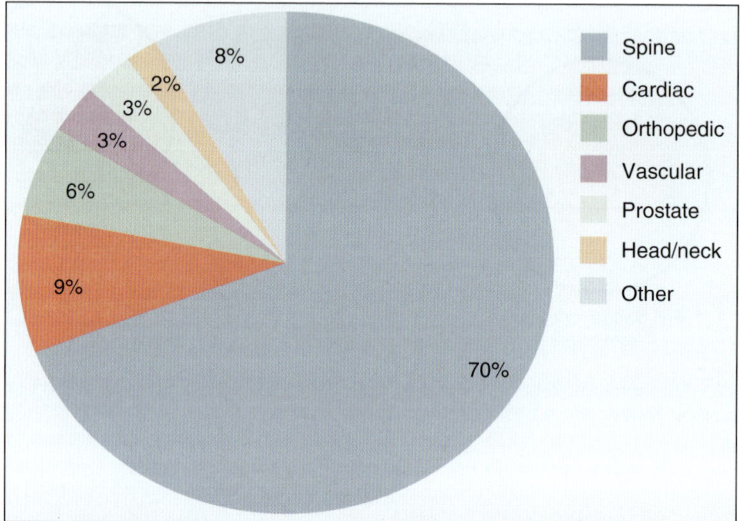

Fig. 16.9 Surgical procedures associated with postoperative vision loss. (Modified from Murray MJ, Rose SH, Wedel DJ, et al. *Faust Anesthesiology Review.* 4th ed. Philadelphia: Elsevier; 2013.)

TEE or precordial Doppler should be used. Surgeon awareness of the concerns should be made with the formulation of treatment plans to occur at any point in the operation.

Postoperative Vision Loss

Postoperative vision loss (POVL) is a rare but devastating complication seen most often after spine surgery (Fig. 16.9). Although compression of the globe can lead to POVL, most cases of POVL in spine surgery are caused by ischemic optic neuropathy, either anterior or posterior, and more rarely by central retinal artery occlusion. Risks for POVL appear to include blood loss greater than 1000 mL and anesthetic duration longer than 6 hours (these are the two most common). Other risks for POVL include preexisting vascular disease (e.g., diabetes, hypertension, CAD, peripheral vascular disease), tobacco use, obesity, and anemia. Reducing the risk of POVL includes having strict blood pressure goals. (The degree of hypertension, CAD, and renal disease must be taken into account when making these goals, including the use of vasopressors.) Management of intraoperative fluids, especially in cardiac patients with preexisting ischemia or depressed LV function, should consider CVP monitoring. CVP or dynamic measures of preload can help guide the use of crystalloid, colloid, blood products, and vasopressors. Although an exact hemoglobin threshold for POVL has not been established, hemoglobin monitoring should regularly occur with treatment of severe anemia, especially when accompanied by low CVP and systemic hypotension. Postoperatively, spine patients should have their visual acuity assessed. If evidence of visual loss is present, immediate consultation with an ophthalmologist should occur.

Hypotension in Beach Chair Position

The beach chair position is commonly used for positioning patients requiring shoulder surgery. (Emergency shoulder surgery could include dislocation with neurovascular compromise or septic joint.) Hypotension is common in this position, especially in cardiac patients. The sitting position the beach chair uses causes decreased venous return and decreased preload. In addition, GA, which decreases SVR further, and occasionally a regional anesthetic block (interscalene block for shoulder surgery) further contribute to hypotension. Cardiac patients may also be β-blocked or on other antihypertensives (especially ACE inhibitors), even further exacerbating hemodynamic instability.

Regarding blood pressure monitoring and cuff placement, for every 2.5 cm increase in the height of patient head positioning versus the cuff, the blood pressure drops 2 mm Hg. For example, if the circle of Willis is 20 cm above the heart, then the blood pressure at that level will be 15 mm Hg less than what the cuff reads. This should be taken into account to ensure adequate cerebral perfusion. For patients with CAD, hypertension, valvulopathy, or depressed ejection fraction, consideration should be given for using different surgical positioning to minimize severe hypotension intraoperatively.

CARDIAC PATIENTS REQUIRING EMERGENCY OTOLARYNGOLOGIC SURGERY

Introduction

Otolaryngologic (ENT) surgery encompasses a wide range of procedures, from the relatively simple tonsillectomy and ear tube placement to the much more complicated tracheal resection, radical neck dissection, and mandibular reconstruction (which may have >12 hours of operative time). However, the majority of truly emergent ENT surgeries (including emergency tracheostomy, posttonsillectomy hemorrhage, emergencies of airway compromise [Ludwig angina, postoperative hematoma, acute epiglottitis, angioedema]) involve processes that immediately threaten the patient's airway or CNS. Some surgeries, such as posttonsillectomy hemorrhage, are exceedingly rare in the cardiac patient population because these procedures typically occur in childhood or young adulthood. Other procedures, such as postoperative hematoma from thyroid or neck dissection surgery, are much more common in patients with potential cardiac comorbidities.

Epidemiology

Emergency tracheostomy surgery occurs for a variety of reasons, including airway trauma or blockage, infectious (e.g., Ludwig angina) or neoplastic processes (oropharyngeal cancer), inability to intubate orally, upper airway burns, and severe facial fractures.

Posttonsillectomy hemorrhage affects 2% to 3% of patients undergoing tonsillectomy surgery, and respiratory compromise affects 9% of these patients. Again, tonsillectomy most often is performed in children and young adults, so this complication rarely affects a patient with cardiac morbidity. Emergencies of airway compromise may be caused by multiple processes as listed earlier. Ludwig angina, which in the preantibiotic era had a 50% mortality rate, is caused by odontogenic infections 90% of the time. Infection occurs in the floor of the mouth and neck and occasionally proceeds to the mediastinum, all of which can cause airway compromise. Postoperative hematoma can occur from any number of surgeries, including thyroidectomy, radical neck dissection, carotid endarterectomy, and several others. Acute epiglottitis obstructs the airway and can be caused by bacteria (*Haemophilus influenzae*, β-hemolytic streptococcus, *Staphylococcus aureus*), viruses (herpes simplex), and atypical organisms (*Aspergillus, Candida,* and *Klebsiella* spp.). Angioedema includes abrupt onset of nonpitting, nonpruritic edema affecting the lips, periorbital area, extremities, abdominal viscera, and genitalia.

Malignant otitis externa (MOE) involves infection of the external auditory canal, temporal bone, and surrounding structures (CNS). It has a mortality rate of 50% to 80% and most often occurs in immunocompromised individuals (up to 90% of patients have diabetes). Medical management remains a mainstay of treatment, but surgery to remove dead or damaged tissue may be needed.

Anesthetic Management of Cardiac Patients Requiring Emergency Otolaryngologic Surgery

Preoperative Evaluation

Emergency ENT surgery ranges in acuity from the need for operative management in minutes to seconds (emergency tracheostomy, postoperative hematoma compressing the airway) to potentially several hours (posttonsillectomy hemorrhage, MOE). When possible, especially regarding the cardiac patient, as much preoperative information should be gathered as possible. This includes performing a thorough history and physical examination, obtaining laboratory values, and obtaining other studies (ECG, chest radiography, echocardiography if available). Although the focus on cardiac issues remains prudent in cardiac patients, many ENT emergencies involve loss of the airway. A quick but thorough discussion should occur between the anesthesiologist and the ENT surgeon regarding the status of the patient's airway and how best to secure it. In situations involving imminent loss of the airway requiring an emergency tracheostomy, minimal preoperative information may be available, so extra vigilance into potential cardiac anomalies should occur. Vigilance regarding hemodynamic stability in patients with hemorrhage should occur because these patients may require large-bore IV access, invasive blood pressure management, vasoactive medications, and blood product transfusion.

Anesthetic Technique

Most urgent airway compromise cases require an awake tracheostomy placement performed under a MAC technique. Patients with true airway compromise and obstruction (e.g., from tracheal stenosis or oropharyngeal cancers) ideally should receive the smallest amount of sedation possible during awake tracheostomy placement. These patients often have very high work of breathing, and even small amounts of sedative can render a patient hypercarbic and hypoxic, which can quickly lead to ischemia in a cardiac patient. Minimal sedation with surgeon-supplied local anesthesia works well for an awake tracheostomy followed by the initiation (if needed) of general inhaled anesthesia after the tracheostomy tube is in place and secured.

446

Aside from patients requiring an awake tracheostomy, the other ENT surgical emergencies typically require GA. Although immediate focus and attention should fall on the patient's airway status and how to secure it, in hemorrhaging patients, hemodynamics must be tended to as well. Often large-bore IV or central venous access may be required for blood transfusion and vasoactive medication administration. In cardiac patients, invasive blood pressure management via arterial catheter should be placed after the airway is stable and secured. In patients with MOE, antibiotic therapy should be continued or initiated in the OR as well.

Induction and Maintenance of Anesthesia

Induction of GA carries great risk in cardiac patients, especially in an emergency ENT setting. Although focus will be on the patient's airway, induction and maintenance of anesthesia medications can depress cardiac function, decrease blood pressure, and decrease sympathetic tone. Instrumentation of the airway can lead to tachycardia and hypertension, which may not be tolerated by cardiac patients. For patients with severe CAD, a moderate opioid-based induction may be more cardiostable; however, opioids may severely decrease sympathetic tone, which bleeding or infected patients may be relying on to maintain normal hemodynamics. For these reasons, in cardiac patients, a preoperative arterial catheter for blood pressure monitoring should be placed if possible. Blood products for transfusion and coagulation management, as well as vasoactive medications, should be immediately available. Maintenance of anesthesia can occur via inhalation agents, IV anesthetic agents, or a combination of both. Although some ENT literature suggests that TIVA may lead to less blood loss during certain ENT procedures, such as functional endoscopic sinus surgery, there are little data regarding TIVA and emergency ENT patients regarding blood loss.

Emergence From Anesthesia

Discussions must occur between the anesthesiologist and the ENT surgeon regarding postoperative disposition of the cardiac patient requiring emergency ENT surgery. For surgeries such as awake tracheostomy, severe postoperative hemorrhage with airway compromise, or MOE with CNS involvement, postoperative ventilation in the ICU may be required. For patients deemed safe to be awakened and extubated, care should be taken to prevent large swings in hemodynamics, which could cause ischemia, worsening heart failure, or arrhythmia in cardiac patients. Medications, including β-blockers, other antihypertensives (e.g., nicardipine), and vasoactive medications, should be on hand to treat large swings if they occur. Close attention to the patient's airway should continue, with concerns being passed on to postanesthesia care unit personnel. In bleeding patients, the arterial catheter should be continued for blood pressure management and laboratory blood draws.

Unique Considerations for Cardiac Patients and Otolaryngologic Surgery

Airway Fires

Airway fires have the potential for occurring any time electrocautery is used on or near the airway with a high fraction of inspired oxygen (F_IO_2) present. Fig. 16.10 details OR fires in general but includes details of airway fires as well. Minimizing F_IO_2 during electrocautery should help reduce the incidence of airway fire. An airway fire is a sentinel event in the OR and would be poorly tolerated by a patient with cardiac compromise.

16

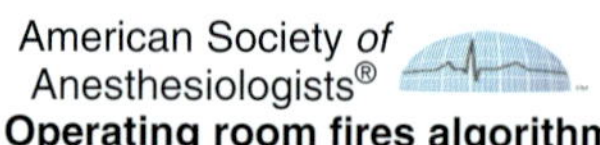

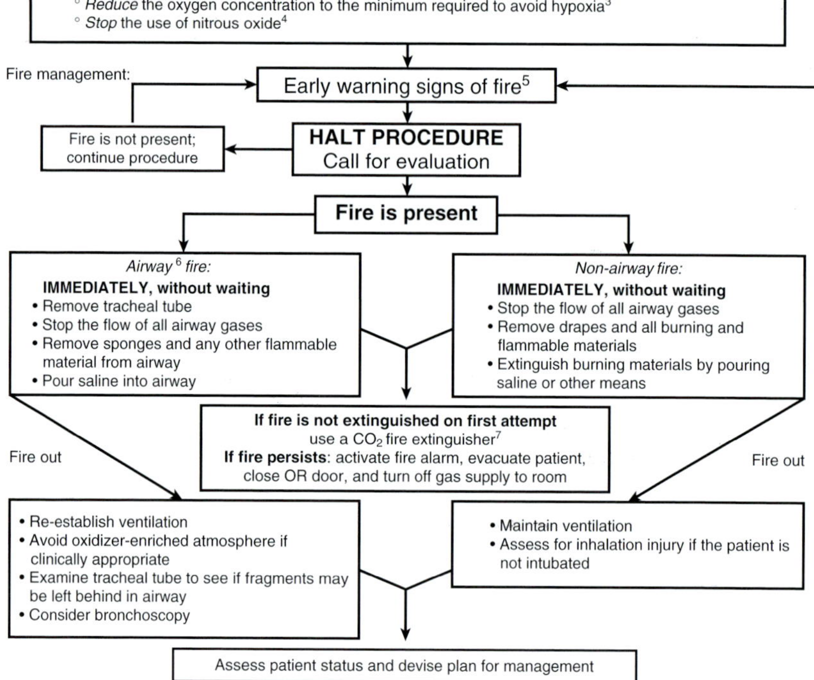

Fig. 16.10 American Society of Anesthesiologists operating room fires algorithm. (Modified from Murray MJ, Rose SH, Wedel DJ, et al. *Faust Anesthesiology Review.* 4th ed. Philadelphia: Elsevier; 2013.)

CARDIAC PATIENTS REQUIRING EMERGENCY OPHTHALMOLOGIC SURGERY

Types of Surgical Ophthalmologic Emergencies

Introduction

Ophthalmologic emergencies (including ruptured globe, acute closed-angle glaucoma, retinal tears or detachments, central retinal artery occlusion, chemical burns, and endophthalmitis) occur relatively infrequently on the spectrum of emergency surgery; however, these patients often require prompt operative intervention to preserve vision in the affected eye. Patients requiring emergency eye surgery have most often sustained trauma to the eye (ruptured globe) or have been affected by an ongoing or suddenly acute disease process (acute glaucoma, retinal detachment, infection). Patients with cardiac disease occasionally have these ailments and require anesthesia for repair.

Epidemiology

More than 2 million eye injuries occur annually in the United States, with more than 40,000 resulting in some measure of permanent visual impairment. Trauma to the globe accounts for nearly 3% of all ED visits in the United States. One-third of all cases of childhood blindness result from ocular trauma. The ruptured globe can occur from blunt, penetrating or perforating trauma. The male-to-female incidence of ruptured globe is nine to one, with the male average age being 36 years and female average age being 73 years.

Regarding nontraumatic eye injuries, glaucoma is the second leading cause of blindness in the United States and accounts for 5.1 million cases of blindness worldwide. Retinal detachment occurs in 1 in 10,000 people annually. Risk factors can include high myopia (>6 diopters) and aphakia (cataract removal without lens implant), and trauma. Most occur in patients aged 40 to 70 years. Endophthalmitis can occur from spontaneous infections, often in immunocompromised individuals, but also occurs after intraocular surgery (e.g., cataract extraction). Posttraumatic endophthalmitis occurs in 4% to 13% of penetrating eye injuries. Vision loss can be a complication requiring enucleation at that point. The very elderly (age >85 years old) are the most common to have this condition.

Pathophysiology

An acutely ruptured globe can occur from blunt, penetrating, or perforating trauma to the eye. This results in a full-thickness injury to the cornea, sclera, or both, causing expulsion of intraocular contents. Globe rupture carries a high frequency of visual loss; however, many eyes can be salvaged with prompt surgical intervention.

Normal intraocular pressure (IOP) ranges from 12 to 22 mm Hg. Glaucoma is a disease process that results in persistently elevated IOP and eventual optic nerve damage. Primary open-angle glaucoma occurs gradually over time as a result of slow eye drainage from the anterior eye chamber. Acute closed-angle glaucoma occurs when drainage from the anterior eye chamber is fully and acutely blocked, resulting in very high IOPs (e.g., 80 mm Hg). This can be a vision-threatening emergency requiring prompt intervention by an ophthalmologist.

Retinal detachment refers to separation of the inner layers of the retina from the underlying retinal pigment epithelium. Causes include previous surgery, trauma to the globe, and extreme nearsightedness. Endophthalmitis is an inflammatory condition of the intraocular chambers usually caused by infection. This condition often requires prompt surgical as well as systemic treatment (antibiotics).

Anesthetic Management of Cardiac Patients Requiring Emergency Eye Surgery

Preoperative Evaluation

Even for true vision-threatening situations, time should be taken to complete a full preoperative evaluation. The patient's anesthetic history, allergy list, medication list, NPO status, and general health history should be obtained. Focus should be on the cardiac history, functional status, and any given diagnoses (e.g., CAD, arrhythmia, valvulopathy, cardiomyopathy, heart failure, pacemaker or automatic implantable cardioverter-defibrillator status). Preoperative laboratory values, electrocardiograms, and echocardiograms should be reviewed if available. IV access must be obtained; two IV lines or central access may be necessary if vasoactive medication is required. An awake arterial catheter should be considered for patients with severe CAD, valvulopathy (e.g., aortic stenosis), or depressed cardiac function (e.g., low ejection fraction). Initial positioning may be challenging in patients with severe CHF and orthopnea. Gastrointestinal prophylaxis should be considered because some patients have a full stomach, leading to a higher risk of aspiration. In addition, a full physical examination, including the airway, should be performed.

Anesthetic Technique

Some eye procedures can be performed with very little to moderate sedation. Occasionally, the anesthesiologist or surgeon will elect to place an eye block (retrobulbar, peribulbar, topical anesthesia).

Many of the ophthalmologic emergencies discussed require GA. Repairs of ruptured globe, retinal detachment, and glaucoma most often require GA for patient comfort. Other reasons for GA include complete patient immobility (minimal coughing, moving, or disinhibition), better control of hemodynamic changes, or contraindication to a regional block (anticoagulation, open globe, increased IOP).

Induction and Maintenance of Anesthesia

Induction of anesthesia carries high risk for cardiac patients. Many anesthetic medications depress cardiac function, blood pressure, and sympathetic tone. Instrumentation of the airway for intubation can lead to the opposite of these parameters, causing massive shifts in hemodynamics. For this reason, a second peripheral IV or even central venous access may be beneficial for vasoactive medication administration. An arterial catheter also may be required for close management of blood pressure during the operation. The use of a paralytic prevents patient coughing, which may cause large swings in IOP, leading to extrusion of intraocular contents. Eye surgery itself tends to be less stimulating in inducing significant blood pressure and HR shifts (aside from potentially triggering the oculocardiac reflex; see later discussion). Therefore maintenance of anesthesia can be performed with a volatile anesthetic and usually minimal opioid. A total IV anesthetic technique can also be used.

Emergence From Anesthesia

Care must be taken during emergence from anesthesia to prevent large swings in hemodynamics that could cause worsening cardiac ischemia (especially in patients with CAD or aortic stenosis) or worsening arrhythmia (avoiding tachycardia). Excessive coughing or bucking should be mitigated because this can put strain on the freshly repaired globe and can lead to suture dehiscence. The use of a laryngotracheal anesthesia lidocaine injection (LTA) or IV lidocaine may help prevent this coughing, as may IV opioids titrated carefully. β-Blockers and vasopressors should be on hand to combat hyper- or hypotension on emergence. Decompressing the stomach via oral-gastric tube before wake up can be done as well.

Unique Considerations for Cardiac Patients and Eye Surgery

Oculocardiac Reflex (Fig. 16.11)

The oculocardiac reflex (OCR) is a reflex resulting in severe bradycardia caused by traction applied to the extraocular muscles (especially the medial rectus muscle), pressure on the globe, ocular trauma, traction on the conjunctiva, or occasionally by placement of a retrobulbar block. The afferent stimulus travels via the ophthalmic branch of cranial nerve V (trigeminal nerve), and the efferent stimulus travels via cranial nerve X (vagus nerve), which leads to severe bradycardia and potentially hypotension, atrioventricular block, ventricular ectopy, and rarely asystole. Treatment involves immediate cessation of the stimuli. If the reflex recurs, IV atropine (glycopyrrolate likely will not provide a strong enough anticholinergic boost) or lidocaine infiltration of the extraocular muscles should be considered. For cardiac patients, this reflex may be poorly tolerated, leading to severely decreased CO and hypotension requiring IV epinephrine or external pacing. Prevention of the reflex can be facilitated

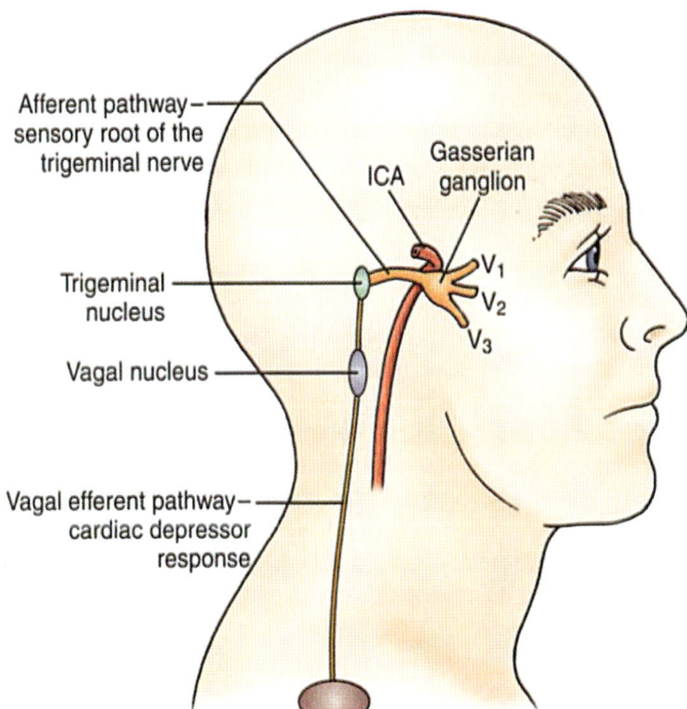

Fig. 16.11 The oculocardiac reflex pathway. Divisions of the trigeminal nerve: V_1, ophthalmic; V_2, maxillary; and V_3, mandibular. *ICA*, Internal carotid artery. (Modified from Murray MJ, Rose SH, Wedel DJ, et al. *Faust Anesthesiology Review*. 4th ed. Philadelphia: Elsevier; 2013.)

by injecting IV atropine; however, this can lead to severe tachycardia and ischemia, so this must be done with extreme caution. Somewhat paradoxically, a retrobulbar block, which has been implicated in causing the oculocardiac reflex, can help prevent the reflex as well by eliminating the stimulation sensed by the eye during traction or pressure.

SUGGESTED READING

American Society of Anesthesiologists Task Force on Perioperative Blood Management. Practice guidelines for perioperative blood management: an updated report by the American Society of Anesthesiologists Task Force on Perioperative Blood Management. *Anesthesiology*. 2015;122:241.

Anton JM, McHenry ML. Perioperative management of lower extremity revascularization. *Anesthesiol Clin*. 2014;32(3):661–676.

Arora V, Velanovich V, Alarcon W. Preoperative assessment of cardiac risk and perioperative cardiac management in noncardiac surgery. *Int J Surg*. 2011;9(1):23–28.

Baehner T, Ellerkmann RK. Anesthesia in adults with congenital heart disease. *Curr Opin Anaesthesiol*. 2017;[Epub ahead of print].

Christos S, Naples R. Anticoagulation reversal and treatment strategies in major bleeding: update 2016. *West J Emerg Med*. 2016;17(3):264–270.

Das S, Forrest K, Howell S. General anaesthesia in elderly patients with cardiovascular disorders: choice of anaesthetic agent. *Drugs Aging*. 2010;27:265.

Ellard L, Djaiani G. Anaesthesia for vascular emergencies. *Anaesthesia*. 2013;68(suppl 1):72–83.

Fleisher LA, Fleischmann KE. 2014 ACC/AHA guideline on perioperative cardiovascular evaluation and management of patients undergoing noncardiac surgery: a report of the American College of Cardiology/American Heart Association Task Force on Practice Guidelines. *J Am Coll Cardiol*. 2014;64(22):e77–e137.

Hope K, Nickols G, Mouton R. Modern anesthetic management of ruptured abdominal aortic aneurysms. *J Cardiothorac Vasc Anesth*. 2016;30(6):1676–1684.

Kristensen SD, Knuuti J. New ESC/ESA guidelines on noncardiac surgery: cardiovascular assessment and management. *Eur Heart J*. 2014;35:2344.

Lee CZ, Young WL. Anesthesia for endovascular neurosurgery and interventional neuroradiology. *Anesthesiol Clin*. 2012;30(2):127–147.

Leonard A, Thompson J. Anaesthesia for ruptured abdominal aortic aneurysm. Continuing education in anaesthesia. *Crit Care Pain*. 2008;8(1).

Meltzer J, Guenzer JR. Anticoagulant reversal and anesthetic considerations. *Anesthesiol Clin*. 2017;35(2):191–205.

Moll FL, Powell JT. Management of abdominal aortic aneurysms clinical practice guidelines of the European Society for Vascular Surgery. *Eur J Vasc Endovasc Surg*. 2011;41(suppl 1):S1–S58.

Murthy S, Hepner DL, Cooper Z, Bader AM, Neuman MD. Controversies in anaesthesia for noncardiac surgery in older adults. *Br J Anaesth*. 2015;115.

Ouanes JPP, Tomas VG, Sieber F. Special anesthetic consideration for the fragility fracture patient. *Clin Geriatr Med*. 2014;30(2):243–259.

Oyetunji TA, Chang DC, Crompton JG, et al. Redefining hypotension in the elderly: normotension is not reassuring. *Arch Surg*. 2011;146(7):865–869.

Peden C, Scott MJ. Anesthesia for emergency abdominal surgery. *Anesthesiol Clin*. 2015;33(1):209–221.

Raphael J. Physiology and pharmacology of myocardial preconditioning. *Semin Cardiothorac Vasc Anesth*. 2010;14:54.

Stoneham M, Murray D, Foss N. Emergency surgery: the big three–abdominal aortic aneurysm, laparotomy and hip fracture. *Anaesthesia*. 2014;69(suppl 1):70–80.

Valentine EA, Ochroch EA. 2016 American College of Cardiology/American Heart Association guideline on the management of patients with lower extremity peripheral artery disease: perioperative implications. *J Cardiothorac Vasc Anesth*. 2017.

Woll MM, Maerz LL. Surgical critical care for the trauma patient with cardiac disease. *Anesthesiol Clin*. 2016;34(4):669–680.

Chapter 17

Cardiac Considerations During Orthotopic Liver Transplantation

Ron Barak, MD • Ruth S. Waterman, MD

Key Points

1. Cardiomyopathy and ischemic coronary artery disease are the most common cardiac conditions in liver transplant candidates.
2. There are no clear recommendations for the assessment of cardiac status before liver transplantation, but each patient must be individually evaluated.
3. Indications for liver transplant have shifted, which has resulted in more patients with underlying cardiac disease presenting for liver transplantation.
4. Pulmonary hypertension and hepatopulmonary syndrome are two conditions that can impact liver transplantation.
5. Intraoperative hemodynamic instability is greatest while the hepatic vein is occluded and during reperfusion.
6. Postreperfusion management focuses on warming the patient, treating coagulopathies, maintaining acid–base balance, and optimizing oxygen delivery via transfusion and the management of hemodynamics.

CARDIAC CONDITION IN LIVER DISEASE

Liver transplant places extreme metabolic and physiologic demands on the heart, which is why knowledge of the patient's baseline cardiac status is imperative. Among cardiac conditions, cardiomyopathy and coronary artery disease (CAD) are most prevalent in this cohort. Estimates indicate that more than 50% of liver transplant recipients will have heart failure (HF) posttransplant, and cardiovascular disease is the third leading cause of death; however, it is unclear which patients should be excluded from liver transplantation based on their initial cardiac status.

Preoperative Cardiac Assessment

Because symptoms related to overt liver disease are often similar to those that are present in cardiac conditions (e.g., shortness of breath, lightheadedness, peripheral edema), preoperative assessment of the patient is challenging. Couple this with the fact that liver transplant candidates are subject to pulmonary hypertension and hepatopulmonary syndrome (HPS), and preoperative cardiac assessments become even more important. Although many tests can help determine the cardiac status of these patients, there are no definitive recommendations. Echocardiography

<table>
<tr><td colspan="2">Table 17.1   Comorbidities Present in Liver Transplant Recipients and Associated Effects</td></tr>
<tr><td>Comorbidity</td><td>Effect</td></tr>
<tr><td>Alcoholism</td><td>Left ventricular dysfunction and disruption of myofibrillary system</td></tr>
<tr><td>Advanced age</td><td>Increased prevalence of atherosclerosis</td></tr>
<tr><td>Nonalcoholic fatty liver disease</td><td>Associated with metabolic syndrome and cardiac disease</td></tr>
<tr><td>Hemochromatosis</td><td>Deposits iron into myocardium: conduction abnormalities and heart failure</td></tr>
<tr><td>Familial amyloid polyneuropathy</td><td>Induces heart disease caused by amyloid deposition: cardiomyopathy and conduction disturbances</td></tr>
</table>

and electrocardiography are routinely performed at most institutions; however, there is variability among centers regarding additional cardiac workup and CAD screening.

The comorbidities that accompany liver disease lead to myriad issues that affect the cardiovascular system, including increased inflammatory mediators, impaired repolarization, reduced vascular resistance, bradycardia, and myocardial depression. If liver disease is secondary to alcohol, the myocardium often thickens because of myocardial toxicity, which results in poor left ventricular function. As more and more patients are being transplanted for nonalcoholic fatty liver disease (NAFLD), there has been an associated increase in cardiac complications postoperatively. The increase in postoperative complications may be attributable to higher rates of CAD in the NAFLD patient population because NAFLD is a component of the metabolic syndrome. The increase in the average age of liver transplant recipients also brings with it greater risk of coronary atherosclerosis (Table 17.1).

The Child-Pugh score is widely used to assess prognosis in liver cirrhosis. For reference, the Child-Pugh score is a model frequently used to predict perioperative risk in patients with cirrhosis. It takes into account serum bilirubin, ascites, albumin, and prothrombin time (PT), as well as the extent of hepatic encephalopathy. The higher the cumulative score (class C being higher than class A), the greater the surgical risk and worse overall prognosis.

Alternatively, the Model for End-stage Liver Disease (MELD) score is occasionally used for risk stratification. Although this scoring system was originally designed to predict death after transjugular intrahepatic portosystemic shunt (TIPS), its use has expanded considerably. The MELD score uses serum bilirubin, creatinine, and international normalized ratio (INR), and the MELDna adds serum sodium to the calculation. Higher cumulative scores correlate with worse disease and greater surgical risk. The MELD score is widely used to rank the priority of liver transplantation candidates.

Pulmonary Hypertension and Circulatory Syndromes

Liver disease often causes direct effects on the circulatory system, with the three most common conditions being pulmonary hypertension, HPS, and hepatorenal syndrome (HRS).

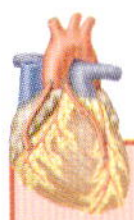

Pulmonary Hypertension

Because liver transplant patients are five times more likely to have pulmonary hypertension, an echocardiogram before surgery is strongly suggested. Although liver transplant recipients are more likely to have pulmonary hypertension, the severity of pulmonary hypertension does not correlate with the severity of the liver disease.

There are no definitive recommendations on the time frame within which an echocardiogram should be obtained, but because the underlying disease can change quickly, it is best to have one done close to surgery. If the preoperative echocardiogram was not completed in a time frame that encompasses the patient's current disease state, it should be repeated.

Although the pathophysiology of pulmonary hypertension in liver disease is not fully understood, the contributing factors include neurohumoral activation, vasoconstriction within the pulmonary arteries, genetic predisposition, a hyperdynamic arterial circulatory system, and increased pressure within the venous system (Box 17.1). A patient is considered to have pulmonary hypertension when the pulmonary artery systolic pressure (PASP) by echocardiography is greater than 30 mm Hg. Severity is based on the PASP with mild pulmonary hypertension being 31 to 44 mm Hg, moderate 45 to 59 mm Hg, and severe greater than 60 mm Hg. It is well documented that there is a decrease in survival for patients displaying severe pulmonary hypertension. Therefore a widely accepted absolute contraindication to liver transplantation is a PASP greater than 50 mm Hg.

It is strongly recommended that any patient with moderate to severe pulmonary hypertension by echocardiography undergo a right heart catheterization. If the right heart catheterization shows a mean pulmonary artery pressure (PAP) greater than 25 mm Hg and a pulmonary capillary wedge pressure 15 mm Hg or less, then the liver transplant can proceed. If the mean PAP is 35 to 45 mm Hg, the patient should be referred to a pulmonologist for management. If the patient has a good response to vasodilatory therapy, then the outcome after liver transplant is comparable to that of other candidates. Any patient who has a mean PAP greater than 45 mm Hg will require initial medical management and should not receive an immediate transplant (Table 17.2).

Hepatopulmonary Syndrome

Hepatopulmonary syndrome is defined by arterial hypoxemia that is attributable to pulmonary vasculature changes in the setting of advanced hepatic disease (Box 17.2). The pathogenesis is unclear. It has been proposed that the damaged liver's inability

Table 17.2 Pulmonary Hypertension and Right Heart Catheterization

Severity	Mean Pulmonary Artery Pressure (mm Hg)	Pulmonary Capillary Wedge Pressure (mm Hg)	Action
Mild	>25	<15	Proceed with liver transplant
Moderate	35–45	<15	Proceed with liver transplant; pulmonary pressures responds to vasodilator therapy
Severe	>45	<15	Medical management

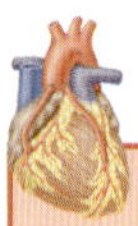

BOX 17.2 *Diagnostic Criteria for Hepatopulmonary Syndrome*[a]

- Presence of liver disease (with or without portal hypertension)
- Arterial hypoxemia
- Pulmonary vascular changes

[a]All three criteria are required.

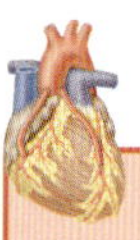

BOX 17.3 *Grading System for Hepatopulmonary Syndrome*

- Mild: PaO_2 >80 mm Hg on room air
- Moderate: PaO_2 <80 mm Hg on room air
- Severe: PaO_2 between 50 and 60 mm Hg on room air
- Very severe: PaO_2 <50 mm Hg on room air *or* PaO_2 <300 mm Hg on F_IO_2 of 1.0

F_IO_2, Fraction of inspired oxygen; *PaO_2*, arterial partial pressure of oxygen.

to clear mediators of pulmonary vasodilation such as nitric oxide, tumor necrosis factor-α, and heme-oxygenase–derived carbon monoxide all contribute to pulmonary capillary dilation with occasional direct arteriovenous (AV) connections.

Irrespective of the pathogenesis, there are three principal mechanisms of arterial hypoxemia in HPS: ventilation/perfusion (V/Q) mismatch, diffusion limitation, and less frequently, anatomic shunt. V/Q mismatch leads to the transit of deoxygenated mixed venous blood straight into the systemic circulation, which depresses arterial saturation (i.e., high venous admixture). Diffusion limitation is the result of enlarged alveolar capillaries, which leads to a reduction in alveolar surface area relative to capillary cross-sectional area. The driving pressure (i.e., partial pressure of oxygen from alveoli to blood) is inadequate to equilibrate with the blood in the center of the enlarged capillary. Unlike a true shunt, this form of hypoxemia responds to increasing fraction of inspired oxygen (F_IO_2) because this will increase the driving pressure of oxygen from the alveoli to the capillary. The severity of HPS is based on the arterial partial pressure of oxygen. Finally, direct anatomic shunt from pulmonary artery (PA) capillaries to pulmonary venous capillaries is rare and like most forms of pure shunt is refractory to increasing F_IO_2 (Box 17.3).

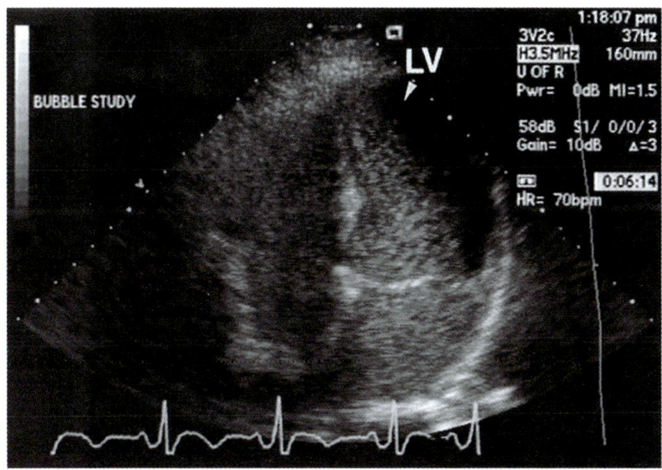

Fig. 17.1 Two-dimensional contrast echocardiogram illustrating delayed right-to-left passage of saline contrast with pulmonary arteriovenous fistula. Dense opacification of left atrium and left ventricle (LV) from intrapulmonary shunting. (From Gudavalli A, Kalaria VG, Chen X, et al. Intrapulmonary arteriovenous shunt: diagnosis by saline contrast bubbles in the pulmonary veins. *J Am Soc Echocardiogr*. 2002;15:1012-1014.)

The diagnosis of HPS is made via both clinical examination and diagnostic testing. Aside from dyspnea and hypoxemia in the setting of advanced hepatic disease, there are two unusual markers of HPS on clinical examination: platypnea and orthodeoxia. These are worsening dyspnea and arterial hypoxemia in the upright position, which improve by transitioning to the recumbent position. Clinically, this contrasts with most other causes of hypoxemia and dyspnea, which improve in the upright position. Mechanistically, this occurs because the majority of HPS-related vascular changes occur in the base of the lungs. Moving to the upright position forces a higher proportion of the cardiac output into these pathologic regions and worsens gas exchange.

Diagnostic testing for intrapulmonary AV shunt is done, in part, via echocardiography, again assuming this is completed in an appropriate time frame. During the echocardiogram, a bubble study can be completed to detect an intrapulmonary AV shunt, patent foramen ovale, or atrial septal defect (Fig. 17.1). The late appearance of bubbles in the left atrium (e.g., 6–10 beats) is consistent with HPS and an AV shunt. In contrast, the early appearance of bubbles in the left atrium (e.g., within 2–3 beats) or a defect in the interatrial septum appreciated on two-dimensional imaging may be indicative of a patent foramen ovale or atrial septal defect.

Hepatorenal Syndrome

Hepatorenal syndrome is acute renal failure secondary to the physiologic sequelae of hepatic dysfunction. It is a diagnosis of exclusion defined by acutely worsening renal function in the setting of advanced hepatic disease once other causes of acute kidney injury have been excluded (Box 17.4). The disease is categorized into severe (type 1) and less severe (type 2), which are largely defined by the rate of rise in creatinine.

The pathogenesis of HRS is secondary to cardiovascular and humoral changes associated with end-stage liver disease. As liver function declines, there is a global drop in systemic vascular resistance (SVR) secondary to increases in vasoactive mediators such as nitric oxide. The drop in SVR leads to increases in cardiac output, but a drop in systemic blood pressure. Paradoxically, the renal vascular beds often display localized

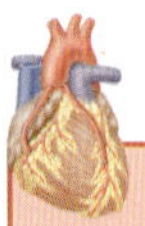

> ## BOX 17.4 *Diagnostic Criteria for Hepatorenal Syndrome*
>
> - Cirrhosis with ascites + AKI
>   - KDIGO criteria for AKI commonly used: creatinine increase >0.3 mg/dL in <48 hours or increase in serum creatinine >50% in <7 days
> - Absence of shock state
>   - Confounded by the fact that spontaneous bacterial peritonitis or another infection is often a precipitant of HRS
> - Absence of hypovolemia
>   - Often defined as off diuretics or given a volume challenge
> - Absence of precipitating or nephrotoxic medications
> - Absence of parenchymal renal disease
>   - Minimal hematuria or minimal proteinuria
>
> *AKI,* Acute kidney injury; *HRS,* hepatorenal syndrome; *KDIGO,* Kidney Disease: Improving Global Outcomes.

increases in vascular resistance brought on by hypotension-induced increases in circulating catecholamines and activation of the renin-angiotensin-aldosterone pathway. Combined with sequestration of large volumes of fluid within the splanchnic vasculature, as well as intravascular fluid losses due to ascites and edema, this leads to profound decreases in renal blood flow and progressive renal failure. In other words, it shares pathophysiologic mechanisms similar to prerenal-type renal failure.

Hepatorenal syndrome, especially type 1, is associated with a very high mortality rate if the underlying hepatic disease is not reversed or the patient is not transplanted. Temporizing therapies are directed at improving renal perfusion. Common treatment modalities include intravascular volume expansion with exogenous albumin, while concurrently increasing perfusion pressures with vasoactive medications such as norepinephrine, vasopressin, or terlipressin. In addition, it is common for these patients presenting for liver transplantation to require continuous renal replacement therapy. This has practical implications for the transplant anesthesiologist, including vascular access limitations, hemodynamic perturbations with fluid shifts, electrolyte imbalances, and the need for support staff to manage the dialysis machine intraoperatively.

PREOPERATIVE TESTING

Stress Test

Because CAD is more prevalent in liver transplant candidates, patients who possess three or more relevant risk factors should have a stress test. Such risk factors include smoking, diabetes mellitus, hypertension, hyperlipidemia, age older than 60 years, left ventricular hypertrophy, or any history of cardiovascular disease.

When undergoing a stress test, it is important that the patient reach a target heart rate for the test to be of value. Most liver transplant patients cannot perform an exercise stress test because of the limitations of their disease state. Additionally, dobutamine stress tests are 56% conclusive in this patient population because many patients are on β-blockers or have chronotropic incompetence. Therefore the utility of a stress test can be limited.

Cardiac Catheterization

Any positive stress test result must be confirmed by catheterization. Even though liver transplant patients are often coagulopathic, catheterizations can be performed with only a slightly increased risk of bleeding. For patients with symptomatic angina that is refractory to medical management, percutaneous coronary intervention (PCI) should be performed before transplant. If stent placement is indicated, bare-metal stents may be used to avoid a prolonged period of dual-antiplatelet therapy. Patients with significant CAD not amenable to medical management or PCI may require coronary artery bypass grafting. The suitability of this surgery depends on the severity of the liver disease (i.e., the greater the Child-Pugh score, the lower the chance of survival at 1 year).

Echocardiography

This examination is warranted in each liver transplant patient to evaluate overall cardiac function and to grade the severity of pulmonary hypertension, if present. If pulmonary hypertension is found and determined to be moderate or severe on echocardiography, then validation via cardiac catheterization is warranted. As previously mentioned, echocardiography with agitated saline can also detect intrapulmonary AV shunts, which are the hallmark of the HPS.

INTRAOPERATIVE MONITORING

Transesophageal Echocardiography

An orthotopic liver transplant places severe stress on the cardiovascular system. Transesophageal echocardiography (TEE) is particularly useful in evaluating the rapid hemodynamic changes the heart endures, helps guide fluid management, and evaluates ventricular dysfunction and wall motion. Additionally, it can be used to guide the placement of a pulmonary artery catheter (PAC), which can be useful not only intraoperatively, but postoperatively as well. Although liver transplant patients often possess esophageal varices, TEE probe placement has generally been considered safe in this patient population with the benefits outweighing the risks.

Intraoperatively, the majority of information required for a liver transplant can be obtained from the midesophageal four-chamber view. This is advantageous because minimizing probe movement may also reduce the chance of esophageal injury. The midesophageal views reveal any sequelae of pulmonary hypertension, such as a dilated or dysfunctional right heart (Fig. 17.2), as well as aid in the management of cardiac function or volume status throughout the case. In addition, TEE is extremely useful during reperfusion. For example, TEE can identify venous microemboli, air emboli, and paradoxical embolization, which may have hemodynamic or systemic sequelae.

Arterial Catheters

For liver transplantation, two arterial catheters are placed: one in the radial artery and another in the femoral artery. Although the mean arterial pressures above and below the abdomen typically do not vary significantly, there can be a difference after perfusion, with the radial artery being significantly lower than the femoral artery pressure. This is a result of decreased blood pressure, heart rate, and SVR. As the hemodynamic and metabolic issues resolve, the mean arterial pressure readings at the two sites will equilibrate.

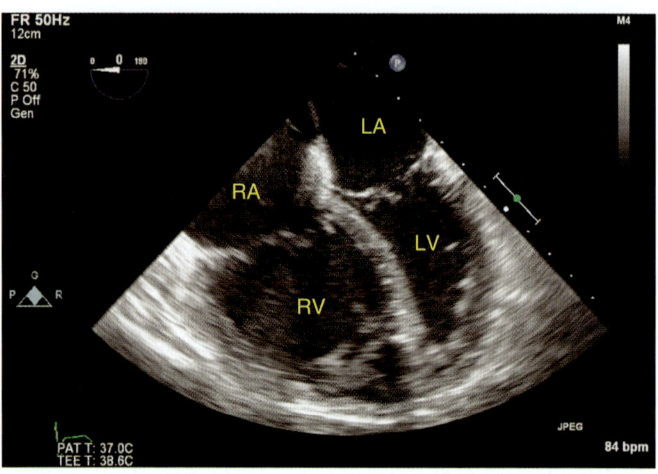

Fig. 17.2 Midesophageal four-chamber view with the probe turned to the patient's right side, bringing the right atrium (RA) and right ventricle (RV) into view. Note that the RV appears larger in area than the LV, which indicates severe right ventricular enlargement. *LA,* Left atrium; *LV,* left ventricle. (From Kaplan JA, Augoustides JGT, Maneck GR, et al. *Kaplan's Cardiac Anesthesia for Cardiac and Noncardiac Surgery.* 7th ed. Philadelphia: Elsevier; 2017:457.)

Central Venous Pressure

Because intrahepatic pressure is entirely dependent on central venous pressure (CVP), it is important to maintain a low CVP (e.g., <5 cm H_2O) to minimize blood loss during the procedure. This is occasionally accomplished by a nitroglycerin infusion, which lowers the CVP through relaxation of the vascular smooth muscle. However, a reduced CVP is not without risk. For example, low CVP can increase the risk for air embolism via lacerations in the hepatic veins.

Pulmonary Artery Catheter

Although still placed in many institutions, PACs are being used less because randomized studies have shown that they do not reduce mortality rates. Although a PAC can measure cardiac output via intermittent thermodilution, the return of cold blood during reperfusion and large fluid volumes can cause thermal noise that underestimates the cardiac output. Another benefit to a PAC is its ability to measure mixed venous oxygen saturation (SvO_2); however, because changes in the SvO_2 are not necessarily correlated with cardiac output, particularly during reperfusion, its accuracy and usefulness are questionable. Despite this, PACs are considered necessary in patients with HPS because they are the only monitor available that can directly measure pulmonary arterial pressures.

Continuous Cardiac Output

Although newer cardiac output monitors that use self-calibrating arterial pulse contour are convenient and easy to follow, their utility during liver transplantation is not accurate secondary to the rapid changes in hemodynamics. Likewise, determining continuous cardiac output via PAC is also not ideal because of changes in temperature, swift administration of fluids, and hemodynamic effects associated with reperfusion. Additionally, because none of these tools has been found to affect outcome, there is currently no preferred monitor for measuring continuous cardiac output during liver transplantation.

INTRAOPERATIVE HEMODYNAMICS

Pre-Anhepatic Phase

Before the inferior vena cava and hepatic vein are clamped, careful attention must be paid to perfusion pressure and optimization of the patient's hemodynamic status. Various strategies may be used to balance volume loading with elevated filling pressures. If the filling pressures or PAP is elevated, increased bleeding and reduced right ventricular (RV) output may ensue. Therefore inotropes or vasopressors (e.g., norepinephrine, phenylephrine, dopamine) may be required to achieve an optimal stroke volume.

Anhepatic Phase

One of the most critical times in orthotopic liver transplantation occurs when the hepatic vein is clamped, leading to the anhepatic phase. This is associated with an increase in peripheral vascular resistance and a drop in preload, which is often exacerbated by third-space fluid losses, hemorrhage, and inadequate volume replenishment. Although the stress of the surgery alone impairs the myocardium and decreases contractility, all of these factors contribute to a reduction in cardiac output. To combat hypotension during the anhepatic phase, phenylephrine and norepinephrine are often used to maintain SVR and to augment venous return via action on venous capacitance vessels. During this phase, it is generally estimated that 4 L of fluid are required to maintain hemodynamic stability. The consequences of clamping the inferior vena cava are largely dependent on the presence or absence of variceal collateralization, which can provide alternative routes of venous return to the heart. After the vascular clamps are removed, preload improves, and the splanchnic circulation returns to the liver. The patient can often be gradually weaned from any supportive medications.

Neohepatic Phase

After the liver is successfully implanted, reperfusion occurs. The vena cava clamps are released first and examined for patency. The hepatic vein is then unclamped. This results in a reduction in SVR and a slow increase in PAPs. At this time, patients with preexisting pulmonary hypertension or poor RV function are at risk of acute decompensation. If right HF ensues, there is a risk of graft failure caused by unfavorable pressure gradients between the portal and central circulations. Reduced left ventricular preload secondary to depressed right heart function can also result in low cardiac output, which may further limit perfusion of the graft.

Reperfusion also brings metabolic derangements. These derangements can lead to postperfusion syndrome, which is defined as a 30% drop in mean arterial pressure from baseline that lasts for at least 1 minute within 5 minutes of reperfusion. It is unclear whether baseline cardiac function has a role in this syndrome. More likely it is secondary to inherent cytokine levels such as interleukin-6, which can have proinflammatory effects. These can unmask the latent systolic dysfunction of cirrhotic cardiomyopathy, leading to HF. Inflammation coupled with an increase in metabolic demand can also lead to arterial plaque rupture and myocardial infarction.

Treatment of postperfusion syndrome can include epinephrine, atropine, calcium chloride, and sodium bicarbonate. In severe cases, methylene blue can be used to

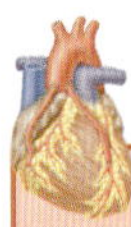

BOX 17.5   *Management Concerns for the Postanhepatic Phase*

- Replete electrolytes
- Transfuse to maintain hematocrit 25%–30%
- Maintain normothermia
- Correct coagulopathies
- Maintain acid-base balance

attenuate the associated hemodynamic changes. Because methylene blue inhibits the nitric oxide pathway, it may increase the systemic blood pressure when administered as a bolus of 1.5 mg/kg before graft reperfusion.

Additional goals for this phase include normothermia, correction of any coagulopathies, optimization of hematocrit and oxygen delivery, repletion of electrolytes, and maintenance of acid–base balance. Therefore it is common to obtain a thromboelastogram, complete blood count, and basic metabolic panel within 15 minutes of reperfusion to guide management. Some institutions also draw liver function tests to evaluate the transplanted liver's viability (Box 17.5).

HEPATIC COAGULOPATHY AND THROMBOSES

Traditionally, end-stage liver disease has been the prototypical model of hypocoagulable medical states associated with bleeding. This is largely based on routinely used laboratory parameters such as PT and INR, which are often grossly elevated in cirrhotic states. Furthermore, patients with end-stage liver disease frequently present with bleeding diathesis such as gastrointestinal bleeding. In addition, liver transplants historically required huge volumes of transfusions, which were seen as evidence of a hypocoagulable state. The reality is much more complex, and as understanding of the coagulation system and hepatic dysfunction has evolved, this paradigm has shifted.

Although it is true that the classic coagulation pathway, which is heavily dependent on hepatic synthesis, is impacted in cirrhotic states, it is equally true that the body's native anticoagulation pathways are also degraded. Examples of this include decreases in protein C and S, decreases in antithrombin III, and increases in circulating factor VIII and von Willebrand factor. In fact, studies have shown that plasma from cirrhotic patients can generate as much thrombin as healthy patients. The net effect of this imbalance is an unpredictable milieu of procoagulation and anticoagulation tendencies.

Clinically, this can play out in the form of intraoperative thrombosis, specifically involving the portal and caval vessels, as well as intracardiac thrombosis. In addition to the possible hypercoagulable state of end-stage liver disease, liver transplantation activates the remaining components of the Virchow triad, including endothelial injury (i.e., surgical incision and inflammation) and stasis (i.e., vascular clamps and catheters). Intraoperative thrombi are believed to occur in approximately 1% to 6% of adult liver transplantations, most frequently during the neohepatic stage when the patient's physiology and the graft's survival are most tenuous. Thrombi may form in the portal or caval structures adjacent to clamp and suture lines and travel upstream to the heart. Alternatively, thrombi may form independently within cardiac structures with vascular access lines potentially acting as a nidus for clot formation. Thrombi within the venous structures pose a serious risk to graft survival because they can occlude venous return to the heart, which increases backpressure on the new liver, causing engorgement and a reduction in perfusion pressure. Intracardiac thrombi, irrespective of the source, may cause intracavitary occlusion or migrate distally becoming pulmonary thromboemboli with resultant RV failure and hemodynamic collapse.

Although suspicion for an intracardiac thrombus is likely to be raised by deteriorating hemodynamics, the diagnosis can be confirmed by TEE. Three TEE views offer the best perspective to detect and monitor for intracardiac and distal caval thromboemboli. The inferior vena cava can be scanned by starting in the midesophageal bicaval view and advancing the probe to the level of the liver. The midesophageal RV inflow-outflow view can be used to identify any right-sided intracardiac thrombi and assess the RV for dilation and dysfunction. Last, the midesophageal ascending aorta short-axis view can be used to interrogate the bifurcation of the main PA and right PA for pulmonary thromboemboli.

The clinical question becomes how to treat acute intraoperative thrombi. In the nontransplant setting, thromboembolic events resulting in hemodynamic deterioration are often treated with aggressive anticoagulation, evacuation, or thrombectomy. However, in the setting of a liver transplant, with the potential for massive bleeding, this becomes a much more risky proposition. There is a growing body of evidence, largely based on case reports, for the use of low-dose anticoagulation in the setting of intraoperative thrombi. A reasonable approach is to escalate therapy as the clinical situation warrants. For example, serial monitoring via TEE can be used in patients who are hemodynamically stable and possess small (e.g., <1 cm) clots that do not propagate. Larger clots that propagate but do not significantly impact hemodynamics can be treated with a heparin bolus followed by an infusion. However, when hemodynamics are compromised, it is prudent to escalate care and low-dose alteplase (e.g., 1–2 mg per administration, up to 4 mg) can be given to aid in clot dissolution. Ultimately, in the event of cardiovascular collapse more aggressive maneuvers including Advanced Cardiac Life Support and extracorporeal membrane oxygenation may be warranted.

In summary, end-stage liver disease can be associated with a propensity to bleed and form excessive clots at the same time. Liver transplantation, with its activation of all three components of the Virchow triad, increases the risk for both massive bleeding and life-threatening thrombi. TEE can be invaluable in not only the diagnosis but also the management of intraoperative thrombi, which may entail anticoagulation despite the risk of bleeding in select patients.

POSTOPERATIVE MANAGEMENT

Cardiovascular and hemodynamic challenges extend into the posttransplant period. Typically, SVR will not normalize for 24 to 48 hours, and pulmonary pressures may take 4 days to normalize in patients who exhibited pulmonary hypertension preoperatively. Of all the hemodynamic instabilities, arterial hypertension is the most common and is often a side effect of immunosuppressive drugs, which vasoconstrict the systemic and renal circulation. Other contributors to hypertension include intense pain or hypervolemia. Depending on the etiology, pain medications, calcium channel blockers, or diuretics may be necessary along with vasodilators.

Abnormalities in serum sodium, potassium, calcium, and magnesium, which can be attributed to reperfusion and the stress of surgery, must be addressed immediately because cardiac arrhythmias may result. Bradycardia is the most frequent arrhythmia after liver transplant, but it is rarely symptomatic. Atrial fibrillation and other supraventricular arrhythmias appear less frequently but have greater clinical consequences. When electrolyte abnormalities are resistant to standard treatments, then additional etiologies such as renal failure, liver failure, or acidosis should be excluded.

Myocardial infarction is always a concern after liver transplantation, especially in individuals with preexisting CAD. Factors contributing to myocardial ischemia or infarction postoperatively include a high cardiac output state that can persist for up to 1 year posttransplant, hemodynamic perturbation associated with reperfusion, coagulation abnormalities, and plaque rupture.

A common complication of liver transplantation is HF. Postoperative HF can be categorized as early onset (<30 days) or late onset (>30 days). The cause of early-onset HF is rooted in the surgical stress on the myocardium, perioperative hemodynamic fluctuations, or underlying cirrhotic cardiomyopathy. Alternatively, late-onset HF often presents in patients with preexisting CAD or metabolic syndrome. Proper fluid management, diuretic administration, afterload reduction, inotropes, and vasopressors are typically used in management; however, in extreme cases biventricular assist devices or ECMO has been used. Therefore patients with a history of ischemia or valvular heart disease require careful attention because they may quickly decompensate postoperatively.

SUMMARY

Before liver transplantation, all patients should have their cardiac function thoroughly assessed and their surgical risk determined by all the cardiovascular risk factors identified. Identifying high-risk patients (e.g., pulmonary hypertension, HPS) will help determine the best anesthetic approach with regard to monitoring and the management of hemodynamic changes during critical parts of the operation. Despite careful selection and management, postoperative cardiovascular events are frequent in liver transplant recipients. Therefore careful attention must be paid to any cardiovascular risk factor that can be controlled.

SUGGESTED READING

Fouad TR, Abdel-Razek WM, Burak KW, et al. Prediction of cardiac complications after liver transplantation. *Transplantation*. 2009;87(5):763–770.

Garg A, Armstrong WF. Echocardiography in liver transplant candidates. *JACC Cardiovasc Imaging*. 2013;6:105–119.

Ho V. Current concepts in the management of hepatopulmonary syndrome. *Vasc Health Risk Manag*. 2008;4(5):1035–1041.

Koelzow H, Gedney JA, Baumann J, et al. The effect of methylene blue on the hemodynamic changes during ischemia reperfusion injury in orthotopic liver transplantation. *Anesth Analg*. 2002;94(4): 824–829.

Lau C, Martin P, Bunnapradist S. Management of renal dysfunction in patients receiving a liver transplant. *Clin Liver Dis*. 2011;15(4):807–820.

Lentine KL, Costa SP, Weir MR, et al. Cardiac disease evaluation and management among kidney and liver transplantation candidates: a scientific statement from the American Heart Association and the American College of Cardiology Foundation: endorsed by the American Society of Transplant Surgeons, American Society of Transplantation, and National Kidney Foundation. *Circulation*. 2012;126:617–663.

Maddur H, Bourdillon PD, Liangpunsakul S, et al. Role of cardiac catheterization and percutaneous coronary intervention in the preoperative assessment and management of patients before orthotopic liver transplantation. *Liver Transpl*. 2014;20(6):664–672.

McElroy LM, Daud A, Davis AE, et al. A meta-analysis of complications following deceased donor liver transplant. *Am J Surg*. 2014;208(4):605–618.

Nicolau-Raducu R, Gitman M, Ganier D, et al. Adverse cardiac events after orthotopic liver transplantation: a cross-sectional study in 389 consecutive patients. *Liver Transpl*. 2015;21(1):13–21.

Peiris P, Pai SL, Aniskevich S 3rd, et al. Intracardiac thrombosis during liver transplant: a 17-year single-institution study. *Liver Transpl.* 2015;21(10):1280–1285.

Planinsic RM, Nicolau-Raducu R, Eghtesad B, et al. Diagnosis and treatment of intracardiac thrombosis during orthotopic liver transplantation. *Anesth Analg.* 2004;99(2):353–356.

Ripoll C, Yotti R, Bermejo J, et al. The heart in liver transplantation. *J Hepatol.* 2011;54:810–822.

Tachotti Pires LJ, Cardoso Curiati MN, Vissoci Reiche F, et al. Stress-induced cardiomyopathy (takotsubo cardiomyopathy) after liver transplantation-report of two cases. *Transplant Proc.* 2012;44:2497–2500.

Testro AG, Wongseelashote S, Angus PW, et al. Long-term outcome of patients treated with terlipressin for types 1 and 2 hepatorenal syndrome. *J Gastroenterol Hepatol.* 2008;10:1535–1540.

Chapter 18

The Pregnant Patient With Cardiac Disease

Menachem M. Weiner, MD • Joshua Hamburger, MD •
Yaakov Beilin, MD

Key Points

1. The rate of maternal heart disease is increasing and complicates up to 4% of pregnancies. It is a leading cause of maternal, fetal, and neonatal morbidity and mortality.
2. The diagnosis of new cardiovascular disease during pregnancy may be challenging because both symptoms and physical signs often overlap with normal healthy pregnancy.
3. The preferred test during pregnancy to screen for structural cardiac abnormalities and to monitor ventricular and valvular functions and pulmonary pressures is transthoracic echocardiography.
4. A woman with known preexisting cardiac disease should receive preconception assessment and counselling with a rigorous, standardized risk assessment to make informed decisions regarding pregnancy. A number of risk assessment tools have been developed.
5. The normal physiologic hemodynamic changes of pregnancy increase myocardial oxygen demand as a result of increases in heart rate and preload and decrease myocardial oxygen supply caused by a decrease in coronary perfusion pressure, dilutional anemia, and a shortening of diastole.
6. The severity of the valvular heart disease and the prepregnancy New York Heart Association functional class are the main predictors of adverse maternal and fetal outcomes.
7. Because of the enormous risk of maternal morbidity and mortality, women with pulmonary hypertension should be advised against pregnancy.
8. During labor, uterine contractions, pain, anxiety, and exertion from pushing during the second stage further increase heart rate, arterial blood pressure, and left atrial pressure stressing a cardiovascular system already strained by the hemodynamic changes of pregnancy, which can lead to heart failure.
9. When a pregnant woman with significant cardiac disease requires nonobstetric surgery, both the mother and fetus are at a greater risk, the extent of which depends on the specific cardiac disease, its interaction with the hemodynamic changes of pregnancy, and its interaction with the hemodynamic changes caused by the surgery and anesthesia.
10. The primary anesthetic goals in peripartum cardiomyopathy are avoidance of drug-induced myocardial depression, maintenance of normovolemia, prevention of increased or rapidly decreased ventricular afterload, and blunting of the sympathetic stimulation induced by pain and anxiety.
11. Resuscitation of a pregnant woman is a rare event, which contributes to a lack of knowledge about the unique modifications to the Advanced Cardiac Life Support (ACLS) guidelines.

12. Modifications to ACLS in pregnancy include performing chest compressions higher on the sternum and with manual left uterine displacement. Intravenous access should be placed above the diaphragm.
13. Voltage for defibrillation and doses of medications during ACLS should not be altered.

INTRODUCTION

Maternal heart disease complicates up to 4% of pregnancies and is a leading cause of maternal, fetal, and neonatal morbidity and mortality. The prevalence of cardiovascular diseases in women of childbearing age is increasing for a number of reasons. As the management and treatment of patients with congenital heart disease (CHD) have improved, there are a growing number of women with palliated or corrected CHD surviving into adulthood who may become pregnant. Advanced maternal age along with other risk factors such as obesity has led to an increase in women presenting with ischemic heart disease. Furthermore, although the incidence of rheumatic heart disease has decreased in developed countries, it remains significant in developing countries and in immigrants from these countries. Cardiomyopathy presenting during pregnancy or in the first few months after delivery is uncommon but accounts for approximately 10% of maternal deaths.

The anesthesiologist involved in the perioperative care of these complex patients must be well versed both in the physiology of pregnancy and the pathophysiology of cardiovascular disease and their interactions to optimize anesthetic management and improve patient outcome. Successful management requires early diagnosis and advanced planning by a multidisciplinary team of obstetricians, cardiologists, anesthesiologists, intensivists, and nurses to optimize outcome.

This chapter reviews the expected hemodynamic changes of pregnancy; the etiology, underlying pathophysiology, and peripartum risk of obstetric patients with cardiovascular disease; and the management issues faced by the anesthesiologist caring for these patients who present for noncardiac surgery during the pregnancy and for labor and delivery.

DIAGNOSIS OF HEART DISEASE DURING PREGNANCY

Diagnosis Including Cardiovascular Imaging

The diagnosis of cardiovascular disease during pregnancy may be challenging because symptoms and physical signs often overlap with the physiologic changes of pregnancy. Pregnant women frequently complain of dyspnea and fatigue, and exercise tolerance is often decreased. Tachypnea, peripheral edema, and lower extremity venous stasis also may occur during pregnancy in women without cardiac disease. Even in women with known preexisting cardiovascular disease, it is important to differentiate expected pregnancy changes from pathologic exacerbations of underlying disease. The distinction is extremely important because it may trigger unnecessary modifications in management on the one hand or may lead to a failure to change management on the other.

A pregnant woman who presents with symptoms consistent with possible cardiovascular disease or exacerbation of known cardiovascular disease requires a careful medical history, family history, and physical examination (Box 18.1) interpreted in

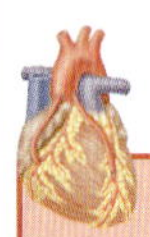

> **BOX 18.1** *Abnormal Physical Examination Findings During Pregnancy*
>
> - Heart rate >100 beats/min or <50 beats/min at rest
> - Pulmonary rales
> - Systolic murmur louder than 3/6, especially with palpable thrill
> - Any diastolic murmur
> - Murmur that persists beyond 6 weeks postpartum
> - Asymmetric lower extremity edema

the context of the physiologic changes of pregnancy. Many disorders such as cardiomyopathy, Marfan syndrome, CHD, or Brugada syndrome can be identified by taking a careful personal and family history. In women who are already in the second trimester, blood pressure should be measured either upright or in the left lateral position to prevent compression of the inferior vena cava and aorta. The pulse often has a rapid upstroke and collapse (a "bounding" character) because of the reduced systemic vascular resistance (SVR) and increased cardiac output. Resting heart rate is generally increased in pregnancy, but rates greater than 100 beats/min or bradycardia (heart rate <50 beats/min) require further evaluation for an underlying cause. Jugular venous pressure should be normal, so elevated jugular venous pressure and pulmonary rales are the most reliable signs of heart failure. A loud and widely split S_1 heart sound caused by the early closure of the mitral valve and the presence of a third heart sound (S_3) are normal in pregnancy. Soft ejection systolic murmurs are heard in more than 90% of pregnant women, usually over the left upper sternal border and the right side of the heart, because of increased cardiac output and increased flow through cardiac valves. These murmurs generally disappear by about 6 weeks postpartum. However, very loud murmurs or a palpable thrill suggest underlying pathology. Furthermore, diastolic murmurs are almost always caused by a pathologic process. The murmurs of aortic and mitral regurgitation commonly decrease during pregnancy because of the decrease in SVR, but the murmurs of mitral or aortic stenosis increase because of increased flow through the valves. Auscultation of new or changed murmurs is a reason for further investigation. Oximetry is an important diagnostic tool in patients with cyanotic CHD or patent shunt lesions. Many pregnant women show some degree of peripheral edema and lower extremity venous stasis because of uterine compression of the inferior vena cava impeding venous return. However, it should be symmetric and decrease with leg elevation and the left lateral decubitus position.

A woman with suspicious findings in the history and physical examination will often need cardiovascular testing during pregnancy. Additionally, pregnant women with known cardiac disease may need testing to judge how they are handling the added stress imposed by pregnancy. Pregnancy may impact the safety, application, and interpretation of several diagnostic cardiac procedures. Additionally, choosing the optimal diagnostic procedure requires consideration of safety for the mother and the fetus. Imaging modalities that do not use ionizing radiation are preferred as long as the required diagnostic information can be obtained. If the necessary information requires a study that uses ionizing radiation, the radiation dose to the fetus should be kept as low as possible.

The electrocardiogram (ECG) often changes during pregnancy. These changes may include a 15- to 20-degree left-axis deviation caused by diaphragmatic elevation, nonspecific ST-segment and T-wave changes (e.g., T-wave inversion in leads III and aVF and ST depression), supraventricular and ventricular ectopic beats, and the presence of small Q waves in lead aVF. If a pregnant woman has a suspected arrhythmia not captured on an ECG or in women with previous documented symptomatic arrhythmias and in women with palpitations, a Holter monitor is indicated because it is noninvasive and safe to use in pregnancy. It is important, however, to correlate symptoms with any abnormality and not treat asymptomatic arrhythmias during pregnancy because the treatments may be detrimental to the fetus. Exercise testing may be useful in the context of early pregnancy to establish functional capacity and assess heart rate, blood pressure, and ischemic changes to exercise. Exercise testing should be used with caution in women with an incompetent cervix, bulging membranes, recent vaginal bleeding, placenta previa or abruption, or preeclampsia. Women with symphyseal-pubic dysfunction, common during pregnancy, may be unable to perform the test because of limited movement. The procedure must be stopped if hypotension develops because this can lead to fetal distress. Performing submaximal exercise tests to reach 80% of predicted maximal heart rate in asymptomatic pregnant patients with suspected cardiac disease does not increase the risk of spontaneous abortion. Dobutamine stress tests should be avoided in pregnant women because there are limited data on their safety in pregnancy.

The preferred test during pregnancy to screen for structural cardiac abnormalities and to monitor ventricular and valvular functions and pulmonary pressures is transthoracic echocardiography (TTE). Many echocardiographic measurements require adjustment for pregnancy, including measurement of chamber dimensions, left ventricular (LV) mass, and in quantifying velocities across valves as these will all be increased in pregnancy. The use of transesophageal echocardiography (TEE) allows for more detailed examination but is more invasive than TTE and may be associated with pulmonary aspiration, which is a greater risk during pregnancy than in the nonpregnant state. TEE may still be indicated in the diagnosis of endocarditis, mechanical valve thrombosis, and complex CHD. However, the use of general anesthesia with tracheal intubation may be necessary to protect the airway.

Although it is preferable not to perform chest radiography during pregnancy because of the ionizing radiation risks, if other tests fail to diagnose the cause of dyspnea or cough, it may be necessary. The chest radiography findings in pregnancy may have a number of seemingly pathologic changes, including prominent vascular markings, a horizontal position of the heart, a flattened left heart border, and a raised diaphragm caused by the gravid uterus. Pulmonary edema, however, should not be seen.

In the setting of suspected acute pulmonary embolus, a computed tomography pulmonary angiogram should be performed because the risk to the fetus is outweighed by the danger of missed pulmonary emboli and can be minimized by lead shielding. Although echocardiography may aid in the diagnosis by identifying raised pulmonary artery pressures and impairment and dilatation of the right ventricle, it is less specific.

Cardiac magnetic resonance imaging (MRI) can provide information on cardiac anatomy and function without the use of ionizing radiation. However, it is generally only used if other investigations such as echocardiography cannot provide the relevant information because the safety of MRI in the early stages of pregnancy has not yet been determined. The safety of gadolinium during pregnancy has not been demonstrated and should be avoided if possible.

The use of cardiac catheterization for visualization of coronary arteries and measurement of intracardiac pressures gives high radiation exposure to the fetus and should only be used if absolutely clinically required. However, it is the diagnostic tool of choice in the management and treatment for ST-segment elevation myocardial infarction (MI) in pregnancy. To reduce fetal radiation exposure, catheterization via the radial artery is preferred to the femoral artery approach, and lead shielding of the uterus should be used. Although heparin is required for the procedure, an activated clotting time not exceeding 300 seconds is preferable to minimize risk of placental bleeding.

It is unclear what dose of radiation constitutes a danger to fetuses, but there is likely a very low risk of congenital malformations, neurobehavioral or intellectual abnormalities, fetal growth restriction, or pregnancy loss at doses of radiation less than 50 mGy (milligray) (10 mGy = 1 rad).

CARDIAC RISK STRATIFICATION DURING PREGNANCY

Ideally, a woman with known preexisting cardiac disease should undergo a preconception evaluation and counseling with a rigorous, standardized risk assessment (see later) to make informed decisions regarding pregnancy, to adjust to the possibility of not having a pregnancy, and to address any correctable lesions before pregnancy. Evaluation should include a careful history, physical examination, assessment of New York Heart Association (NYHA) functional class, a 12-lead ECG, and TTE. A right heart catheterization may be necessary for women with CHD or pulmonary hypertension. Medications that are contraindicated during pregnancy should be discontinued or changed to acceptable alternatives when possible. Many women present after they are already pregnant and should undergo immediate cardiac evaluation as already described. Although women found to be at low risk can often be managed by their primary cardiologist and obstetrician; women who are considered to be at medium or high pregnancy risk should be referred to a tertiary care referral center with expertise in pregnancy and cardiac disease for highly specialized management by a multidisciplinary team.

Several risk assessment tools have been proposed to stratify cardiac risk during pregnancy. Using these risk scores, it may be possible to predict whether the woman will tolerate the pregnancy. Three risk assessment tools commonly used to predict maternal cardiovascular events during pregnancy are the CARPREG (Cardiac Disease in Pregnancy) (Table 18.1), the ZAHARA (Zwangerschap bij vrouwen met een Aangeboren HARtAfwijking-II, translated as Pregnancy in Women With Congenital Heart Disease II) (Table 18.2), and one developed by the World Health Organization (WHO) (Table 18.3). It is also important to note that pregnancy-related risks are additive, meaning that a patient with a cardiac condition who is considered low risk (WHO 1 or 2) may move up a risk category if there are other cardiac or noncardiac risk factors such as poor ventricular function or diabetes to consider. Serum levels of the biomarker brain natriuretic peptide early on in pregnancy may also be used to stratify risk. It is important to stratify risk based on specific lesions as the risks of pregnancy depends on the specific cardiac condition and ranges from as high as a 50% risk of death for women with severe pulmonary hypertension to about equal to the general population for some minor lesions.

Because maternal cardiac disease is associated with an increased incidence of neonatal complications such as prematurity, intrauterine growth retardation, and fetal death, it is necessary to also determine the fetal risk of the pregnancy (Box 18.2). Neonatal complications occur in 20% to 28% of pregnant women with heart disease. Neonatal risks increase with NYHA functional class greater than II, presence of a mechanical valve prosthesis, cyanosis, anticoagulation use during pregnancy, multiple gestation, smoking during pregnancy, aortic or mitral stenosis, and use of cardiac medications before pregnancy.

Table 18.1	CARPREG (CARdiac Disease in PREGnancy) System for Predicting Maternal Cardiovascular Events[a]

1. Prior cardiac event (1 point)
   a. Heart failure
   b. Transient ischemic attack
   c. Cerebrovascular accident
   d. Arrhythmia
2. NYHA class >II or cyanosis (1 point)
3. Mitral valve area <2 cm^2 (1 point)
4. Aortic valve area <1.5 cm^2 (1 point)
5. Left ventricular outflow tract gradient >30 mm Hg (1 point)
6. Ejection fraction <40% (1 point)

CARPREG Points	Cardiac Complication Rate (%)
0	5
1	27
2	75

[a]Points are added, and the total score reflects the predicted cardiac event rate.
NYHA, New York Heart Association.
Modified from Siu SC, Sermer M, Colman JM, et al. Prospective multicenter study of pregnancy outcomes in women with heart disease. *Circulation.* 2001;104:515-521; and Chestnut DH, Wong CA, Tsen LC, et al, eds. *Chestnut's Obstetric Anesthesia: Principles and Practice.* 5th ed. Philadelphia: Elsevier; 2014.

Table 18.2	ZAHARA (Zwangerschap bij vrouwen met een Aangeboren HARtAfwijking) for Predicting Maternal Cardiovascular Events[a]

1. History of arrhythmia (1.5 points)
2. Use of cardiac medications before pregnancy (1.5 points)
3. NYHA class >II (0.75 point)
4. Left-sided heart obstruction (peak gradient >50 mm Hg or aortic valve area <1.0 cm^2) (2.5 points)
5. Systemic atrioventricular valve regurgitation (moderate or severe) (0.75 point)
6. Pulmonic atrioventricular valve regurgitation (moderate or severe) (0.75 point)
7. Mechanical valve prosthesis (4.25 points)
8. Repaired or unrepaired cyanotic heart disease (1.0 point)

ZAHARA Points	Cardiac Complication Rate (%)
0–0.5	2.9
0.51–1.50	7.5
1.51–2.50	17.5
2.51–3.50	43.1
≥3.51	70.0

[a]Points are added, and the total score reflects the predicted cardiac event rate.
NYHA, New York Heart Association.
Modified from Drenthen W, Boersma E, Balci A, et al. Predictors of pregnancy complications in women with congenital heart disease. *Eur Heart J.* 2010; 31:2124-2132; and Chestnut DH, Wong CA, Tsen LC, et al, eds. *Chestnut's Obstetric Anesthesia: Principles and Practice.* 5th ed. Philadelphia: Elsevier; 2014.

18

Table 18.3 Modified World Health Organization Cardiac Risk Assessment

Class I (No Increase or a Mild Increase in Morbidity From the General Population; Follow-up During Pregnancy May Usually Be Limited to One or Two Visits)
1. Mild pulmonic valve stenosis
2. PDA
3. Mitral valve prolapse with minimal mitral regurgitation
4. Repaired ASD, VSD, PDA, anomalous pulmonary venous return
5. Atrial or ventricular ectopic beats, isolated

Class II (Small Increase in Maternal Mortality; Moderate Increase in Maternal Morbidity; Follow-up Every Trimester Is Indicated)
1. Unrepaired ASD or VSD
2. Repaired tetralogy of Fallot
3. Most arrhythmias
4. Mild left ventricular dysfunction
5. Hypertrophic cardiomyopathy
6. Marfan syndrome without aortic dilation
7. Bicuspid aortic valve with aortic diameter <45 mm
8. Repaired coarctation
9. Heart transplantation

Class III (Significant Increase in Maternal Mortality and Severe Increase in Maternal Morbidity; Expert Cardiac and Obstetric Care Required Prepregnancy, Antenatal, and Postnatal; Women Need Frequent [Monthly or Bimonthly] Follow-up During Pregnancy, Both by a Cardiologist and an Obstetrician)
1. Mechanical valve(s)
2. Systemic right ventricle
3. Fontan circulation
4. Unrepaired cyanotic heart disease
5. Complex congenital heart disease
6. Marfan syndrome with aortic dilation 40–45 mm
7. Bicuspid aortic valve with aortic dilation 45–50 mm

Class IV (Pregnancy Is Not Recommended or Is Contraindicated Because of an Extremely High Risk of Maternal Morbidity and Mortality; Termination Should Be Discussed if Already Pregnant but When a Patient Chooses to Carry on With the Pregnancy, her Follow-up Is Similar as for Women With WHO Class III)
1. Pulmonary artery hypertension of any cause
2. Severe left ventricular dysfunction
3. Previous peripartum cardiomyopathy with residual left ventricular dysfunction
4. Severe mitral stenosis
5. Severe aortic stenosis
6. Marfan syndrome with aortic dilation >45 mm
7. Bicuspid aortic valve with aortic dilation >50 mm
8. Severe unrepaired aortic coarctation
9. Severe systemic ventricular dysfunction (LVEF <30%)

ASD, Atrial septal defect; *LVEF,* left ventricular ejection fraction; *PDA,* patent ductus arteriosus; *VSD,* ventricular septal defect; *WHO,* World Health Organization.

Modified from Thorne S, MacGregor A, Nelson-Piercy C. Risks of contraception and pregnancy in heart disease. *Heart.* 2006; 92:1520-1525; Regitz-Zagrosek V, Blomstrom Lundqvist C, Borghi C, et al. European Society of Cardiology guidelines on the management of cardiovascular diseases during pregnancy. *Eur Heart J.* 2011; 32:3147-3197; and Regitz-Zagrosek V, Gohlke-Bärwolf C, Iung B, Pieper PG. Management of cardiovascular diseases during pregnancy. *Curr Probl Cardiol.* 2014;39:85-151; and Chestnut DH, Wong CA, Tsen LC, et al, eds. *Chestnut's Obstetric Anesthesia: Principles and Practice.* 5th ed. Philadelphia: Elsevier; 2014.

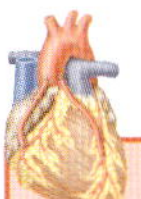

BOX 18.2 *Factors Associated With Significantly Increased Fetal Morbidity in Women With Cardiac Disease*

- New York Heart Association functional class >II
- Presence of a mechanical valve prosthesis
- Cyanosis (oxygen saturation <85%)
- Anticoagulation use during pregnancy
- Multiple gestation
- Smoking during pregnancy
- Aortic or mitral stenosis
- Use of cardiac medications before pregnancy

Table 18.4 Cardiovascular Changes in Pregnancy

Variable	Change[a]
Blood volume	+35%–50%
Plasma volume	+40%–45%
Heart rate	+15%–20%
Stroke volume	+30%
Cardiac output	+30%–50%
Contractility	Variable
Central venous pressure	Unchanged
Pulmonary vascular resistance	−15%
Pulmonary arterial pressure	Unchanged
Pulmonary capillary wedge pressure	Unchanged
Systemic vascular resistance	−15% to 20%
Systemic blood pressure	−5%
Myocardial oxygen demand	Increased
Systolic flow murmur	2/6

[a]Peaks in the early third trimester (at about 32 weeks' gestation).

PREGNANCY AND CARDIAC DISEASE

Cardiovascular Physiologic Changes of Pregnancy, Labor, and Delivery

Cardiovascular physiologic changes of pregnancy are summarized in Table 18.4.

Coronary Artery Disease

The incidence of significant coronary artery disease (CAD) in pregnancy is not known, although the incidence of acute myocardial infarction (AMI) during pregnancy or the postpartum period is 3 to 6 per 100,000 deliveries, with a 5% to 37% mortality rate. Fetal death after maternal AMI is 12% to 34%.

Whereas myocardial oxygen demand is increased during pregnancy because of increases in heart rate and preload, myocardial oxygen supply is decreased secondary to a decrease in coronary perfusion pressure, dilutional anemia, and shortening of diastole. This will present a challenge to women with known or previously undiagnosed

CAD. This challenge becomes greater during labor and delivery and especially immediately after delivery because of further increases in cardiac output. Although CAD
in pregnancy is relatively uncommon, it has increased with the increasing maternal
age and increased risk factors such as hypertension, diabetes, obesity, and smoking
among women of reproductive age.

Pregnancy-related hypertensive diseases are also associated with an increased
incidence of AMI. Additionally, the hypercoagulable state of pregnancy may lead to
coronary thrombosis or embolism in women without underlying CAD. Severe
postpartum hemorrhage may result in myocardial ischemia, and the use of methylergonovine for postpartum bleeding can cause coronary vasospasm.

The diagnostic principles for myocardial ischemia during pregnancy are the same
as for the nonpregnant patient and are based on angina symptoms, ECG changes,
and increase in cardiac biomarkers (e.g., troponin). Creatine phosphokinase and its
MB isoenzyme may not be helpful in the diagnosis of myocardial ischemia during
pregnancy because these enzymes are often elevated during pregnancy, particularly
during labor. The differential diagnosis of chest pain includes common pregnancy
symptoms (e.g., gastroesophageal reflux disease, nausea and vomiting), musculoskeletal
pain, aortic dissection, and preeclampsia.

The hemodynamic goals with an acute coronary syndrome during pregnancy are
to prevent further ischemia by avoiding increases in myocardial oxygen demand or
decreases in supply. Medical management is similar to nonpregnancy, with medical
therapy consisting of β-blockers for tight heart rate control and low-dose aspirin,
both of which have been found safe and effective in pregnancy. However, angiotensin-
converting enzyme (ACE) inhibitors, angiotensin receptor blockers (ARBs), and statins
are known teratogens and should be avoided in pregnancy. The preferred approach
for women with either acute ST-segment elevation MI (STEMI) or non–ST segment
elevation MI (NSTEMI) with risk factors is percutaneous coronary angiography with
intervention and reperfusion through stenting if needed. The radiation exposure to
the fetus when shielding is used is minimal, and the benefits outweigh the risks.
Clopidogrel should only be used for the shortest duration as possible because of the
risk of placental bleeding during pregnancy and postpartum, and thus the use of
bare-metal stents is preferred over drug-eluting stents. If clopidogrel is still being
used at the time of vaginal or cesarean section delivery, the possibility of increased
postpartum bleeding must be anticipated. The use of coronary artery bypass grafting
is rarely needed during pregnancy and is associated with high fetal mortality rate. In
women with NSTEMI without risk factors, conservative management with medical
therapy and watchful waiting can be applied. Women with CAD should have the
early institution of neuraxial anesthesia during labor to prevent pain and the increase
myocardial oxygen demand that accompanies it. In the case of an AMI, labor and
delivery should be delayed for at least 2 weeks if possible because maternal mortality
rates are significantly increased during this time.

Valvular Heart Disease

The most common causes of valvular heart disease (VHD) in women of childbearing
age are rheumatic heart disease and CHD (e.g., bicuspid aortic valve), with mitral
stenosis the most common lesion encountered. VHD is a significant cause of maternal
cardiac disease because rheumatic heart disease accounts for more than 90% of maternal cardiac disease cases worldwide. Pregnant women with VHD have an increased
incidence of adverse maternal and fetal outcomes, with severe mitral stenosis forming
a particularly high-risk group, with a reported maternal mortality rate of greater than
10% and a cardiac event rate of 67%. The most commonly encountered maternal

cardiac complications are congestive heart failure and arrhythmias, and the most common fetal complications are prematurity and intrauterine growth retardation.

Women with known VHD before pregnancy should undergo preconception counseling. Women with moderate or severe mitral stenosis unless corrected before pregnancy or with moderate or severe aortic stenosis who are symptomatic or have LV dysfunction should be advised against pregnancy. Women at high risk who have a desire to pursue pregnancy should be managed by a multidisciplinary team in centers with expertise in the management of these patients. The hemodynamic changes of pregnancy can exacerbate mild symptoms. Symptoms tend to worsen with increasing gestational age. The severity of VHD and the prepregnancy NYHA functional class are the main predictors of adverse maternal and fetal outcomes. Many women with VHD are first diagnosed during pregnancy when the hemodynamic changes of pregnancy precipitate symptoms.

In general, regurgitant lesions are much better tolerated in pregnancy than stenotic ones because the decrease in SVR favors forward flow. In the absence of LV dysfunction, these lesions pose only a minor threat. Symptomatic patients may be treated with diuretics and afterload reduction with close monitoring for uteroplacental insufficiency. Afterload reduction should be provided with nitrates and hydralazine because ACE inhibitors and ARBs are contraindicated in pregnancy. However, the increases in preload, cardiac output, and heart rate during pregnancy cause a significant increase in the transvalvular gradient produced by stenotic lesions. In the case of mitral stenosis, it also compromises LV filling and increases left atrial pressure, which is then transmitted to the pulmonary veins. The decrease in LV filling and the increase in pressure in the pulmonary veins lead to deterioration in functional class with increased dyspnea, decreased exercise tolerance, and possibly pulmonary edema. Atrial arrhythmias (e.g., atrial fibrillation) associated with ventricular rate acceleration are a common cause of worsening symptoms and must be treated aggressively with rate control and possibly cardioversion.

In general, mitral stenosis is more of a management challenge than aortic stenosis because in aortic stenosis the increase in pressure is reflected initially to the hypertrophied left ventricle rather than the pulmonary veins as in mitral stenosis. Women with mild or moderate aortic stenosis generally tolerate pregnancy well. Medical therapy for stenotic lesions in symptomatic women consists of heart rate control with β-blockers and restriction of physical activity and preload reduction with diuretics. Metoprolol is the preferred β-blocker because atenolol has been linked to adverse fetal outcomes, including intrauterine growth retardation and preterm delivery. Heart rate control leads to improved LV filling and lower left atrial pressure. Diuretic use, in particular, must be accompanied by monitoring for signs of uteroplacental insufficiency. Patients with mitral or aortic stenosis who are refractory to medical therapy may be candidates for percutaneous balloon valvuloplasty, which should be done with abdominal shielding and delayed until after the first trimester if possible to minimize the radiation risks to the fetus.

Women with valve replacements, particularly mechanical prostheses, are at an increased risk for pregnancy complications and pose a particular challenge because of the risk of valve thrombosis and anticoagulation management. The presence of a mechanical prosthesis, particularly in the mitral position, is a contraindication to pregnancy. Warfarin should be continued until 36 weeks' gestational age with the possible exception of weeks 6 to 12 because it is teratogenic, when a changeover to either unfractionated or low-molecular-weight heparin (LMWH) may be recommended, particularly if the dose of warfarin is greater than 5 mg/day. After 36 weeks, a changeover to heparin is recommended. Alternatively, these women can be switched from warfarin to LMWH from the beginning of pregnancy. These women require weekly monitoring of a postdose anti-Xa level.

Pulmonary Hypertension

The incidence of pulmonary hypertension in pregnancy is approximately 1.1 in 100,000 pregnancies. The hemodynamic changes of pregnancy are not well tolerated by women with pulmonary hypertension, with an overall mortality rate of 25% to 38%. The risk of maternal morbidity and mortality in women with pulmonary hypertension from any cause makes pregnancy particularly dangerous in these women, who should be advised against pregnancy. Those who present already pregnant should be offered termination. Death generally occurs in late pregnancy or in the first month after delivery and results from right heart failure, pulmonary hypertensive crisis, pulmonary thromboembolism, or arrhythmias. Although there is some evidence of better outcomes in women with mild pulmonary hypertension (pulmonary artery systolic pressure <50 mm Hg), there is no specific safe cutoff. Furthermore, pulmonary hypertension generally is exacerbated by the physiologic hemodynamic changes of pregnancy, including increased cardiac output and circulating blood volume and decreased SVR because the vascular remodeling present in women with pulmonary hypertension prevents them from being able to compensate with the pulmonary vasodilatory mechanisms of pregnancy. This results in increased pulmonary vascular resistance (PVR), overload of the right ventricle, and right ventricular strain with even mild forms of pulmonary hypertension possibly becoming severe.

When termination is refused and the patient chooses to continue with the pregnancy, care should be managed in a facility with expertise in high-risk pregnancies and pulmonary hypertension management under the care of a multidisciplinary team. Recent treatment advances and the use of a multidisciplinary team have led to an improvement in survival. Management during pregnancy involves finding a balance between systemic and pulmonary pressures because decreased systemic pressures compromise right ventricular perfusion. Pulmonary hypertension therapy should generally be continued other than the endothelin-1 receptor blocker, bosentan, which is teratogenic in animal studies. Prostacyclin analogs such as epoprostenol, inhaled nitric oxide, and phosphodiesterase-5 inhibitors such as sildenafil have not been found teratogenic. Initiating women who were not previously on targeted therapies at the beginning of the third trimester of pregnancy is recommended. It is also critically important to avoid conditions that will increase the pulmonary vascular pressures, including hypoxia, hypercarbia, acidosis, and sympathetic stimulation, because they may lead to right ventricular failure. Inotropic support may be needed in the setting of right ventricular failure. Maternal hemodynamic decompensation will generally occur in the second or third trimesters and shortly after delivery of the fetus. Early planned delivery, usually at 32 to 34 weeks' gestational age, may contribute to improved outcomes.

Congenital Heart Disease

Congenital heart disease has become the most prevalent chronic maternal heart disease in pregnancy, accounting for 66% to 80% of cases. This has stemmed from an increased number of patients with CHD living into their childbearing years because of advances in surgical repair and palliation procedures. Although many women with CHD tolerate the expected hemodynamic changes of pregnancy, maternal cardiovascular complications occur in approximately 5% to 25% of such pregnancies. The most common complications are congestive heart failure, thromboembolism, and arrhythmias.

Because most women with CHD are known before pregnancy, preconception counseling with a thorough risk assessment (see previous section) is indicated. CHD encompasses a wide array of diseases from mild to extremely complex, so the risk of pregnancy varies greatly and also depends on if the congenital defect has been repaired and if permanent damage occurred before the repair. Pregnancy should not be discouraged in patients who have had successful surgical repair with good exercise tolerance and functional status because they have only a very small increased risk, provided no mechanical valve has been implanted. Patients who have moderate or complex disease who choose to continue with pregnancy should be managed in a facility with expertise in high-risk pregnancies and CHD under the care of a multidisciplinary team.

In the absence of pulmonary hypertension, women with repaired shunt lesions, including atrial septal defect, ventricular septal defect, atrioventricular canal defect, and patent ductus arteriosus tolerate pregnancy well without a significant increase in cardiovascular risk. They are, however, at increased risk for preeclampsia. With unrepaired shunt lesions, there is a risk of paradoxical embolism, particularly during labor, when a Valsalva maneuver is used during the second stage of labor. Patients with unrepaired atrioventricular canal defects are at greater cardiovascular risk than those with either atrial septal defects or ventricular septal defects because severe atrioventricular valve regurgitation or ventricular dysfunction may cause failure during pregnancy. Additionally, if patients with unrepaired shunt lesions develop Eisenmenger syndrome, the maternal mortality rate increases to 28% to 52%, with a fetal mortality rate of 28%. The reduction in SVR exacerbates the right-to-left shunt and increases cyanosis while the increase in cardiac output leads to heart failure. Severe cyanosis (oxygen saturation <85%) makes the chance of a live birth extremely unlikely. Management goals include maintenance of SVR and PVR, with strict avoidance of hypoxia, acidosis, hypercarbia, and sympathetic stimulation.

Women who have unrepaired cyanotic heart disease such as tetralogy of Fallot should be counseled against pregnancy because these pregnancies have a maternal complication rate greater than 30%. Complications include heart failure, thromboembolism, and arrhythmias. When maternal resting oxygen saturation is less than 85%, the maternal risk is extremely high, and the chance of a live birth is only 12%. Such women should be advised against pregnancy. Women with corrected tetralogy of Fallot generally tolerate pregnancy fairly well, with cardiac complications such as arrhythmias and heart failure in 12% of patients. Risk factors for complications are preexisting right ventricular dysfunction or dilation, pulmonary hypertension, severe pulmonic valve regurgitation, and right ventricular track outflow obstruction.

The presence of a systemic right ventricle, such as in congenitally corrected transposition of the great arteries, after an atrial switch operation for complete transposition of the great arteries, or in hypoplastic left heart syndrome after a Fontan operation, is independently associated with adverse cardiac and pregnancy outcomes. These patients are at increased risk for heart failure and life-threatening arrhythmias. Women with severe right ventricular dysfunction or severe atrioventricular valve regurgitation or who are NYHA class III or IV patients should be counseled against pregnancy. Women with Fontan physiology are at risk to experience deterioration in functional status. Hemodynamic goals should include the maintenance of pulmonary blood flow by minimizing PVR and maintaining intravascular volume, SVR, and sinus rhythm.

MANAGEMENT OF LABOR AND DELIVERY IN WOMEN WITH CARDIAC DISEASE

Importance of Multidisciplinary Planning

The period of labor and delivery is a critical time for women with heart disease because abrupt hemodynamic changes make compensation more difficult. Uterine

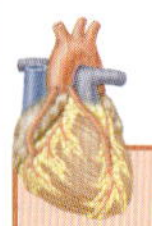

> **BOX 18.3** *Questions for the Multidisciplinary Team to Address*
>
> 1. What is the best timing for delivery?
> 2. What should be the mode of delivery?
> 3. What is the optimal location for delivery (labor and delivery suite, cardiac operating room)?
> 4. Should a cardiac surgeon and cardiopulmonary bypass capabilities be on standby?
> 5. When should the mother be admitted for predelivery optimization and possible antenatal corticosteroid administration?
> 6. Is any further diagnostic testing necessary?
> 7. What type of anesthesia or analgesia should be planned for the patient?
> 8. What type of monitoring should be used?
> 9. Where will the patient be monitored after delivery? For how long?
> 10. Which oxytocic drugs will be given?
> 11. What is the contingency plan if the mother presents urgently in labor or in acute decompensation?
> 12. Are there any other specific needs, precautions, or concerns?

contractions, pain, anxiety, and exertion from pushing further increase heart rate, arterial blood pressure, and left atrial pressure, stressing an already compromised cardiovascular system. Cardiac output increases steadily from 15% in early labor to 50% to 60% (~11 L/min) during pushing efforts to an 80% increase in the immediate postpartum period because of the relief of inferior vena cava obstruction. Furthermore, each uterine contraction increases cardiac output by 20% by autotransfusing blood into the central blood volume. This can result in heart failure and acute pulmonary congestion. As a result, the management of labor and delivery requires a skilled collaborative effort that includes a multidisciplinary team of cardiologists, obstetricians, anesthesiologists, and for the highest risk patient, a cardiac surgeon with the availability of cardiopulmonary bypass (Box 18.3).

Delivery should generally be planned so the team can be present rather than allowing spontaneous labor. The timing of delivery should be individualized because there is a lack of prospective data and individual patient characteristics will influence the decision. Women with complex cardiac lesions, severe congestive heart failure, or severe pulmonary hypertension often require an early planned delivery before maternal and fetal decompensation.

Mode of Delivery

The mode of delivery depends on both obstetric indications and the maternal hemodynamic status. If a decision is made that the delivery needs to take place significantly before term because of a deteriorating maternal cardiac status, then a cesarean delivery will be necessary because the induction of labor will likely be unsuccessful. For women who are able to continue the pregnancy to term, vaginal delivery is favored because it poses less cardiac risk because it is associated with less blood loss and fluid shifts and has a decreased risk of venous thrombosis. Vaginal delivery can be assisted by vacuum or forceps to shorten the second stage of labor and minimize maternal pushing efforts and Valsalva maneuvers, thus avoiding further increases in cardiac output in women who will not be able to tolerate them. Cesarean delivery is generally reserved for obstetric indications. However, there are certain lesions in which vaginal delivery may be contraindicated (Box 18.4). These include women in severe heart

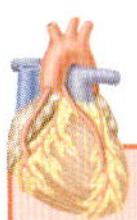

> **BOX 18.4** *Conditions in Which Cesarean Delivery Should Be Strongly Considered*
>
> - Planned early delivery in which induction is unlikely to succeed
> - Acute or severe heart failure; poor functional class
> - Severe mitral or aortic stenosis
> - Severe pulmonary hypertension
> - Aortic dilation >40 mm in Marfan syndrome
> - Women on anticoagulation secondary to risk of fetal intracranial hemorrhage

failure, those on oral anticoagulants because of the risk of neonatal intracranial bleeding, and patients in whom the stress of labor and delivery put them at greater risk for aortic dissection (e.g., Marfan syndrome with an aortic diameter >45 mm) and should be considered when the aortic diameter is >40 mm. Cesarean delivery may also be favored for women with severe stenotic valvular lesions, severe pulmonary hypertension, poor functional class, and acute heart failure. The trend has tilted in favor of cesarean delivery because it is believed that this allows for greater control of the timing of delivery as well as hemodynamics.

The choice of uterotonic agents is also important in these patients. Most women are able to tolerate a slow intravenous (IV) infusion of oxytocin postpartum to prevent maternal hemorrhage. However, oxytocin causes an increase in PVR and tachycardia. Methylergonovine should be avoided in most women with significant cardiac disease because of the risk of coronary vasoconstriction and both systemic and pulmonary hypertension. Carboprost can also cause both systemic and pulmonary hypertension and should be avoided. Furthermore, although misoprostol (administered either buccally or rectally) has no known cardiac side effects, its efficacy as a uterotonic agent is not clear and is generally used as the last uterotonic agent. On the other hand, the avoidance of these medications is also not without risk because maternal hemorrhage and the concomitant need for rapid infusion of fluid and blood products are also poorly tolerated in these women.

Anesthetic Options and Monitoring

Anesthetic options differ depending on mode of delivery, the specific cardiac disease, and patient functional status. An understanding of the specific cardiac disease and its severity along with the hemodynamic goals will guide the choice of individualized anesthetic technique. Care should be used when considering neuraxial anesthesia techniques for women on anticoagulation.

For women who will be undergoing labor, there should be an early institution of analgesia to decrease sympathetic stimulation secondary to pain that would in turn increase heart rate and cardiac output. Continuous lumbar epidural analgesia with low dose of local anesthetic along with an opioid (e.g., bupivacaine 0.0625% with 2 µg/mL fentanyl) will provide excellent analgesia with attenuation of the increases in heart rate and cardiac output with minimal changes in SVR. The addition of an opioid to the local anesthetic solutions enhances the quality of the analgesia without increasing the sympathetic blockade. This can be supplemented with the use of a short-acting β blocker (e.g., esmolol) if needed. A careful titration providing a slow onset of sympathetic blockade allows for the ability to have tighter control over hemodynamic changes. However epidural block, with the use of local anesthetic, even in low concentrations, will still reduce SVR, causing hypotension, a decreased cardiac preload, and reflex tachycardia that may be poorly tolerated in women with mitral or aortic stenosis, CAD, pulmonary hypertension, or severe heart failure. A decrease in SVR in women with an intracardiac shunt also has the potential to reverse the direction of flow, leading to decreased pulmonary blood flow and hypoxia. Careful titration and close monitoring are necessary to avoid these complications. Patients with hypotension should be aggressively treated with a vasopressor, and any hint of heart failure should be treated with inotropic support. Patients who are particularly at risk for decompensation and heart failure may benefit from the prophylactic institution of a dobutamine infusion (2–3 µg/kg per minute) to assist the heart in dealing with the autotransfusion associated with delivery. Although women who are critically ill generally undergo cesarean delivery, if labor is chosen, the use of neuraxial opioids without local anesthetics will provide analgesia without any decrease in SVR and thus avoid cardiovascular effects. This can be accomplished with the use of a continuous spinal technique because epidural analgesia typically requires some local anesthetic to provide analgesia. Women with uncorrected tetralogy of Fallot, severe pulmonary arterial hypertension, and severe hypertrophic cardiomyopathy may be unable to tolerate any decreases in SVR or cardiac preload so neuraxial blockade should be used with extreme caution. Invasive monitoring of arterial, central venous, and pulmonary arterial pressures is reserved for women who have poor functional status or who have severe valvular stenosis or other hemodynamically significant lesions. This invasive hemodynamic monitoring should be continued into the postpartum period because the large intravascular volume shifts may precipitate pulmonary edema even in women in whom the conduct of labor had been without hemodynamic insult.

Anesthetic options for women undergoing cesarean delivery include neuraxial and general anesthesia. The advantages of regional anesthesia include an attenuation of sympathetically mediated increases in heart rate and cardiac output and minimal alteration in hemodynamics when carefully titrated. It also avoids the abrupt changes in hemodynamics associated with induction of general anesthesia, laryngoscopy, tracheal intubation, and extubation, although these can be blunted with suitable pharmacologic agents (e.g., IV opioids or β-blockers).

General anesthesia has the advantage of airway control and the use of TEE monitoring for real-time assessment of cardiac function and volume status. Care must be taken to avoid situations that will increase PVR, including hypercarbia, hypoxemia, hypothermia, and sympathetic stimulation. Women who are in the highest risk category should be seen antepartum by a cardiac surgeon and preparation for lifesaving cardiac support (extracorporeal membrane oxygenation or ventricular assist device) should be available during the cesarean delivery in case maternal decompensation occurs.

If general anesthesia is chosen, it is particularly important that an adequate depth of anesthesia be maintained throughout the intraoperative period to avoid tachycardia and hypertension. Large concentrations of volatile anesthetic agents should be avoided to prevent uterine atony. A high-dose opioid technique is associated with stable hemodynamics but can cause fetal respiratory depression. This can be minimized with the use of a short-acting opioid, remifentanil, which although it does cross the placenta, its effects will be short lived. Although standard American Society of Anesthesiologists monitoring including noninvasive blood pressure, ECG, and pulse oximetry is usually adequate for vaginal delivery, cesarean delivery often requires more invasive monitoring for tight hemodynamic control. Most patients require invasive arterial blood pressure monitoring, with central venous and pulmonary artery catheter monitoring reserved for critically ill women and for women in whom the need for use of vasoactive medications is likely. The hemodynamic perturbations of delivery continue into the postpartum period, so monitoring should continue for at

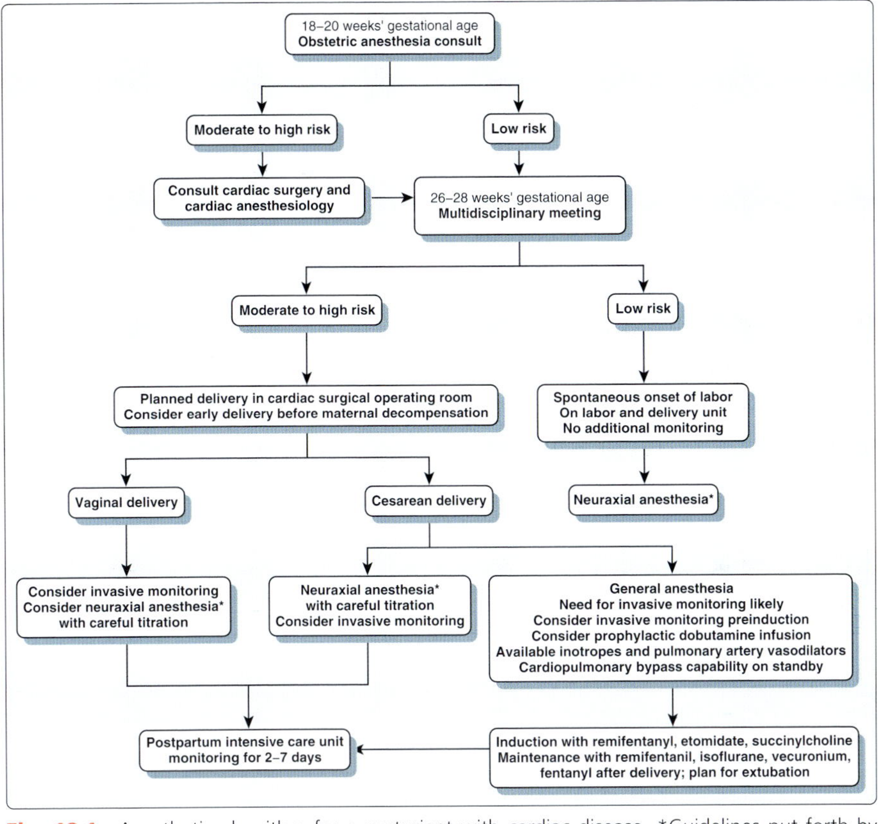

Fig. 18.1 Anesthetic algorithm for a parturient with cardiac disease. *Guidelines put forth by the American Society of Regional Anesthesia must be strictly adhered to.

least 48 hours in an intensive care unit. Cardiac status takes 2 to 6 weeks postpartum to gradually return to baseline.

An algorithm for the anesthetic care of these patients is presented in Fig. 18.1.

NONCARDIAC SURGERY DURING PREGNANCY IN WOMEN WITH CARDIAC DISEASE

Nonobstetric surgery during pregnancy is one of the few times that the anesthesiologist has to care for two patients simultaneously with sometimes conflicting goals. When the mother has significant cardiac disease, the risks are even greater. Preoperatively, the anesthesiology team should be in close communication with the patient's cardiologist and obstetrician as part of a multidisciplinary perioperative planning team. A multidisciplinary intraoperative team should include the anesthesiologist, primary proceduralist, obstetrician, neonatologists, and two teams of surgical technicians: one for the mother and the baby in case a cesarean delivery is required. It is self-evident that all nonurgent operations should be delayed until after delivery. Furthermore, any patient requiring a procedure should be managed in a specialized center with the expertise and capability to care for both the mother with cardiac disease and its possible consequences and be prepared for urgent delivery and subsequent care of the fetus.

Maternal and Fetal Monitoring

Patients with significant cardiac disease require increased monitoring during surgery, which may include arterial, central venous or pulmonary artery pressure monitoring, and TEE depending on the specific cardiac lesion, surgery, and the planned anesthetic technique. Patients with poor functional status and surgeries that involve large fluid shifts require the greatest amount of monitoring.

The fetal heart rate (FHR) should be monitored if at all possible. It is the best way to assure maintenance of a normal physiologic milieu for the baby. This is even more important in women with significant cardiac disease because the fetus is at greater risk because of the higher risk of decreased cardiac output and hypotension leading to uterine hypoperfusion. Monitoring and interpretation should be performed by an obstetrician or someone other than the anesthesiologist with expertise in FHR interpretation. Regardless of the decision to perform intraoperative FHR monitoring, the FHR and uterine contractions should be monitored before and after the surgery.

Anesthetic Considerations

The anesthetic plan should focus on optimizing the mother's cardiac condition while protecting the developing fetus. A complete discussion of anesthetic considerations for pregnant women undergoing nonobstetric surgery is beyond the scope of this chapter. Focused situations in which there are specific considerations for the pregnant woman with cardiac disease are presented here.

Organogenesis is complete by week 8, and it is therefore prudent to delay surgeries until after this critical period of development. None of the anesthetic agents are known teratogens, and the incidence of congenital defects is not greater after surgery with either general or neuraxial anesthesia. There is, however, an increased risk of spontaneous abortions in the first and second trimester when mothers undergo surgery, but it is not possible to determine which is the cause, the pathophysiology requiring surgery, the surgery itself, or the anesthetic. The basic principle when anesthetizing a pregnant woman is to optimize uteroplacental blood flow by optimizing cardiac output and avoiding hypoxia, hypercarbia, acidosis, and hypotension.

In healthy parturients, uterine blood flow is primarily determined by the perfusion pressure, which is directly related to maternal arterial pressure. Conditions that reduce maternal arterial pressure decrease uterine perfusion pressure. These include hypovolemia, which can be relative from sympathetic blockade or actual from hemorrhage, myocardial depressants such as general anesthetics, and mechanical obstruction caused by aortocaval compression by the gravid uterus. Decreases in uterine blood flow from aortocaval compression can be prevented by tilting the mother to the left.

In women with heart disease, uterine perfusion pressure is at risk of being compromised. In low cardiac output states such as systolic heart failure or critical aortic stenosis, the uterine blood flow may be compromised by diversion of blood to critical organs. With right-sided failure or pulmonary hypertension, the normally low pressure venous system may become congested so that forward flow to the uterus can be compromised.

An increase in uterine vascular resistance can also decrease uterine blood flow. This can occur under anesthesia as a result of catecholamine release or initiation of vasopressors, and women with cardiac disease are likely to require vasopressors. The most common agents used in healthy parturients are phenylephrine and ephedrine. The effects of epinephrine and norepinephrine on uterine blood flow and outcome have not been fully elucidated. However, the danger of not initiating vasopressor or inotropic support in a woman who needs it is great. Therefore the clinician should not hold back from starting them because of this concern.

Severe hypoxia and hypercarbia also decrease uterine blood flow, and even mild hypoxia and hypercarbia directly affect the oxygen tensions and acid-base status of neonatal blood. Supplemental oxygen and end-tidal carbon dioxide monitoring should always be used when sedating this patient population.

The anesthetic technique—regional or general anesthesia—should depend on the type of cardiac disease and the extent of surgery. In noncardiac patients, there is no evidence that one technique is superior to the other in regard to either maternal or neonatal outcomes. However, there are cardiac disease states in which neuraxial techniques may be relatively contraindicated or need very careful titration.

Laparoscopic surgery is safe during pregnancy, but those with cardiac disease may not be as able to tolerate the reduced preload or the rise in carbon dioxide partial pressures from insufflation. Uterine blood flow should be maximized with left uterine displacement and lowering insufflation pressures to no more than 10 to 15 mm Hg and, of course, monitoring maternal end-tidal carbon dioxide to avoid acidosis.

Glycopyrrolate is commonly given in conjunction with neostigmine for reversal of nondepolarizing neuromuscular agents to prevent anticholinesterase-induced bradycardia or asystole. However, as a quaternary amine, glycopyrrolate does not readily cross the uteroplacental barrier, but neostigmine does, which may lead to iatrogenic fetal bradycardia. Therefore some prefer to use atropine, which does cross the placenta. However, the effects of atropine with the possibility of inducing tachycardia must be considered in women with cardiac disease.

PERIPARTUM CARDIOMYOPATHY

Definition

Peripartum cardiomyopathy (PPCM) (Table 18.5) is defined as the development of an (1) idiopathic life-threatening cardiomyopathy with strict echocardiographic criteria including a left ventricular ejection fraction (LVEF) less than 45% or M-mode fractional shortening less than 30% (or both), and end-diastolic dimension greater than 2.7 cm/m^2; (2) in the last month of pregnancy or within the first 5 months postpartum in women; and (3) without recognizable preexisting heart disease. The importance of adhering to the timeline provided in the definition was emphasized to exclude other acquired preexisting causes of cardiomyopathy, which may be unmasked earlier in pregnancy (second trimester) because of the cardiovascular changes of pregnancy. PPCM is a distinct form of cardiomyopathy resulting from pregnancy, not an exacerbation of an underlying idiopathic dilated cardiomyopathy.

Incidence

Peripartum cardiomyopathy is a relatively rare disease, with an estimated incidence of less than 0.1% of pregnancies, although its incidence varies both according to race and geographic region. (The incidence of PPCM in the United States is about 1 in 3200.)

Risk Factors

Risk factors for PPCM include multiparity (parity of ≥4), advanced maternal age (>30 years old), multifetal pregnancy, preeclampsia, gestational hypertension, HELLP (hemolysis, elevated liver enzymes, and low platelet count) syndrome, and African American race. The prolonged use of tocolysis has also been associated with

Table 18.5	**Peripartum Cardiomyopathy**		
Definition	**Echocardiographic Criteria**	**Possible Etiologies**	**Risk Factors**
Idiopathic No recognizable heart disease Occurs in the last month of pregnancy or in the first 5 months postpartum[a]	Left ventricular ejection fraction <45%, M-mode fractional shortening <30%, or both Left ventricular end-diastolic dimension >2.7 cm/m^2	Oxidative stress Autoimmunity Inflammatory Myocarditis	Multiparity Advanced maternal age Multifetal pregnancy Preeclampsia African American race Prolonged use of tocolysis Family history

[a]The Working Group on PPCM from the Heart Failure Association of the European Society of Cardiology removed time frames from the definition because it thought they were arbitrary and led to underdiagnosis.

development of PPCM. Other risk factors that have been identified include hypertension, diabetes, smoking, and severe anemia. There also appears to be a genetic susceptibility because a number of cases of PPCM have been found among patients with a family history of dilated cardiomyopathy.

Etiology

The pathophysiology of PPCM remains poorly understood. Several causes have been proposed:

1. **Oxidative stress:** The most recent hypothesis is that PPCM develops as a result of oxidative stress, which enhances activity by the protease cathepsin-D, leading to increased cleavage of the hormone prolactin, resulting in an N-terminal 16-kDa prolactin fragment (also called *vasoinhibin*), which is a potent antiangiogenic, proapoptotic, and proinflammatory factor. This leads to massive endothelial damage, capillary dissociation, and vasoconstriction and results in myocardial dysfunction. Consistent with these findings, a novel specific therapeutic approach through inhibition of prolactin secretion by bromocriptine, a dopamine D2 receptor agonist, prevented the development of PPCM in an animal model of PPCM, and the first human clinical experience was promising at leading to better survival and improvement of LV function.
2. **Autoimmunity:** In a phenomenon called *fetal microchimerism,* cells from the fetus take up residence in the mother, provoking a cardiotoxic autoimmune component. Treatment of PPCM with therapies proven successful in graft-versus-host disease and organ rejection may be useful.
3. **Inflammatory process:** Proinflammatory serum markers such as tumor necrosis factor-α, sFas/Apo1 (a plasma marker of apoptosis), C-reactive protein, interferon-γ, and interleukin-6 have been found to be significantly elevated in women with PPCM. This mechanism is underscored by the survival benefit of the antiinflammatory agent pentoxifylline.

4. **Myocarditis:** Myocarditis has been found on the endomyocardial biopsy specimens of the right ventricle of women with PPCM. Immunosuppressive drug therapy should be considered when active myocarditis has been confirmed by endomyocardial biopsy.

Clinical Presentation and Diagnosis

Fewer than 10% of cases of PPCM occur at the end of pregnancy; 78% present in the first 4 months postpartum. The diagnosis of PPCM requires a high index of suspicion because symptoms of PPCM can be confused with the physiologic changes of pregnancy and the early postpartum period. Consequently, women with PPCM generally are diagnosed relatively late when they are already NYHA class III or IV, resulting in higher rates of morbidity and mortality.

Most patients present with signs and symptoms similar to other forms of heart failure and reflect reduced cardiac output, resulting in tissue hypoperfusion and pulmonary edema from congestive heart failure. They include dyspnea on exertion, cough, orthopnea, hemoptysis, and paroxysmal nocturnal dyspnea. Additional symptoms include nonspecific fatigue, malaise, palpitations, chest (pleuritic chest pain can be presenting symptoms of pulmonary embolism) and abdominal discomfort (secondary to hepatic congestion), and postural hypotension.

On physical examination, signs of heart failure may be present, including tachycardia, displacement of the apical impulse, presence of an S_3 third heart sound, and evidence of mitral or tricuspid regurgitation. Elevated jugular venous pressure, pulmonary rales, hepatomegaly, and pedal edema may also be present. Women may have difficulty lying flat for the examination.

The differential diagnosis for suspected PPCM includes malignant hypertension, diastolic dysfunction, sepsis, pulmonary embolus, and obstetric complications such as preeclampsia, eclampsia, and amniotic fluid embolism.

If PPCM is suspected, a complete blood count, electrolytes, liver function tests, C-reactive protein, arterial blood gases, and troponin should be performed, which may be helpful in ruling out MI. Disease-specific biomarkers include prolactin and factors involved in the prolactin cleavage pathway. Levels of B-type natriuretic peptide and N-terminal pro-B-type natriuretic peptide can help in confirming the diagnosis.

An ECG may be normal or may show sinus tachycardia and nonspecific ST-segment and T-wave abnormalities, conduction abnormalities such as prolonged PR and QRS intervals, and LV hypertrophy. A chest radiograph often shows cardiomegaly and pulmonary venous congestion, and sometimes demonstrates pulmonary edema and pleural effusion. An echocardiogram is the key to diagnosis and will show moderate to severe LV systolic dysfunction. Doppler evaluation may show moderate to severe mitral and tricuspid valve regurgitation and pulmonary hypertension.

Outcomes and Predictors of Recovery

Peripartum cardiomyopathy is a potentially life-threatening condition accounting for up to 11% of maternal deaths. It has a highly variable clinical course, and rapid progression to end-stage heart failure may occur within days and spontaneous and complete recovery may also occur. Recovery from PPCM is defined as recovery to an LVEF greater than 50% or improvement by 20%. End stage heart failure is seen in 10% to 23% of patients and recovery to an LVEF greater than 50% is seen in 35% to 50% of patients.

A number of factors have been associated with recovery or nonrecovery. Predictors of recovery include white race, LVEF greater than 30%, LV end-diastolic diameter smaller than 5.5 cm, and postpartum diagnosis. Factors associated with lack of recovery are an LV end-diastolic dimension greater than 5.6 cm, LVEF less than 30%, the presence of LV thrombus, and African-American race.

Recovery usually occurs between 2 and 6 months postpartum but might occur as late as 48 months postpartum. Delayed diagnosis, greater NYHA functional class, black race, LV thrombus, multiparity, and coexisting medical illnesses are associated with delayed recovery.

The mortality rate in women with PPCM seems to be decreasing as the treatment for heart failure has improved. The risk increases with older age, LVEF less than 25%, multiparity, African-American ethnicity, and delayed diagnosis.[114] The estimated mortality rate of PPCM in the United States varies from 0% to 16.5%; worldwide, the mortality rate ranges from 1.4% to 32%. Race, ethnicity, and environmental differences as well as access to medical care may be responsible for the varying results.

There seems to be an elevated risk of PPCM in a subsequent pregnancy, particularly if the LVEF has not recovered to baseline. Almost 50% of such women were reported to have suffered heart failure during or after the subsequent pregnancy. In general, the severity of PPCM in a subsequent pregnancy increases. Any woman with an LVEF of less than 25% at previous diagnosis or in whom the LVEF has not normalized should be advised against a subsequent pregnancy. All patients should be informed that pregnancy can have a negative effect on cardiac function, and development of heart failure and death may occur.

Management During Pregnancy, Labor and Delivery, and Postpartum

When it occurs in the peripartum period, PPCM requires a well-coordinated multidisciplinary approach that involves obstetricians, cardiologists, perinatologists, neonatologists, anesthesiologists, and cardiac surgeons to manage a pregnant woman with heart failure. Both the heart failure condition and the heart failure treatment in PPCM may result in placental insufficiency, leading to intrauterine fetal death or premature birth. If the patient can be stabilized with medical therapy, continuation of pregnancy to allow for fetal maturity may be possible with close monitoring. However, if the mother deteriorates, the consideration for an urgent premature delivery with a timely use of corticosteroids for fetal lung maturation should be discussed to rescue both the mother and child. Termination of pregnancy often results in improvement of both symptoms and cardiac function and should be considered in patients with worsening symptoms or cardiac function.

The medical management of PPCM is similar to that of other types of heart failure that focus on reducing preload and afterload and increasing cardiac inotropy. However, it varies depending if the patient is still pregnant or is postpartum because the medication safety profiles during pregnancy or lactation must be considered, and their side effects must be closely monitored and managed. The first aim is to improve symptoms, and the second is to attempt to manage the disease through the administration of targeted therapies. Rapid treatment may be necessary when the patient has pulmonary edema or is hypoxic. When women with PPCM have hypotension, worsening heart failure, altered mental status, and increased work of breathing, they should be treated in the hospital. Medications should be continued until there is improved or resolved LV dysfunction.

Treatment for the acute symptomatic management of PPCM should be with oxygen and heart failure medications, mainly β-blockers and afterload-reducing agents such as ACE inhibitors or ARBs, with the addition of loop diuretics if necessary.

β-Blockers, such as metoprolol and carvedilol, have been approved for use in PCCM, are considered safe for use during pregnancy, and they improve survival. They are also crucial for long-term management of systolic dysfunction, if present. β_1-Selective blockers such as metoprolol and carvedilol are preferred over nonselective β-blockers such as propranolol to avoid the antitocolytic action induced by β_2-receptor blockade. Carvedilol combined with an afterload-reducing agent has been shown effective in PPCM. Newborns born to mothers on β-blockers are at risk for bradycardia, hypoglycemia, and respiratory depression and should be monitored for 48 to 72 hours.

Angiotensin-converting enzyme inhibitors and ARBs are considered first-line drugs for heart failure management and have been shown to improve survival. However, they are contraindicated in pregnancy because of their teratogenicity that may cause oligohydramnios, renal agenesis, and fetal death. These medications are the mainstay of treatment of PPCM after delivery for afterload reduction. They are secreted in breast milk, so breastfeeding must be stopped before commencing therapy. Prenatally, the preferred afterload reducer that is safe to use is hydralazine. More severe cases necessitate the use of IV nitroglycerin. Nitroprusside is not recommended because of the potential for cyanide toxicity.

Diuretics are used to treat symptomatic volume overload, including pulmonary congestion and peripheral edema. Both hydrochlorothiazide and furosemide are safe during pregnancy and lactation. However, the benefit of symptomatic relief must be weighed against the risk of diuretic-induced reduction in intravascular volume that can result in uteroplacental hypoperfusion. For patients on furosemide, fetal amniotic fluid volume should be measured regularly. Although the potassium-sparing diuretic spironolactone has been used successfully to treat heart failure, there are insufficient data regarding its use during pregnancy.

The use of inotropic agents such as epinephrine, dobutamine, or milrinone should be confined to cases of severe low cardiac output and those with congestion that persists despite optimal medical therapy with vasodilators and diuretics. The patient should be weaned from them as soon as hemodynamically stable, adequate organ perfusion is restored, and congestion is reduced.

When inotropes are insufficient to restore cardiac output or in patients who present in cardiogenic shock, temporary circulatory support with an intraaortic balloon pump, extracorporeal membrane oxygenation, or implantation of an LV assist device as a bridge to recovery or even as a bridge to heart transplantation will be necessary. After there is clinical and echocardiographic evidence of recovery of cardiac function, weaning from the device may be attempted. Bridging to recovery with LV assist devices has helped to dramatically decrease the percentage of PPCM patients requiring transplantation. However, if weaning is not successful, transplantation should be considered.

Heart failure and pregnancy are independent risk factors for thromboembolism. Therefore, although the incidence of thromboembolic complications in pregnant women with cardiomyopathy is not known, patients with PPCM should receive therapeutic anticoagulation, particularly if the LVEF is less than 35%. The administration of heparin or LMWH during pregnancy and postpartum is recommended. Warfarin is teratogenic and must be avoided during pregnancy. Warfarin is considered safe during breastfeeding.

Ventricular arrhythmias are common in patients with PPCM, causing a significant percentage of PPCM deaths. The decision on implantation of an ICD is particularly difficult in patients with PPCM, because many experience an improvement in LV function within the first few months after delivery. Temporary use of a wearable defibrillator should be considered until a final decision is made.

The timing and mode of delivery in PPCM and its anesthetic management should be a multidisciplinary decision that will be dependent on both the clinical status of the mother and the unborn child. A plan for the mode of delivery, type of anesthesia, and need for any invasive hemodynamic monitoring should be identified before the commencement of labor. The use of invasive hemodynamic monitoring before labor and delivery allows for optimization of the hemodynamic status before delivery and for monitoring during and after the delivery.

Labor is best accomplished in an institution where there is experience in managing pregnancies with cardiac disease and should be induced at a time when all necessary medical and surgical teams are present in the hospital. Labor and delivery produce hemodynamic challenges, including increased cardiac output, and blood loss. Women need to be carefully monitored during labor, delivery, and the postpartum period. In addition to continuous ECG monitoring, continuous pulse oximetry, and noninvasive blood pressure monitoring, the use of an arterial line for continuous blood pressure monitoring and a central line in anticipation of the need for inotropes and vasopressors should be considered, particularly in women at high risk for decompensation. In general, medications such as β-blockers should be continued, and diuretics and vasodilators should be used on an individual basis. Vaginal delivery is preferred in stable patients. Aggressive pain management is pivotal for controlling heart rate and SVR. Nevertheless, an elective planned cesarean delivery is preferable to better control hemodynamic fluctuations for women who are critically ill and in need of inotropic therapy or mechanical support. Furthermore, a cesarean delivery will be necessary if a preterm delivery is necessary because inducing labor will likely be unsuccessful.

Anesthetic technique must be individualized and is dependent on understanding the physiology of pregnancy and its interaction with the individual patient's pathophysiology. Anesthesia during labor and delivery can cause rapid hemodynamic changes, including hypotension caused by rapid lowering of the SVR, which can be challenging for women with cardiomyopathy. The primary anesthetic goals are avoidance of drug-induced myocardial depression, maintenance of normovolemia, prevention of increased or rapidly decreased ventricular afterload, and blunting of the sympathetic stimulation induced by pain and anxiety. Careful use of either general or regional anesthesia can effectively meet these goals. Regional anesthesia may not be possible if the mother has been placed on anticoagulation. Furthermore, the use of general anesthesia provides the additional benefit of allowing for the use of TEE monitoring. Because alterations in hemodynamic status continue to occur for the first 24 hours after delivery, adequate cardiovascular monitoring must be maintained into the postpartum period.

A therapeutic algorithm for acute patients with severe PPCM has recently been published (Fig. 18.2).

Management During Noncardiac Surgery

Patients with heart failure require continuous optimization of cardiac status before, during, and after all surgeries. They generally do not tolerate any sudden increases or decreases in sympathetic tone leading to increases or decreases in preload and afterload, hypoxia, or hypercarbia that will increase PVR. Patients with severe dysfunction can rapidly decompensate with even small changes in hemodynamic parameters. The combination of a pregnant woman with heart failure requires an individualized approach that keeps hemodynamic goals in mind. Invasive monitoring with intraarterial

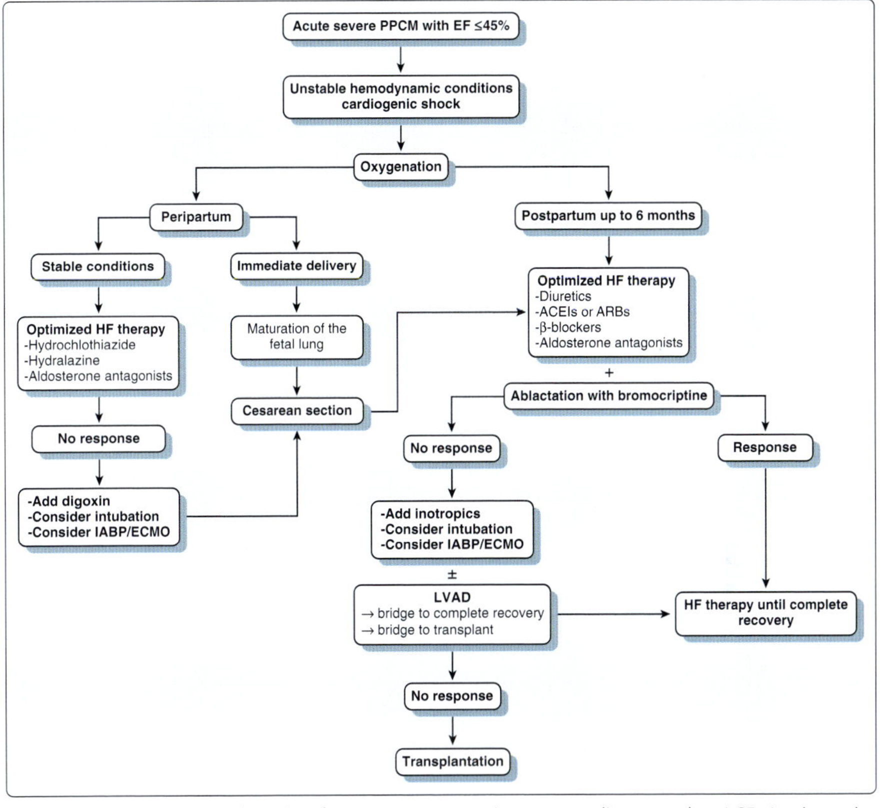

Fig. 18.2. Therapeutic algorithm for acute severe peripartum cardiomyopathy. *ACE,* Angiotensin-converting enzyme; *ARB,* angiotensin receptor blocker; *ECMO,* extracorporeal membrane oxygenation; *EF,* ejection fraction; *HF,* heart failure; *IABP,* intraaortic balloon pump; *LVAD,* left ventricular assist device. (From Bachelier-Walenta K, Hilfiker-Kleiner D, Sliwa K. Peripartum cardiomyopathy: update 2012. *Curr Opin Crit Care.* 2013;19(5):397-403.)

and central catheters for the ability to rapidly titrate inotropes and vasopressors are recommended, particularly in women with severe dysfunction and for procedures with rapid fluid shifts. The use of intraoperative TEE monitoring can be invaluable for early detection of decompensation.

ADVANCED CARDIAC LIFE SUPPORT IN PREGNANT WOMEN

Cardiac arrest in the pregnant woman is challenging to the healthcare team as they try to resuscitate two patients, the mother and the unborn baby. Maternal cardiac arrest is rare, with the most common causes being hemorrhage, heart failure, amniotic fluid embolism, or sepsis. Because the incidence is rare, most healthcare professionals will never need to provide Advanced Cardiac Life Support (ACLS) to a pregnant woman.

The basic tenets of ACLS are similar between pregnant and nonpregnant women, with some modifications primarily related to the physiologic and anatomic changes in pregnant women. These modifications, however, may mean the difference between a successful and unsuccessful resuscitation.

Table 18.6	Modifications to ACLS Protocol for the Pregnant Woman	
ACLS Intervention	**Modifications**
Activation of cardiac arrest:	Notifying multiple specialty teams (e.g., anesthesiologists, obstetricians, pediatricians, neonatologists, and nurses)
Patient position	Manual left uterine displacement
Chest compressions	Hand placement higher on the sternum than normal
Airway	Difficult intubation so laryngoscopy by most experienced person
	Application of cricoid pressure until airway is secured
Defibrillation	Removal of fetal monitor before defibrillation if possible
Medications	IV access placed above the diaphragm
Cause of cardiac arrest	BEAUCHOPS: **b**leeding/DIC, **e**mbolism, **a**nesthetic complications, **u**terine atony, **c**ardiac disease, **h**ypertension or preeclampsia, **o**ther (differential diagnosis for standard ACLS guideline), **p**lacental issues, and **s**epsis
PMCD	Begin cesarean within 4 minutes of cardiac arrest and delivery by 5 minutes
	Cesarean delivery equipment on crash cart

ACLS, Advanced Cardiac Life Support; *DIC,* disseminated intravascular coagulation; *IV,* intravenous; *PMCD,* perimortem cesarean delivery.

This section reviews the modifications to ACLS in pregnant patients and the reasons for the changes (Table 18.6).

1. **Activation of cardiac arrest alarm:** Most hospitals have a system in place to activate a cardiac arrest alarm, such as "code blue" or "team 7000." In addition to the "typical" resuscitation team, successful resuscitation of the pregnant woman and neonate requires multiple specialty teams that must arrive at the onset of the arrest. The team includes anesthesiologists, obstetricians, pediatricians, neonatologists, and nurses. Successful resuscitation may require expeditious delivery of the neonate that should be started within 4 minutes of the arrest and completed within 5 minutes (see later section on perimortem resuscitation). This requires advanced planning and a means of alerting the resuscitation team that a pregnant woman has arrested because the additional personnel (e.g., obstetricians, pediatricians, and neonatologists) do not routinely participate in adult resuscitation. This is particularly important if the arrest occurs in a location other than the labor floor.

2. **Patient position:** Aortocaval compression in the supine position occurs by the 20th week of pregnancy and even earlier in some pregnant women. In the supine position, inferior vena cava compression will decrease venous return, resulting in reduced cardiac output during chest compressions. Also, placental blood flow is reduced in the supine position, leading to fetal acidosis. Tilting the patient on her left side will improve cardiac output and improve uteroplacental perfusion. However, tilting the patient to the left may reduce the effectiveness of chest compressions, with greater degrees of tilt decreasing the maximum resuscitative force. Left uterine displacement should be performed with either a human wedge (knees of the resuscitator under the patient's right side) or manual displacement of the uterus rather than full body tilt to maximize chest compression force. It should be performed in anyone with an obvious gravid uterus regardless of gestational age.

3. **Chest compressions:** Hand placement for chest compressions should be slightly higher on the sternum than normal to account for cephalad movement of the diaphragm from the gravid uterus.

4. **Airway:** Anatomic changes to the airway, including laryngeal and pharyngeal edema, can make ventilation and tracheal intubation more difficult. Decreases in functional residual capacity in conjunction with increases in cardiac output, metabolic rate, and oxygen consumption lead to the development of arterial hypoxemia at a faster rate than in the nonpregnant woman. Also, a decrease in gastric emptying along with a decrease in lower esophageal sphincter tone place pregnant women at risk for pulmonary aspiration. Therefore tracheal intubation to maximize oxygen delivery should occur as soon as possible after cardiac arrest and performed by the most experienced anesthesiologist. Also, a smaller than usual tracheal tube should be used. Although the efficacy of applying cricoid pressure to reduce pulmonary aspiration is controversial, cricoid pressure should be applied until tracheal intubation is confirmed to reduce the risk of pulmonary aspiration. However, if applying cricoid pressure makes ventilation or tracheal intubation more difficult, it should be released.

5. **Defibrillation:** Voltage administered for defibrillation in a pregnant woman should be the same as for a nonpregnant patient. There is theoretical concern that electrical current could induce burns in the fetus or mother if FHR monitors are being used. This is highly unlikely because the electrical current is being administered to the maternal thorax. However, it is prudent to remove any fetal monitors before defibrillation if possible. However, defibrillation should not be delayed for removal of the monitors. Additionally, there is a theoretical risk of inducing fetal arrhythmias, but the risk is small, and defibrillation should not be delayed or avoided for this reason.

6. **Medications:** Aortocaval compression could increase the time or completely impede medications from reaching the heart. Therefore IV access should be placed above the diaphragm. Although during pregnancy intravascular volume and volume of distribution increase and protein binding decreases, the timing and doses of medications during ACLS should not be altered from the nonpregnant woman.

7. **Cause of cardiac arrest:** The American Heart Association has suggested the mnemonic BEAUCHOPS to help remember the possible causes of maternal cardiac arrest. The mnemonic stands for **b**leeding or disseminated intravascular coagulation, **e**mbolism, **a**nesthetic complications, **u**terine atony, **c**ardiac disease, **h**ypertension or preeclampsia, **o**ther (differential diagnosis for standard ACLS guidelines), **p**lacental issues, and **s**epsis. Reversible and treatable causes of cardiac arrest should be sought and include magnesium sulfate toxicity, amniotic fluid embolism, hemorrhage, and anesthetic complications such as local anesthetic toxicity and total spinal anesthesia. Magnesium sulfate toxicity should be treated by stopping the infusion and administering calcium. Amniotic fluid embolism has a high fatality rate, but with aggressive treatment survival has increased. Hemorrhage requires aggressive replacement of blood and blood products. Local anesthetic toxicity should be treated with Intralipid, and total spinal anesthesia should be treated with tracheal intubation and management of hemodynamic instability.

8. **Perimortem cesarean delivery (PMCD):** PMCD refers to cesarean delivery that is performed after the start of resuscitation and may increase the survival rate for both the mother and baby. If there is no return of spontaneous circulation within 4 minutes, cesarean delivery should commence, and delivery should occur within 5 minutes. PMCD should be performed at the location of the cardiac arrest, and there should not be an attempt to move the patient to the operating room.

SUGGESTED READING

Bachelier-Walenta K, Hilfiker-Kleiner D, Sliwa K. Peripartum cardiomyopathy: update 2012. *Curr Opin Crit Care.* 2013;19:397–403.

Bedard E, Dimopoulos K, Gatzoulis MA. Has there been any progress made on pregnancy outcomes among women with pulmonary arterial hypertension? *Eur Heart J.* 2009;30:256–265.

Canobbio MM, Warnes CA, Aboulhosn J, et al. Management of pregnancy in patients with complex congenital heart disease: a scientific statement for healthcare professionals from the American Heart Association. *Circulation.* 2017;135:e50–e87.

Cobb B, Lipman S. Cardiac arrest: obstetric CPR/ACLS. *Clin Obstet Gynecol.* 2017;60:425–430.

Drenthen W, Boersma E, Balci A, et al. Predictors of pregnancy complications in women with congenital heart disease. *Eur Heart J.* 2010;31:2124–2132.

Drenthen W, Pieper PG, Roos-Hesselink JW, et al. Outcome of pregnancy in women with congenital heart disease: a literature review. *J Am Coll Cardiol.* 2007;49:2303–2311.

Elkayam U, Jalnapurkar S, Barakat M. Peripartum cardiomyopathy. *Cardiol Clin.* 2012;30:435–440.

Jeejeebhoy FM, Zelop CM, Lipman S, et al. Cardiac arrest in pregnancy: a scientific statement from the American Heart Association. *Circulation.* 2015;132:1747–1773.

Kealey A. Coronary artery disease and myocardial infarction in pregnancy: a review of epidemiology, diagnosis, and medical and surgical management. *Can J Cardiol.* 2010;26:185–189.

Kuczkowski KM. Labor analgesia for the parturient with cardiac disease: what does an obstetrician need to know? *Acta Obstet Gynecol Scand.* 2004;83:223–233.

Nanna M, Stergiopoulos K. Pregnancy complicated by valvular heart disease: an update. *J Am Heart Assoc.* 2014;3:e000712.

Obican SG, Cleary KL. Pulmonary arterial hypertension in pregnancy. *Semin Perinatol.* 2014;38:289–294.

Regitz-Zagrosek V, Blomstrom Lundqvist C, Borghi C, et al. European Society of Cardiology guidelines on the management of cardiovascular diseases during pregnancy. *Eur Heart J.* 2011;32:3147–3197.

Regitz-Zagrosek V, Gohlke-Barwolf C, Iung B, Pieper PG. Management of cardiovascular diseases during pregnancy. *Curr Probl Cardiol.* 2014;39:85–151.

Selle T, Renger I, Labidi S, Bultmann I, Hilfiker-Kleiner D. Reviewing peripartum cardiomyopathy: current state of knowledge. *Future Cardiol.* 2009;5:175–189.

Simpson LL. Maternal cardiac disease: update for the clinician. *Obstet Gynecol.* 2012;119:345–359.

Sliwa K, Hilfiker-Kleiner D, Petrie MC, et al. Current state of knowledge on aetiology, diagnosis, management, and therapy of peripartum cardiomyopathy: a position statement from the Heart Failure Association of the European Society of Cardiology Working Group on peripartum cardiomyopathy. *Eur J Heart Fail.* 2010;12:767–778.

Westhoff-Bleck M, Podewski E, Hilfiker A, Hilfiker-Kleiner D. Cardiovascular disorders in pregnancy: diagnosis and management. *Best Pract Res Clin Obstet Gynaecol.* 2013;27:821–834.

Windram JD, Colman JM, Wald RM, et al. Valvular heart disease in pregnancy. *Best Pract Res Clin Obstet Gynaecol.* 2014;28:507–518.

Wolff GA, Weitzel NS. Management of acquired cardiac disease in the obstetric patient. *Semin Cardiothorac Vasc Anesth.* 2011;15:85–97.

Chapter 19

Goal-Directed Fluid Therapy, Perioperative Pain Management, and Enhanced Recovery

Gerard R. Manecke Jr, MD • Engy T. Said, MD

> **Key Points**
>
> 1. The costs of healthcare are escalating. Goal-directed fluid therapy (GDT) and multimodal pain relief are ways to control cost while improving quality.
> 2. GDT is an integral part of enhanced recovery programs (ERPs), as is multimodal pain management.
> 3. The traditional, liberal approach to perioperative fluid management has no sound evidence base and causes perioperative fluid and salt overload. "Zero fluid balance" is recommended using a goal-directed approach. ERPs emphasize avoidance of salt and water overload.
> 4. GDT involves cardiovascular monitoring such as minimally invasive cardiac output and application of an algorithm or guidelines specific to fluid and hemodynamic management.
> 5. GDT and ERPs increase quality by decreasing variability in practice with evidence-based management. Decreased cost results from less perioperative morbidity and streamlined care delivery.
> 6. Various monitors may be used for GDT, ranging from invasive (e.g., pulmonary artery catheter) to noninvasive (e.g., finger cuff cardiac output). The choice of monitor is based on the clinical situation and individual or institutional preference. The most common monitors used are esophageal Doppler and arterial pulse-wave analysis systems.
> 7. ERPs are multidisciplinary, multifactorial care pathways. They incorporate optimal preoperative preparation, careful intraoperative management of fluid status and temperature, antibiotic administration, minimally invasive surgery, multimodal pain relief, postoperative nausea and vomiting control, and early mobilization.
> 8. Multimodal perioperative pain relief using opiate-sparing techniques facilitates early mobilization and patient comfort and decreases opiate-related complications. Effective multimodal pain management is essential for ERPs.

With recent advances in expensive diagnostic and treatment modalities, the costs of healthcare have skyrocketed. The need to care for increasing numbers of patients undergoing procedures while controlling cost has pushed healthcare systems to devise increasingly efficient ways to deliver care. The "throughput" of patients is often stymied by prolonged hospital stays and readmission after procedures. Inefficient systems, inconsistent care, and perioperative complications cause delays, poor patient and provider satisfaction, and high cost.

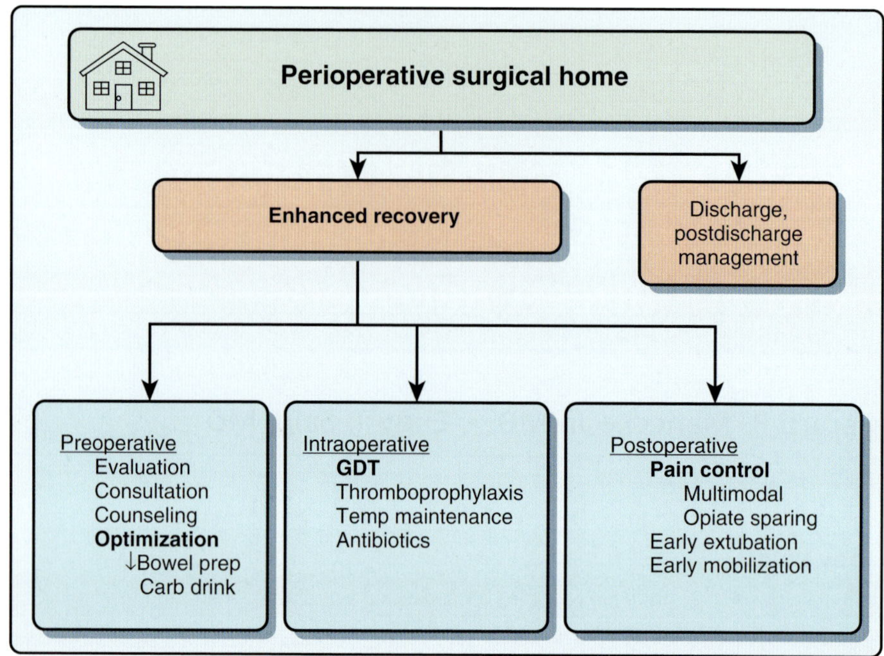

Fig. 19.1 Goal-directed fluid therapy (GDT) is part of enhanced recovery programs, which lie under the perioperative surgical home umbrella.

Goal-directed fluid therapy (GDT), enhanced recovery programs (ERPs), and the perioperative surgical home (PSH) are three related approaches to patient care that have emerged to provide optimal outcomes for patients undergoing surgery. GDT refers to fluid and hemodynamic management targeting optimal cardiovascular performance using monitoring beyond standard noninvasive monitors. ERPs are designed to incorporate patient management processes, such as preoperative optimization, multimodal pain management, and early mobilization after surgery, so as to facilitate recovery. PSH is a construct consisting of a coordinated, multidisciplinary team using best-evidence guidelines and protocols to guide patients through the entire perioperative experience as seamlessly as possible. Fig. 19.1 shows GDT as a component of ERPs and both under the PSH umbrella. GDT and multimodal pain relief are two approaches that facilitate early ambulation, patient comfort, and enhanced recovery. These approaches are particularly important in patients with cardiovascular illness.

GOAL-DIRECTED FLUID THERAPY

Traditional, liberal fluid management, which entailed a cookbook-type approach, is now outmoded. This involved calculation of maintenance fluid requirement based on body weight, calculation of a deficit based on the period during which the patient has not had any fluid (e.g., nothing by mouth [NPO]), presumed effects of a bowel prep, and estimation of third-space losses based on the invasiveness of the surgery. Typically, for major abdominal surgery, 6, 8, 10, or even 12 mL/kg per hour of crystalloid would be administered to replace insensible losses and loss to the third space. The concept of a "third space" has been called into question. What has been referred to

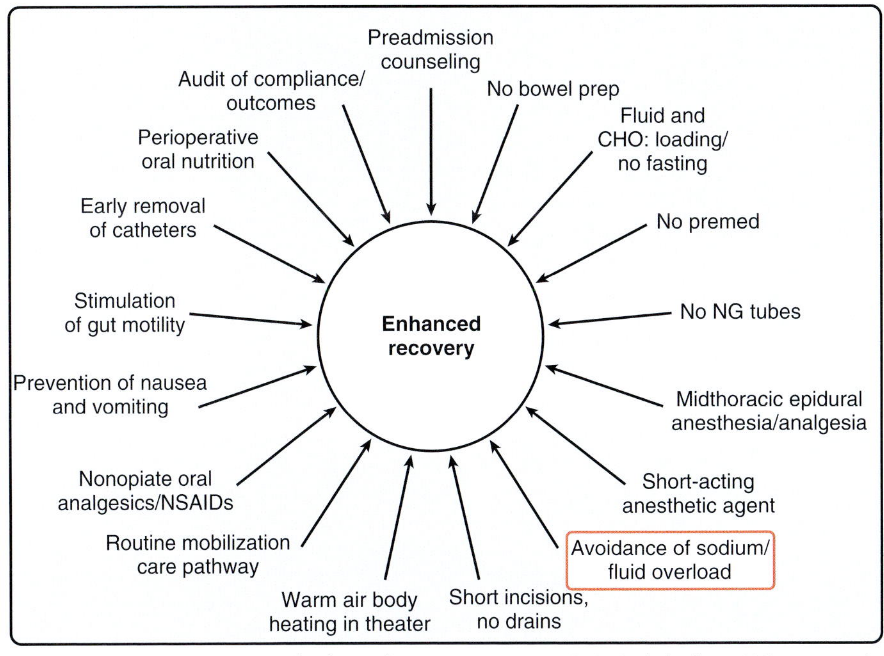

Fig. 19.2 Major components of enhanced recovery programs. *CHO,* Carbohydrate; *NG,* nasogastric; *NSAIDs,* nonsteroidal antiinflammatory drugs.

as fluid loss to the third space likely represents translocation of administered fluid out of the vascular space, resulting in intracellular and extracellular edema.

Excess salt and fluid in the perioperative period is potentially harmful. Fluid and salt excess can lead to airway edema, increased lung water, tissue edema, and cardiac failure. Relative fluid restriction results in shorter hospital lengths of stay, improved wound healing, fewer surgical infections, and fewer cardiovascular and pulmonary complications. It is sometimes argued that excess perioperative fluid and salt are acceptable because, with time, the patient will mobilize the fluid. However, the potential airway problems, prolonged ventilation, increased complication rate, and extra time in recovery associated with excess fluid and salt administration are neither necessary nor acceptable. Avoidance of fluid and salt overload in major surgery is now a standard component of ERPs (Fig. 19.2).

Overaggressive fluid restriction can have negative consequences as well, with hypovolemia leading to hypotension, tachycardia, organ ischemia, and vital organ failure. Morbidity rates are higher in the setting of either hypovolemia or hypervolemia (Fig. 19.3). Targeting no perioperative change in body weight, fluid restriction protocols do allow modest fluid administration with a background rate (e.g., 1–4 mL/ kg per hour) and fluid boluses to maintain hemodynamic stability. Likewise, blood products are used as needed to maintain adequate hemoglobin concentration and coagulation.

A goal-directed, protocol-based approach to fluid and hemodynamic management has grown out of accumulating evidence that optimizing hemodynamic status improves outcome and that accurate assessment of volume and hemodynamic status using only standard, noninvasive monitors is often impossible. Tachycardia, hypotension, and oliguria can result from either hypovolemia or hypervolemia (i.e., heart failure).

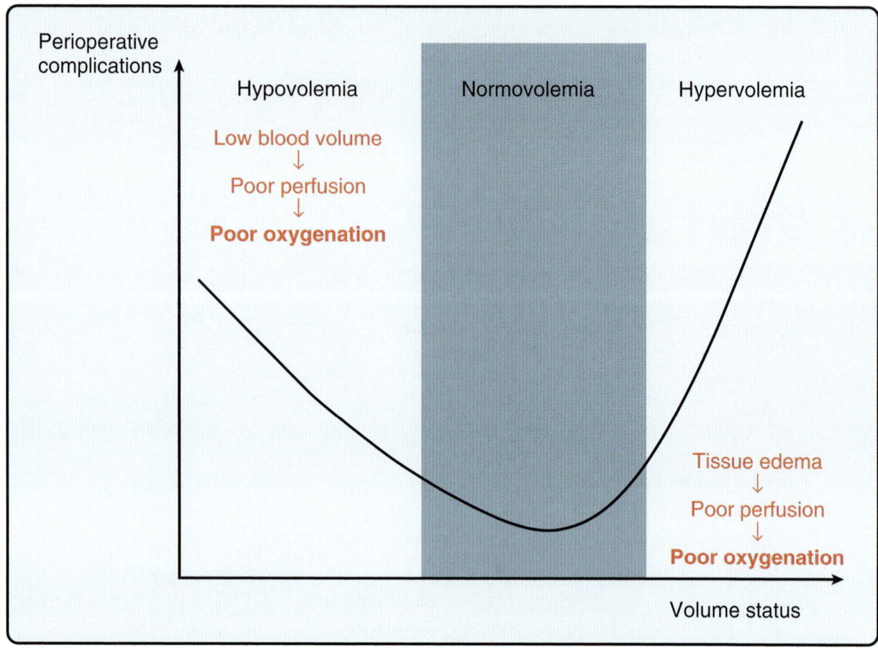

Fig. 19.3 Either hypervolemia or hypovolemia may cause impaired tissue perfusion and poor outcome. (From Bellamy MC. Wet, dry or something else? *Br J Anaesth.* 2006;97:755-757.)

GDT adoption has also resulted from recognition that decreasing variability of practice using a best-evidence approach improves outcome. Decreasing process variability is essential to creating high-performance systems.

Some perioperative GDT grows out of current approaches to critically ill patients. Early, aggressive fluid and hemodynamic management of septic patients is an integral factor leading to dramatic improvements in mortality rate. This work, published in 2001, revolutionized the initial management of patients with sepsis, such that the vast majority of tertiary care centers now have a sepsis protocol that incorporates an early, goal-directed approach.

In 2002, Gan and colleagues studied 100 patients undergoing major elective surgery, randomly assigning them to receive either "standard" therapy or GDT based on esophageal Doppler parameters. The GDT group experienced shorter hospital stays (5 ± 3 days vs. 7 ± 3 days), less nausea and vomiting, and earlier return of bowel function. Numerous studies of a wide variety of surgical populations using various GDT algorithms and monitors followed, with the vast majority showing benefit. Large meta-analyses have subsequently confirmed the benefits of using thoughtful, informed fluid administration, often with the use of algorithms with sound bases in physiology.

Goal-Directed Fluid Therapy and Cost Reduction

With its decreased morbidity and hospital length of stay, GDT reduces cost. Perioperative complications, in addition to being distressing to patients and healthcare delivery teams, dramatically increase healthcare costs. This increased cost results from increased

Table 19.1 Mortality Rate, Hospital Length of Stay (LOS), and Direct Costs of Patients With No Surgical Complications vs. Those With ≥1 Complication

	No Complications	≥1 Complication	P Value
Mortality rate	1.4%	12.4%	<.001
Hospital LOS (days)	8.1 ± 7.1 days	20.5 ± 20.1 days	<.001
Direct costs (mean)	$17,408 ± $15,612	$47,284 ± $49,170	<.001

Modified from Manecke GR, Asemota A, Michard F. Tackling the economic burden of postsurgical complications: would perioperative goal-directed fluid therapy help? *Crit Care*. 2014;18:566.

utilization of expensive resources (e.g., intensive care unit and hospital beds, diagnostic tests, medical and surgical therapies) and lost opportunity as fewer patients can be cared for in the system. A single complication in a major surgery patient can cost many thousands of dollars, and by decreasing the incidence of such complications, GDT dramatically reduces cost. The mortality rate, hospital length of stay, and direct costs for patients with at least one complication versus those with no complications are shown in Table 19.1.

Monitoring for Goal-Directed Fluid Therapy

Various monitors have been used successfully in GDT, ranging from invasive (e.g., pulmonary artery catheter) to noninvasive (e.g., finger plethysmographic waveform). The data provided supplements standard monitoring (i.e., heart rate and blood pressure) with parameters tracking overall cardiac performance such as cardiac output and stroke volume (SV), or indexes of potential fluid responsiveness such as stroke volume variation (SVV), pulse pressure variation (PPV, arterial pulse-wave analysis systems), and corrected flow time (FTc, esophageal Doppler). Continuous monitoring of central venous oxygenation also has been used to assess adequacy of circulation. Assessment of tissue perfusion by means of gastric tonometry has been used in GDT, and attempts at evaluating tissue oxygenation (e.g., near-infrared spectroscopy) have been made as well.

Each monitoring system has strengths and weaknesses, and monitoring should be tailored to individual situations and institutional preference. Although the accuracy of minimally invasive cardiac output monitors such as arterial waveform systems and esophageal Doppler has been questioned, the ability of the systems to assess and trend cardiovascular performance appears to be adequate for perioperative GDT. In critically ill or unstable patients, invasive monitors such as pulmonary artery catheters and transesophageal echocardiography should be considered. Monitors used for GDT are presented in Table 19.2.

The most studied monitor for GDT is esophageal Doppler (CardioQ Deltex Medical). This system consists of a small probe placed in the esophagus that insonates the descending thoracic aorta. Estimation of the cross-sectional area of the aorta is made based on patient characteristics (e.g., age, height, gender, and weight) and the area under the velocity time is calculated, with the terms velocity time integral (VTI) and

Table 19.2	Monitors for Goal-Directed Fluid Therapy (GDT)				
Invasiveness	Technology	Device	Parameters for GDT	Strengths	Weaknesses
Invasive	Thermodilution, CO, pulmonary artery and central pressure	Pulmonary artery catheter	CO	Clinical gold standard CO measurement; vast amount of potentially useful data, including RV function	Invasive, requires central venous access
	Transpulmonary thermodilution	PiCCO (Pulsion Medical Systems) central arterial catheter	Pulmonary artery and central venous pressure	Vast amount of potentially useful data, including thoracic blood volume and extravascular lung water	Invasive; requires central arterial access
	Fiberoptic oximetry	Precep Catheter (Edwards Lifesciences)	Mixed venous and venous oxygen saturation	Assessment of global oxygen balance and extraction ratio	No direct information about cardiac performance or fluid responsiveness

Minimally invasive	Doppler flow measurement, descending aorta	CardioQ (Deltex Medical)	CO	Most common monitor successfully used for GDT	Requires skill (placement)
			Corrected flow time (preload, afterload), peak velocity	Newer systems incorporate arterial pressure wave	Inaccurate in aortic crossclamping, aortic aneurysm, aortic regurgitation
	Pressure wave pulsatility	Vigileo/FloTrac (Edwards Lifesciences)	CO, SVV (fluid responsiveness)	Easy to use SVV is a powerful parameter combined with CO	Inaccurate in aortic crossclamping, aortic regurgitation, cirrhosis, and sepsis
Noninvasive	Finger cuff	Clearsight (Edwards Lifesciences)	CO, SVV (fluid responsiveness)	Noninvasive	Potential accuracy issues; relatively unstudied in GDT
	Finger plethysmography	Pulse oximetry (Masimo)	Waveform variation, pleth variability index	Noninvasive	Potential accuracy issues; relatively unstudied in GDT; no CO data
	Thoracic electrical impedance, bioreactance, velocimetry	NICOM (Cheetah Medical), ICON (Cardiotronics)	CO	Noninvasive	Potential accuracy issues; relatively unstudied in GDT

CO, Cardiac output; RV, right ventricular; SVV, stroke volume variation.

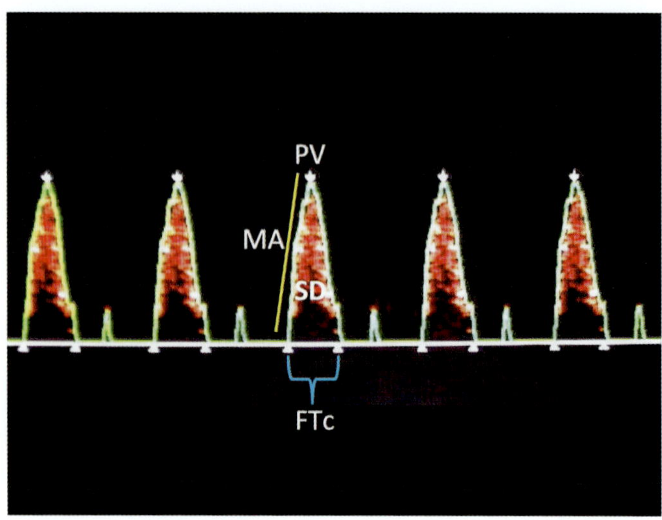

Fig. 19.4 Esophageal Doppler velocity-time waveform. *FTc,* Corrected flow time; *MA,* mean acceleration; *PV,* peak velocity; *SD,* stroke distance.

stroke distance (SD) used interchangeably. SD is multiplied by the aortic cross-sectional area to obtain SV:

$$SV = SD \times Aortic\ cross\text{-}sectional\ area \qquad \textbf{Eq 1}$$

Because of its common use and its track record of utility in GDT, a number of algorithms have been developed for use with esophageal Doppler. These may use SV and FTc for volume responsiveness and afterload. Other potentially useful parameters include peak velocity and mean acceleration (contractility assessment) (Fig. 19.4). Experienced users are able to recognize waveform changes that reflect changes in hemodynamics (Fig. 19.5). Newer esophageal Doppler systems can incorporate arterial pressure waveform analysis when an arterial catheter is used, allowing the added assessment of SVV and PPV. Proper placement and use of the esophageal Doppler require practice, particularly in optimizing the velocity-time waveform. About 15 practice sessions are required to gain facility.

The FloTrac/Vigileo system is the most commonly used arterial pressure–based system used for GDT. An arterial catheter is required, and the arterial wave is digitized by a proprietary transducer. The SV is determined by the pulsatility of the wave (standard deviation of the arterial wave), and a resistance-compliance factor, K, is calculated using patient characteristics and characteristics of the waveform:

$$SV = K \times Pulsatility \qquad \textbf{Eq 2}$$

A list of potential monitors for GDT is presented in Table 19.2.

Noninvasive cardiac output monitoring systems are available that use pressure waveform analysis from either the finger or the wrist. They are very promising in concept because they do not involve intravascular catheters or esophageal probes. Electrical impedance and cardiometry devices are available as well. Their use for GDT has yet to be firmly established, but it is likely that they will undergo further development, becoming valuable tools.

In certain situations, particularly in critically ill patients, minimally invasive systems are inadequate to provide the detailed information that invasive ones such as pulmonary artery catheterization with thermodilution, transpulmonary thermodilution, and

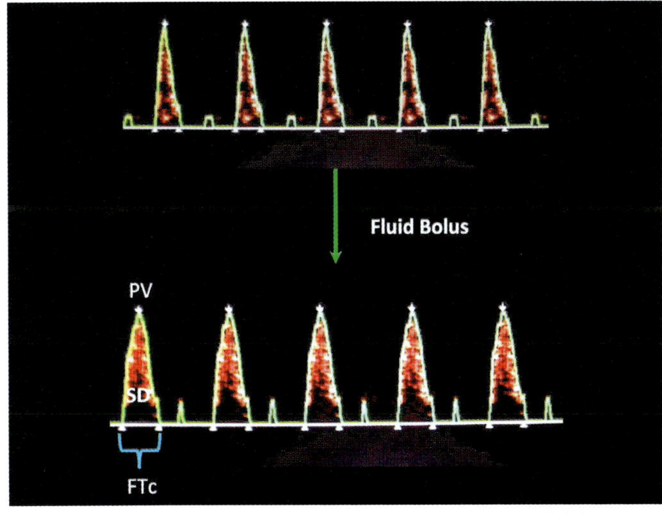

Fig. 19.5 Visual waveform inspection reveals a positive response to a fluid bolus, with increases in peak velocity (PV), corrected flow time (FTc), and stroke distance (SD).

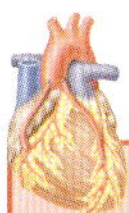

BOX 19.1	***High-Risk Surgeries in Which Goal-Directed Fluid Therapy Is Recommended***

- Exploratory laparotomy
- Large bowel resection, colectomy
- Whipple pancreato-duodenectomy
- Hepatectomy
- Splenectomy
- Kidney transplant
- Radical neck dissection
- Aortofemoral, popliteal, or axillary bypass
- Open hysterectomy, total abdominal or bilateral salpingo-oophorectomy
- Hyperthermic or interperitoneal chemotherapy
- Laminectomy fusion with instrumentation (more than three levels)
- Arthroplasty of the hip, knee, or elbow
- Burn excision
- Cystoprostatectomy with ileal conduit
- Radical cystectomy

transesophageal echocardiography can provide. These advanced monitors provide the necessary information for GDT and allow for complex hemodynamic and cardiac problem solving as well.

Patient Selection for Goal-Directed Fluid Therapy

Goal-directed fluid therapy is recommended for major procedures in which substantial blood loss or fluid shifts are anticipated (Box 19.1). These may include major general, vascular, urologic, or orthopedic surgery (e.g., pancreatectomy, open colectomy, radical cystectomy). Major patient comorbidities such as cardiac disease or a debilitated state should prompt the use of GDT as well. Many patients with cardiac disease are sensitive to fluid administration (e.g., patients with diastolic dysfunction), so use of specific guidelines for fluid administration that are based on physiologic parameters is beneficial for them. GDT has been studied in cardiac surgery with some positive results. Cardiac anesthesiologists and surgeons apply goals, hemodynamic monitoring, and interventions in managing their patients perioperatively. However, GDT, as discussed here, has not been widely adopted in cardiac surgery.

Algorithms in Goal-Directed Fluid Therapy

Numerous algorithms have been used successfully in GDT, with application of SV and preload responsiveness parameters such as PPV, SVV, and FTc. An algorithm based solely on the patient's SV response to fluid bolus is attractive because of its simplicity (Fig. 19.6), but it can be associated with fluid overload. Algorithms based solely on SVV have been used, but application of SVV as a primary parameter are limited to patients without significant arrhythmias receiving controlled positive-pressure ventilation. Likewise, Doppler FTc has been used as a preload responsiveness parameter. A synthesis of the above approaches, with use of blood pressure as an additional parameter to facilitate hemodynamic problem solving is available (Fig. 19.7).

A physiologic approach to GDT and hemodynamic problem solving can be achieved using a four-quadrant plot of blood flow (*x*-axis) versus blood pressure (*y*-axis), with chosen target hemodynamics in the center of the plot. Deviations from the target

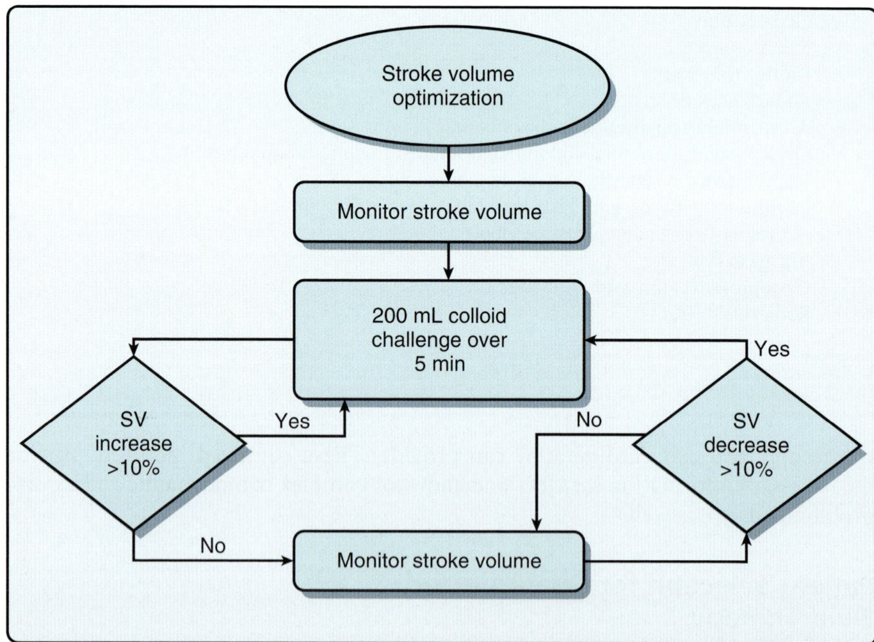

Fig. 19.6 A simple goal-directed fluid therapy algorithm based on responses to fluid bolus. *SV,* Stroke volume.

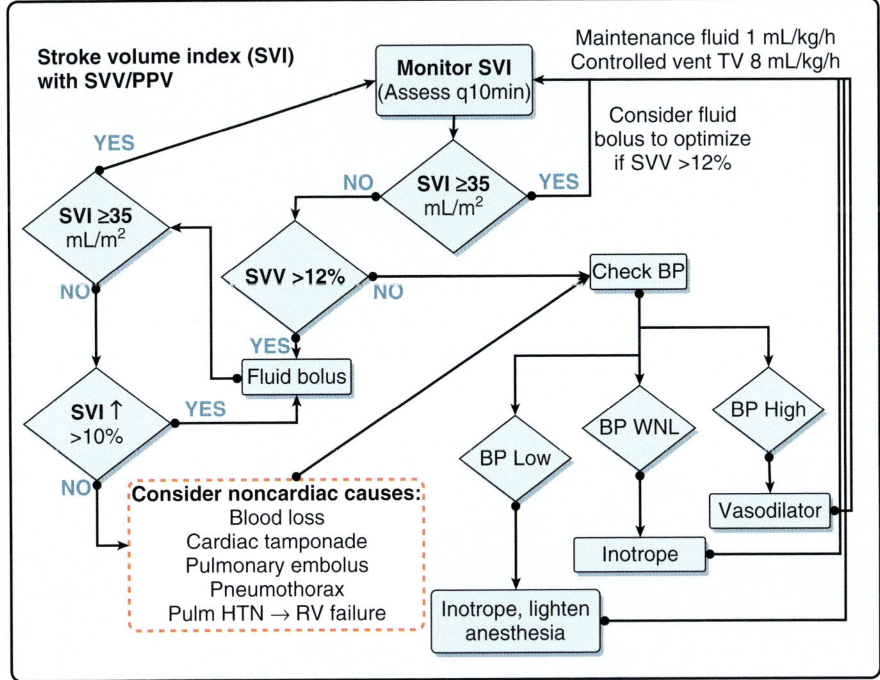

Fig. 19.7 Goal-directed fluid therapy algorithm used at the University of California, San Diego. Stroke volume index (SVI) is the primary parameter, and the values of the targets can be adjusted according to clinical circumstances. Corrected flow time (FTc) can be substituted for stroke volume variation (SVV) for esophageal Doppler use, and an algorithm for use when SVV or FTc cannot be applied is available as well. *BP,* Blood pressure; *HTN,* hypertension; *PPV,* pulse pressure variation; *Pulm,* pulmonary; *RV,* right ventricular; *TV,* tidal volume; *Vent,* ventilation; *WNL,* within normal limits.

zone, depending on the quadrant, are associated with a differential diagnosis and recommended management. This approach facilitates understanding of the hemodynamics, leading to accurate, prompt diagnosis and management (Fig. 19.8).

Most important, using a logical, physiologically based algorithm in a thoughtful way results in improved outcomes. The choice of algorithm depends on the monitors available, the clinical situation, and institutional preferences. Using a systematic approach to fluid and hemodynamic management with particular emphasis on avoiding fluid and salt overload results in improved outcome and with enhanced recovery for patients undergoing major noncardiac surgery (Box 19.2).

ENHANCED RECOVERY

Enhanced recovery after surgery programs have gained acceptance as a multifactorial, evidence-driven multidisciplinary way of managing patients undergoing surgery. The main goal of these programs is to facilitate rapid, complete, comfortable recovery after procedures by minimizing physiologic perturbations and stress response. Care pathways for a variety of surgeries, primarily general and orthopedic, have been shown to achieve this goal, and emphasis is placed on minimizing the invasiveness of the surgery (e.g., laparoscopic, small incision). ERPs not only decrease complications

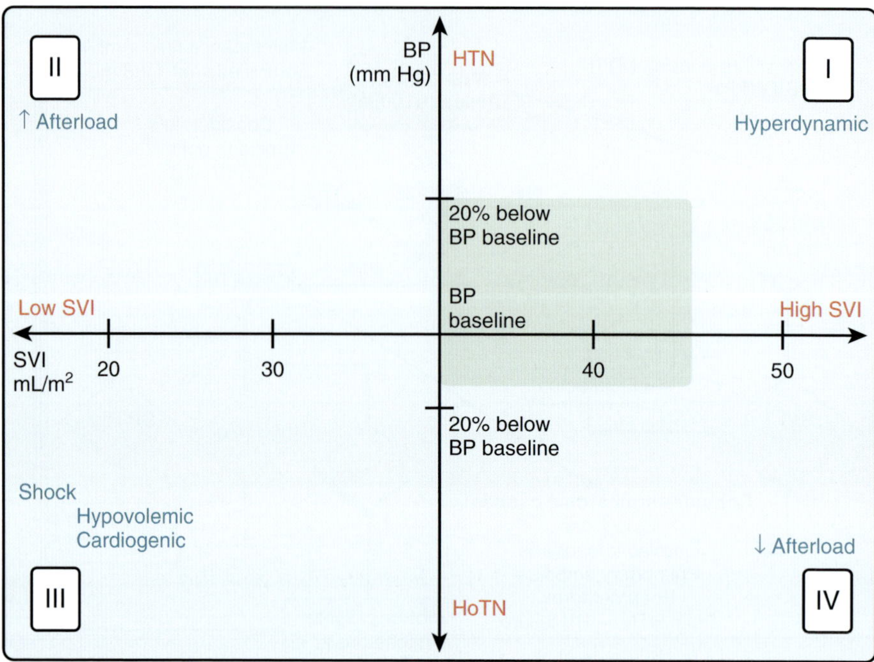

Fig. 19.8 A four-quadrant plot can be created by plotting the stroke volume index (SVI) on the *x*-axis and mean arterial pressure on the *y*-axis. A target zone *(green)* can be created, and deviations from the target zone are associated with hemodynamic aberrations specific to each quadrant. Point-of-care guidance for each quadrant can be provided. *BP,* Blood pressure; *HoTN,* hypotension; *HTN,* hypertension.

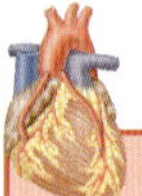

BOX 19.2   *Goal-Directed Fluid Therapy*

- Standardizes fluid and hemodynamic management
- Aims to avoid fluid and salt overload while avoiding hypovolemia
- Is based on parameters beyond heart rate and blood pressure, such as
  - Minimally invasive or invasive cardiac output
  - Stroke volume variation
  - Pulse pressure variation
  - Doppler-corrected flow time
  - Central venous oxygen saturation

Many algorithms have been used successfully. The algorithm should have physiologic basis and be easy to use.

---

but also facilitate return to baseline function even in the absence of complications. The main components of ERP programs are careful preoperative optimization; optimization of intraoperative management, particularly with regard to fluid and temperature management; multimodal opiate-sparing pain management; and early mobilization (see Fig. 19.2 and Box 19.3).

Enhanced recovery programs preoperative fasting guidelines call for fasting periods of 2 hours for clear liquids, 6 hours for a light meal, and a preoperative carbohydrate

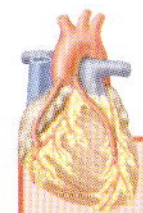

drink shortly before surgery. These guidelines, along with reduced bowel preparation, result in improved volume and metabolic status at the time of surgery.

There is accumulating, strong evidence that ERPs decrease complication rates and the length of hospital stay. Enhanced recovery quality improvement projects at institutional and national levels are now common, with the National Health Service Enhanced Recovery Partnership in the United Kingdom being an example.

PERIOPERATIVE ACUTE PAIN MANAGEMENT

Although associated with many disadvantages, in many centers, opioid analgesics remain the mainstay treatment of postoperative pain. Adverse effects of opiates can be both distressing and dangerous, including pruritus, constipation, nausea and vomiting, urinary retention, oversedation, and respiratory depression. Likewise, high intraoperative doses of opioids are associated with hyperalgesia and significant increases in acute pain postoperatively. Furthermore, opioids are now responsible for more deaths than the number of deaths from both suicide and motor vehicle crashes or deaths from cocaine and heroin combined. These adverse effects, along with the magnitude of the opioid crisis in the United States, have led to a greater emphasis on developing strategies for multimodal analgesic regimens.

The use of multimodal analgesia limits the amount of opioids consumed and provides more effective pain control than opioids alone. Practice guidelines for perioperative pain management recommend that multimodal therapy should be standard of care and used in all postsurgical patients (American Society of Anesthesiologists [ASA] Task Force). Multimodal regimens may include combinations of nonopioid adjuvant analgesic drugs, peripheral nerve blocks, and neuraxial anesthesia with opiate availability as back-up.

Pharmacologic Opioid-Sparing Analgesics

Pregabalin

The use of gabapentinoids as adjuvants perioperatively for acute pain management has gained vast attention recently for its opioid-sparing effects. Pregabalin is an anticonvulsant agent that improves postoperative analgesia in comparison with placebo, with a 25% opioid-sparing rate at 24 hours. The optimal dose or frequency in this setting remains unclear, varying from 75 to 300 mg orally preoperatively, with no difference in acute pain outcomes between single and multiple dosing. Side effects may include increased sedation and visual disturbances.

Intravenous Lidocaine

Although lidocaine is most commonly used for local anesthesia infiltration and peripheral nerve blocks, systemic administration has analgesic effects. A recent meta-analysis of perioperative intravenous (IV) lidocaine infusions, during and after abdominal surgery, has shown decreases in ileus duration, pain, nausea and vomiting, and length of hospital stay. Likewise, for patients undergoing outpatient laparoscopic procedures, IV lidocaine results in less opioid consumption and thus improved quality of recovery. The efficacy of IV lidocaine for nonabdominal surgery has yet to be demonstrated.

Nonsteroidal Antiinflammatory Drugs

Nonsteroidal antiinflammatory drugs (NSAIDs) play an important role in multimodal analgesia. Besides their antiinflammatory properties, NSAIDs reduce opioid consumption and decrease nausea and vomiting. Preoperative administration of cyclooxygenase II NSAIDs (coxibs) is frequently encountered on ERPs. Despite positive results, use of NSAIDs continues to be limited by concerns over perioperative bleeding, anastomotic leaks in colorectal surgery, and renal toxicity. Although ketorolac is often administered intravenously in the postoperative period as an adjuvant therapy, it is limited by its duration of use (5 days).

Acetaminophen

Acetaminophen is a well-known peripherally and centrally acting analgesic with antipyretic properties. With a minimal adverse effects profile, few contraindications, and recent IV availability, acetaminophen has become an integral part of multimodal acute pain management regimens. Recommended dosing for adults weighing more than 50 kg is not to exceed 4000 mg/day to minimize the risk of hepatic toxicity.

Ketamine Infusion

Ketamine is an N-methyl-D-aspartate receptor antagonist most commonly known for its dissociative anesthetic properties and used in the treatment of refractory pain in patients with cancer or depression and in acute pain management. Given that its mechanism of action differs from opioids, ketamine is considered a useful adjuvant in multimodal therapy. Ketamine exhibits its analgesic properties in subanesthetic doses at 0.2 to 0.5 mg/kg per hour intravenously. Psychomimetic side effects (e.g., hallucinations, vivid dreams, dysphoria) occasionally limit its use. Nausea and vomiting, dizziness, and diplopia may occur as well. Low-dose benzodiazepines may be used to control dysphoria, and haloperidol is often given to manage any associated hallucinations or delirium.

Dexamethasone

Glucocorticoids are often administered for their antiinflammatory benefits and are frequently administered intraoperatively for the prophylactic prevention of nausea and vomiting. A small single dose of dexamethasone intraoperatively is recommended as part of a multimodal opioid-sparing regimen. The most notable side effect of dexamethasone is hyperglycemia.

Dexmedetomidine

Dexmedetomidine is an α_2-agonist with sedative and analgesic properties. Minimal impact on respiratory function is one of its unique attributes, although cardiovascular side effects such as bradycardia and hypotension may limit its usage. Studies of perioperative administration have shown decreased postoperative pain, opioid requirement, and incidence of nausea. Typical dosing for dexmedetomidine is a 0.5 μg/kg IV bolus followed by 0.2 to 0.7 μg/kg per hour infusion.

Nonpharmacologic Opioid-Sparing Analgesics

Thoracic Epidural Analgesia

Thoracic epidural analgesia (TEA), by providing profound analgesia, plays an important role for patients undergoing open abdominal and thoracic procedures. TEA reduces postoperative ileus duration after major abdominal surgery by an average of 36 hours. The mechanism by which TEA shortens the duration of ileus may include decreases in sympathetic tone, stress response inflammatory processes, and systemic opiate administration. Epidural analgesia provides superior postoperative analgesia, decreased perioperative pulmonary-cardiac morbidity, and earlier return of gastrointestinal tract function compared with systemic analgesia.

Transversus Abdominis Plane Block

The transversus abdominis plane (TAP) block has also gained momentum as part of a multimodal approach to enhanced recovery, especially in patients undergoing minimally invasive abdominal surgery and for those who are not epidural candidates. TAP blocks have the advantages of being relatively safe and simple and providing reduced postoperative opioid consumption as well as decreased nausea and vomiting. Superior analgesia is most notable with pain at rest and less so with pain with movement. Likewise, preoperative administration of a TAP block, compared with postoperative, may be efficacious.

PERIOPERATIVE SURGICAL HOME

The PSH is an organizational umbrella under which ERPs may function. Emphasizing the continuum that is required in ERPs and seamless care before, during, and after surgery, PSHs are now being formed as part of quality improvement and cost containment strategies. PSH has the strong backing and support of national organizations such as the ASA. Challenges in creating PSHs include the complexity of the perioperative care, communication and coordination among many team members, and institutional resistance to change. It is likely that anesthesiologists, with their wide scope of influence and organizational skills, will enhance their value to their health systems by increasing their involvement in the implementation and management of ERPs and PSHs (Box 19.4).

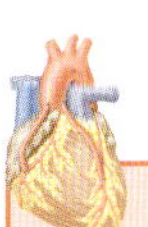

BOX 19.4   *Perioperative Surgical Home Requirements*

- Multidisciplinary, coordinated effort
- Team leader
- Understanding and navigation of organizational complexities and politics
- Understanding the surgical and medical aspects of care
- Integration of enhanced recovery pathways
- Maintenance and close quality monitoring

SUGGESTED READING

Arkin DB, Saidman LJ, Benumof JL. Hypotension following cardiopulmonary bypass. *Anesth Analg.* 1977;56:720–724.

Bell RF, et al. Peri-operative ketamine for acute post-operative pain: a quantitative and qualitative systematic review (Cochrane review). *Acta Anaesthesiol Scand.* 2005;49(10):1405–1428.

Bellamy MC. Wet, dry or something else? *Br J Anaesth.* 2006;97:755–757.

Blaudszun G, Lysakowski C, Elia N, Tramer N. Effect of perioperative systemic α2 agonists on postoperative morphine consumption and pain intensity: systematic review and meta-analysis of randomized controlled trials. *Anesthesiology.* 2012;116(6):1312–1322.

Chappell D, Jacob M, Hofmann-Kiefer K, Conzen P, Rehm M. A rational approach to perioperative fluid management. *Anesthesiology.* 2008;109:723–740.

Corcoran T, Rhodes JE, Clarke S, Myles PS, Ho KM. Perioperative fluid management strategies in major surgery: a stratified meta-analysis. *Anesth Analg.* 2012;114:640–651.

De Oliveira GS Jr, Castro-Alves LJ, Nader A, Kendall MC, McCarthy RJ. Transversus abdominis plane block to ameliorate postoperative pain outcomes after laparoscopic surgery: a meta-analysis of randomized controlled trials. *Anesth Analg.* 2014;118:454–463.

Gan TJ, Soppitt A, Maroof M, et al. Goal-directed intraoperative fluid administration reduces length of hospital stay after major surgery. *Anesthesiology.* 2002;97:820–826.

Greco M, Capretti G, Beretta L, et al. Enhanced recovery program in colorectal surgery: a meta-analysis of randomized controlled trials. *World J Surg.* 2014;38:1531–1541.

Hamilton MA, Cecconi M, Rhodes A. A systematic review and meta-analysis on the use of preemptive hemodynamic intervention to improve postoperative outcomes in moderate and high-risk surgical patients. *Anesth Analg.* 2011;112:1392–1402.

Johns N, O'Neill S, Ventham NT, et al. Clinical effectiveness of transversus abdominis plane (TAP) block in abdominal surgery: a systematic review and meta-analysis. *Colorectal Dis.* 2012;14(10):e635–e642.

Jørgensen H, Wetterslev J, Møiniche S, Dahl JB. Epidural local anaesthetics versus opioid-based analgesic regimens on postoperative gastrointestinal paralysis, PONV and pain after abdominal surgery. *Cochrane Database Syst Rev.* 2000;(4):CD001893.

Kain ZN, Vakharia S, Garson L, et al. The perioperative surgical home as a future perioperative practice model. *Anesth Analg.* 2014;118:1126–1130.

Macario A, Royal MA. A literature review of randomized clinical trials of intravenous acetaminophen (paracetamol) for acute postoperative pain. *Pain Pract.* 2011;11:290–296.

Manecke GR, Asemota A, Michard F. Tackling the economic burden of postsurgical complications: would perioperative goal-directed fluid therapy help? *Crit Care.* 2014;18:566.

Mythen MG, Webb AR. Perioperative plasma volume expansion reduces the incidence of gut mucosal hypoperfusion during cardiac surgery. *Arch Surg.* 1995;130:423–429.

NHS Enhanced Recovery Care Pathway. National Health Service, 2015. Available at http://www.nhsiq.nhs.uk/8846.aspx.

Nisanevich V, Felsenstein I, Almogy G, et al. Effect of intraoperative fluid management on outcome after intraabdominal surgery. *Anesthesiology.* 2005;103:25–32.

Pearse R, Dawson D, Fawcett J, et al. Early goal-directed therapy after major surgery reduces complications and duration of hospital stay. A randomised, controlled trial [ISRCTN38797445]. *Crit Care.* 2005;9:R687–R693.

Pearse RM, Harrison DA, MacDonald N, et al. Effect of a perioperative, cardiac output-guided hemodynamic therapy algorithm on outcomes following major gastrointestinal surgery: a randomized clinical trial and systematic review. *JAMA.* 2014;311:2181–2190.

Pronovost PJ, Armstrong CM, Demski R, et al. Creating a high-reliability health care system: improving performance on core processes of care at Johns Hopkins Medicine. *Acad Med.* 2015;90:165–172.

Rivers E, Nguyen B, Havstad S, et al. Early goal-directed therapy in the treatment of severe sepsis and septic shock. *N Engl J Med.* 2001;345:1368–1377.

Waldron HA, Jones CA, Gan TJ, Habib AS. Impact of perioperative dexamethasone on postoperative analgesia and side-effects: systematic review and meta-analysis. *Br J Anaesth.* 2013;110(2):191–200.

Section III
Critical Care Medicine

Chapter 20

Management in the Postanesthesia Care Unit of Complications in Cardiac Patients

Albert P. Nguyen, MD • E. Orestes O'Brien, MD •
Ulrich H. Schmidt, MD, PhD, MBA

Key Points

1. The postanesthesia care unit (PACU) is a specialized unit designed to monitor for early postanesthesia and surgical adverse events.
2. Early cardiac decline after noncardiac surgery requires prompt evaluation, early intervention, and cardiologist consultation for advanced care.
3. Neurohormonal changes and sympathetic nervous system activation can impair cardiac function in patients with cardiac disease.
4. Anesthetic management can be used to suppress adverse effects related to surgical trauma.
5. Fluid resuscitation, medication administration, and underlying comorbidity are areas of consideration for the source of respiratory distress in PACU patients.
6. Whereas neuromuscular blockade reversal with neostigmine and glycopyrrolate has unpredictable effects on blood pressure and heart rate, sugammadex has no adverse hemodynamic effects.
7. Postsurgical hemorrhage may have a subtle presentation, requiring high clinical suspicion and frequent patient evaluation.
8. Thromboelastography is a rapid point-of-care device that is used in the measurement of hemostasis.
9. Direct oral anticoagulants are new medications with more predictable therapeutic effects compared to warfarin and have new reversal agents.

The postanesthesia care unit (PACU) traces its origin back to 1942 at the Mayo Clinic. This specialized unit is usually managed by the department of anesthesiology. During its daily operation, a designated anesthesiologist has the responsibility for making final medical decisions in the unit. PACU nurses have training in airway and basic life support management, as well as skill in the care of surgical wounds and drainage systems. The purpose of the PACU is to provide dedicated, centralized monitoring and nursing care to patients immediately after their operations before transferring them to a ward or intensive care unit (ICU) bed. A 1:1 patient-to-nurse ratio is required during the initial 15 minutes of a patient's arrival to the PACU. During this crucial period, the patient has the highest risk for anesthesia-related complications.

Table 20.1 Modified Aldrete Scoring System for Postanesthesia Care Unit Discharge[a]

Discharge Criteria	Score
Activity: Ability to Move to Command or Spontaneously	
Four-extremity movement	2
Two-extremity movement	1
Zero-extremity movement	0
Respiration	
Able to deeply breathe or spontaneously cough	2
Dyspnea, shallow breathing, or limited breathing	1
Apnea	0
Circulation	
Blood pressure ± 20 mm Hg of baseline	2
Blood pressure ± 20–50 mm Hg of baseline	1
Blood pressure ± 50 mm Hg of baseline	0
Consciousness	
Fully awake	2
Arousal to sound or stimulation	1
Nonresponsive	0
Oxygen Saturation	
Maintains SpO_2 >92% on room air	2
Requires supplemental O_2 to keep SpO_2 >90%	1
O_2 saturation <90% despite supplemental O_2	0

[a]A score of ≥9 is required for postanesthesia care unit discharge.

Discharge from the PACU to an ICU or ward is based on the modified Aldrete scoring system, a checklist in which a score of greater than 9 is required to transfer the patient (Table 20.1).

Every patient admitted to the PACU requires an assessment for pain, airway patency, respiratory rate, oxygen saturation, heart rate and rhythm, and blood pressure. Depending on the severity of the patient's condition, these vital signs are recorded every 5 minutes for the first 15 minutes and liberalized to every 15 minutes if the patient's condition is favorable. The PACU is capable of providing more in-depth care if the patient's condition warrants it. Arterial blood pressure monitoring with pulse-wave contour analysis can be performed to manage the causes of hemodynamic instability. Pulmonary artery pressure monitoring and transthoracic echocardiography can be performed at the bedside to assess volume status and cardiac function. Essentially, the PACU environment is capable of providing the highest level of care to meet the patient's changing condition.

Postanesthesia care of patients with cardiac diseases is a complex and important topic that does not get the attention it deserves. Many patients with significant cardiac disease present for surgical procedures other than cardiac surgery. The type of operation and perioperative management influence the likelihood of postoperative cardiac complications in those with preexisting cardiac comorbidities. It is estimated that cardiac complications, such as myocardial infarctions (MIs) and cardiac arrests, can occur in up to 5% of patients undergoing noncardiac or nonvascular surgeries and up to 8% in vascular operations. The objective of this chapter is to address the common postoperative complications, their diagnoses, and management.

SURGERY, ANESTHESIA, AND THE HEART

The intention of surgery is often to alleviate suffering, but its very process induces trauma. This controlled injury induces an inflammatory and stress response in the patient and leads to sympathetic nervous system activation, both of which may be detrimental to the patient with preexisting cardiac disease. The inflammatory process is driven by cytokines, including interleukin (IL)-1, IL-6, and tumor necrosis factor-α (TNF-α), which are released from activated macrophages after injury. During the acute phase of inflammation, there are increases in vascular dilation and permeability that are mediated by the release of histamine, serotonin, prostaglandin E_2, leukotriene B4, and nitric oxide. This increased permeability allows for migration of plasma fluid that contains factors responsible for immunity, wound healing, and clotting. Depending on the severity of the inflammatory response, relative hypovolemia and hypotension can occur during and after surgery, with attendant risks to the patient.

During surgical stress, the neuroendocrine process is responsible for mediating volume and electrolyte balance. The posterior pituitary releases the hormone arginine vasopressin, which acts on the AVPR2 receptors in the kidneys, resulting in a rise in permeability at the distal collecting tubules and collecting ducts, allowing for increased water reabsorption and concentrated urine. Renin secretion results in aldosterone release, which enhances sodium and water reuptake in the distal collecting tubules. Together these neuroendocrine processes result in increased fluid retention and potentially increased circulating volume.

In addition to hormonal stimulation, the sympathetic autonomic nervous system is activated. The hypothalamus is responsible for stimulating catecholamine release from the adrenal medulla and presynaptic nerve terminals. The sympathetic effects of the released epinephrine and norepinephrine result in hypertension and tachycardia. The culmination of the inflammatory and sympathetic responses to stress leads to variations in hemodynamic and cardiac function (e.g., hypotension, hypertension, and tachycardia). In patients with cardiac disease, an unregulated response can precipitate myocardial ischemia or infarction, which often is first diagnosed in the PACU.

Inherent to surgery is the risk of blood loss, and to compensate for acute blood loss, the body has developed several adaptations. The systemic vascular resistance increases to maintain an appropriate mean arterial perfusion pressure, but this increase in afterload may come at the cost of decreased stroke volume and cardiac output in cardiac patients with poor left ventricular function. Blood flow is redistributed unequally, preferentially favoring high oxygen-extracting organs such as the heart and brain. During periods of anemia, the coronary arteries can increase their blood flow up to five times normal flow. Patients with heart disease, however, may not be capable of such compensation and may develop ischemia from oxygen deficit. Anemia caused by acute blood loss does not cause an immediate rightward shift of the oxygen dissociation curve (e.g., unloading of oxygen from hemoglobin). To decrease oxygen's affinity for hemoglobin, it takes upwards of 12 hours for 2,3-DPG to be synthesized and produce a rightward shift of the curve. The decision to transfuse a patient should not be based solely on the value of the hemoglobin. A holistic view of the cardiac patient's condition including ongoing blood loss, end-organ dysfunction, and increases in oxygen demand should guide the need to transfuse.

POSTANESTHESIA CARDIAC COMPLICATIONS IN CARDIAC PATIENTS

Acute Coronary Syndrome

In patients with preexisting coronary artery disease (CAD), the narrowing of the coronary arteries is most commonly the result of atherosclerotic plaques. The size of the arterial occlusion will reduce the maximal flow of coronary blood to meet oxygen demand. When coronary oxygen demand outstrips oxygen delivery, angina pain can arise, and myocardial necrosis begins to occur. The postoperative period is a particularly dangerous time for patients with CAD because oxygen consumption can increase up to 50% from baseline, and the incidence of MI is as high as 5%.

Acute coronary syndrome is the term used to describe an acute reduction in coronary perfusion that results in cardiac impairment. The events that define this syndrome are unstable angina (UA)/non–ST segment elevation myocardial infarction (NSTEMI), and ST-segment elevation myocardial infarction (STEMI).

Unstable Angina/Non–ST Segment Elevation Myocardial Infarction

The development of UA/NSTEMI in the perioperative period is a result of multiple factors: a nonocclusive thrombus can form from plaque rupture, hypothermia can trigger coronary vasospasm that leads to impaired coronary blood flow, and myocardial ischemia can be precipitated from tachycardia as a result of pain, anemia, hypovolemia, and fever. The diagnosis of UA/NSTEMI is based on patient complaints, electrocardiography (ECG), and cardiac biomarkers. Patients presenting with UA/NSTEMI in the PACU may complain of substernal chest pain or pressure, with radiation to the jaw or arm or may have only subtle complaints, including midepigastric discomfort. What differentiates these symptoms from stable angina is that these symptoms occur spontaneously and are unprovoked, and there is an increase in frequency and severity. The 12-lead ECG is a critical diagnostic tool in this scenario. A finding of a prominent R wave with ST-segment depression of more than 0.5 mm or a T-wave inversion measuring greater than 1 mm in two contiguous leads is suggestive of UA/NSTEMI. The presence of cardiac biomarkers further differentiates angina pain caused by NSTEMI from UA. The creatine kinase-MB (CK-MB) has been a traditional biomarker for myocardial necrosis. It is, however, less sensitive than cardiac troponins because low levels of CK-MB have been detected in healthy humans and are also released when skeletal muscles are damaged. The troponin T and troponin I are specific to cardiac muscle. A rise in either troponin T or troponin I can be detected as early as 2 hours after the onset of symptoms or change in the ECG. Unlike CK-MB, the troponin levels can remain elevated for up to 14 days.

The medical treatment for UA/NSTEMI in the PACU is targeted toward the causes of increased oxygen demand. Supplemental oxygen should be administered to increase available systemic oxygenation. Shivering, which can increase total body oxygen consumption by up to 400%, should be treated with meperidine, if not contraindicated, along with surface-warming devices. Aggressive analgesic regimens should be used to treat acute postsurgical pain–induced hypertension and tachycardia. Acute blood loss and hypovolemia-induced ischemia should be treated with blood product administration and judicious fluid resuscitation. Stress-mediated tachycardia not caused by hypovolemia can be treated with β-blockade that allows for increased coronary perfusion time. Sublingual or intravenous (IV) nitroglycerin has been used for coronary vasodilation and to improve blood flow and relieve angina. Care should be taken in reducing systemic afterload and coronary perfusion pressure when administering nitrates. In addition, antiplatelet and anticoagulation therapy is aimed at preventing further coronary thrombus formation and can be used if surgical bleeding is not a concern. Aspirin is a first-line antiplatelet therapy in the treatment of UA/NSTEMI and can be started immediately. Clopidogrel is an alternative agent if patients are unable to tolerate aspirin therapy. Immediate dual-antiplatelet therapy with aspirin and clopidogrel or aspirin and ticagrelor is warranted if an invasive coronary intervention is planned. The American Heart Association/American College of Cardiology also recommends including anticoagulation therapy for the first 48 hours of symptom manifestation. Enoxaparin and unfractionated heparin are the first-line agents recommended, but fondaparinux is preferred for patients with increased risk of bleeding. Thrombolytics are contraindicated in the treatment of UA/NSTEMI because they have been associated with increased mortality rates. The administration of anticoagulation must be done with caution, being aware of the risks of anticoagulation in the setting of recent surgery, particularly in closed spaces (e.g., intraocular surgery). Multidisciplinary efforts including anesthesiology, cardiology, and surgery are essential for successful management (see Chapter 22).

Changes in the ECG tracing and positive cardiac biomarkers warrant cardiology consultation and close follow-up. Patients who are older than 65 years, present with prolonged chest pain, and have preexisting coronary stents, hemodynamic instability, or moderate renal insufficiency are considered to be at high risk for death. In these patients, there is benefit from early coronary angiography and intervention for obstructing lesions. In contrast, for lower risk patients, stress test evaluation in the form of an exercise stress test, radionucleotide myocardial perfusion scan, or pharmacologic stress test can be performed on a nonurgent basis. Coronary angiography in this group is done only if significant ischemia is seen during stress testing.

ST-Segment Elevation Myocardial Infarction

ST-segment elevation MI occurs when there is an abrupt cessation of coronary blood flow. The most common cause of an STEMI is lipid-rich atherosclerotic plaque rupture. This triggers the local release of serotonin, adenosine diphosphate, and epinephrine. These agents stimulate platelet aggregation and lead to coronary vessel obstruction. Coagulation factor activation forms fibrin-enhanced clots in the vessels that become resistant to thrombolysis. Thromboxane A_2 release further exacerbates MI through its powerful vasoconstricting properties. Less common causes of STEMI are severe coronary spasm, coronary arterial emboli, and coronary stent thrombosis.

The diagnosis of STEMI is based on the patient's physical symptoms, ECG changes, rise in cardiac biomarkers, and echocardiography. The physical symptoms that patients in PACUs may exhibit are severe unrelenting substernal chest pain, anxiety, diaphoresis, and pallor. New rales may be auscultated in the lung fields, as well as new cardiac murmurs. The biomarkers CK-MB, troponin I, and troponin T all rise within 3 hours of the onset of the STEMI. A perioperative MI usually produces a rise in troponin to more than five times the top normal value of the laboratory. The degree of troponin I and troponin T rise is correlated with the degree of myocardial injury. ST-segment elevation on the ECG is considered significant if the height of the ST segment after the J-point is greater than 0.2 mV in men or 0.15 mV in women in the anterior leads or greater than 0.1 mV in all other leads. The location of the ST-segment elevation on a 12-lead ECG is useful in determining the culprit lesion(s) (Table 20.2). Echocardiography also is helpful in the diagnosis of STEMI. Transthoracic echocardiography is capable of detecting regional wall motion abnormalities in acute MI, contractility dysfunction, and the presence of pericardial effusion.

The detection of STEMI requires immediate cardiology consultation for emergent coronary angiography and reestablishment of coronary blood flow. The immediate medical treatment is similar to the treatment of UA/NSTEMI. IV opioids should be

Table 20.2	STEMI Electrocardiogram Diagnosis Criteria[a]		
STEMI Type	**Affected Coronary**	**ST-Segment Elevation Leads**	**Reciprocal Leads**
Anterior	Left anterior descending	V_1–V_6	None
Posterior	Right circumflex	V_7, V_8, V_9	R in V_1–V_3, ST depression in V_1–V_3
Inferior	Right coronary	II, III, aVF	I, aVL
Lateral	Left circumflex	I, aVL, V_5, V_6	II, III, aVF
Septal	Left anterior descending: septal arterial branches	V_1–V_4, absent Q wave in V_5, V_6	None
Right ventricle	Right coronary	V_1, reversed V_4	I, aVL

[a]The most common type of ST segment elevation myocardial infarction (STEMI) is the inferior myocardial infarction (MI), with an incidence of 58%; the second most common is anterior MI, occurring 39% of the time.

used to treat angina pectoris and to reduce the sympathetic stress response that can increase myocardial oxygen demand. Dual-antiplatelet therapy with either aspirin and clopidogrel or aspirin and prasugrel is used to reduce thrombus formation, if not surgically contraindicated. In STEMI patients without evidence of cardiogenic shock, administration of β-blockers can reduce infarct size, suppress arrhythmias, and relieve chest pain from increased myocardial oxygen demand. Thrombolytic therapy with tenecteplase or tissue plasminogen activator is reserved for centers that lack immediate access to a coronary catheterization laboratory. It is recommended that therapy be initiated within 12 hours of the onset of symptoms. In immediate postsurgical patients, the risks of thrombolytic therapy should be strongly considered. Surgical site bleeding, gastrointestinal bleeding, and most devastating of all, intracranial hemorrhage can arise from this therapy.

Coronary angiography and percutaneous coronary intervention (PCI) should occur within 90 minutes of the diagnosis of STEMI. PCI with drug-eluting stents is indicated for patients presenting with two or fewer culprit lesions. Presently, some interventional cardiologists perform PCI on patients with left main CAD because the safety profile has been shown to be comparable to coronary artery bypass grafting (CABG). Patients in cardiogenic shock can be supported temporarily with percutaneous mechanical support. The intraaortic balloon pump (IABP) has been in use since the 1960s and is able to reduce myocardial oxygen demand by increasing coronary perfusion pressure, reducing arterial systemic afterload, and providing up to 0.5 L/min of cardiac output. The Abiomed Impella is a percutaneous ventricular assist device that is inserted retrograde through the femoral artery, traverses the aortic valve, and sits in the left ventricle (LV). A small axial pump pulls blood from the LV and expels up to 4 L/min of flow into the ascending aorta. For patients with biventricular failure after a STEMI, venoarterial extracorporeal membrane oxygenation (VA-ECMO) can be used to deliver 5 L/min of oxygenated blood. All of these devices can be inserted in the catheterization laboratory during coronary angiography and intervention.

In patients found to have three or more coronary arteries diseased, CABG has been found to be superior to PCI for long-term survival. Referral for emergent CABG can occur when coronary angioplasty has failed, coronary dissection occurs during percutaneous intervention, or MI-induced ventricular septal rupture or mitral

515

regurgitation and posterior wall MI are present. Although CABG has been shown to have superior long-term survival rates compared with PCI, emergent surgical revascularization has significantly higher mortality rates in the first week after surgery.

Acute Decompensated Heart Failure

Decompensated heart failure (HF) is defined as the heart's inability to deliver oxygenated blood to meet the body's metabolic needs. For patients in the PACU presenting with acute decompensated HF, the causes include volume overload, pressure overload, and acute contractility dysfunction. Increases in preload from fluid administration may precipitate HF symptoms (shortness of breath, hypoxemia, pulmonary congestion, peripheral edema, alteration in mental status, and end-organ dysfunction) from the inability of the LV to increase stroke volume caused by reduced myocardial contractility. Sympathetic stress responses from surgical pain lead to arterial vasoconstriction and result in an increase in afterload. The LV in patients with reduced myocardial contractility is unable to overcome the high resistance, leading to a reduction in stroke volume and symptoms of acute HF. The causes of new-onset contractility failure can be the result of MI and cardiac valve impairment.

The diagnosis of acute HF can be made by presenting symptoms, biochemical findings, and imaging studies. A PACU patient with acute-onset HF may complain of dyspnea or orthopnea and require an increase in supplemental oxygen. Physical findings are notable for rales on pulmonary auscultation, presence of jugular venous distention, and cold and clammy extremities from decreased perfusion. The biomarkers B-type natriuretic peptide (BNP) and N-terminal fragment pro-BNP (NT-proBNP) are used in the diagnosis of HF because values of 500 pg/mL or greater and 300 pg/mL or greater, respectively, have a 90% positive predictive value. Obtaining a complete metabolic panel is helpful in assessing liver and renal dysfunction from venous congestion and poor perfusion. In addition, the laboratory findings are helpful in the identification of electrolyte abnormalities such as hyponatremia and hypokalemia. Transthoracic echocardiography is a powerful imaging tool that provides real-time information both visually and numerically of the heart's chamber size, thickness, and systolic and diastolic function, as well as the presence of any structural abnormality. This information can provide a diagnosis as well as guide therapy. Chest radiography may demonstrate pulmonary venous congestion, interstitial edema, and cardiomegaly. It should be noted, however, that these findings may not manifest while the patient is in the PACU. Radiographic findings generally are delayed by up to 12 hours from the onset of clinical symptoms.

The treatment of acute HF in the PACU is directed to its cause. Agents such as loop diuretics reduce preload and diastolic ventricular wall stress and can optimize myocardial contractility. For patients with signs of volume overload, diuretics provide symptomatic relief by quickly reducing pulmonary and peripheral congestion. For patients with pressure overload–induced HF symptoms, afterload-reducing agents such as nicardipine, clevidipine, nitroprusside, and hydralazine will lower the resistance against which the heart must contract. As a result of vascular smooth muscle relaxation, stroke volume and cardiac output will increase. The inodilators dobutamine and milrinone should be considered in patients with worsening HF symptoms who have been refractory to the treatments described. These agents are able to increase contractility and reduce systemic vascular resistance, leading to improved cardiac output and systemic perfusion. In acute HF, care should be taken to avoid any agents that can reduce contractility, such as β-blockers. When there is an escalation in symptoms or treatment, a cardiologist should be consulted, as well as consideration for transferring to a facility with a higher level of care (i.e., ICU), if needed.

Medical therapy can be considered a failure should patients continue with altered mental status; cold, clammy extremities; rising lactate level; and worsening end-organ dysfunction. In this situation, temporary percutaneous mechanical circulatory support is necessary with such devices as the IABP, Abiomed Impella, and VA-ECMO. Each device is capable of providing left ventricular support during cardiogenic shock from acute HF. VA-ECMO is unique in that it can provide biventricular support. In patients with acute renal failure and fluid overload, consultation with a nephrologist for renal replacement therapy and volume removal also is prudent.

Arrhythmias

The heart's conduction system is composed of a network of excitable cells that transmit electrical impulses, resulting in organized and rhythmic contractions. Abnormalities in impulse generation and conduction are responsible for the development of arrhythmias. The ECG remains the most essential tool in the diagnosis and management of these electrical abnormalities (see Chapter 9).

Tachyarrhythmias are cardiac rhythms that have a rate greater than 100 beats/min. Sinus tachycardia is the most common arrhythmia, with a heart rate ranging from 100 to 160 beats/min. This arrhythmia is a sympathetic-mediated hastening of the sinoatrial node. Pain, hypovolemia, and stimulants can trigger this rhythm. On ECG, the QRS complex is normal, and the sole abnormality is a fast rate. Treatment is directed toward the triggering cause of the sinus tachycardia.

Supraventricular tachycardia (SVT) is a paroxysmal, regular, and narrow-complex tachycardia (QRS <140 ms) with a rate between 140 and 280 beats/min. The most common form of SVT is atrioventricular nodal reentrant tachycardia (AVNRT). In AVNRT, the functional reentry circuit occurs within the atrioventricular (AV) node. Patients in the PACU presenting with this arrhythmia often complain of rapid palpitations, dyspnea, and presyncopal events. The treatment for SVT depends on the patient's condition. In a hemodynamically stable PACU patient (defined as a mentally alert patient with a perfusing heartbeat, and a mean arterial pressure sufficient to perfuse end organs), vagal maneuvers in the form of a Valsalva or carotid massage can be attempted. If these maneuvers fail or the patient is unstable, adenosine, a transient AV nodal blocking agent, should be administered intravenously. Secondary options for chemical treatment include an IV calcium channel blocker, diltiazem, or β-blocker such as metoprolol or esmolol.

Atrial fibrillation is an irregularly irregular narrow-complex tachycardia with rates between 110 to 180 beats/min. On ECG, there is an absence of a P wave, and the QRS complex is narrow and has an irregular rhythmic pattern. The aberrant conduction abnormality occurs in the atria and in portions of the pulmonary vein caused by reentrant circuits and electrical spiral waves in which the tissue lacks a refractory period. Risk factors for the development of atrial fibrillation include cardiac ischemia, hyperthyroidism, mitral valve disease, excessive alcohol use, pericarditis, and pulmonary embolism. In patients presenting with new-onset atrial fibrillation who are hemodynamically stable, the goal is to achieve ventricular rate control, targeting a rate of less than 110 beats/min. Agents such as metoprolol and diltiazem are effective pharmacologic therapy to achieve this goal. Pharmacologic cardioversion using an IV amiodarone bolus followed by a continuous infusion for 24 hours has a conversion to sinus rhythm success rate ranging from 55% to 95%. Patients presenting with new-onset atrial fibrillation and hemodynamic instability should immediately receive direct-current synchronized cardioversion set to 100 to 200 J. A transesophageal echocardiogram should be obtained to confirm the absence of an atrial thrombus before electrical cardioversion. Sedation or anesthesia should be considered in the PACU.

Atrial flutter presents with a sawtooth pattern on ECG caused by the presence of rapid P-waves. The QRS complex can appear regular or irregular depending on the presence of an AV conduction block. During atrial flutter, the atrial rate can be as high as 350 beats/min. The ventricular rate can be as high as 150 beats/min. A reentrant circuit in the atria is responsible for the triggering of the arrhythmia and is strongly associated with the presence of structural heart disease. The therapeutic agents used in atrial fibrillation are helpful in reducing the ventricular rate in atrial flutter but have a poor success rate in converting the patient to sinus rhythm. Electrical cardioversion is reserved for the hemodynamically unstable patient.

Premature ventricular contractions (PVC) originate from foci below the AV node. Stress, pain, stimulants, hypomagnesemia, and hypokalemia can trigger a PVC. In isolation, a PVC is benign. With multiple PVCs, the PACU patient may complain of palpitations and near syncope. A PVC occurring on the T wave, corresponding with ventricular repolarization, can trigger ventricular fibrillation or torsades de pointes, requiring immediate corrective action (i.e., defibrillation and magnesium sulfate administration). The initial treatments of PVCs consist of replacing electrolytes and discontinuation of proarrhythmic drugs. If the symptoms persist, lidocaine, β-blockers, and amiodarone are effective therapeutic agents.

Ventricular tachycardia (VT) is defined as three or more consecutive PVCs occurring at a heart rate of greater than 120 beats/min. On ECG, repetitive wide QRS complex and absent P waves are the typically observed features. VT may occur spontaneously in patients with systolic ejection fractions of 35% or less as a result of QT–prolonging medications or electrolyte depletion or in ischemic and structural heart disease. In patients with VT who are hemodynamically stable, medical therapy with amiodarone is appropriate. Further therapies should be targeted toward removing triggers. Patients who present in unstable monomorphic VT require immediate cardioversion. Synchronized cardioversion decreases the risk of the monomorphic VT degenerating to ventricular fibrillation. In polymorphic VT and pulseless VT, Advance Cardiac Life Support (ACLS) should begin immediately, with defibrillation at 360 J with a monophasic defibrillator.

Ventricular fibrillation (VF) is a lethal rhythm if timely intervention is not performed. VF correlates to unorganized ventricular contraction and the loss of stroke volume and cardiac output. Initial management of VF is to initiate the most current ACLS protocol. Chest compressions should be started immediately for systemic perfusion. Defibrillation should be applied as soon as possible. If electrical therapy fails, alternating doses of IV epinephrine and vasopressin should be administered. During resuscitative efforts, the anesthesiologist should identify and treat the inciting event (e.g., hyperkalemia, iatrogenic drug administration, acidosis, or hypoxemia).

Bradyrhythmias include abnormal conduction with rates less than 60 beats/min. Sinus bradycardia occurs any time a regular heart rhythm is below 60 beats/min. Excessive vagal tone, nodal blocking agents, and neuraxial blockade from a paravertebral block or thoracic epidural can contribute to its manifestation. In asymptomatic patients, no treatment is required. Patients presenting with β-blocker or calcium channel blocker overdose can be reversed with glucagon or β-agonists. Neuraxial blockade–induced bradycardia can be treated with ephedrine. If hypotension, bradycardia, and altered mental status occur, epinephrine or dopamine infusions can alleviate symptoms. A cardiology consultation should be obtained for any PACU patient with persistent and symptomatic bradycardia because cutaneous or transvenous pacing may be required.

Disruption of AV conduction occurs with third-degree heart block. There is complete dissociation of electrical impulses from the atria to the ventricles. As a result, the QRS complex is wide, and the rate is 30 to 45 beats/min. Patients with third-degree heart block may present with weakness, dyspnea, or syncope. Aside from a cardiology consultation, immediate treatment includes transcutaneous or transvenous pacing, depending on the facility's capability, or pharmacologic stimulation with isoproterenol infusion.

RESPIRATORY COMPLICATIONS AFTER NONCARDIAC SURGERY

Acute respiratory failure after noncardiac surgery ranges from 0.4% to 7% and is associated with a mortality rate increase of up to 26%. The main predictors have been identified as American Society of Anesthesiologists classification, emergent surgery, type of surgery, preoperative functional status, and sepsis (see Chapter 21).

Effects of Anesthesia on Respiratory Function

Anesthesia, especially general anesthesia, decreases functional residual capacity by about 20%. This occurs mainly through a loss of chest wall muscle tone as well as an upward movement of the diaphragm. The resulting ventilation/perfusion mismatch can contribute to postoperative hypoxemia. This aberration is aggravated by the fact that most volatile anesthetics inhibit hypoxic pulmonary vasoconstriction, further worsening ventilation-perfusion mismatch.

Dyspnea is one of the hallmarks of patients with chronic HF. Anatomically, the increased heart size decreases the space for the lungs and causes a restrictive respiratory pattern. In addition, increased cardiac filling pressures seen in more advanced HF result in increased pressures in the pulmonary circulation, leading to further airflow obstruction. Patients with advanced HF present with decreased diffusing capacity, further contributing to hypoxemia. These changes in HF happen in addition to the effects of anesthesia on pulmonary function. Fluid administration during surgery may worsen the observed dyspnea in this patient population.

In the postanesthetic period, the residual effects of volatile anesthetics, IV anesthetics, narcotics, and benzodiazepines attenuate the effects of hypercarbia on the ventilatory drive. The hypoxic drive is also blunted. These effects increase the risk of hypoxemia and hypercarbia in the postoperative period.

With the exception of ketamine, IV anesthetics and most volatile anesthetics and narcotics decrease pharyngeal muscle tone. This effect lasts well into the postoperative period and increases the aspiration risk in the PACU.

Respiratory Monitoring, Diagnosis, and Treatment in the Postanesthesia Care Unit

Hypoxemia

Hypoxemia, defined as oxygen saturation lower than 90%, has been observed in up to 55% of PACU patients. Although this is well tolerated in healthy individuals, patients with HF or pulmonary hypertension might not tolerate even mild episodes of hypoxemia. Pulse oximetry can detect these changes quite readily and should be used continuously for all PACU patients.

Detection of hypoxemia should lead to immediate treatment followed by an evaluation of potential causes. Atelectasis is common because of the decrease in functional residual capacity and decrease in chest wall muscle tone during the anesthetic period. Postoperative chest radiography can confirm this diagnosis. In most cases, conservative treatment such as upright positioning and deep breathing is sufficient. Despite its wide use, incentive spirometry has not been shown to be effective for treatment of atelectasis. In more severe cases, noninvasive ventilation has been shown to improve atelectasis rapidly.

Pulmonary edema is common in patients with a history of HF, especially if there are additional increased hydrostatic pressures because of fluid administration. Increased permeability of the capillary membranes as seen in sepsis additionally can contribute to pulmonary edema. This diagnosis can be made by chest radiography. Alternatively, transthoracic ultrasonography will also reveal evidence of pulmonary edema. The first treatment step is to decrease the intrathoracic volume with diuretics; noninvasive ventilation has been shown to improve dyspnea and decrease the rate of intubation. Therefore it should be used in patients with more severe pulmonary edema. Improving cardiac contractility with either inotropes or afterload reduction may be indicated.

Pneumothorax is often iatrogenic, such as in patients after central catheter placement and infraclavicular blocks, as well as surgeries (e.g., renal procedures) that might have injured the diaphragm. The diagnosis in more stable patients can be made by either chest radiography or ultrasonography. Larger pneumothoraces (>1.5 cm) benefit from chest tube placement, but patients with small pneumothoraces can be closely observed.

Pulmonary aspiration in the PACU is often directly observed; the diagnosis can be confirmed by bronchoscopy. In stable patients, no immediate treatment is required. Immediate antibiotics are, however, indicated in patients who aspirated bowel contents, patients with decreased immune status, or patients who are hospitalized.

Pulmonary embolism should be considered in hypoxemic patients in the PACU. Risk factors such as malignancies or long surgeries should increase suspicion. The diagnosis can be made with contrast computed tomography of the chest; however, an echocardiogram can help to determine the severity of disease. Treatment including anticoagulation and thrombolysis needs to be performed in consultation with the surgeon to address the benefits and risks of bleeding.

Hypercarbia and Hypoventilation

Hypoventilation is often caused by the residual effects of anesthetics, benzodiazepines, and opioids. Decreased oxygen saturation is a late sign to detect hypercarbia. Measuring respirations and end-tidal CO_2 will provide an earlier warning sign of hypoventilation. In most cases, the continuation of mechanical ventilation is the treatment of choice. Effects of residual opioids can be treated with naloxone. Given that the half-life of naloxone (30–60 minutes) is shorter than for most narcotics, it is important to closely observe the patient for signs of recurrence. Flumazenil is an antidote to benzodiazepine overdose. Its use is, however, limited by its short half-life and the risk for benzodiazepine withdrawal seizures.

Residual neuromuscular blockade causing ventilatory insufficiency is a frequent cause of respiratory failure in the PACU setting. The most sensitive test is quantitative measurement of train-of-four stimulation. A ratio of greater than 0.9 is a threshold for adequate recovery of neuromuscular function. Clinical tests indicate residual blockade, overall weakness, and the inability for a sustained head lift. Qualitative train-of-four measurements are not very useful to detect residual neuromuscular blockade. Residual paralysis with rocuronium can be reversed with sugammadex. Sugammadex is less effective for the reversal of vecuronium. Notably, sugammadex does not reverse quinolone-based neuromuscular blocking agents. In these cases, neostigmine might be indicated. The unpredictable effects of neostigmine and glycopyrrolate on heart rate carry additional risk in patients with ischemic cardiac disease and patients with arrhythmias. In these patients, reinstitution of mechanical ventilation should be considered.

BLEEDING IN CARDIAC PATIENTS AFTER NONCARDIAC SURGERY

In the United States, ischemic cardiovascular disease, some forms of chronic HF, atrial fibrillation, and other arrhythmias are routinely treated with long-term oral anticoagulation. This treatment can include the administration of oral antiplatelet agents and drugs that affect the coagulation cascade (Table 20.3) at various stages. For chronically anticoagulated patients, invasive procedures often require interruption and sometimes reversal of this therapy. For some cardiac patients, bridging with a shorter acting agent has been recommended before surgery.

Vitamin K Antagonists

Warfarin has been the mainstay of oral anticoagulation for more than 50 years, and it is still a commonly prescribed oral anticoagulation agent for stroke prevention among patients with atrial fibrillation, valvular heart disease, and venous thromboembolism. Warfarin has significant limitations, including a narrow therapeutic range, significant drug-drug interactions, and a requirement for frequent monitoring and dose adjustment. In addition, there is evidence that many patients are outside of the therapeutic range as much as 40% of the time during therapy. Surgery that carries a high bleeding risk requires that warfarin be held before the operative period. These surgeries include hip and knee replacement, neurologic and spine surgery, and general abdominal surgery. Many surgeries that last longer than 45 minutes are generally considered high risk. Frequently, lower risk procedures do not require cessation of anticoagulation therapy. Low-risk surgeries include abdominal hernia repairs, hysterectomies, cholecystectomies, gastrointestinal endoscopy, and arthroscopic surgery lasting less than 45 minutes. Any surgery using neuraxial anesthesia requires that warfarin be discontinued. To accomplish this, warfarin is usually held 5 days before the procedure and a prothrombin time (PT)/international normalized ratio (INR)

Table 20.3	Oral Anticoagulants				
	Mechanism of Action	Plasma Half-Life	Duration of Action	Elimination	Drug Interactions
Warfarin	Vitamin K antagonist	20–60 h	48–96 h	Metabolism	CYP2C9, CYP3A4, CYP1A2
Dabigatran	Direct thrombin inhibitor	12–14 h	48 h	80% renal	P-glycoprotein inhibitors
Apixaban	Xa inhibitor	8–15 h	24 h	25% renal	CYP3Y4, P-glycoprotein inhibitors
Edox-aban	Xa inhibitor	10–14 h	24 h	50% renal	P-glycoprotein inhibitors
Rivaroxiban	Xa inhibitor	7–10 h	24 h	50% renal, 50% hepatic	CYP3A4, P-glycoprotein inhibitors and inducers

is measured on the day before or day of surgery. This duration is chosen because the half-life of warfarin is approximately 36 to 42 hours. Most high-bleeding-risk surgeries require that the INR has fallen to at least 1.4. If the INR remains greater than 1.4, low-dose vitamin K can be administered. Postoperatively, warfarin is usually restarted at the prior dosage approximately 48 hours after the procedure. In patients with a higher baseline INR, earlier discontinuation of warfarin is necessary along with more extensive and frequent testing.

Direct Oral Anticoagulants

Because of the limitations of warfarin, alternatives were sought. This resulted in the recent development of oral anticoagulants with a mechanism that does not involve vitamin K antagonism. These drugs are either direct inhibitors of plasma- and membrane-bound thrombin (dabigatran) or direct inhibitors of free and prothrombinase bound factor Xa (apixaban, edoxaban, and rivaroxaban). Compared with warfarin, they have more rapid onset of action and shorter elimination half-lives in patients with normal renal function. As a result, routine monitoring of coagulation is not required for patients taking direct oral anticoagulants (DOACs). However, the absence of any laboratory tests that can estimate drug plasma concentration means that it is difficult for clinicians to gauge the effectiveness of withholding the drug before an elective surgery. In addition to renal function, DOAC concentration can be affected by other drugs that inhibit or induce P-glycoprotein (P-gp) transporter or, for the factor Xa inhibitors, CYP3A4 activity. For patients after a high-risk noncardiac surgery, either an unrecognized reduction in creatinine clearance or the presence of P-gp or CYP3A4 inhibitor would increase a patient's risk of major bleeding. Most clinicians adhere to the manufacturers' recommendation that DOACs are held in patients with reduced creatinine clearance or who are taking an inhibitor.

For emergent bleeding or in circumstances when discontinuation of an oral anticoagulant is not possible, dabigatran has a reversal agent, idarucizumab, that reverses the anticoagulant. Idarucizumab is a monoclonal antibody fragment that forms a high-affinity bond with the active thrombin binding site of dabigatran with a much larger affinity than thrombin. It displaces dabigatran from thrombin, which allows fibrin generation. For prompt reversal of warfarin, vitamin K—either orally or IV—is usually the first-line agent. The route of administration usually depends on the urgency or the surgery. IV vitamin K can overcome a warfarin effect within 6 to 12 hours, but oral vitamin K can take 24 to 36 hours. For more urgent reversal of warfarin, prothrombin complex concentrates (PCCs) or fresh-frozen plasma (FFP) is recommended, and dosing can be guided by following the INR. Some of the PCCs contain heparin, which is best avoided in patients with heparin-induced thrombocytopenia, but unless otherwise contraindicated, PCCs are usually preferred over FFP. PCCs offer several advantages over FFP for rapid warfarin reversal, including significantly lower volume, standardized coagulation factor content, no requirement to establish ABO compatibility, shorter preparation time, and a lower risk of pathogen transmission or transfusion-related acute lung injury (TRALI). For urgent reversal of warfarin, IV vitamin K is frequently coadministered because both PCC's and FFP's clotting effect diminishes after 6 hours (equivalent to roughly the half-life of factor VII).

Although the rate of major bleeding reported with DOACs was generally lower compared with vitamin K antagonists, the bleeding risk was not negligible. Annual risk was reported as high as 3.6% in patients with atrial fibrillation. A new reversal agent specific to factor Xa inhibitors was recently approved. Andexanet alfa is a recombinant modified human activated factor Xa that binds to factor Xa inhibitors with high affinity but itself does not catalyze any factor conversion. Dosed according to the specific DOAC taken and the interval since the last dose, it has been reported to achieve good or excellent hemostasis in 79% of older adult patients with cardiovascular disease taking factor Xa inhibitors who presented with major bleeding. Among this population, and especially in patients with renal impairment, these reversal agents will likely play a large part in managing major bleeding in the operating room (OR) and PACU.

Antiplatelet Agents

Antiplatelet agents are routinely prescribed to cardiac patients to prevent thrombus formation and ischemic events. Although highly effective for this purpose, these drugs can have a profound impact on hemorrhage risk in the OR and PACU. Three broad categories of agents are most commonly prescribed: acetylsalicylic acid (aspirin), $P2Y_{12}$ receptor antagonists (e.g., clopidogrel, prasugrel, ticagrelor), and glycoprotein IIb/IIIa inhibitors. These agents are frequently combined as dual therapy to reduce thrombotic events.

As with anticoagulants, the risk of postoperative hemorrhage depends on the inherent bleeding risk of the operation and the duration of time between the last dose and surgery. Unlike anticoagulants, there are no antagonists for any of the antiplatelet agents, so blood products (e.g., platelets, fibrinogen, factors), desmopressin, and tranexamic acid are the principal agents used to reverse bleeding associated with loss of platelet function. Many patients who present for urgent surgery are receiving antiplatelet agents because they are at high risk of arterial thrombosis. Before withholding antiplatelet agents and administering prothrombotic reversal agents, the risks and benefits should be carefully considered because these actions increase the patient's risk of acute arterial thrombosis. Discontinuation of antiplatelet therapy should be performed in consultation with both the surgeon and cardiologist. This is particularly important in patients with coronary stents because abrupt withdrawal of antiplatelet therapy leaves these patients at risk for acute in-stent thrombosis (see Chapter 3).

Diagnosis and Management of Postoperative Bleeding

Acute major postoperative bleeding is not clinically difficult to detect. Hemodynamic changes including hypotension, tachycardia, hypothermia, changes in pulse pressure variation and stroke volume variation, as well as decreased urine output are frequently observed in the PACU. In addition, rapid filling of indwelling drains or soaking of dressings can make a diagnosis obvious. There are, however, clinical circumstances when a diagnosis of postoperative hemorrhage is less apparent. Occult hemorrhage can be difficult to detect immediately after surgery. Furthermore, intraoperative estimates of blood loss can be inaccurate and an individual hemoglobin may not accurately reflect blood loss at the start of an acute bleeding event. Complicating the diagnosis is the fact that many other conditions can mimic acute blood loss, including inadequate fluid replacement, myocardial dysfunction, anaphylaxis, and septic shock. Usually the diagnosis is made from laboratory tests obtained serially. Hemoglobin is obtained and a restrictive trigger for transfusion (hemoglobin levels <7–8 g/dL) is used in most patients undergoing noncardiac surgery. PT and activated partial thromboplastin time are also obtained, and the trigger for the transfusion of either PCC or FFP is a value greater than 1.5 times the reference. Platelets are also serially followed, but the trigger to transfuse platelets depends on the location of the surgery. Patients who have undergone intracranial procedures and intraspinal procedures or who have known platelet dysfunction are usually transfused when the level falls below 100,000/μL. In most other cases, 50,000/μL is the threshold. Fibrinogen level is also routinely measured, and cryoprecipitate or fibrinogen concentrate is administered when it falls below 100 mg/dL.

Several clinical conditions complicate large-volume transfusions in cardiac patients after surgery. First, the time to obtain laboratory values is often 45 to 90 minutes. In the case of rapid blood loss, the results can be substantially inaccurate by the time they are reported. Thromboelastography (TEG) can shorten diagnostic times in ongoing hemorrhage and accurately graph the kinetics of clot formation. This test can effectively guide blood product transfusion and identify blood product abnormalities, preventing the administration of unnecessary products. TEG can identify factor deficiencies, platelet dysfunction, and fibrinolysis, and in many centers, TEG is routinely used for trauma resuscitation and to manage bleeding after liver transplantation.

Second, in patients with reduced vascular and chamber compliance, transfusion-associated circulatory overload can confer mortality risk via pulmonary edema. The benefits of anemia correction in patients with underlying cardiac disease have to be balanced against the risks of volume overload. In a patient requiring substantial resuscitation in the PACU, invasive cardiac monitoring is often essential. Pulse pressure and stroke volume variation from invasive arterial cannulae can be used as a dynamic measure of volume status, and central venous access and monitoring of central venous pressure can be used to estimate right atrial pressure and right ventricular response to volume administration. Additionally, the central access allows for repeated sampling of central venous blood gases. During resuscitation in patients with diminished left ventricular systolic or diastolic function, volume overload can result in worse end-organ perfusion even if anemia and coagulopathy are corrected. These two competing endpoints require prolonged vigilance to optimize outcomes in cardiac patients who are bleeding postoperatively. Toward this end, PCCs and fibrinogen concentrates are frequently used in patients for whom excess circulating volume is poorly tolerated. In addition, there is often a low threshold to administer noninvasive positive-pressure ventilation and diuretics to optimize gas exchange during resuscitation. Warming of blood products and maintenance of calcium homeostasis during transfusion in cardiac patients are essential to prevent hypothermia- and hypocalcemia-related arrhythmias, hypotension, and cardiac dysfunction.

Like all patients receiving blood products, those with underlying cardiac disease are at risk for complications associated with blood product transfusion, including transfusion-related lung injury (TRALI), bacterial and viral transmission, and immunologically mediated acute transfusion reactions. Among patients with underlying HF, however, the presentation of these events can overlap with an acute exacerbation of HF. In circumstances when the diagnosis is unclear, additional monitoring including transthoracic echocardiography and pulmonary artery catheterization may assist in management of volume status and guide exogenous inotropic support.

In summary, patients with underlying cardiac disease who are bleeding in the PACU require some special considerations. This is related to their chronic exposure to various anticoagulants and antiplatelet agents and, in addition, many have diminished cardiovascular tolerance of acute anemia, hypovolemia, and blood product resuscitation. In these patients, prompt reversal of anticoagulation can be lifesaving, and deliberately managed blood product resuscitation is essential to prevent worsening end-organ injury. Bleeding patients with cardiac disease in the PACU present many challenges that are best confronted with a thoughtful plan to correct anemia and coagulopathy while optimizing pump function and systemic perfusion.

SUGGESTED READING

American Society of Anesthesiologists Task Force on Perioperative Blood Management. Practice guidelines for perioperative blood management: an updated report by the American Society of Anesthesiologists Task Force on Perioperative Blood Management. *Anesthesiology*. 2015;122:241.

Brueckmann B, Sasaki N, Grobara P, et al. Effects of sugammadex on incidence of postoperative residual neuromuscular blockade: a randomized, controlled study. *Br J Anaesth*. 2015;115(5):743–751.

Canet J, Gallart L. Postoperative respiratory failure: pathogenesis, prediction, and prevention. *Curr Opin Crit Care*. 2014;20(1):56–62.

Connolly SJ, Milling TJ, Eikelboom JW, et al. Andexanet Alfa for acute major bleeding associated with factor Xa inhibitors. *N Engl J Med*. 2016;375:1131–1141.

Farkouh ME, Domanski M, Sleeper LA, et al. Strategies for multivessel revascularization in patients with diabetes. *N Engl J Med*. 2012;367:2375–2384.

January CT, Wann LS, Alpert JS, et al. 2014 AHA/ACC/HRS guideline for management of patients with atrial fibrillation: executive summary. *Circulation*. 2014;130(23):2071–2104.

Koenig-Oberhuber V, Filipovic M. New antiplatelet and new oral anticoagulants. *Br J Anaesth*. 2016;117(S2):ii74–ii84.

Nava S, Hill N. Non-invasive ventilation in acute respiratory failure. *Lancet*. 2009;374:250–259.

Neumar RW, Shuster M, Callaway CW, et al. 2015 American Heart Association guidelines update for cardiopulmonary resuscitation and emergency cardiovascular care. *Circulation*. 2015;132:S315–S367.

Salmonson T, Dogne JM, Janssen H, et al. Non-vitamin-K oral anticoagulants and laboratory testing: now and in the future. *Eur Heart J Cardiovasc Pharmacother*. 2017;3:42–47.

Sasaki N, Meyer MJ, Malviya SA, et al. Effects of neostigmine reversal of nondepolarizing neuromuscular blocking agents on postoperative respiratory outcomes a prospective study. *Anesthesiology*. 2014;121(5):959–968.

Thiele H, Zeymer U, Neumann FJ, et al. Intraaortic balloon support for myocardial infarction with cardiogenic shock. *N Engl J Med*. 2012;367:1287–1296.

Wikkelsø A, Wetterslev J, Møller AM, Afshari A. Thromboelastography (TEG) or thromboelastometry (ROTEM) to monitor haemostatic treatment versus usual care in adults or children with bleeding. *Cochrane Database Syst Rev*. 2016;CD007871.

Yancy CW, Jessup M, Bozkurt B, et al. 2017 ACC/AHA/HFSA focused update of the 2013 ACCF/AHA guidelines for the management of heart failure: a report of the American College of Cardiology/ American Heart Association task force on clinical practice guidelines and the Heart Failure Society of America. *Circulation*. 2017;136(6):e137–e161.

Chapter 21

Postoperative Care of the Critically Ill

Jeffrey Katz, MD • Torin Shear, MD •
Steven B. Greenberg, MD

Key Points

1. Cerebrovascular accidents are some of the most significant perioperative complications because they increase long-term disability, hospital length of stay, and mortality.
2. Recent stroke is associated with a 1.8-fold increased risk of death in noncardiac surgery.
3. There are a broad spectrum of critical care issues involving the pulmonary system, ranging from chronic diseases to surgical and anesthesia complications.
4. Postoperative respiratory failure can be defined as unplanned intubation and mechanical ventilation within 48 hours of noncardiac surgery.
5. Postoperative pulmonary edema can be either cardiogenic (e.g., heart failure) or noncardiogenic (e.g., negative pressure–induced) in origin.
6. Massive transfusion in the perioperative period is still a significant cause of morbidity and mortality. The exact ratio of plasma to platelets to red blood cells has yet to be delineated.
7. High-risk patients may have up to a 6% risk of developing venous thromboemboli in the postoperative period. Both deep venous thrombosis and pulmonary emboli require anticoagulation if it is not contraindicated by surgery.
8. The initial treatment of sepsis revolves around three concepts: source control of infection, antibiotics, and early goal-directed resuscitation.

This chapter focuses on postoperative care of critically ill surgical patients and complications from surgery. It is organized by organ system and is intended to be an introduction to the topics that it covers. This is not an exhaustive review of critical illness. The Suggested Reading section is provided for a more in-depth review of the topics that are covered. Consultation with a specialist should be considered when clinically appropriate.

NEUROLOGIC SYSTEM

Perioperative Cerebrovascular Accident

Cerebrovascular accident (CVA) is one of the most significant perioperative complications. The incidence of perioperative CVA in the general surgical population depends on the type of procedure and associated perioperative risk factors, but it remains low at approximately less than 0.7%. CVA, however, is responsible for a substantial increase in long-term disability, longer intensive care unit (ICU) and hospital stay, and mortality. The etiology is primarily embolic, and it is far more common than those related to hypoperfusion. Noncardiac surgery induces a hypercoagulable state, and tissue trauma enhances formation of thrombus and inflammation. Surgical stress is marked by decreased levels of tissue plasminogen activator (tPA), increased fibrinogen degradation products, increased thrombin-antithrombin complexes, and increased D-dimers. These prothrombotic changes coupled with dehydration, bed rest, general anesthesia, and cessation of anticoagulants increase the risk for postoperative CVA. The majority of CVAs occur on the second postoperative day and are typically related to the development of atrial fibrillation or myocardial ischemia.

Common perioperative risk factors are listed in Tables 21.1 and 21.2. Modifiable risk factors may be addressed in the preoperative period to reduce morbidity and mortality.

Preventive strategies for perioperative CVA are not well defined. Decreasing surgical time may reduce risk for CVA, but this may be difficult to modify. Patients with symptomatic carotid artery stenosis may benefit from carotid revascularization before undergoing major surgery. However, at least one study of 2000 high-risk patients

Table 21.1	Modifiable Factors Affecting Cerebrovascular Accident Risk	
Preventive		**Therapeutic**
Decreased surgical time		Intravenous tissue plasminogen activator: higher risk of bleeding
Carotid artery revascularization in symptomatic patient		Supportive care: intubation for airway protection and mechanical ventilation
β-Blockers		
Statins		Intraarterial thrombolysis: questionable efficacy
Glycemic control		
Continuation of anticoagulants when safe		Endovascular mechanical clot disruption: questionable efficacy
Consider delaying elective surgery for >9 months after cerebrovascular accident		

Table 21.2	Cerebrovascular Accident Risk Factors		
Preoperative		**Intraoperative**	**Postoperative**
Patient age >70 years		Surgery type	Heart failure
Female sex		Type of anesthesia (general vs. local)	Low ejection fraction
History of cerebrovascular accident or transient ischemic attack		Duration of surgery	Myocardial infarction
History of symptomatic carotid artery stenosis		Manipulation of proximal aortic lesions	Arrhythmias
Atherosclerosis of the ascending aorta		Arrhythmias	Dehydration
History of hypertension		Hyperglycemia	Blood loss
Diabetes		Hypotension	Hyperglycemia
Creatinine >2 mg/dL		Hypertension	
History of cardiac disease			
Peripheral vascular disease			
Ejection fraction <40%			
Smoking			

undergoing noncardiac surgery suggested no association between carotid artery stenosis and perioperative stroke. Preliminary studies suggest a small reduction in perioperative stroke risk with perioperative β-blockers, statins, and glycemic control. Timing of elective noncardiac surgery in patients with a prior stroke is important. A large database study suggested that a recent stroke is associated with a 1.8-fold increase risk of death in patients undergoing noncardiac surgery less than 3 months after a stroke, which stabilizes at approximately 9 months. The perioperative care team might consider delaying elective noncardiac surgery when feasible.

Perioperative anticoagulation should be continued whenever the risk of bleeding is deemed low by the surgical team. Cessation of anticoagulation may result in an increased risk of perioperative CVA. Discontinuing aspirin is likely to exacerbate the already increased hypercoagulable state of surgery. Guidelines suggest continuing aspirin in all perioperative situations except for those with very low cardiac risk or in situations in which even minor bleeding may be catastrophic. Warfarin and clopidogrel are often stopped several days before surgery. Cessation of these medications should be based on each unique clinical situation. Bridging anticoagulation with heparin or low-molecular-weight heparin may be considered in patients at high perioperative risk of stroke and when hemorrhage is also a concern. If oral anticoagulants must be held before surgery, it is prudent for the managing service to restart these drugs as soon as appropriate in the postoperative period. Consultation with a specialist may be prudent.

Therapies for perioperative CVA are few. Recent guidelines suggest that early diagnosis and management in a stroke unit with general supportive care is paramount. Intravenous (IV) tPA is a proven therapy for ischemic CVA but is relatively contraindicated after major surgery because of bleeding risk. Each case should be evaluated by the perioperative team and, if possible, an expert in the field of CVA. Other modalities such as intraarterial thrombolysis and endovascular mechanical clot disruption may be appropriate for those who have undergone recent major noncardiac surgery, but the benefit remains unproven.

PULMONARY SYSTEM

There are a broad spectrum of critical care issues involving the pulmonary system in the perioperative settings. These may arise from primary pulmonary disease, such as chronic obstructive pulmonary disease (COPD), or secondary manifestations such as cardiogenic pulmonary edema or neuromuscular weakness. This section focuses on key perioperative respiratory diseases, including pulmonary edema, COPD exacerbations, and acute lung injury or acute respiratory distress syndrome (ARDS) as well as management strategies for these syndromes in the perioperative setting.

Respiratory Failure

Respiratory failure can be categorized into two broad types, which are described next (Table 21.3).

Type 1 Respiratory Failure: Hypoxemic

Hypoxemic respiratory failure is typically associated with parenchymal lung diseases that affect oxygen exchange at the alveolar level. It is defined as a PaO_2 less than 50 mm Hg on room air. Five pathophysiologic mechanisms can explain hypoxemia—low oxygen admixture, ventilation/perfusion (V/Q) mismatch, shunting, diffusion impairment, and alveolar hypoventilation. Shunt physiology is unique because it is nonresponsive

Table 21.3 Types of Respiratory Failure

Type	Definition	Mechanism	Common Diseases and Risk Factors
1	Hypoxemic	Low O_2 admixture V/Q mismatch Shunting Diffusion impairment Alveolar hypoventilation	Cardiogenic pulmonary edema ARDS PE Pneumonia Shunts (right to left)
2	Hypercarbic	Central respiratory depression Respiratory system mechanical failure Respiratory muscle fatigue	Neuromuscular disorders (e.g., ALS, Guillain-Barré syndrome) COPD

ALS, Amyotrophic lateral sclerosis; *ARDS,* acute respiratory distress syndrome; *COPD,* chronic obstructive pulmonary disease; *PE,* pulmonary embolism; *V/Q,* ventilation/perfusion.

to supplemental oxygen. Pulmonary edema and ARDS are two examples of hypoxemic respiratory failure and are discussed later in this chapter.

Type 2 Respiratory Failure: Hypercarbic With or Without Hypoxemia

Hypercapnic respiratory failure is associated with ventilatory failure and inadequate carbon dioxide elimination. It occurs when the arterial partial pressure of carbon dioxide ($PaCO_2$) increases above 50 mm Hg in patients without chronic CO_2 retention and may be associated with hypoxemia. There are three main causes of ventilation failure: depression of the respiratory centers in the brainstem, mechanical dysfunction of the respiratory muscles and associated structural tissues (e.g., the chest wall and diaphragm), and respiratory muscle fatigue associated with increased work of breathing. Depressed respiratory drive from medication effects (e.g., narcotics, inhalation anesthetics) is a classic cause of hypercapnic respiratory failure in the perioperative period. COPD is the most common cause of type 2 respiratory failure. Rare neuromuscular diseases (i.e., amyotrophic lateral sclerosis, muscular dystrophy, and myasthenia gravis) may lead to chronic hypercapnic respiratory failure.

Postoperative Respiratory Failure

Postoperative respiratory failure may be defined as unplanned intubation and mechanical ventilation within 48 hours of surgery. It is a serious complication associated with an 18-fold increased risk of death. Postoperative respiratory failure may be either hypoxemic or hypercarbic depending on the underlying pathophysiology. Patients may also require intubation for impending respiratory failure before hypercarbia or hypoxemia develops. Risk factors for postoperative respiratory failure are either patient related or procedure or anesthesia related. Patient factors include American Society of Anesthesiologists score greater than 3, older age, ethanol use, tobacco use, COPD, insulin-dependent diabetes mellitus, heart failure, hypertension, cancer, liver dysfunction, cachexia and weight loss, and morbid obesity (body mass index >40). Surgical and anesthesia factors include emergency surgery, medium- to high-risk surgery, surgery for sepsis, surgical location (upper abdominal or thoracic surgery), and surgery lasting longer than 2 hours. General anesthesia may pose a higher risk of postoperative respiratory failure versus regional or neuroaxial anesthesia, although this remains controversial. Residual neuromuscular blockade is an important risk factor for immediate perioperative respiratory failure.

Respiratory Failure in Circulatory Shock

Circulatory shock–associated respiratory failure develops when an imbalance between respiratory muscle oxygen supply and demand occurs. Respiratory compensation for a metabolic acidosis requires an increased minute ventilation to decrease the $PaCO_2$. Increased work of breathing requires greater oxygen supply, which is compromised in shock. Respiratory muscles fatigue and fail when the oxygen supply is insufficient to maintain the higher respiratory workload.

Pulmonary Edema

Starling forces control the net flow of fluid across the alveolar membrane and are proportional to the permeability and surface area of the alveolar membrane, as well as the balance between hydrostatic and oncotic pressures of both the capillaries and alveoli. In a normal lung, the extravasation of fluid from the capillaries into the alveoli is matched by the lymphatic system's ability to drain the lung water. Imbalances in the Starling forces cause pulmonary edema and occur primarily from a high hydrostatic pressure in cardiogenic pulmonary edema or increased alveolar capillary permeability in noncardiogenic pulmonary edema. Restoration of the normal ebb and flow of alveolar lung water is often rapid in cardiogenic pulmonary edema because the elevated hydrostatic forces are normalized with diuresis and a negative fluid balance. In contrast, the resolution of noncardiogenic pulmonary edema can be prolonged and requires the restoration of the integrity of the alveolar membrane. A patient with pulmonary edema typically presents with tachypnea, dyspnea, and hypoxemia.

Cardiogenic Pulmonary Edema

Cardiogenic pulmonary edema can present with slowly progressive dyspnea or an acute dyspnea referred to as flash pulmonary edema. Slowly progressive edema is caused by a decline in cardiac function and progressive accumulation of intravascular and extravascular fluid. Contributing factors include medication effects (noncompliance or inadequate dose), renal dysfunction, and respiratory infection. Flash pulmonary edema is caused by abrupt physiologic derangement such as a sudden increase in blood pressure, acute myocardial ischemia, acute myocarditis, acute valve dysfunction (e.g., mitral regurgitation), or arrhythmia. Elevated filling pressures in the left heart cause an increase in pulmonary venous pressures and increased hydrostatic pressure in the pulmonary capillary bed. These changes force a transudative edema fluid into the interstitium and the alveoli when the left atrial pressure increases above 18 mm Hg. Alveolar fluid impairs oxygen exchange and results in hypoxemia.

Evaluation of the patient with pulmonary edema should focus on the severity of the respiratory distress and required respiratory support then shift to an assessment of etiology. Chest radiography and 12-lead electrocardiography are cornerstones of management, and laboratory evaluation should include cardiac troponins, complete blood count (CBC), complete metabolic panel (CMP), and brain natriuretic peptide level. Transthoracic echocardiography may be considered for better definition of cardiac structure and function.

Urgent treatment of pulmonary edema focuses on correction of hypoxemia and stabilization of respiratory distress. Patients with mild to moderate dyspnea and hypoxemia can often be treated with supplemental oxygen via nasal cannula; however, more severe dyspnea may require noninvasive or invasive mechanical ventilation. Noninvasive ventilation (NIV) may lead to quicker resolution of respiratory symptoms and decreased need for intubation. After respiratory stabilization, diuresis and afterload reduction should be considered. Loop diuretics are the mainstay of therapy for volume overload. Hypoxemia and respiratory distress improve as pulmonary edema resolves with a negative fluid balance. Afterload reduction with vasodilators reduces cardiac workload and may hasten recovery. Inotropes and advanced mechanical heart failure therapies may also be considered in the appropriate clinical setting.

Noncardiogenic Pulmonary Edema

The most important cause of noncardiogenic pulmonary edema is acute respiratory distress syndrome (ARDS). Less common etiologies of noncardiogenic pulmonary edema include neurogenic, diffuse alveolar hemorrhage, medication induced (e.g., naloxone), and negative-pressure pulmonary edema. Initial treatment includes stabilization of the respiratory distress with oxygen therapy, NIV, or invasive mechanical ventilation. Loop diuretics are often used for a negative fluid balance depending on patient stability.

Negative-Pressure Pulmonary Edema

Negative-pressure pulmonary edema occurs when extreme negative intrathoracic pressure (deep breath) occurs against an obstructed airway. The obstruction can be caused by an obstructed endotracheal tube, laryngospasm, or an upper airway obstruction. The large negative inspiratory force against an obstructed airway creates a vacuum effect and draws fluid into the alveoli, resulting in pulmonary edema characterized by pink, frothy sputum. The presentation can be immediate or delayed. There is misconception that negative-pressure pulmonary edema is typically associated with individuals who are capable of generating significant negative intrathoracic force; however, many of the patients who develop this disorder have preexisting cardiac disease.

Acute Respiratory Distress Syndrome

Acute respiratory distress syndrome is a common cause of respiratory failure, affects approximately 200,000 people a year, and is associated with 15% of all ICU admissions. ARDS is characterized by diffuse alveolar damage leading to increased alveolar capillary permeability, resulting in pulmonary edema, hypoxemia, and respiratory distress. The most common causes are pneumonia (viral or bacterial), sepsis, trauma, gastric aspiration, transfusion related, medications, and pancreatitis. The diagnosis of ARDS requires hypoxemia, bilateral opacities on chest radiographs, and pulmonary edema associated with a clinical insult and *not* fully explainable by cardiac function. ARDS severity is measured by the degree of hypoxemia using PaO_2/F_IO_2 (fraction of inspired oxygen) ratio of mild, 200 to 300; moderate, 100 to 200; and severe, less than 100, correlating with increasing mortality rate (26%–35%). The cause of death in ARDS is most often related to multisystem organ failure and bacterial sepsis.

Treatment of ARDS is supportive and requires treatment of the underlying condition (e.g., antibiotics and source control for sepsis). The mainstay of therapy for ARDS is lung-protective ventilation and conservative fluid management. Lung-protective ventilation consists of low tidal volume ventilation (6 mL/kg), maintaining plateau pressures less than 30 cm H_2O, and permissive hypercapnia to avoid ventilator-induced lung injury (volume trauma and barotrauma). Conservative fluid therapy in ARDS begins after circulatory shock has resolved (no longer requiring fluid boluses or vasopressors for 12 hours). The goal for conservative fluid therapy is a net negative fluid balance of 500 mL/day achieved through diuresis and has led to decreased ventilator-dependent days and ICU length of stay. Several adjuvant therapies may lead to an additional decrease in mortality rate from severe ARDS, including short-term paralysis with cisatracurium, prone positioning in the ICU, and extracorporeal membrane oxygenation. Consultation with critical care specialists is recommended.

Chronic Obstructive Pulmonary Disease

Chronic obstructive pulmonary disease is a very common disorder and is projected to be the third leading cause of death by 2020. Smoking is the leading risk factor, and 70% of patients with COPD have a cardiovascular comorbidity. COPD causes a constant, low-grade inflammatory response that accelerates atherosclerosis and is associated with a two- to threefold increased risk of cardiovascular death. Not surprisingly, COPD is a major risk factor for postoperative complications, including pneumonia, respiratory failure, myocardial infarction, cardiac arrest, sepsis, reoperation, and kidney injury or failure.

Chronic obstructive pulmonary disease is characterized as chronic and progressive airflow limitations from damage to the lung parenchyma or inflammation of the airways. Symptoms include dyspnea, respiratory signs of distress (i.e., accessory muscle use), increased sputum production, and chronic cough. Exposure to tobacco smoke is nearly universal, although there are other risk factors such as environmental exposures and rare genetic defects (α_1-antitrypsin). Common physical examination findings include expiratory wheezing, increased expiratory time, diminished breath sounds, and a barrel chest. Diagnosis is confirmed with spirometry. COPD severity is important because it directly relates to increased risk of exacerbation. The Global Initiative for Chronic Obstructive Lung Disease has developed a simple disease severity scale based on forced expiratory volume in 1 second (FEV_1) with the assumption that the patient has an FEV_1/FVC (forced vital capacity) ratio less than 0.7. An FEV_1 less than 80% predicted value is mild, FEV_1 of 50% to 79% is moderate, FEV_1 of 30% to 49% is severe, and FEV_1 less than 30% is very severe. Other risk factors for exacerbation include gastroesophageal reflux disease, asthma, heart failure, cancer, and respiratory infections.

It is important for the anesthesiologist to recognize the severity of COPD in patients presenting for surgery. Preoperative pulmonary function testing should be considered for those who are at risk for COPD or have an established diagnosis of COPD. A specific level of functional status and spirometric data points have not been established for COPD patients who require an operation. Consultation with a pulmonologist should be considered. Standard medical therapies for COPD include smoking cessation and inhalers for symptom alleviation. Bronchodilator therapy with a β_2-agonist (i.e., albuterol, salmeterol) and/or an antimuscarinic (i.e., tiotropium) are commonplace, as are inhaled corticosteroids. Oxygen therapy is added when patients develop resting hypoxemia, pulmonary hypertension, or heart failure. It is beneficial that these medications are continued in the perioperative period.

Exacerbations of COPD are characterized by worsening of symptoms ranging from increased wheezing to hypercarbic respiratory failure. Treatment includes respiratory support with oxygen, noninvasive or invasive mechanical ventilation, and medical management. Noninvasive mechanical ventilation is the mainstay of therapy in severe COPD exacerbations and has been shown to decrease mortality rates, the need for intubation, and hospital length of stay. In the perioperative period, the anesthesiologist should be cognizant of the relative contraindications to NIV such as diminished mental status, ability to protect the airway or aspiration risk, recent and severe facial surgery or trauma, hemodynamic instability, and upper gastrointestinal (GI) surgery. After NIV has been initiated, frequent patient assessment is required. NIV failure is defined as no improvement or worsening of the respiratory acidosis within 1 hour of initiation, and intubation should be considered. Declining mental status and increased work of breathing are additional signs of NIV failure, suggesting that intubation and mechanical ventilation may be needed. Pharmacotherapy for acute COPD exacerbations includes antibiotics for respiratory infection, inhaled β-agonists (e.g., albuterol), and anticholinergic agents (e.g., ipratropium). Systemic corticosteroids also are recommended.

HEMATOLOGY

Many aspects of perioperative medicine and anesthesia critical care involve the hematologic system. In the perioperative period, clinicians are often challenged by perturbations in the hematologic system, which may impair oxygen delivery or the coagulation cascade. This hematology section focuses on two clinical challenges that anesthesiologists may face in all phases of the perioperative period: massive hemorrhage and venous thromboembolism (VTE).

Massive Hemorrhage

Massive hemorrhage is a significant cause of morbidity and mortality worldwide. The anesthesiologist is confronted by massive hemorrhage in a variety of clinical settings, including trauma, obstetric hemorrhage, GI bleeding, and major surgery (e.g., cardiac, spine, transplantation). Massive hemorrhage is defined as the need for greater than 10 units of packed red blood cells (PRBCs) or approximately a patient's total blood volume in 24 hours, transfusion of greater than 4 units of PRBCs in 1 hour, or replacement of more than 50% of total blood volume in 3 hours. Coagulopathy of massive transfusion can develop quickly from hypothermia, dilutional coagulopathy, platelet dysfunction, fibrinolysis, and hypofibrinogenemia. The pathophysiologic changes associated with massive transfusion have led to clinical interest in higher ratios of blood product transfusion (plasma:platelets:red blood cells [RBC] ratio, such as 1:1:1) and have been shown to be effective in preventing early death (within 24 hours) of trauma patients. The exact ratio of plasma to platelets to RBCs has not yet been delineated, and a large study of trauma patients comparing a ratio of 1:1:1 to 1:1:2 showed no difference in mortality rate at 24 hours or 30 days. Meta-analysis studies have showed no strong evidence to use a precise blood product transfusion ratio. It is unclear if the high platelet:plasma:RBC ratios are generalizable to other patient populations.

The treatment of massive hemorrhage relies on a multidisciplinary approach fostering excellent communication and efficiency between the care team and supportive services such as the blood bank and laboratory. Massive transfusion protocols have been developed to overcome institutional barriers and help facilitate the care of these critically ill patients. Multiple protocols exist and vary in the ratio of platelets:plasma:RBCs, but are related in their formula-based approach (no laboratory tests) to coordinate care between departments and improve efficiency. Adherence to formula-driven massive transfusion protocols has been associated with improved survival from massive hemorrhage. Laboratory-driven transfusion protocols have been created, but they are limited by long laboratory turnaround times and subsequent relevance of the laboratory tests. Massive transfusion protocols based on point-of-care testing such as thromboelastography (TEG) and thromboelastometry (TEM) have been shown to be noninferior to formula-driven protocols. TEG- and TEM-based protocols may actually decrease the amount of blood product administration, which may lead to decreases in transfusion-related morbidity and mortality.

Complications of Massive Transfusion

One of the main complications of massive hemorrhage is death by exsanguination or inadequate transfusion, which accounts for approximately 40% of associated deaths. The coagulopathy of massive transfusion and the treatment is addressed in the preceding section. Transfusion-related reactions can also account for significant morbidity and include hemolytic and nonhemolytic reactions; immunologic reactions such as transfusion-associated acute lung injury; circulatory effects such as transfusion-associated circulatory overload; and metabolic effects, including hypocalcemia, hypomagnesemia, hyperkalemia, metabolic acidosis from hypoperfusion, and hypothermia. Complications are more likely in patients with preexisting comorbidities, including patients with cardiac disease.

Venous Thromboembolism Prophylaxis and Treatment in the Perioperative Setting

Venous thromboembolism is a common and serious complication in the postoperative setting. The overall risk of VTE with appropriate prophylaxis is approximately 1%, but can be as high as 2.5% in high-risk procedures such as those undergoing joint replacement. Risk factors include age older than 60 years, history of VTE or thrombophilia, cancer, comorbid medical conditions such as heart failure or infection, bed bound or decreased activity level for 3 or more days, obesity, and ICU admission. High-risk patients may have as much as a 6% risk of VTE. Guidelines from the American College of Chest Physicians regarding VTE prophylaxis fall into four patient categories, including very low, low, moderate, and high risk, with corresponding risk of VTE at less than 0.5%, 1.5%, 3%, and 6%, respectively. Very-low-risk patients require no pharmacologic or mechanical VTE prophylaxis. Sequential compression boots are recommended for low-risk patients. Moderate-risk patients should receive sequential compression boots and pharmacologic prophylaxis with a heparinoid. The recommendation for high-risk patients is mechanical and pharmacologic prophylaxis that is extended 4 weeks postoperatively. Patients undergoing joint arthroplasty are at especially high risk of VTE complications postoperatively, and it is recommended that chemoprophylaxis of VTE be extended to 35 days with low-molecular-weight heparin (LMWH), warfarin, dabigatran, apixaban, or rivaroxaban. Inferior vena cava (IVC) filters may be considered for patients at high risk of VTE with contraindications to anticoagulation.

Treatment of VTE can be separated into two subsets: isolated deep venous thrombosis (DVT) and pulmonary embolism (PE). Both scenarios require anticoagulation in the absence of contraindication; however, PE with major impact on cardiovascular and pulmonary systems may benefit from thrombolytic therapy. The Chest Guidelines for initial therapy of DVT and PE recommend IV anticoagulation (e.g., heparin, or argatroban in heparin-induced thrombocytopenia) or oral rivaroxaban. Treatment of initial VTE should be for 3 months with LMWH, fondaparinux, or warfarin. The NOACs also have gained approval for VTE treatment. Patients who have VTE but are unable to be anticoagulated may benefit from an IVC filter.

The presentation of PE consists of dyspnea, chest pain, and occasionally hemoptysis. Massive PE is defined as PE associated with hypotension (systolic blood pressure <90 mm Hg) and shock. It occurs in approximately 4.5% of all PEs and is associated with a very high mortality rate (~50%). The gold standard diagnostic tool of PE is pulmonary angiography, but it is typically not required because computed tomography angiography (CTA) of the chest has high sensitivity and specificity. V/Q nuclear medicine scan is occasionally used for diagnosis of patients with suspected PE who are hemodynamically stable but have contraindications to CTA. Echocardiography for PE may be useful in hypotensive patients who are unable to have CTA of the chest. Echocardiography is neither sensitive nor specific, but new right ventricular dilation and dysfunction are suggestive of massive PE in the setting of suspected PE. Thrombus may be identified in the right-sided heart structures or in the pulmonary artery. Furthermore, a normal right ventricle in a hypotensive patient makes PE an unlikely etiology.

Hemodynamically stable PE requires no additional treatment beyond anticoagulation. Treatment of massive PE focuses on reperfusion of the lung and dissolution of the thrombus and systemic thrombolytic therapy as recommended by the Chest Guidelines and European Society of Cardiology. If contraindications exist to systemic thrombolytic therapy, then catheter-guided thrombolytic therapy, catheter-guided embolectomy, or surgical embolectomy should be considered because of the high mortality rate. If evidence of thrombus is found in the right ventricle, surgical embolectomy may be preferred to catheter-guided embolectomy. Supportive care includes respiratory support with intubation and mechanical ventilation and hemodynamic therapy with vasopressors and inotropes.

Sepsis

Infection and sepsis account for approximately 21% of all admissions to the ICU with approximately 750,000 cases per year. The most common sites of infection are respiratory, bloodstream, genitourinary, abdominal, and prosthetic device infections. The mortality rate from severe sepsis has improved significantly but remains approximately 18% to 30%. Anesthesiologists encounter patients with sepsis in several settings, including the operating room for source control of the infection (e.g., ureteral stents for pyelonephritis or hydronephrosis, exploratory laparotomy for GI-derived sepsis), offsite locations (e.g., diagnostic radiology, interventional radiology, GI laboratory for endoscopic retrograde cholangiopancreatography [ERCP]), and the ICU for supportive procedures and management (e.g., intubation, vascular access procedures, arterial catheter placement).

Sepsis is defined along a spectrum that requires suspected or confirmed infection and the systemic inflammatory response syndrome (SIRS). SIRS criteria include temperature dysregulation (>38.3°C or <36.0°C), tachycardia (heart rate >90 beats/min), tachypnea (respiratory rate >20 breaths/min), and leukocytosis or leukopenia. Severe sepsis includes the criteria for sepsis and objective evidence of organ dysfunction. Septic shock is vasodilatory shock unresponsive to aggressive fluid resuscitation. It must be reiterated that sepsis is a syndrome, and its presentation can vary as widely as the infections that cause sepsis. Presentation also depends on associated organ system dysfunction and preexisting medical conditions such as cardiac disease and COPD.

The initial treatment of patients with sepsis revolves around three concepts: source control, antibiotics, and early goal-directed resuscitation. Initial evaluation of patients with suspected sepsis should focus on anatomic etiology of the infection. A detailed history and physical examination can help guide the diagnostic workup. IV access should be obtained, and laboratory inquiries, including blood cultures, CBC, CMP, lipase, coagulation parameters, and lactate. Radiographic workup will likely involve chest radiography and may involve more advanced imaging such as CT. If an anatomic infection is identified, then source control by surgery, interventional radiology, or ERCP may be required.

Empiric broad-spectrum antibiotics should be started early for a patient with suspected sepsis. Antiviral and antifungal agents should be considered in patients at risk for such infections. Targeted antibiotic therapy should be delayed until a causative organism is identified and sensitivities to antibiotics are determined.

The Surviving Sepsis Campaign recommends protocolized resuscitation in patients presenting with sepsis-associated hypotension and elevated blood lactate levels. Treatment goals include a central venous pressure of 8 to 12 mm Hg by aggressive

21

crystalloid administration, a mean arterial pressure of 65 mm Hg by vasopressors as needed, urine output greater than 0.5 mL/kg per hour, and a central venous oxygen saturation of 70% by RBC transfusion for hematocrit greater than 30%. Inotropic support should be considered as needed. Early goal-directed therapy improves mortality rates and decreases organ system dysfunction. Norepinephrine is considered the vasopressor of choice in septic shock and vasopressin is often added as a second-line agent if needed. Lactate clearance is also a well-defined goal of sepsis resuscitation.

It must be noted that the protocolized resuscitation recommendations from the Surviving Sepsis Campaign have been questioned with emerging data from large randomized controlled trials comparing nonprotocolized care to protocolized early goal-directed therapy in early sepsis patients and found no differences in mortality rate, length of hospital stay, or duration of organ system support. In light of this new information, the sepsis guidelines may be modified.

Sepsis presents a major challenge for patients with preexisting cardiac disease because the vasodilatory state places increased workload on the heart. Patients with compromised hearts may have significant difficulty meeting this demand, and the mortality rate of patients with heart failure in sepsis may be as high as 70%. Furthermore, it is well established that the septic state includes potent myocardial depression. Advanced hemodynamic monitoring with a pulmonary artery catheter, echocardiography, transpulmonary thermodilution, or pulse-waveform analysis may be useful for hemodynamic optimization.

Perioperative anesthetic management of patients includes all of the considerations discussed earlier, including antibiotics and resuscitation with IV fluids and vasopressors. The induction and maintenance of anesthesia can be a considerable challenge because most agents are vasodilatory in nature. Consideration can be given to ketamine and etomidate, although concern about adrenal suppression after single-dose etomidate exists. If propofol is used, dose reduction should be strongly considered. The minimum alveolar concentration of anesthetic gases is decreased in sepsis. Hemodynamic monitoring with arterial and central venous catheters, pulmonary artery catheter, pulse pressure variation, or transesophageal echocardiography may be considered. Recovery in the ICU and postoperative intubation may also be considered.

SUGGESTED READING

Acute Respiratory Distress Syndrome Network. Ventilation with lower tidal volumes as compared with traditional tidal volumes for acute lung injury and the acute respiratory distress syndrome. *N Engl J Med*. 2000;342:1301–1308.

Amsterdam EA, Wenger NK, Brindis RG, et al. 2014 AHA/ACC guideline for the management of patients with non-ST-elevation acute coronary syndromes: a report of the American College of Cardiology/American Heart Association Task Force on Practice Guidelines. *J Am Coll Cardiol*. 2014;64:e139–e228.

Angus DC. The acute respiratory distress syndrome. *JAMA*. 2012;307.

ARISE Investigators, ANZICS Clinical Trials Group, Peake SL, Delaney A, et al. Goal-directed resuscitation for patients with early septic shock. *N Engl J Med*. 2014;371:1496–1506.

Brueckmann B, Villa-Uribe JL, Bateman BT, et al. Development and validation of a score for prediction of postoperative respiratory complications. *Anesthesiology*. 2013;118:1276–1285.

Eissa D, Carton EG, Buggy DJ. Anaesthetic management of patients with severe sepsis. *Br J Anaesth*. 2010;105:734–743.

Fleisher LA, Fleischmann KE, Auerbach AD, et al. 2014 ACC/AHA guideline on perioperative cardiovascular evaluation and management of patients undergoing noncardiac surgery: a report of the American College of Cardiology/American Heart Association Task Force on Practice Guidelines. *Circulation*. 2014;130:e278–e333.

Guérin C, Reignier J, Richard J-C, et al. Prone positioning in severe acute respiratory distress syndrome. *N Engl J Med*. 2013;368:2159–2168.

Gupta H, Ramanan B, Gupta PK, et al. Impact of COPD on postoperative outcomes. *Chest*. 2013;143:1599.

Guyatt GH, Akl EA, Crowther M, et al, American College of Chest Physicians Antithrombotic Therapy and Prevention of Thrombosis Panel: Executive summary: antithrombotic therapy and prevention of thrombosis, 9th ed: American College of Chest Physicians Evidence-Based Clinical Practice Guidelines. *Chest*. 2012; 141:pp 7S–47S.

Hawn MT, Graham LA, Richman JS, et al. Risk of major adverse cardiac events following noncardiac surgery in patients with coronary stents. *JAMA*. 2013;310:1462–1472.

Konstantinides SV, Torbicki A, Agnelli G, et al. 2014 ESC guidelines on the diagnosis and management of acute pulmonary embolism: The Task Force for the Diagnosis and Management of Acute Pulmonary Embolism of the European Society of Cardiology (ESC). Endorsed by the European Respiratory Society (ERS). *Eur Heart J*. 2014;35:3033–3037.

Matthay MA. Resolution of pulmonary edema. Thirty years of progress. *Am J Respir Crit Care Med*. 2014;189:1301–1308.

Mebazaa A, Pang PS, Tavares M, et al. The impact of early standard therapy on dyspnoea in patients with acute heart failure: the URGENT-dyspnoea study. *Eur Heart J*. 2010;31:832–841.

National Heart, Lung, and Blood Institute Acute Respiratory Distress Syndrome (ARDS) Clinical Trials Network, Wiedemann HP, Wheeler AP, et al. Comparison of two fluid-management strategies in acute lung injury. *N Engl J Med*. 2006;354:2564–2575.

Papazian L, Forel J-M, Gacouin A, et al. ACURASYS study investigators: neuromuscular blockers in early acute respiratory distress syndrome. *N Engl J Med*. 2010;363:1107–1116.

Pham HP, Shaz BH. Update on massive transfusion. *Br J Anaesth*. 2013;111(suppl 1):i71–i82.

ProCESS Investigators. A randomized trial of protocol-based care for early septic shock. *N Engl J Med*. 2014;370:1683–1693.

Chapter 22

Reducing Major Adverse Cardiac Events and All-Cause Mortality in Noncardiac Surgery: Perioperative Strategies

Antonio Pisano, MD • Michele Oppizzi, MD • Stefano Turi, MD • Giovanni Landoni, MD

Key Points

1. Major adverse cardiac events (MACEs) are relatively common in patients undergoing noncardiac surgical procedures. The incidence of perioperative myocardial infarction (PMI) is about 0.9%. However, a larger percentage of patients experiences a perioperative increase in cardiac troponins without other criteria for myocardial infarction (myocardial injury after noncardiac surgery [MINS]).
2. Preventive and therapeutic strategies for acute coronary syndromes are well established in the nonsurgical setting, but clear evidence about the impact of such strategies on both the incidence and outcomes of perioperative myocardial injury or PMI is lacking. Many therapeutic interventions that have cardioprotective properties may be difficult to apply, or even harmful, in the perioperative period.
3. Factors associated with an increased risk of MACE are patient specific (advanced age, high American Society of Anesthesiologists (ASA) class, kidney disease, anemia) and surgery specific (type of procedure, urgency, complexity, intraoperative complications). Several scoring systems allow clinicians to predict, both preoperatively (e.g., Revised Cardiac Risk Index, National Surgical Quality Improvement Program) and intraoperatively (e.g., ANESCARDIOCAT), the risk of cardiac adverse events and to identify patients who need preventive measures and strict intraoperative and postoperative monitoring.
4. Risk stratification is pivotal in patients with PMI or MINS because therapeutic options also depend on a careful balance between the risk of mortality associated with the cardiac complications and the risks (primarily bleeding) of therapeutic strategies (dual-antiplatelet therapy, percutaneous coronary interventions [PCIs]).
5. The Thrombolysis in Myocardial Infarction and Global Registry of Acute Cardiac Events scores allow reliable prediction of 30-day, 6-month, and 12-month mortality rates in patients with ST-segment elevation MI (STEMI) and non–ST segment elevation MI (NSTEMI), respectively. Conversely, the risk of bleeding may be predicted according to the type of surgical procedure and patient-related factors (CRUSADE [Can Rapid Risk Stratification of Unstable Angina Patients Suppress Adverse Outcomes With Early Implementation of the ACC/AHA Guidelines] score).
6. NSTEMI is the most common type of PMI. Unlike STEMI, it is often caused by an impaired balance between myocardial oxygen supply and demand in the absence of complete

occlusion of a coronary vessel. Accordingly, the need for urgent revascularization is less stringent compared with STEMI, but prevention or prompt treatment of anemia, hypotension, hypoxia, pain, and tachycardia is of primary importance.

7. PCI should always be considered in patients with perioperative STEMI, especially in patients with good life expectancy and moderate to large infarctions. Probably, only patients at low risk of death and at high risk of bleeding should be treated with medical therapy alone.

8. Aspirin and low-dose oral β-blockers should be initiated within 24 hours in all patients with MINS unless contraindicated. A platelet receptor $P2Y_{12}$ inhibitor (clopidogrel, prasugrel, ticagrelor) may be added when bleeding risk is decreased sufficiently. Angiotensin-converting enzyme inhibitors should be started in patients with an ejection fraction of less than 40%, hypertension, or diabetes, including those with stable chronic kidney disease.

9. A novel Web-enabled, "democracy-based" approach to consensus building has been used to summarize the best-quality and most widely agreed-on evidence about mortality reduction in different settings, including the noncardiac surgical perioperative period.

10. Hemodynamic optimization, noninvasive ventilation, neuraxial anesthesia, selective decontamination of the digestive tract, and avoidance of β-blocker initiation shortly before surgical procedures may improve survival in patients undergoing noncardiac operations. Tranexamic acid may also be considered to reduce mortality rates, but further investigations are needed.

11. Intraaortic balloon pump, volatile anesthetic agents, leukocyte-depleted red blood cell transfusions, protective ventilation, and vacuum-assisted closure therapy have been shown to reduce mortality rates in other settings, especially in cardiac surgical procedures. It is reasonable to assume that these interventions will have similar beneficial effects in noncardiac surgical settings.

12. Further strategies that deserve to be investigated for a possible impact on survival in patients undergoing noncardiac surgery include nutritional support and vitamin supplementation, sedation, inspired oxygen fraction, high-flow nasal cannula oxygen, early renal replacement therapy, extracorporeal mechanical circulatory support, and point-of-care coagulation testing.

Despite technical improvements, major surgical procedures currently remain associated with high mortality and morbidity rates. In Europe, an overall 30-day mortality rate of 4% has been reported after major noncardiac operations, and the rate can reach 6% in high-risk populations.

About half of these deaths are attributable to *major adverse cardiac events* (MACEs) including nonfatal cardiac arrest, acute myocardial infarction (AMI), congestive heart failure (HF), or new cardiac arrhythmias. Cardiac complications are the most common causes of postoperative morbidity and death; they occur in up to 5% of adult patients undergoing surgical procedures and have a major impact on both length and costs of hospitalization. Perioperative myocardial infarction (PMI) is the most dangerous cardiac complication, and coronary artery disease (CAD) is a major determinant of both early and late mortality rates.

PERIOPERATIVE MYOCARDIAL INFARCTION OR INJURY

According to the third universal definition, *myocardial infarction* (MI) is defined as a rise and fall in cardiac troponin (cTn) with at least one value above the 99th percentile upper reference limit (>0.014 ng/mL), together with at least one of the following:

- Ischemic chest pain
- New and significant electrocardiographic (ECG) changes such as ST segment or T-wave changes, left bundle branch block, or Q waves

- New regional wall motion abnormalities (echocardiography)
- Intracoronary thrombus (angiography or autopsy)

Myocardial injury after noncardiac surgery (MINS) is defined as (1) an elevation of postoperative troponin with an ischemic origin, (2) without other criteria of PMI, (3) that is prognostically relevant. Two different mechanisms lead to PMI: PMI type 1 is caused by rupture of a vulnerable coronary plaque or, uncommonly, by severe coronary vasospasm, leading to platelet aggregation, occlusive (ST-segment elevation [STEMI]) or nonocclusive (ST-segment depression [NSTEMI]) thrombus formation, and prolonged myocardial ischemia resulting in cell death. Plaque disruption is demonstrated in autopsy studies in approximately 50% of patients who died of PMI. PMI type 2 usually results from a sustained imbalance between myocardial oxygen supply (decreased) and demand (increased) combined with the presence of significant, obstructive, but not occlusive, CAD. Most patients with PMI type 2 have ST-segment depression (NSTEMI). Patients undergoing major operations are particularly prone to ischemic adverse events because of the surgery-associated inflammation and hypercoagulable state, as well as perioperative factors that increase the risk of plaque rupture (pain, hypertension, elevated levels of catecholamines), increase myocardial oxygen demand (hypertension, tachycardia, elevated left ventricular [LV] diastolic pressure), or decrease myocardial oxygen supply (blood loss, anemia, hypotension, hypoxia, tachycardia, coronary vasoconstriction). NSTEMI is the most common type of PMI. Compared with patients with STEMI, patients with NSTEMI are generally older, have multivessel or left main CAD more frequently, and often have multiple risk factors and comorbidities.

Epidemiology of Perioperative Myocardial Infarction

Perioperative myocardial infarction occurs in 0.88% of patients hospitalized for major noncardiac surgery. However, the incidence is widely variable according to the different populations, the type of surgical procedures (major or minor, vascular or nonvascular), the different definitions, and the troponin cutoff values used. Overall, the rate of PMI (especially STEMI) has declined in the past few years, thanks to many factors, including a careful risk stratification, more appropriate medical treatment and preoperative myocardial revascularization of higher risk patients, wider use of less invasive surgical approaches, and optimization of perioperative care. Most PMIs (≈80%) occur on the ward, especially 48 to 72 hours postoperatively; only 20% of PMIs develop in the operating room. However, the risk remains elevated during the first 2 postoperative weeks in patients undergoing orthopedic surgical procedures. Patients usually exhibit the strongest stress reaction within 72 hours postoperatively. Several factors may affect the myocardial oxygen delivery (DO_2)–myocardial oxygen consumption (MVO_2) balance, including discontinuation of medications or decreased doses, preoperative diet, electrolyte disorders, pain, anxiety, stress reactions, bleeding, neuroendocrine changes (increased catecholamine release triggered by postoperative pain and other stresses), and alterations in the coagulation mechanism.

Diagnosis of Myocardial Ischemia and Infarction

The diagnosis of myocardial ischemia may be overlooked in the perioperative period. Indeed, some patients with myocardial injury do not meet the diagnostic criteria for PMI. Typical anginal symptoms occur in less than half of the patients, and the symptoms are often masked by analgesics, advanced age, and diabetes. Some patients experience vague chest pain, shortness of breath, hemodynamic instability, and palpitations. Whereas ST segment depression is quite common, occurring in approximately 30% of patients, 20% of patients have T-wave inversion, and 10% have ST-segment elevation. Conversely, ECG changes may be only minor or transient in approximately 40% of patients. However, continuous ECG monitoring is not widely used, and its implementation is difficult.

Because neither clinical symptoms nor ECG changes can guarantee early recognition of PMI, the best diagnostic tool is cTn, which is also a strong independent predictor of short-term and intermediate-term mortality. However, the interpretation of cTn increase can be troublesome in some cases because of the interference of renal dysfunction, cerebral disease, and inflammation.

Risk Stratification and Prevention

The treatment of patients who develop a cardiac ischemic complication during or after noncardiac surgical procedures starts with prevention through the identification of factors and markers that can predict a complicated course. Variables significantly associated with an increased risk of MACE are (1) patient specific: old age, high American Society of Anesthesiologists (ASA) class and cardiac risk indexes, kidney disease, and anemia and (2) surgery specific: type of procedure (emergency or urgent, major operation, particularly vascular) and intraoperative complications (severe hypotension, serious bleeding, increased heart rate).

Patient's Age

The risk of PMI and MINS is nearly doubled in patients older than 70 years, especially in men with cardiovascular (CV) risk factors. Mortality and death from CAD are strongly associated with age. As a consequence of the aging population, it is estimated that this problem will increase in future decades. Older patients are more frail, have multiple comorbidities, and exhibit more severe CAD. They also tend to present greater technical challenges during percutaneous coronary intervention (PCI) because of heavier coronary artery calcification, tortuous anatomy in coronary and peripheral arteries, increased risk of procedure-related complications (e.g., contrast-induced nephropathy, vascular or neurologic complications), and reduced tolerance to bleeding.

Cardiac Risk Indexes

Two clinical indexes are used to estimate patients' risk of perioperative cardiac complications. The Revised Cardiac Risk Index (RCRI) incorporates six independent variables that predict the risk of cardiac complications: history of ischemic heart disease, HF, cerebrovascular disease, diabetes mellitus, chronic kidney disease (serum creatinine >2 mg/dL), and major operations (suprainguinal vascular, intrathoracic, and intraperitoneal). Perioperative risk of both cardiac complications (e.g., nonfatal AMI and nonfatal cardiac arrest) and death increases with index scores. For example, in a large cohort study including 782,969 patients, the in-hospital mortality rates were 1.4% for RCRI of 0, 2.2% for RCRI of 1, 3.9% for RCRI of 2, 5.8% for RCRI of 3, and 7.4% for RCRI of 4 and greater.

The RCRI is currently the most widely used cardiac risk stratification tool. However, it has several limitations, including its relatively low discriminative ability. In fact, although the RCRI has a moderately good ability to discriminate patients who will develop cardiac events from those who will not after mixed noncardiac surgical procedures (area under the curve [AUC] 0.75), it is less accurate in patients undergoing vascular surgical procedures (AUC, 0.64), and it is less able to predict all-cause mortality (median AUC, 0.62).

To overcome these limitations of RCRI, the National Surgical Quality Improvement Program (NSQIP) score was developed and validated on 211,410 surgical patients. This model includes age, ASA class, functional status, abnormal serum creatinine, and a novel and more appropriate organ-based categorization of surgery. Risk may be quantified by a risk calculator on the Internet. The discriminative or predictive ability of the NSQIP score is significantly better as compared with RCRI (AUC, 0.88), and it works well also in vascular surgical patients.

Kidney Disease

The most important comorbidity associated with poor postoperative outcome is chronic kidney disease (CKD). The rate of adverse cardiac events and the length of hospital stay increase significantly in patients with impaired renal function, especially in those with CKD from stage 3b onward (estimated glomerular filtration rate <45 mL/min).

Most of the CV disease risk factors, such as older age, diabetes mellitus, systolic hypertension, and low levels of high-density lipoprotein cholesterol, in addition to an inflammatory and thrombogenic milieu, are highly prevalent in patients with CKD. CAD and valvular disease are more common and severe in these patients, with half of deaths resulting from cardiac causes. CKD-associated anemia also reduces myocardial oxygen supply and is associated with cardiomyopathy. LV hypertrophy increases myocardial demand and evolves toward diastolic dysfunction, impairing subendocardial perfusion, and may be complicated by diastolic HF (the stiff ventricle is more vulnerable to preload and afterload changes, tachycardia, and loss of atrial kick during atrial fibrillation or other arrhythmias).

Some precautions may be useful to reduce the risk of perioperative cardiac events in patients with CKD. Stress testing can identify patients with CAD. Discontinuation of angiotensin-converting enzyme (ACE) inhibitor therapy for at least 10 hours before general anesthesia is recommended to reduce the risk of postinduction hypotension. Anemia may require preoperative blood transfusion, supplementation with iron, or administration of erythropoietin. Patients with end-stage kidney disease should undergo dialysis the day before the operation.

The main goals during surgical procedures include a mean arterial pressure greater than 65 mm Hg (or higher for the uncontrolled hypertensive patient) and adequate volume status. Particular attention should be paid to analgesic requirements in the perioperative period. Opioids may accumulate in patients with CKD, with increased risk of respiratory depression, but nonsteroidal antiinflammatory drugs are not recommended because of the risk of worsening renal function.

In patients with renal impairment, it is appropriate to measure baseline values of troponin to compare them with the postoperative values. Troponin values may be elevated in the setting of even mild kidney disease, probably reflecting microinfarctions or LV hypertrophy.

Anemia and Blood Transfusion

The prevalence of preoperative anemia is increasing in the surgical population, especially in older patients. In a large (39,309 patients) European study, anemia (defined according to the WHO criteria, e.g., hemoglobin [Hb] <13 g/dL in men and <12 g/L in non-pregnant women) was found in 31% of men and 26% of women. Preoperative anemia is commonly associated with comorbidities such as kidney disease, CAD, HF, diabetes mellitus, and hepatic cirrhosis and is known to be associated with increased mortality rates. In fact, anemia reduces DO_2, increases heart rate, and may be complicated by hypotension.

After adjustment for major confounders including transfusion, preoperative anemia was strongly associated with a more than twofold increase in 90-day mortality rates, as well as increased postoperative intensive care unit (ICU) admission and greater use of ICU resources (hemodynamic monitoring, mechanical ventilation, inotropic and vasoactive agents). In particular, in-hospital mortality rates increase linearly with hematocrit reduction.

Although anemia is associated with mortality, transfusions may contribute to increased mortality rates (according to the "second hit" theory). However, recent data suggest that blood transfusions in the perioperative period may not necessarily be harmful and, particularly, that more liberal transfusion strategies are associated with reduced mortality rates in certain settings.

Patients at risk for anemia who are undergoing elective surgical procedures should be screened 4 to 8 weeks preoperatively, and the causes of anemia (e.g., blood loss, nutritional deficiencies, kidney disease, chronic or inflammatory diseases) should be identified and treated. Iron supplementation (oral or intravenous [IV], depending on iron status or tolerance and timing of the operation) is recommended (grade 1C recommendation) in patients with iron deficiency (serum ferritin <30 µg/L). The efficacy of iron supplementation in raising Hb concentration and decreasing perioperative transfusion rate is well demonstrated. If iron deficiency is ruled out, erythropoietin-stimulating agents administered up to an Hb concentration of 12 to 13 g/dL are suggested (grade 2A recommendation). The need for blood transfusions has been shown to be reduced by approximately 50% in patients treated with these drugs (data from pooled studies including mainly orthopedic surgical patients). The risk of thrombotic complications, particularly in patients with CAD, coronary stenting, or risk of venous thrombosis, should be considered.

Type of Surgical Procedure

The type of surgical procedure is a strong risk factor for MACE and death. Urgent or emergency operation has been well recognized as the strongest predictor of death, with an increase of more than three times in 30-day mortality rates. Unfortunately, this is a largely unmodifiable risk factor.

Perioperative myocardial infarction is more common in patients who are urgently hospitalized, particularly those undergoing vascular, thoracic, and noncardiac transplant surgery (which are all independent risk factors for PMI) compared with elective hospital admissions (adjusted odds ratio [OR], 2.38).

Vascular surgical procedures are associated with a two- to fourfold higher risk of adverse cardiac events (PMI, cardiac death) compared with other types of noncardiac operations. In fact, CAD is more common among patients undergoing vascular surgical procedures (with a prevalence ranging from 37% to 78%) than in other noncardiac surgical patients. Aortic cross-clamping and declamping, abrupt changes in systemic arterial pressure, fluid shifts, hypoxia induced by one-lung ventilation, acute anemia secondary to major bleeding, and inflammatory or hypercoagulable states induced by both surgical procedures and transfusions can trigger perioperative ischemia and MI, especially in patients with CAD, acute HF, or LV dysfunction.

In a recent retrospective investigation, surgical priority was found to be the only preoperative risk factor independently associated with PMI among patients undergoing major open vascular surgery (OR, 1.70). In this cohort of patients, the only postoperative variables associated with PMI were the nadir hematocrit and postoperative transfusion, thus suggesting that minimizing intraoperative blood loss and prioritizing early intraoperative transfusion may be potential ways for preventing myocardial damage.

The vascular procedure with the highest associated mortality rate is surgery for abdominal aortic aneurysmal rupture, followed by elective thoracoabdominal aortic replacement, lower extremity arterial bypass, and carotid endarterectomy. Patients requiring lower extremity amputation also have diffuse and severe CAD (up to 92% in a pathologic study). Accordingly, perioperative risk is high in these patients, with reported 30-day mortality rates of up to 17% and PMI as the leading cause of postprocedural death. Conversely, endovascular aortic repair (EVAR) procedures are associated with reduced myocardial stress and, accordingly, with a decreased incidence of perioperative myocardial damage. However, an increase in troponin levels after EVAR was associated with a higher long-term incidence of adverse cardiac events (49 vs. 15% in a follow-up period of 3 years).

Altered Preoperative Coagulation

A recent substudy of an international prospective cohort investigation of perioperative CV events in noncardiac surgery (VISION) found that the preoperative elevation of blood markers of hypercoagulability was associated with an increased risk of MINS in patients undergoing vascular surgery. In particular, as compared with patients with no myocardial injury, patients with MINS showed a significantly higher concentration of factor VIII (186 vs 155%; $P = .006$), von Willebrand factor activity (223 vs 160%; $P < .001$), von Willebrand factor concentration (317 vs 237%; $P = .02$), fibrinogen concentration (5.6 vs 4.2 g/L; $P = .03$), D-dimer (1680.0 vs. 1090.0 ng/mL; $P = .04$), plasmin-antiplasmin complex (747 vs 512 ng/mL; $P = .002$), and C-reactive protein (10 vs 4.5 mg/L; $P = .02$).

Cardiac Biomarkers

Preoperative Troponin

Cardiac troponin has high sensitivity for detection of small amounts of myocardial necrosis. Increased cTn levels indicate the presence of, but not the underlying reason for, myocardial injury. Besides AMI, troponin release may be associated with many other disorders, including HF, sepsis, and end-stage kidney disease (Box 22.1). Regardless of the cause of cTn release, elevated cTn levels almost always imply a poor prognosis. Elevated preoperative cTn values are found in a variable proportion of patients undergoing vascular surgical procedures. In the largest trial available, the preoperative finding of increased cTn (high-sensitive troponin T, hsTnT) was present in up to 24% of patients, and it was independently associated with a significantly higher risk of PMI, cardiac death, and all-cause death. Moreover, hsTnT showed an additive value (AUC, 0.80) in association with cardiac risk index (AUC, 0.65) and natriuretic peptide levels (AUC, 0.76). A combined endpoint (including all-cause death, PMI, acute HF, and cardiac arrest) occurred in 9.4% of patients with hsTnT levels higher than 0.014 ng/mL compared with 1.9% in patients with hsTnT levels of up to 0.014 ng/mL ($P < .001$). Possible causes of elevated cTn associated with adverse outcomes include silent myocardial ischemia or microinfarction, LV dysfunction, cerebrovascular disease, renal impairment, sepsis, pulmonary hypertension, and pulmonary embolism. The need to add cTn to routine preoperative tests performed in high-risk surgical patients is still debated. According to the 2014 European Society of Cardiology/European Society of Anaesthesiology (ESC/ESA) guidelines, the assessment of cTn in high-risk patients, both before and 48 to 72 hours after major surgical procedures, may be considered (class IIb, level B), even if the suboptimal specificity of this test should be taken into account. A practical approach in patients with preoperatively increased troponin levels involves a baseline transthoracic echocardiogram (primarily assessing ventricular function and regional wall motion), a cardiology consultation, and when feasible, deferral of surgery until the troponin levels fall (Fig. 22.1). If it is not possible to postpone the procedure, a less-invasive surgical approach, targeted perioperative

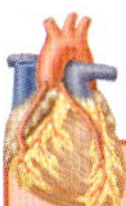

BOX 22.1	*Causes of Troponin Elevation in the Absence of Myocardial Ischemia*

Cardiac Causes

- Heart failure
- Cardiac arrhythmias
- Cardioversion
- Implantable cardioverter-defibrillator shock
- Myocarditis
- Pericarditis
- Cardiac amyloidosis

Noncardiac Causes

- Sepsis and septic shock
- Pulmonary embolism
- Primary pulmonary hypertension
- Pulmonary edema
- Chronic kidney disease
- Stroke
- Subarachnoid hemorrhage
- High dose of chemotherapy
- Sympathomimetic drugs

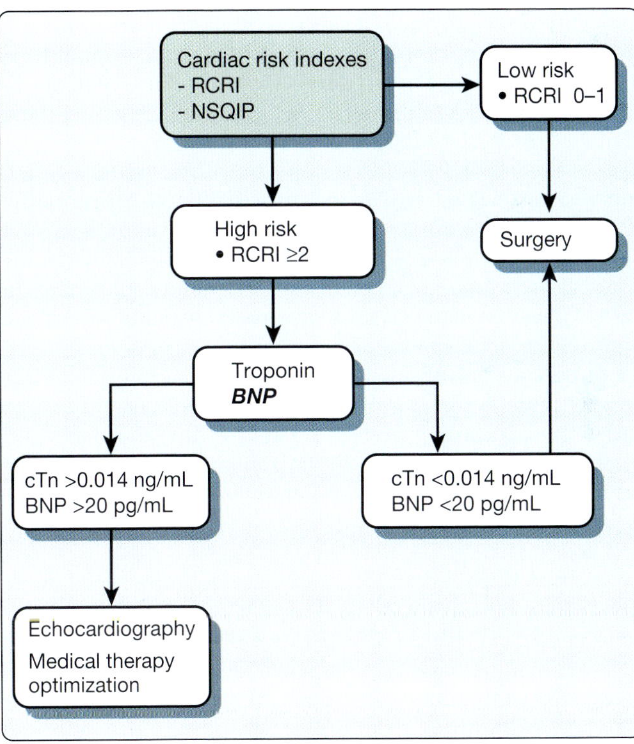

Fig. 22.1 Preoperative risk stratification. *BNP,* Brain natriuretic peptide; *cTn,* cardiac troponin; *NSQIP,* National Surgical Quality Improvement Program; *RCRI,* Revised Cardiac Risk Index.

monitoring, and careful cardiac optimization should be recommended. Moreover, patients should be informed about the increased risk.

Postoperative Troponin

Evaluation of peak cTn level during the first 3 days after noncardiac surgical procedures improves the ability to identify patients with myocardial damage, even in the absence of symptoms or ECG changes. Moreover, this value is an independent predictor of 30-day mortality. In a recent large international cohort study involving 15,065 patients aged 45 years or older from five continents, an abnormal value of TnT ($\geq$0.04 ng/mL) was found in 8% of patients within 3 days after noncardiac surgical procedures and was an independent predictor of 30-day mortality rates (9.8% vs 1.1%; adjusted ratio, 4.82). In another cohort study including 2216 participants older than 60 years of age who were undergoing medium-risk to high-risk noncardiac surgical procedures, an elevation of cTnI (>0.06 ng/mL) was recorded in 19% of patients. The 30-day mortality rate in these patients was 8.6% compared with 2.2% in patients without cTnI elevation ($P < .001$). The relative risk of death was 2.4 for patients with lower increases in cTnI (0.07–0.59 ng/mL) and 4.2 for patients with higher increases ($\geq$0.60 ng/mL). The median time to death was 12 days.

A recent meta-analysis of 11 studies including, overall, 2193 patients undergoing noncardiac, nonvascular surgery, found that postoperative troponin elevation was strongly associated with MACE at 30 days (OR, 5.92) and 1 year after surgery (adjusted OR, 3.0) and was a predictor of 30-day mortality (OR, 3.52) and an independent predictor of 1-year mortality (adjusted OR, 2.53).

A strong association between postoperative cTn elevation and both short- and long-term mortality was confirmed in two recent large observational investigations. Among 21,842 patients who underwent noncardiac surgery, multivariate analysis showed that peak postoperative hsTnT levels were correlated with 30-day mortality; in particular, 30-day mortality rates were 3%, 9.1%, and 29.6% in patients with an hsTnT value of 20 to 64 ng/L (hazard ratio [HR], 23.63), 65 to 999 ng/L (HR, 70.34), and 1000 ng/L or greater (HR, 222.01), respectively. An absolute hsTnT change of 5 ng/L or higher was associated with an increased risk of 30-day mortality (HR, 4.69).

A gradual association between postoperative TnT elevation and both short- and long-term mortality rates was also found among 12,882 vascular surgery patients, with the greatest hazard ratio for mortality within the first 10 months after surgery.

Postoperative cTn surveillance is cost effective in patients older than 45 years of age. According to the abovementioned evidence, it seems to be useful for early identification of patients at increased risk of myocardial injury and death and may also allow prompt initiation of appropriate therapeutic interventions. Optimization of perioperative care, including prevention of hypotension, tachycardia, anemia, hypoxia, pain, hypoglycemia, and hypothermia, may prevent postoperative troponin elevation and major cardiac events and potentially reduce mortality rates.

B-Type (Brain) Natriuretic Peptides

B-type (brain) natriuretic peptides (BNPs) are released from myocardium in response to multiple physiologic stimuli, including ischemia, myocardial stretch, inflammation, and other neuroendocrine triggers. Preoperative BNP levels are strong independent predictors of adverse short-term CV outcome. The preoperative addition of BNPs to the widely used risk stratification systems (RCRI and functional capacity assessment) leads to a significantly improved risk discrimination (AUC from 65% to 80%). The predictive value of N-terminal pro–brain natriuretic peptide (NT-proBNP) seems to be higher as compared with BNP, probably because it is more indicative of baseline conditions and is less affected by transient fluctuations in concentrations, given its longer half-life.

The optimal cutoffs of BNPs to predict CV events after surgical procedures are approximately 20 to 30 pg/mL for BNP (with 95% sensitivity and 44% specificity) and approximately 125 pg/mL for NT-proBNP. In a relatively small prospective study in high-risk patients undergoing major noncardiac operations, a preoperative BNP level greater than 40 pg/mL allowed identification of patients with an almost sevenfold increased risk of cardiac events. In particular, each 100-pg/mL increase in BNP levels was associated with a 35% increase in the relative risk of death. The utility of BNP testing in patients with kidney disease is controversial.

Finally, the negative predictive value of normal BNP levels (<20 pg/mL) to indicate a favorable postoperative outcome is as high as 96%, a finding suggesting that patients with normal levels of BNPs may proceed directly to surgery with no additional preoperative cardiac testing.

Postoperative (days 1–3) measurement of BNPs in addition to preoperative values significantly improve the prediction of death or nonfatal MI at both 30 days (OR, 3.7) and more than 180 days. An individual patient data meta-analysis including 2051 patients demonstrated that patients with postoperative BNP values of 0 to 250 pg/mL, greater than 250 to 400 pg/mL, and greater than 400 pg/mL reached a composite endpoint, including 30-day death and nonfatal MI at a rate of 6.6%, 15.7%, and 29.5%, respectively.

No prospective, randomized, controlled trials (RCTs) investigated the use of BNP-guided management in perioperative medicine. Nevertheless, according to a meta-analysis of RCTs that showed a 48% reduction in all-cause mortality rates with BNP-guided therapy in nonsurgical patients with HF, the following approach seems reasonable (Fig. 22.1). In the presence of clinical risk factors and/or reduced physical capacity, measurement of BNPs should be performed 4 to 5 weeks before a scheduled major operation. If BNP levels are lower than the optimal cutoff (20 pg/mL), the patient can proceed with the surgical procedure without the need for further testing. Conversely, if BNP levels are higher than this threshold, further testing, primarily echocardiography and (BNP-guided) optimization of medical therapy (e.g., fluid restriction, diuretics, ACE inhibitors, nitrates, β-blocking agents) may be recommended. At the same time, worsening of renal function and hypotension, sometimes also induced by ACE inhibitors themselves, must be prevented. Specific therapeutic interventions may be considered in selected cases, for example, cardiac resynchronization therapy in patients with symptomatic NYHA functional class III disease with an LV ejection fraction (LVEF) of less than 35% and a large QRS complex (>120 ms) or transcatheter mitral clip implantation in patients with severe functional mitral regurgitation. Repeating assessment of BNPs shortly before the surgical procedure may allow for adjustment of perioperative treatment strategies (e.g., choice of surgical and anesthetic techniques, perioperative monitoring, fluid, drugs, and management of devices).

Perioperative Risk Indices

Intraoperative factors identified as independent predictors of adverse postoperative cardiac events are related to the surgical intervention (vascular surgical procedures), complexity (e.g., duration of the procedure, need for blood transfusions), and urgency, as well as to physiologic insults (tachycardia, prolonged hypotension or hypertension, hypothermia).

A meta-analysis of 14 studies, including mainly nonrandomized evidence, found a strong association between the need for blood transfusions and postoperative cardiac events. Unfortunately, it was not possible to define an accurate point estimate associated with the risk of adverse cardiac events. CV physiologic variables (e.g., >20 mm Hg fall in mean arterial pressure lasting >60 min, >30% increase in baseline systolic pressure, tachycardia in the recovery room, and transmitral flow propagation <45 cm/s) were shown to be independently associated with adverse outcomes in some of the included studies. In the only investigation that controlled for blood transfusions, the aforementioned association was not observed. This finding suggests that changes in

22

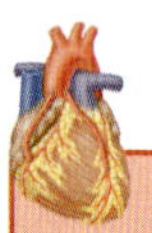

BOX 22.2	*Seven ANESCARDIOCAT Score Factors*[a]

- History of CAD
- History of chronic CHF
- History of cerebrovascular disease
- Chronic kidney disease
- Preoperative abnormal ECG (LV hypertrophy, LBBB, ST-T abnormalities)
- Intraoperative hypotension (≥20 mm Hg or ≥20% fall in MAP for >1 hour)
- Blood transfusion

[a]Risk of major adverse cardiac and cerebrovascular events: 0 factors, 1.5%; 1 factor, 4.5%; 2 factors, 8.9%; ≥3 factors, 20.6%.

CAD, Coronary artery disease; *CHF*, congestive heart failure; *ECG*, electrocardiogram; *LBBB*, left bundle branch block; *LV*, left ventricular; *MAP*, mean arterial pressure.

From Sabaté S, Mases A, Guilera N, et al. Incidence and predictors of major perioperative adverse cardiac and cerebrovascular events in noncardiac surgery. *Br J Anaesth*. 2011;107:879–890.

physiologic variables (e.g., hypotension, tachycardia, and hypothermia) may jointly contribute with anemia to the increased cardiac risk observed in patients needing blood transfusions; however, these variables become independently predictive only in the absence of the need for blood transfusions.

The ANESCARDIOCAT score (Box 22.2) stratifies patients undergoing elective or emergency noncardiac interventions of intermediate to high surgery-specific risk in four groups with different (very low, low, intermediate, and high) degrees of risk of major adverse cardiac and cerebrovascular events (MACCE). This scoring system is based on the following factors: intraoperative hypotension, defined as 1 hour of a 20 mm Hg or greater decrease or a 20% change in mean arterial pressure; need for blood transfusion; history of CAD, HF, or cerebrovascular disease; CKD; and baseline ECG abnormalities, including LV hypertrophy, left bundle branch block, and ST-segment and T-wave abnormalities. The predicted rate of MACCE is 1.5% if none of these factors is present (very low risk), 4.5% in the presence of one factor (low risk), 8.9% in the presence of two factors (intermediate risk), and 20.6% when three or more factors are present (high risk). Among the foregoing predictors of postoperative adverse cardiac events, physiologic variables (and, to a certain extent, transfusions) are the main factors potentially modifiable by anesthesiologists and may thus offer an opportunity to improve patients' outcomes.

Postoperative Management

In patients at high risk for PMI, an electrocardiogram and a blood sample for troponin should be obtained at baseline, immediately postoperatively, and after 6 and 12 hours, as well as once a day for the first 3 postoperative days to detect early myocardial damage. As mentioned, ECG abnormalities such as ST-segment depression, transient ST-segment elevation, or prominent T-wave inversions may be present, but they are not required for the diagnosis of PMI or perioperative myocardial injury. Consultation with a cardiologist is always appropriate. Echocardiography is helpful for detecting the site and extension of regional wall motion abnormalities and to quantify global cardiac function.

Adequate analgesia and sedation are pivotal to prevent or minimize the deleterious effects of sympathetic stimulation on myocardial ischemia. Of course, hemodynamic stability plays a key role in preventing adverse cardiac events; adequate DO_2 should be maintained by adequate Hb levels (≥ 8 g/dL at least, although higher Hb values, e.g., between 9 and 10 g/dL, may be desirable to improve outcome).

Finally, active prevention of infection may help reduce the incidence of PMI, given both the "hemodynamic" changes induced by sepsis, or simply by fever (e.g., tachycardia), and the myocardial dysfunction associated with sepsis and septic shock.

MEDICATIONS AND PERCUTANEOUS INTERVENTIONS TO PREVENT AND TREAT PERIOPERATIVE MAJOR ADVERSE CARDIAC EVENTS

Few RCTs evaluated the efficacy of medical or interventional treatments in reducing in-hospital and long-term outcomes after PMI in noncardiac surgical procedures. Accordingly, the following considerations about drug therapy and PCI for PMI are mainly extrapolated from evidence on management of acute coronary syndromes in the nonsurgical setting by adapting the strategies generally used in the coronary care unit (CCU) to the scenario of the perioperative ICU.

Statins

Statins (3-hydroxy-3-methyl-glutaryl–coenzyme A reductase inhibitors) contribute to plaque stability by means of reducing plaque size (through lipid lowering), modifying the physicochemical properties of the lipid core, and decreasing oxidative stress and inflammation (by inhibition of macrophage accumulation and metalloprotease production).

Among the drugs used for the treatment of PMI, statins are the easiest to handle. Indeed, contraindications (e.g., pregnancy, acute hepatic injury, porphyria) are uncommon, and high doses are usually safe (rhabdomyolysis and myopathy are infrequent) and well tolerated. However, critically ill patients with a complicated course should be closely monitored because they represent a population at increased risk of important statin side effects or drug interactions that may go unnoticed. In patients who require treatment with drugs that increase the plasma concentration of statins through interaction with CYP3A4 (e.g., calcium channel blockers, antifungal agents, and macrolides), the use of pravastatin or fluvastatin may be preferable because these statins are not primarily metabolized by CYP3A4. Conversely, rifampicin, phenobarbital, carbamazepine, and phenytoin induce both CYP3A4 and CYP2C9, thus leading to increased metabolism of liver-metabolized statins. Accordingly, the lipid-lowering effect of statins can be reduced by concomitant use of these drugs. Finally, when statin therapy is initiated or whenever any change in statin use occurs (except for pravastatin), careful monitoring of the international normalized ratio (INR) is recommended in patients taking warfarin because of the potential risk of bleeding complications.

Although the perioperative initiation of high-dose statins to prevent PMI seemed to be reasonable until recently, especially before vascular surgical procedures, new evidence suggests that such a strategy could be ineffective, if not even harmful. In the LOAD trial, 648 statin-naive patients at risk for cardiac events undergoing medium- to high-risk noncardiac surgery were randomized to receive atorvastatin 80 mg within 18 hours before surgery and 40 mg/day during the next 7 days, or placebo. No significant differences were observed in all-cause 30-day mortality, nonfatal MI, myocardial injury, and stroke. Although this trial was limited by lack of adequate statistical power and by high event rates, similar results have been recently found in cardiac surgery patients (see later) in whom the perioperative initiation of statins, in addition to being ineffective in preventing myocardial damage, was found to increase the risk of acute kidney injury. Adequately designed and powered RCTs should investigate the effectiveness of different statin regimens (e.g., longer preoperative courses) in preventing MACE after noncardiac surgery to draw a definitive conclusion about this topic.

β-Blockers

It is generally accepted that patients previously treated with β-blockers should receive these drugs in the perioperative period. β-Blocker therapy can be a double-edged sword, however. β-Blockers exert a cardioprotective effect by reducing MVO_2, the rate of atrial and ventricular arrhythmias, and mechanical stress on vulnerable plaques. However, they may cause hypotension and hinder an increase in cardiac output (CO) when it is required. Probably because of this ambivalence, in a large trial (POISE) the *intraoperative* use of β-blockers in *unselected patients* was shown to lead to a reduction in PMI, as well as to dangerous increases in stroke and mortality rates.

The rationale for the use of β-blockers in patients with ongoing MI is twofold: in the early hours, these drugs reduce infarct size; in the following days, they have an antiremodeling effect. Regarding the use of β-blockers in the CCU, the recommendations of the American Heart Association (AHA) and those of the ESC differ.

American Heart Association guidelines suggest that it is reasonable to administer IV β-blockers at admission, unless they are contraindicated, in patients with MI who are hypertensive or have ongoing ischemia, and that an oral β-blocker should be initiated in any patient without contraindications within the first 24 hours (class 1, level A). The main contraindications to β-blocker therapy include symptomatic HF, low-output states, a PQ interval greater than 0.24 ms, second- or third-degree atrioventricular block without a cardiac pacemaker, active asthma, and the presence of risk factors for cardiogenic shock (e.g., late diagnosis [>12 h] of AMI, age >70 years, systolic arterial pressure <120 mm Hg, heart rate <60 beats/min, and heart rate >110 beats/min).

European Society of Cardiology guidelines are less categorical because most trials were conducted before the advent of modern reperfusion strategies. The role of routine early IV β-blocker administration is less clearly established, and higher IV doses may be associated with early hazard and increased mortality rates.

β-Blocker use has been associated with reduction of adverse events, including death, in patients who do not undergo reperfusion. Conversely, in patients who underwent myocardial revascularization, the benefits are limited to reductions of MI and angina, but at the price of increased risks of HF and cardiogenic shock.

Anemia is a cause for concern, particularly in older adults, when using β-blockers. In a large, single-center, propensity-matched cohort study including 4387 patients and focusing on acute surgical anemia, β-blocker therapy was found to be associated with a greater incidence of MACE (relative risk [RR], 2.38; 95% confidence interval [CI], 1.43–3.96; $P = .0009$) only when Hb levels dropped by more than 35% from baseline. Anemia may worsen the perioperative adverse effects of β-blockade by further limiting DO_2. Conversely, the ability of the heart to increase stroke volume (SV) at an Hb value between 9 and 10 g/dL is rate dependent. Given the circulatory abnormalities of older patients, anemia and decreased CO are among the potential mechanisms for the increased stroke rate found in the POISE trial.

Perioperative β-Blocker Strategy

β-Blockers may be started in ICU patients with PMI and without contraindications. However, some precautions should be taken to make the use of these drugs safer.

Oral administration of β-blockers is indicated in all patients not undergoing PCI because of the antiischemic effect of these drugs. Oral β-blocker therapy is also indicated, in association with ACE inhibitors and aldosterone antagonists, in patients who have undergone coronary revascularization with a moderate-to-large MI (LVEF <40%), to achieve an antiremodeling effect. It is advisable to start 2 or 3 days postoperatively with low doses of a β_1-selective antagonist (bisoprolol 1.25 mg/day, metoprolol 25 mg twice daily [bid]) or an α_1/β-antagonist (carvedilol 6.25 mg bid) and gradually titrate doses over time. A recent large cohort study found no differences in both mortality and the risk of MACE after noncardiac surgery with respect to the β-blocker subtype administered (metoprolol, carvedilol, or atenolol) except for a reduced all-cause mortality in patients with prior MI treated with carvedilol.

Early IV administration should be limited to patients with tachycardia and hypertension (to decrease MVO_2) and to patients with atrial fibrillation when rate control is needed. The indication for use is more compelling in patients not undergoing PCI. Before IV administration of β-blockers, any risk condition that may underlie (compensatory) tachycardia should be excluded or treated. Patients with acute anemia may need blood transfusion rather than (or before) β-blockers. Echocardiography should be performed to rule out severe impairment of LV function, particularly if associated with functional mitral regurgitation or right ventricular dysfunction. An attractive choice, because of its very short half-life, is esmolol (a test dose of 20 mg; bolus injection of 0.5–1 mg/kg over 30 s; followed by continuous infusion of 50 μg/kg per minute, up to 300 μg/kg per minute).

Ivabradine

Oral (2.5–5 mg bid) or IV (5 mg bolus followed by 5 mg infusion over 8 h) ivabradine, a cardiac pacemaker "funny channel" (I_f) inhibitor, could be an attractive alternative to β-blockers for patients at risk of hypotension. The efficacy and safety of IV ivabradine administration in STEMI were demonstrated in a pilot study of 124 patients treated with PCI, in which heart rate was reduced by 22 beats/min, on average without hypotension, and LV volumes were lowered (anti–adverse remodeling effect) as compared with patients not receiving ivabradine.

Angiotensin-Converting Enzyme Inhibitors and Aldosterone Antagonists

Angiotensin-converting enzyme inhibitors and aldosterone antagonists (spironolactone, eplerenone) are highly recommended (class 1, level A) in patients with a large PMI, reduced LV systolic function (LVEF <40%), or diabetes mellitus. ACE inhibitors can be used safely in patients with stable kidney disease (up to a creatinine level of 3 mg/dL). Aldosterone blockade is contraindicated in patients with severe renal dysfunction (creatinine >2.5 mg/dL in men and >2 mg/dL in women; or serum potassium levels >5 mEq/L). In patients who are intolerant of ACE inhibitors (cough), the angiotensin receptor antagonist valsartan (80 mg bid, up to 160 mg bid) is recommended and well tolerated. During the first weeks of treatment, serum potassium and creatinine levels should be monitored closely. The greatest benefits in patients with large MI (antiremodeling effect) are obtained when administration of ACE inhibitors is started within 24 hours. However, the hemodynamic impact of aggressive ACE inhibitor (as well as β-blocker) therapy in the early postoperative period remains to be investigated.

Nitrates

Nitrates such as nitroglycerin reduce MVO_2 by decreasing LV preload and afterload, and they increase coronary blood flow by dilating capacitance vessels. However, the main limitations of nitrate therapy are the reflex increases in heart rate and contractility induced by peripheral vasodilation that reduces the hemodynamic benefits of nitrates on MVO_2, the early occurrence of tolerance, and the lack of proven benefits on MACE. For these reasons, IV administration of nitrates is indicated for a short period (usually <24 hours) and only for the treatment of persistent myocardial ischemia (ST-segment elevation or depression), particularly when complicated by systemic hypertension or HF. Nitroglycerin should not be administered to patients with myocardial ischemia and hypotension unless it is used concomitantly with an arterial vasoconstrictor such as phenylephrine, and it should be used with caution in patients with right ventricular infarction (as a result of the preload dependence of pulmonary output). Because no improvement in outcomes has been shown, long-term (oral or transdermal) administration of nitrates should be restricted to patients with HF who cannot tolerate ACE inhibitors.

Antithrombotic Agents

Antiplatelet drugs comprise the cornerstone of management of acute coronary syndromes in the nonsurgical setting. Early and aggressive treatment with dual-antiplatelet therapy (DAPT) is routinely used to prevent complete coronary occlusion or stent thrombosis after revascularization. Whereas adverse cardiac events have been shown to be significantly reduced with DAPT, the absence of antithrombotic therapy is an independent risk factor for death. However, this therapeutic strategy has the untoward effect of increasing the risk of bleeding events, especially gastrointestinal (GI) bleeding, as a result of direct damage to the gastric mucosa and inhibition of prostaglandin production, and it may be particularly hazardous in the perioperative period. Aspirin is the established first-line therapy (class 1 recommendation; level of evidence: A). The initial loading dose is 162 to 325 mg/day, subsequently reduced to a maintenance dose of 81 to 162 mg to minimize the risk of bleeding. A platelet receptor $P2Y_{12}$ inhibitor is usually administered in addition to aspirin because DAPT has been shown to be superior to aspirin alone in reducing adverse events. Approved $P2Y_{12}$ inhibitors (class 1 recommendation) include the following:

- Clopidogrel, 600 mg loading dose, then 75 mg/day (level of evidence: B in the United States, C in Europe)
- Prasugrel, 60 mg loading dose, then 10 mg/day (level of evidence: B)
- Ticagrelor, 180 mg loading dose, then 90 mg twice daily (level of evidence: B)

Compared with aspirin alone, clopidogrel was found to reduce the incidence of a composite endpoint of CV death, nonfatal MI, and stroke at 30 days by 20%. The efficacy of clopidogrel, however, is limited by the delayed onset of its effect (several hours after ingestion), secondary to the slow biotransformation from prodrug to the active metabolite, as well as by the substantial interpatient variability in the response to the drug. Another limitation of clopidogrel is its irreversible platelet inhibition. Ticagrelor and prasugrel have a faster onset of action and provide greater and more consistent platelet inhibition. These pharmacokinetic and pharmacodynamic advantages translate to greater outcome improvement. In fact, compared with clopidogrel, ticagrelor and prasugrel were found to reduce the same composite endpoint by 16% and 24%, respectively. Ticagrelor has some advantages over prasugrel. Prasugrel is not recommended (at the dose of 10 mg/day) in patients with a history of transient ischemic attack or stroke because of an increased risk of fatal intracranial bleeding, and it has neither clinical benefit nor greater sensitivity to bleeding in patients with a body weight of less than 60 kg or in patients older than 75 years. In patients older than 75 years or patients weighing less than 60 kg, a dose of 5 mg/day of prasugrel can be given, but its efficacy and safety have not been prospectively assessed. Moreover, administration of prasugrel before coronary angiography in patients with NSTEMI did not lead to a reduction in the primary endpoint compared with the drug's administration at the time of PCI.

Consistent with the more pronounced antiplatelet effects, major bleeding is more common with ticagrelor and prasugrel than with clopidogrel. Nevertheless, the balance between safety (bleeding) and efficacy (reduction of adverse outcomes) favors prasugrel and ticagrelor.

Unfortunately, PMI usually occurs within 3 days after surgical procedures, and this timeline limits the early and widespread use of these drugs in the postoperative ICU setting because they may lead to significant bleeding both at the surgical site and in the GI tract. To date, no specific studies have addressed the risks of surgical bleeding in patients treated with antiplatelet agents for PMI. Available data mostly come from investigations performed in cardiac surgical patients in stable condition and without PMI who are treated with antiplatelet drugs shortly after surgical procedures because of previous coronary stents; these investigations showed an increased risk of bleeding, reexploration, and transfusions. In the large POISE-2 study involving 10,010 noncardiac surgical patients (65% of whom underwent orthopedic or general surgery with only 6% vascular operations) without PMI, perioperative aspirin administration increased the risk of major bleeding by approximately 20% (4.6 vs 3.8%; HR, 1.23; 95% CI, 1.01–1.49; $P = .04$), without reducing the risk of MI or death.

The decision to administer DAPT, as well as its timing, in patients with PMI is challenging. Perioperative bleeding itself is an independent predictor of adverse outcome. In-hospital mortality rates are approximately 10% to 20% for major bleeding compared with 10% for reinfarction and 3% for stroke. The reason for such high mortality rates is multifactorial and includes the burden of comorbidities, bleeding-related hemodynamic instability, the possible unfavorable impact of blood transfusions on outcome, and the risk of stent thrombosis or reinfarction resulting from discontinuation of antithrombotic agents. Clinical factors that carry additive risk for GI bleeding are advanced age (>70 years), diabetes mellitus, HF, a history of ulcers and previous GI bleeding, alcohol abuse, and kidney disease. Advanced age predisposes patients to a greater risk of bleeding because of vessel injuries caused by aging, but patients with kidney disease have advanced and diffuse arterial disease and coagulation abnormalities, and they are more prone to antithrombotic overdose resulting from reduced clearance.

Antiplatelet Drugs Discontinuation and Bridging

Dual-antiplatelet therapy should be administered for at least 12 months in patients with first-generation drug-eluting stents (DESs) and 6 months in those with second-generation DESs because earlier discontinuation is associated with a high risk of stent thrombosis. Accordingly, unless the surgical team considers the bleeding risks of proceeding without stopping DAPT acceptable, surgery should be opportunely postponed whenever possible in these patients. Furthermore, a recent subgroup analysis of the POISE-2 trial showed that patients who had stents positioned longer than 1 year before surgery have a decreased 30-day risk of MACE, cardiac death, and MI if randomized to perioperative aspirin versus placebo without difference in major bleeding.

If deferral of surgery is not possible or advisable (e.g., cancer patients), bridging with other antithrombotic agents may be considered. In surgical practice, bridging therapy with low-molecular-weight heparin (LMWH), albeit criticized by cardiologists, is frequently used in patients with coronary stents undergoing noncardiac surgery, although the efficacy and safety of this strategy are unclear. A recent retrospective study found a higher rate of AMI, in addition to a higher risk of major bleeding, in patients bridged with LMWH before noncardiac procedures. In patients with a very high risk of stent thrombosis and cardiac events, bridging with IV short-acting antiplatelet drugs such as tirofiban should be considered. Moreover, the role of a tailored approach with the aid of point-of-care (POC) monitoring of antithrombotic therapy should be investigated.

Strategy for Using Antithrombotic Agents While Minimizing the Risk of Bleeding

Several strategies may help prevent bleeding in patients who require antithrombotic therapy, including the following: prophylaxis of GI bleeding with high doses of proton pump inhibitors; tailoring antithrombotic drug doses according to age and renal function; use of fondaparinux or bivalirudin, which are proven to have a lower rate of bleeding complications; and the adoption of radial access, vascular closure devices, and ultrasound-guided femoral access in patients undergoing PCI. In particular, the use of proton pump inhibitors in patients receiving antiplatelet drugs, including clopidogrel, has been associated with significant reductions in the risk of GI bleeding, erosions, and ulcers. As mentioned, the use of POC platelet function monitoring may have the potential to guide antiplatelet therapy in the early perioperative period to optimize the balance between cardiac protection and the risk of bleeding. However, no aggregometry targets have been identified that could be clinically useful for this purpose in the noncardiac surgical perioperative period.

Blood transfusion is reasonable (benefits probably exceed the risks) in patients with hemodynamic instability and hematocrit lower than 25% or Hb lower than 8 g/dL. Controversies still remain for higher Hb concentrations. Restrictive transfusion strategies were formerly thought to be associated with better outcomes, but newer data seem to suggest that more liberal transfusion triggers may reduce mortality rates in perioperative patients. In patients receiving antiplatelet therapy, platelet transfusion may be considered even when the platelet count is normal if hemorrhage continues despite the usual hemostatic techniques.

Postoperative patients admitted to the ICU may be intubated and unable to swallow. In these cases, antiplatelet drugs can be administered through a nasogastric tube after crushing the tablets (and mixing the resulting powder with 50 mL of water). In healthy volunteers, the administration of crushed tablets resulted in faster and greater bioavailability than whole tablets. However, careful attention should be paid to those conditions of reduced enteral absorption or impaired hepatic metabolism that may affect both pharmacokinetics and pharmacodynamics of orally administered antiplatelet drugs.

Percutaneous Coronary Intervention

Early primary PCI with stenting, performed by an experienced team, is the preferred therapeutic option for STEMI. Normal anterograde flow is restored in approximately 90% to 95% of patients. DAPT is mandatory to prevent stent thrombosis, but it increases bleeding risk in the perioperative period. Before excluding PCI because of the risk of bleeding, however, the following data coming from CCU cases should be considered. Compared with thrombolysis, primary PCI resulted in a 25% reduction in mortality rate and in a 64% reduction in reinfarction. Conversely, thrombolytic therapy was shown to reduce hospital mortality rates by 18% (10.7% vs 13%; OR, 0.81) compared with medical therapy (without DAPT). Accordingly, the overall reduction in mortality rates with PCI compared with medical therapy may be estimated to be 50%. Despite the lack of specific evidence, PCI should always at least be considered in patients with perioperative STEMI. However, a recent observational investigation including 281 patients with PMI who underwent PCI after noncardiac surgery showed that mortality of PMI, especially STEMI, remained high despite PCI. Bleeding events after PCI (OR, 4.33), peak cTn (OR, 1.20), and underlying peripheral vascular disease (OR, 4.86) were found to be associated with an increased 30-day mortality after PCI (OR, 4.33, 1.2 and 4.86, respectively), and increasing age (HR, 1.03), bleeding after PCI (HR, 2.31), kidney disease (HR, 2.26), and vascular surgery (HR, 1.48) were all independent predictors of long-term mortality.

Coronary angioplasty without stenting with a medicated balloon (to avoid the immediate need for DAPT) may be an option in patients at high risk of bleeding.

TREATMENT OF PERIOPERATIVE MYOCARDIAL INFARCTION

Treatment should be individualized according to the following: (1) age, comorbidity, and life expectancy of the patient; (2) hemodynamic status; (3) type of PMI (STEMI, NSTEMI) or MINS; and (4) the balance between the risks of death and bleeding (Fig. 22.2). Patients with significant ST-segment changes, hemodynamic or electrical instability, or recurrence of angina are admitted to the ICU or CCU. Low-dose aspirin, when the bleeding risk is acceptable, is recommended in all patients. Currently, about 20% to 25% of patients with PMI are managed invasively, with PCI or stenting performed in more than 50% of patients with STEMI.

Age and Comorbidity

Age is one of the most important predictors of risk with a PMI. Patients older than 75 years of age have a mortality rate at least double that of younger patients. Moreover, the risk of complications of MI increases with age. Older patients are also at higher risk of side effects of medical treatment, particularly bleeding from antithrombotic agents, hypotension and bradycardia from β-blockers, and kidney disease. Accordingly, drugs should be used with caution, generally at lower doses, and adapted to estimated glomerular filtration rate. Nevertheless, older patients have the largest survival benefit from an invasive rather than a conservative strategy, although at the price of an increased risk of major bleeding and need for transfusions. Age therefore should not constitute a contraindication to aggressive treatment. The patient's perspective and the advice of all the members of the clinical team are important to weigh risks and benefits of aggressive versus medical treatment of PMI both for frail elderly patients and for patients with serious comorbidities (e.g., severe hepatic, pulmonary, or kidney disease, active or inoperable cancer).

Patients in Unstable Condition

Patients with PMI and hemodynamic instability require a rapid and aggressive diagnostic and therapeutic approach. First, major surgical bleeding leading to MACE must be excluded as the primary cause of instability. Most cases of PMI complicated by hemodynamic instability are caused by severe ischemic LV dysfunction associated

22

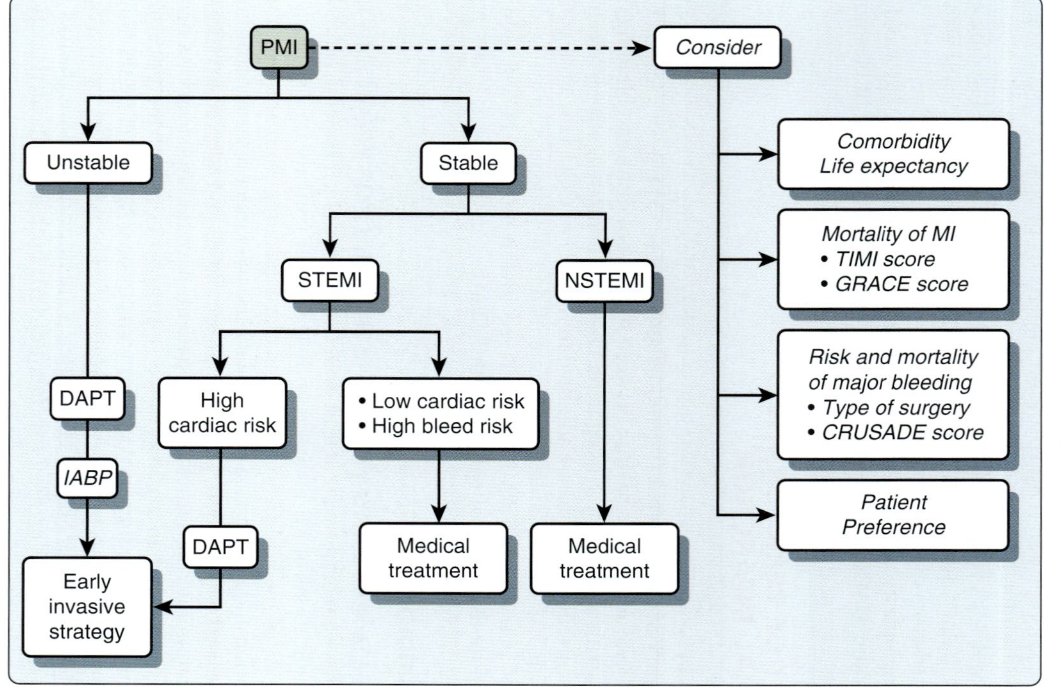

Fig. 22.2 Treatment of perioperative myocardial infarction (PMI): first 24 hours. *CRUSADE,* Can Rapid Risk Stratification of Unstable Angina Patients Suppress Adverse Outcomes With Early Implementation of the ACC/AHA Guidelines; *DAPT,* dual-antiplatelet therapy; *GRACE,* Global Registry of Acute Cardiac Events; *IABP,* intraaortic balloon pump; *MI,* myocardial infarction; *NSTEMI,* non–ST segment elevation myocardial infarction; *STEMI,* ST-segment elevation myocardial infarction; *TIMI,* Thrombolysis In Myocardial Infarction.

with extensive or proximal CAD. Whereas hypotension in the presence of critical coronary artery stenosis dramatically reduces coronary blood flow, tachycardia increases MVO_2, thus creating a vicious cycle that can lead to cardiogenic shock. In-hospital mortality rates can reach 30% to 50%. In view of the high mortality rates with medical treatment, immediate coronary angiography and PCI are recommended after administration of DAPT. PCI in patients in unstable condition may be limited by the no-reflow phenomenon, as well as by the greater risk of stent thrombosis associated with a low-flow state, although in some cases, the improvement in 6-month survival rate, compared with medical therapy, is significant. Patients in cardiogenic shock with multivessel CAD may have the best chance of survival with PCI of all proximal critical stenoses.

The supportive treatment of patients with ongoing ischemia, cardiac dysfunction, and hypotension is particularly difficult because catecholamines may increase infarct size and produce atrial or ventricular arrhythmias, and they are poorly tolerated in patients with right ventricular dysfunction.

Intraaortic balloon pump (IABP) counterpulsation is used in this situation to increase both myocardial perfusion and CO. However, as discussed later, data showing improved survival in noncardiac surgical settings are lacking. The risk-to-benefit ratio of IABP use should be carefully evaluated in patients with aortic aneurysms or peripheral vascular disease. Particular attention should be paid to patients with peripheral vascular disease who are at risk for ischemia of the lower limb. Finally, if an atrial arrhythmia is present in the patient in unstable condition, synchronized electrical cardioversion is mandatory.

Patients in Stable Condition

In hemodynamically stable patients, the choice of the best therapeutic strategy (according to the evidence coming almost entirely from the nonsurgical setting) should take into account the balance between the risk of death from PMI and the risk of major bleeding in the perioperative period. Risk of death can be easily calculated at the bedside (also with the aid of specific mobile phone applications) by using TIMI (Thrombolysis in Myocardial Infarction) or GRACE (Global Registry of Acute Cardiac Events) risk scores (Tables 22.1 to 22.3). These scoring systems, validated in

Table 22.1	TIMI Score (STEMI)

	Points
Age 65–74 years	2
Age ≥75 years	3
Systolic arterial pressure <100 mm Hg	3
Heart rate >100 beats/min	2
Killip class 2–4	2
Anterior STEMI or LBBB	1
Diabetes, hypertension, or angina	1
Weight <67 kg	1
Time to treatment >4 hours	1

LBBB, Left bundle branch block; *STEMI*, ST-segment elevation myocardial infarction; *TIMI*, Thrombolysis in Myocardial Infarction.

Table 22.2   30-Day Mortality Rate According to TIMI Score (STEMI)

Score	30-Day Mortality Rate (%)
0	<1
1	1.6
2	2.2
3	4.4
4	7.3
5	12.4
6	16.1
7	23.4
8	26.8
>8	35.9

STEMI, ST-segment elevation myocardial infarction; *TIMI*, Thrombolysis in Myocardial Infarction.

Table 22.3   GRACE Score and Mortality (NSTEMI)

Risk Category	GRACE Score	Risk of Death	
Low	≤108	<1%	In-hospital
	≤88	<3%	Discharge to 6 months
Intermediate	109–140	1%–3%	In-hospital
	89–118	3%–8%	Discharge to 6 months
High	>140	>3%	In-hospital
	>118	>8%	Discharge to 6 months

Modified from Kristensen SD, Knuuti J, Saraste A, et al. 2014 ESC/ESA guidelines on noncardiac surgery: cardiovascular assessment and management: the Joint Task Force on Noncardiac Surgery: cardiovascular assessment and management of the European Society of Cardiology (ESC) and the European Society of Anaesthesiology (ESA). *Eur Heart J.* 2014;35:2383-2431.

nearly 35,000 patients with both STEMI (TIMI and GRACE) and NSTEMI (GRACE), show a strong predictive ability and an excellent concordance with observed 30-day, 6-month, and 12-month mortality rates. Both TIMI and GRACE scores identify a subgroup of patients at high risk of cardiac death who probably need an aggressive invasive therapeutic strategy despite the risk of bleeding, as well as a subgroup of low-risk patients, who may be managed with medical therapy, especially if the bleeding risk is high.

The risk of bleeding is related to surgical factors and patient factors. With regard to the hemorrhagic risk, surgical interventions can be classified into low-risk, medium-risk, and high-risk procedures (Table 22.4), according to previous studies and expert opinion. A patient's individual risk may be predicted using the CRUSADE (Can Rapid Risk Stratification of Unstable Angina Patients Suppress Adverse Outcomes With Early Implementation of the ACC/AHA Guidelines) bleeding score (Table 22.5 and Fig. 22.3), developed in approximately 89,000 patients with STEMI or NSTEMI.

Table 22.4 Surgical Hemorrhagic Risk

	Low Risk	Medium Risk	High Risk
Surgery	Hernioplasty	Hemorrhoidectomy	Intracranial
	Cholecystectomy	Splenectomy	Intraspinal
	Appendectomy	Gastrectomy	Eye posterior chamber
	Colectomy	Obesity surgery	Open thoracic and
	Gastric resection	Rectal resection	thoracoabdominal aorta
	Intestinal	Thyroidectomy	Major prosthetic (hip or knee)
	resection	Open abdominal	Major trauma (pelvis, long
	Breast surgery	aorta surgery	bones)
	Carotid	Prosthetic	Fractures of the proximal femur
	endarterectomy	shoulder	in an older adult
	Bypass or	surgery	Radical and partial nephrectomy
	endarterectomy	Major spine	Cystectomy and radical
	of lower	surgery	prostatectomy
	extremity	Knee surgery	TURP
	EVAR	Foot surgery	TURBT
	TEVAR	Prostate biopsy	Hepatic resection
	Limb amputations	Orchiectomy	Duodenocefalopancreatectomy
	Hand surgery	Circumcision	
	Shoulder and	Lobectomy	
	knee	Pneumonectomy	
	arthroscopy	Mediastinoscopy	
	Minor spine	Sternotomy	
	surgery	Mediastinal mass	
	Wedge resection	excision	

EVAR, Endovascular aortic repair; *TEVAR,* thoracic endovascular aortic repair; *TURBT,* transurethral resection of bladder tumor; *TURP,* transurethral resection of the prostate.

ST-Segment Elevation Myocardial Infarction

Elevation of ST segments usually results from an acute coronary thrombotic occlusion. In this setting, urgent coronary angiography and PCI lead to a significant reduction in mortality rates. Accordingly, these procedures should always be considered in patients with perioperative STEMI, especially in those with good life expectancy and moderate to large infarctions. In the authors' opinion, only patients at low risk of death (<3%–5%) and, at the same time, at high risk of bleeding should be treated with medical therapy alone.

Infarction size can be quantified by echocardiography and by both clinical and ECG parameters. Signs of large infarctions include the presence of pulmonary rales, ECG changes involving more than three leads, ST-segment elevation in aVR (which suggests left main or proximal left anterior descending artery stenosis), new onset of bundle branch block or arrhythmias in inferior infarction, a reduction of LVEF (<40%), or right ventricular involvement.

Before a PCI procedure, a loading dose of aspirin (162–325 mg), together with a loading dose of a P2Y$_{12}$ inhibitor (clopidogrel 600 mg, prasugrel 60 mg, ticagrelor 180 mg), should be administered as early as possible. Clopidogrel may cause less bleeding, but it is also the least effective. Prasugrel should be avoided in patients with a history of transient ischemic attack or stroke, body weight less than 60 kg, and age older than 75 years.

Table 22.5 Calculation of CRUSADE Score

Predictor	Points
Baseline Hematocrit (%)	
<31	9
31–33.9	7
34–36.9	3
37–39.9	2
≥40	0
Creatinine Clearance (mL/min)	
≤15	39
>15–30	35
>30–60	28
>60–90	17
>90–120	7
>120	0
Heart Rate (beats/min)	
≤70	0
71–80	1
81–90	3
91–100	6
101–110	8
111–120	10
≥121	11
Sex	
Male	0
Female	8
Signs of CHF at Presentation	
No	0
Yes	7
Prior Vascular Disease	
No	0
Yes	6
Diabetes Mellitus	
No	0
Yes	6
Systolic Blood Pressure (mm Hg)	
≤90	10
91–100	8
101–120	5
121–180	1
181–200	3
≥201	5

CHF, Congestive heart failure; *CRUSADE,* Can Rapid Risk Stratification of Unstable Angina Patients Suppress Adverse Outcomes With Early Implementation of the ACC/AHA Guidelines.

Modified from Kristensen SD, Knuuti J, Saraste A, et al. 2014 ESC/ESA guidelines on noncardiac surgery: cardiovascular assessment and management: the Joint Task Force on Noncardiac Surgery: cardiovascular assessment and management of the European Society of Cardiology (ESC) and the European Society of Anaesthesiology (ESA). *Eur Heart J.* 2014;35:2383–2431.

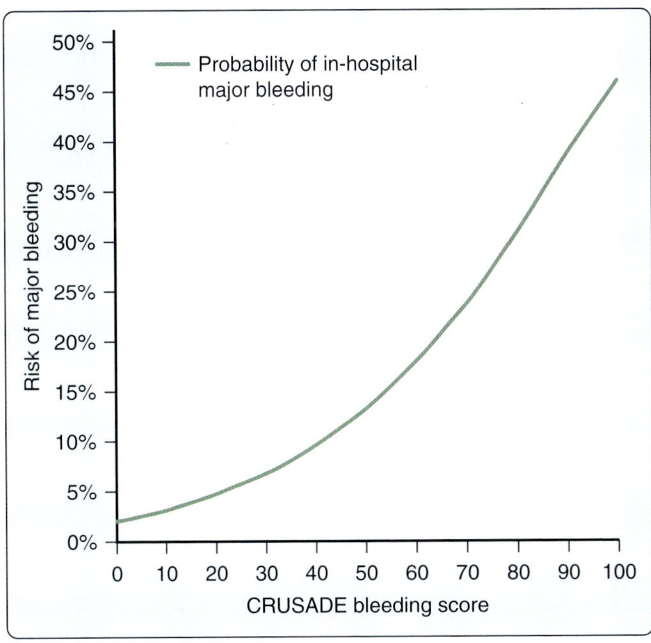

Fig. 22.3 CRUSADE (Can Rapid Risk Stratification of Unstable Angina Patients Suppress Adverse Outcomes With Early Implementation of the ACC/AHA Guidelines) score and risk of major bleeding. (Modified from Kristensen SD, Knuuti J, Saraste A, et al. 2014 ESC/ESA guidelines on non-cardiac surgery: cardiovascular assessment and management: the Joint Task Force on non-cardiac surgery: cardiovascular assessment and management of the European Society of Cardiology (ESC) and the European Society of Anaesthesiology (ESA). *Eur Heart J.* 2014;35:2383–2431.)

Non–ST Segment Elevation Myocardial Infarction

Three characteristics distinguish NSTEMI from STEMI. First, NSTEMI may result from a myocardial oxygen supply–demand mismatch induced by extracardiac causes. The treatment of these causes may reverse ischemic changes. Second, in most cases, no complete thrombotic occlusion of a coronary artery is accountable for the infarction but only a critical stenosis often involving multiple coronary vessels. Accordingly, compared with STEMI, the need for urgent PCI is less compelling, especially if the hemorrhagic risk is high, as in the perioperative period. Finally, the incidence of adverse events at 1-year follow-up is higher in NSTEMI than in STEMI. As a consequence, a strategy of routine invasive therapy before hospital discharge has been shown to be generally superior to medical therapy alone.

Myocardial oxygen supply–demand mismatch is typically induced by hypotension, acute anemia, or hypertension and tachycardia, usually in patients with CAD, LV hypertrophy, or aortic stenosis. Before antiischemic therapy is begun, these causes must be found and treated vigorously. Moreover, anemia from acute bleeding is an absolute contraindication to reperfusion and antiplatelet therapy. After underlying causes are excluded (e.g., pain, anemia, hypoxemia), tachycardia should be treated to reduce infarct size. IV β-blockers are then continued orally to control heart rate and hypertension.

Coronary angiography is recommended before hospital discharge in patients at high cardiac risk (diabetes, kidney disease, significant ST-segment depression, LVEF <40%, previous PCI or coronary artery bypass graft, GRACE risk score >109).

Myocardial Injury After Noncardiac Surgery

Aspirin (325 mg on day 1; then 100 mg/day) and low-dose oral β-blockers (e.g., bisoprolol 1.25 mg/day) should be initiated within 24 hours in all patients without contraindications. High-dose statins (atorvastatin 80 mg/day) are also usually started early after AMI, but their efficacy and safety in the perioperative setting are uncertain. A $P2Y_{12}$ inhibitor (e.g., ticagrelor 90 mg bid) may be added to low-dose aspirin in the postoperative period. ACE inhibitors should be started in patients with an LVEF of less than 40%, hypertension, diabetes, and stable CKD.

An invasive strategy (coronary angiography and PCI) before hospital discharge is indicated in patients in whom angina or hemodynamic or electrical instability develops during mobilization. PCI is also reasonable in patients without severe comorbidities who are asymptomatic but who have a high risk of short-term cardiac events (GRACE score >140). In the remaining low-risk patients, an ischemia provocative test during medical therapy is recommended before discharge; coronary angiography is performed if myocardial ischemia is documented unless the patient has extensive comorbidities.

The hypothesis that providing appropriate therapy to patients with MINS may limit long-term mortality was validated in a study including 667 consecutive patients undergoing major vascular surgical procedures. Patients with postoperative elevated troponin levels but not receiving early evidence-based CV therapy (antiplatelet agents, β-blockers, statins, ACE inhibitors) had a significant increase in MACE (death, AMI, HF, myocardial revascularization) at 12 months (HR, 2.80; 95% CI, 1.05–24.2; $P = .04$).

OUTCOME AFTER PERIOPERATIVE MYOCARDIAL DAMAGE

Perioperative myocardial damage is associated with short-term, midterm, and long-term cardiac morbidity and death. Because perioperative myocardial damage is most often silent, many patients remain untreated. This may also contribute to an increased risk of long-term CV death. Accordingly, perioperative cardiac monitoring should be implemented to allow early diagnosis and treatment.

Despite a significant reduction in the incidence of PMI in the past years, in-hospital mortality remains high ($\approx$15%–20%). Acute HF, cardiogenic or septic shock, and multiorgan failure are the most common causes of death.

As mentioned, invasive management including myocardial revascularization and antithrombotic medical therapy may improve outcomes.

Short-Term Outcome

Patients with PMI are more likely to have life-threatening CV complications, including cardiogenic shock (4.7% vs 0.1%; $P < .0001$) and cardiac arrest (5.2% vs 0.3%; $P < .0001$). Hospital length of stay is significantly longer in patients with AMI, with the potential of an increased risk of common in-hospital complications such as infections, venous thromboembolism, and muscular deconditioning.

Patients treated with invasive management (coronary angiography) have lower in-hospital mortality than those who are treated conservatively (8.9% vs 20.5%, $P < .001$; OR, 0.38), despite higher rates of postoperative bleeding associated with antithrombotic therapy (8.1% vs 5.3%; $P < .001$). Patients undergoing coronary revascularization also have lower mortality rates than patients managed conservatively (10.5% vs 18.7%, $P < .001$; OR, 0.51). Accordingly, the reluctance to refer patients

Table 22.6	Mortality Score in Patients With Myocardial Injury After Noncardiac Surgery[a]	
		Points
Age ≥75 years		1
Anterior ischemic findings		1
ST-segment elevation or new LBBB		2

[a]Expected 30-day mortality rate: 0 points, 5.2%; 1 point, 10.2%; 2 points, 19.0%; 3 points, 32.5%; 4 points, 49.8%.

LBBB, left bundle branch block.

From Botto F, Alonso-Coello P, Chan MT, et al. Myocardial injury after noncardiac surgery: a large, international, prospective cohort study establishing diagnostic criteria, characteristics, predictors and 30 day outcomes. *Anesthesiology.* 2014;120:564–578.

with PMI to coronary angiography, primarily because of the concerns about bleeding, should be overcome.

A simple score including three independent predictors of death—age 75 years or older (1 point), anterior ischemic findings (1 point), ST-segment elevation or new left bundle branch block (2 points)— showed a good correlation with 30-day mortality rates in patients with MINS. According to this scoring system, predicted 30-day mortality ranged from 5.2% if none of the aforementioned predictors were present (0 points) to 49.8% if all of them were present (4 points) (Table 22.6). Patients with MINS have a lower risk of fatal cardiac events than do patients with PMI but a higher risk of death than patients with no elevated cardiac biomarkers. In a large, international study, the 30-day mortality rate among patients with MINS was 9.8%, as opposed to 1.1% among patients without MINS.

Long-Term Outcome

As mentioned, in addition to early adverse events, cTn also predicts late mortality rates. The 1-year mortality rate after vascular surgical procedures is 20% in patients with pathologic troponin increases compared with 4.7% in patients with normal values. Identifiers of outcome include preoperative creatinine level greater than 2.0 mg/dL (OR, 2.55), preoperative history of HF (OR, 1.96), and age older than 70 years (OR, 1.62). These data show that in a homogeneous group of patients with documented CAD who undergo elective vascular surgical procedures, a combination of preoperative risk variables, including age, renal function, and previous HF, along with postoperative elevations in cardiac biomarkers in patients with diabetes, predicts long-term outcome.

PERIOPERATIVE CARE TO REDUCE MORTALITY RATES IN NONCARDIAC SURGICAL PROCEDURES

The all-cause mortality rate after noncardiac surgical procedures has been reported to be 0.8% to 1.5%. However, postoperative mortality rates may greatly increase according to patient-related and procedure-related factors, such as age (≥80 years), ASA physical status (≥3), cancer, surgical specialty (GI, thoracic, and vascular surgical procedures are those at higher risk), and the severity and urgency (expedited, urgent, immediate) of the procedure. Moreover, large differences in mortality rates exist among different countries and even among different centers. With more than 230 million major surgical procedures performed annually worldwide, even small reductions in perioperative mortality rates would result in thousands of lives saved each year.

In their daily clinical practice, anesthesiologists make many choices that can affect clinically relevant outcomes in the (1) preoperative period (drug continuation or discontinuation), (2) operating room (anesthetic technique, airway management, type and amount of fluids administered, hemodynamic monitoring and optimization, type and age of blood products administered and transfusion triggers), and (3) postoperative care (cardiocirculatory support, ventilation, drug prescriptions). However, for nonsurgical interventions (drugs, techniques, strategies), evidence from RCTs and consensus on their impact on postoperative mortality rates are limited.

A novel approach to consensus building developed in the past few years, referred to as "democracy-based medicine," has made it possible to summarize the best-quality and most widely agreed-on evidence about mortality reduction in different settings, including the noncardiac surgical perioperative period.

"Democracy-Based," Web-Enabled Approach to Consensus on Perioperative Mortality Rate Reduction

Physicians should base most of their clinical decisions on the best evidence available in the literature. However, they must always contend with the challenging issue of understanding the meaning, applicability, robustness, and biologic plausibility of clinical evidence coming from published studies. Moreover, although some topics lack high-quality investigations from which to draw conclusions, other topics have a plethora of often contradictory data that do not allow clinically useful synthesis. In both cases, guidelines may be inconclusive or even lacking. Consensus conferences are currently considered the best way to assess evidence systematically and to reach agreement among experts, particularly when no definitive conclusions can be drawn from RCTs or meta-analyses. This approach has some limitations, including the high priority given to expert opinions (with a poor definition of "expertise"), the risk of influences and biases, and the possibility that the resulting recommendations may not be widely applicable.

A "democracy-based" process, feasible thanks to the advent of the Internet, was suggested for the first time in 2010 as a possible alternative to the "traditional" approach to consensus on mortality rate reduction. This method brings together the features of consensus conferences, international surveys, and systematic reviews, thus leading to a rigorous selection of published evidence through an open, dynamic, comprehensive, and easily reproducible process that also provides insightful details on current worldwide clinical practice.

The consensus building takes place through the following steps: (1) systematic literature search and analysis (the identified articles are included in the subsequent step if they fulfill the prespecified criteria of dealing with nonsurgical interventions, reporting a statistically significant effect on mortality rates, being published in a peer-reviewed journal, and including adult patients), (2) consensus meeting (a task force of anesthesiologists, intensivists, surgeons, cardiologists, and epidemiologists meets to discuss and, if necessary, to vote on each topic, finally writing a brief summary statement describing the effects on mortality and the reasons for the inclusion of that topic), (3) web-based survey (the summary statements are listed online, and voters are asked whether they agree with these statements or not and whether they use the presented interventions in their clinical practice; topics receiving a low percentage of agreement are excluded).

From 2010 to present, the consensus method was applied to four different settings: cardiac surgery, the perioperative period of any surgical procedure, acute kidney injury, and critically ill patients. The findings of the democracy-based consensus conference on perioperative mortality, which were updated in 2016, are addressed below.

Results of the Updated Web-Based Consensus Conference on Perioperative Mortality

The article collection was focused on RCTs and meta-analyses of RCTs. Among the 19,633 articles analyzed, only 75 (concerning 29 different interventions) fulfilled all inclusion criteria and were accordingly voted on by 500 physicians from 61 countries. Sixteen topics were excluded during the subsequent steps because of methodologic limitations, inconclusive findings, low agreement at the web poll, or the publication of new high-quality evidence after the conclusion of the consensus process.

Of the 13 interventions that potentially increase or decrease perioperative mortality rates according to the final findings of the consensus process (Fig. 22.4), 7 have been only (or mostly) investigated in the cardiac surgical setting (insulin, IABP, leukocyte depletion, levosimendan, volatile anesthetic agents, remote ischemic preconditioning, avoidance of aprotinin). The remaining topics, concerning noncardiac operations, are discussed in the next sections and are summarized in Box 22.3. In addition, it is reasonable to assume that some of the interventions that conferred survival benefits in other settings such as cardiac surgery and critical care may have a beneficial effect in noncardiac surgical patients as well.

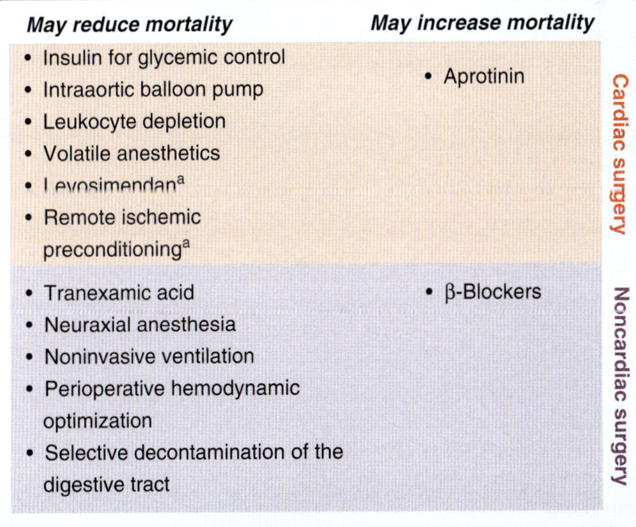

Fig. 22.4 Interventions influencing perioperative mortality rates (any surgical procedure) according to the updated Web-Based Consensus Conference on Perioperative Mortality. [a]Recent randomized evidence does not confirm the survival benefit.

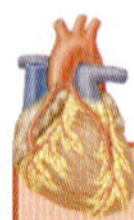

> ## BOX 22.3 *Practical (Evidence-Based) Suggestions to Reduce Mortality Rates in Noncardiac Surgery Patients*
>
> - *Hemodynamic optimization* according to adequate monitoring and flow-related parameters should be pursued in high-risk patients. However, the best monitoring tools, hemodynamic goals, and resuscitation targets are yet to be defined.
> - *Noninvasive ventilation* should be promptly started in patients who develop postoperative acute respiratory failure. Its intraoperative role, although promising, is less clear.
> - *Neuraxial anesthesia*, as well as epidural analgesia in addition to general anesthesia, should be preferred whenever possible, even if physicians' skills and a highly individualized choice of the anesthetic technique are probably pivotal.
> - *Selective decontamination of the digestive tract* may be considered in postoperative intensive care unit patients, but this topic needs further research.
> - *Tranexamic acid* seems to be effective in reducing intraoperative and postoperative blood losses and hemorrhagic complications and is probably safe when administered in the perioperative setting; however, whether this intervention favorably affects mortality rates is still unclear.
> - *Volatile anesthetics, leukocyte depletion, lung-protective ventilation, intraaortic balloon pump, and vacuum assisted closure* have been proven to reduce mortality in other settings, but also might be beneficial in noncardiac surgery patients.
> - *Nutritional support and vitamin supplementation, sedation, inspired oxygen fraction, high-flow nasal cannula oxygen, early renal replacement therapy, extracorporeal mechanical circulatory support, and point-of-care coagulation testing* are among the strategies that should be investigated for a potential role in affecting mortality in the perioperative setting.
> - *β-Blocker* initiation in unselected patients shortly before surgery should be avoided. However, perioperative continuation of β-blockers is recommended in patients already receiving these drugs. This topic needs further research.

Interventions That May Reduce Mortality Rates in Noncardiac Surgical Procedures

Perioperative Hemodynamic Optimization

Referred to as goal-directed therapy (GDT), hemodynamic optimization involves the proactive administration of fluids (associated or not with inotropic drugs) to maintain one or more flow-related hemodynamic parameters within a certain target to match the imbalance that often occurs in the perioperative period between oxygen supply and demand or to prevent tissue hypoxia and organ injury. Six meta-analyses of RCTs found reduced mortality rates with GDT protocols in patients undergoing noncardiac surgical procedures. The trials included in these meta-analyses were highly heterogeneous in both their quality and design. Furthermore, hemodynamic optimization strategies investigated by different studies were extremely varied, including different hemodynamic goals (e.g., CO or cardiac index [CI], DO_2, dynamic parameters such as SV variation or pulse pressure variation [PPV], central or mixed venous oxygen saturation [ScO_2 or SvO_2], and flow time corrected [FTc]), different monitoring devices (pulmonary artery catheter, pulse contour analysis, esophageal Doppler imaging, bioreactance), different resuscitation targets (normal or "supranormal" DO_2 levels), and different therapeutic interventions to achieve these goals and targets (fluids, inotropes, blood

566

transfusions). In two of these meta-analyses (including 2808 noncardiac surgical patients and 4805 patients undergoing any operation, respectively), subgroup analyses revealed that the reduction in mortality rates with GDT protocols (compared with standard therapy) was restricted to studies using a pulmonary artery catheter as the monitoring tool, CO or DO_2 as hemodynamic goals, fluids and inotropes as therapeutic strategies, and "supranormal" resuscitation targets. Moreover, three among the six meta-analyses found that the survival benefit was restricted to patients with an extremely high risk of death ($\geq 20\%$).

In the authors' opinion, it is not difficult to agree with the concept that hemodynamic status should be promptly "optimized" in the perioperative period to prevent the development of an "oxygen debt" and probably to reduce major postoperative complications and mortality rates. Moreover, it is reasonable to assume that flow-based hemodynamic monitoring may provide the greatest advantages. However, the best monitoring tools, hemodynamic targets, therapeutic interventions (including the type of fluids or inotropes), and the most appropriate settings are yet to be clearly defined. In fact, the more recent RCTs investigating the use of GDT protocols based on minimally invasive or noninvasive monitoring devices, which are gradually replacing invasive monitoring in most noncardiac surgical settings, failed to show clinical benefit. In particular, the recent COGUIDE trial, a multicenter RCT of 244 patients undergoing moderate-risk abdominal surgery, found no advantages in terms of postoperative complications with the use of minimally invasive CI and PPV monitoring compared with mean arterial pressure–guided hemodynamic therapy. However, these results are not against a GDT approach at all and are consistent with the findings of the abovementioned meta-analyses, which suggest that the survival benefit may be limited to the higher risk patients.

Noninvasive Ventilation

Several articles reported the perioperative use of noninvasive ventilation (NIV) in nearly all types of surgical procedures including abdominal, thoracic, urologic, orthopedic, obstetric, ophthalmic, and neurosurgical, as well as endovascular cardiac procedures.

Improved outcomes were found with the postoperative use of NIV. One multicenter trial including 209 patients from 15 ICUs showed a reduced rate of tracheal intubation and a lower incidence of complications (infections, sepsis, pneumonia, and anastomotic leaks) in patients in whom postoperative hypoxia developed after abdominal surgical procedures and who were treated with 7.5 cm H_2O continuous positive airway pressure (CPAP) through a helmet compared with standard care.

So far, however, randomized evidence of improved survival with NIV in noncardiac surgical patients comes from only two small RCTs performed in patients undergoing thoracic surgery and solid organ transplantation. Among 48 patients who developed acute hypoxemic lung failure after pulmonary resection, those who received pressure support ventilation through a nasal mask (set to maintain exhaled tidal volumes within 8–10 mL/kg, respiratory rate <25 breaths/min, and arterial oxygen saturation >90%) showed a threefold reduction in 120-day mortality rate compared with those who received standard care (12.5% vs 37.5%; $P = .045$). A similar NIV strategy through a face mask was found to reduce ICU mortality rates from 50% to 20% ($P = .05$) in 40 patients who developed acute lung failure after liver, kidney, or lung transplantation.

Nevertheless, strong indications that NIV may have a key role in reducing perioperative mortality rates derive from the critical care setting. In fact, with as many as nine multicenter RCTs in support, NIV is the therapeutic intervention with the best evidence to have a significant impact on mortality rates in critically ill patients in the history of modern medicine. A meta-analysis of RCTs including 7365 patients confirmed that NIV reduced mortality rates in acute care settings (RR, 0.73; 95% CI, 0.66–0.81; $P < .001$) when it was used to treat or prevent acute respiratory failure but not as a means to allow earlier tracheal extubation. Moreover, the survival benefit is lost when NIV is started too late. Accordingly, NIV should be promptly applied whenever indicated. Most remarkably, the favorable effect of NIV on mortality rate was preserved also when only postoperative patients with acute respiratory failure were considered. This finding indicates that NIV may be pivotal in the treatment of *postoperative* respiratory failure to reduce mortality rates.

Noninvasive ventilation is usually delivered through nasal masks, full-face masks, or helmets and includes different modes (e.g., CPAP, pressure support/positive end-expiratory pressure, or bilevel positive airway pressure ventilation). A recent meta-analysis of 11 RCTs (including 1480 patients with acute hypoxemic nonhypercapnic respiratory failure, overall), in addition to confirming a reduction in both endotracheal intubation rates and hospital mortality with the use of NIV, suggests that the use of a helmet as patient-ventilator interface and the use of bilevel ventilation could both be associated with a survival advantage. However, further research is needed to address this topic, and it is not possible to recommend the use of one interface or one NIV mode with respect to another according to the currently available data.

The role of intraoperative NIV in reducing mortality rates is less clear. NIV may be used in the operating room to treat sudden respiratory distress to allow continuation of the operation without tracheal intubation. More often, it is used as a prophylactic measure in patients with cardiorespiratory diseases who cannot tolerate the supine position or to avoid respiratory failure resulting from deep sedation. Similarly, the use of NIV, through both a face mask and a helmet, has been described in patients undergoing diagnostic procedures (upper digestive endoscopy, fiberoptic bronchoscopy, transesophageal echocardiography) that may induce respiratory distress or require deep sedation. A full-face mask that can be opened is available (Janus Biomedical) and can be positioned without stopping the ongoing endoscopic procedure. Large, randomized trials are needed to assess the impact on mortality rates of intraoperative or intraprocedural use of NIV, both as a prophylactic measure and as a rescue treatment.

Neuraxial Anesthesia

Both spinal anesthesia and epidural anesthesia used alone, as well as epidural anesthesia or analgesia in association with general anesthesia, have been reported to have favorable effects (e.g., antiinflammatory effects, reduction of stress response biomarkers, better functional recovery, lower cancer recurrence) and to reduce the incidence of major postoperative complications (particularly pulmonary complications and venous thromboembolism) in patients undergoing noncardiac surgical procedures. It is reasonable to assume that the use of neuraxial anesthesia techniques in these settings may improve survival, although this is a matter of long-standing debate. In fact, no RCT has been able to show any difference in mortality rates between regional anesthesia and general anesthesia. Moreover, despite several large observational or retrospective studies, mostly involving orthopedic surgical patients, which suggested a mortality rate reduction with neuraxial anesthesia, data coming from recent similar investigations are conflicting.

The results of four meta-analyses (two published in 2000 and two in 2014) suggest postoperative mortality reduction when using neuraxial anesthesia. One of the early meta-analyses included 141 RCTs in which patients (a total of 9559) undergoing all types of surgical procedures (mainly general, gynecologic, obstetric, orthopedic, urologic, and vascular operations) were randomized to receive neuraxial or general anesthesia: a reduction in 30-day mortality rate of approximately one-third was found in patients receiving neuraxial anesthesia (OR, 0.70; 95% CI, 0.54–0.90; $P = .006$), without significant differences among the different types of surgical procedures. The survival benefit observed reflected a trend toward reduction in deaths from several complications including pulmonary embolism, cardiac events, stroke, and infection. The other meta-analysis published in 2000, which was limited to trials involving patients with hip fracture, found a similar reduction in 1-month mortality rate in patients receiving regional anesthesia (OR, 0.66; 95% CI, 0.47–0.96). The meta-analyses conducted thereafter had conflicting results. However, in 2014, an overview of nine Cochrane systematic reviews including RCTs that compared neuraxial anesthesia with general anesthesia alone or combined neuraxial and general anesthesia with general anesthesia alone in patients of any age undergoing any surgical procedures was performed. The investigators confirmed with a moderate level of evidence that neuraxial anesthesia, compared with general anesthesia, was associated with a reduction in up-to-30-day mortality rates (RR, 0.71; 95% CI, 0.53–0.94; heterogeneity index [I^2], 0%) in patients undergoing surgical procedures at intermediate to high cardiac risk. Moreover, whereas neuraxial anesthesia was associated with a lower risk of pneumonia (RR, 0.45; 95% CI, 0.26–0.79; I^2, 0%), the rate of MI was similar with the two techniques.

Finally, another meta-analysis published in 2014 focused on epidural analgesia in addition to general anesthesia, compared with general anesthesia alone, and showed a reduction in mortality rate from 4.9% to 3.1% (OR, 0.60; 95% CI, 0.39–0.93), without significant heterogeneity among data ($P = .44$; I^2, 0%). Moreover, the risk of arrhythmias (atrial fibrillation and supraventricular tachycardia), respiratory depression, deep vein thrombosis, atelectasis, pneumonia, ileus, and postoperative nausea and vomiting was significantly reduced with epidural analgesia, although an increased risk of arterial hypotension, itching, urinary retention, and motor blockade was found.

Unfortunately, in addition to the well-known limitations of meta-analyses, none of these investigations was able to consider the individual skills of anesthesiologists, which probably have a key role in this context. In the authors' opinion, regional anesthesia should be the anesthetic technique of choice in noncardiac surgical procedures whenever possible. However, key factors to improve outcomes and probably to reduce mortality rates are careful and comprehensive risk assessment, anesthesiologists' skills, and a highly individualized choice of anesthetic technique. For example, especially in patients with cardiac diseases, even the degree of patients' anxiety or fear, which may increase the risk of MACE and death, should be taken into account when choosing between general anesthesia and regional anesthesia. Conversely, the indiscriminate use of a technique only because it has been shown to reduce mortality rates in meta-analyses or RCTs may be harmful for the individual patient.

Selective Decontamination of the Digestive Tract

Selective decontamination of the digestive tract (SDD) involves the use of topical and oral nonabsorbable antimicrobial agents (polymyxin E, tobramycin, amphotericin B, and vancomycin in case of endemic methicillin-resistant *Staphylococcus aureus*), possibly in conjunction with parenteral antibiotics (usually cephalosporins) to control the overgrowth of potentially pathogenic microorganisms, as often occurs in critically ill patients. This prophylactic measure has been largely proven to reduce bloodstream and pulmonary infections and mortality rates in ICU patients. The effectiveness of SDD also has been investigated in surgical ICU patients, but evidence is not overwhelming. Until recently, a meta-analysis performed in 1999 including 11 RCTs was the only study showing a survival benefit with SDD in the postoperative setting. The authors found that SDD significantly reduced mortality rates among critically ill surgical patients (OR, 0.70; 95% CI, 0.52–0.93) because of reduced rates of bacteremia and pneumonia. Furthermore, the survival benefit was greater with the use of SDD regimens that included both oral and parenteral antimicrobial agents (OR, 0.60; 95% CI, 0.41–0.88). These findings seem to be confirmed by a recent (2017) individual patient data meta-analysis including six RCTs performed in countries with low levels of antibiotic resistance, which showed reductions in both hospital and ICU mortality rates regardless of the ICU admission type (medical or surgical).

Conversely, the perioperative use of SDD protocols outside the ICU setting has not been shown to reduce mortality rates, although it seemed to be a promising prophylactic measure, especially in patients undergoing upper GI tract surgical procedures.

The use of SDD is not widespread and not generally suggested, even in the critical care setting. The reason is probably multifactorial and mainly reflects concern about development of bacterial resistance to antibiotics, even if SDD seems to be safe from this point of view. A large, multicenter RCT in patients undergoing elective colorectal cancer operations that is evaluating the role of SDD in addition to standard antibiotic prophylaxis and that includes death among its endpoints is currently ongoing. Meanwhile, the role of SDD, both in the perioperative period and in postsurgical ICU patients, as a strategy to improve survival remains uncertain.

Tranexamic Acid

Tranexamic acid (TXA) is the only antifibrinolytic drug that seems to have a favorable effect on perioperative mortality rates. According to a meta-analysis of 129 RCTs including 10,488 patients, strong evidence indicates that tranexamic acid reduces the need for transfusions in surgical patients by more than one-third (RR, 0.62; 95% CI, 0.58–0.65; $P < .001$). However, uncertainty remains about its impact on MI, stroke, deep vein thrombosis, pulmonary embolism, and mortality rates. Although a reduced mortality rate with the use of tranexamic acid was found (RR, 0.61; 95% CI, 0.38–0.98; $P = .04$), statistical significance was lost after restriction of analysis to studies with adequate concealment.

Indirect evidence about a possible beneficial effect of tranexamic acid on mortality rates in the perioperative period comes from the trauma setting, which is similar to that of surgery. The large multicenter RCT CRASH-2 (2010) included 20,211 patients from 274 hospitals and found that a short course of TXA (1 g over 10 minutes, followed by continuous infusion of 1 g over 8 hours, starting within 8 hours from injury) significantly reduced all-cause mortality rates in bleeding trauma patients (RR, 0.91; 95% CI, 0.85–0.97; $P = .0035$), with a greater effect when TXA was started earlier.

At this time, it seems reasonable to assume that TXA can be safely administered perioperatively with the aim of reducing blood losses and hemorrhagic complications, but whether this intervention favorably affects mortality rates is still unclear.

Interventions That May Increase Mortality Rates in Noncardiac Surgical Procedures

Perioperative β-Blockers

Preoperative prescription of β-blockers was formerly thought to be an effective and safe strategy to reduce cardiac risk in patients undergoing noncardiac surgical procedures. However, the evidence about safety of perioperative β-blockade was mainly based on a set of investigations (the DECREASE trials) that were accused of serious scientific misconduct. Conversely, high-dose β-blockers started shortly before noncardiac surgical procedures increased mortality rates significantly in patients with, or at risk for, ischemic heart disease, according to the large multicenter trial POISE, as well as three meta-analyses. In the POISE study (2008), 8351 patients with CV disease, or who were scheduled for major vascular operations, or with at least three of seven risk factors (intrathoracic or intraperitoneal operations, emergency or urgent procedures, previous HF, transient ischemic attack, diabetes, serum creatinine >175 μmol/L, age >70 years) were randomized to receive oral extended-release metoprolol or placebo for 30 days starting 2 to 4 hours preoperatively. Although the rate of MI was reduced by 27% (4.2% vs 5.7%; $P < .0017$), a 33% increase in the overall mortality rate (3.1% vs 2.3%; $P = .0317$) and a 100% increase in the rate of stroke (1.0% vs 0.5%; $P = .0053$) were found, mainly from hypotension.

A meta-analysis of 11 trials in which bisoprolol (three studies), metoprolol (five studies), atenolol (two studies), or propranolol (one study) was started between 37 days and 30 minutes preoperatively and was continued for 5 to 30 days postoperatively was published in 2014. The investigators found a significant increase in all-cause mortality rates with perioperative β-blockers (RR, 1.27; 95% CI, 1.01–1.60; $P = .04$), and they strongly argued for a change in guidelines.

In the revised 2014 ESC/ESA guidelines on noncardiac surgical procedures, the recommendations on perioperative β-blockers were substantially downgraded. Although perioperative *continuation* of β-blockers is still recommended in patients already receiving these drugs, it is suggested that their *initiation* may be considered in patients with recognized ischemic heart disease and in patients undergoing high-risk surgical procedures with ASA grade 3 or higher or with two or more RCRI risk factors (class II; level of evidence: B). Careful dose titration according to individualized heart rate targets is advisable. Although it is suggested that atenolol or bisoprolol may be preferred to metoprolol, a recent large cohort study found no differences in both mortality and the risk of MACE with respect to the β-blocker subtype. Conversely, perioperative initiation of β-blockers is not recommended in patients undergoing low-risk procedures.

Two other meta-analyses were published shortly after the 2014 update of the ESC/ESA guidelines. A Cochrane systematic review of 89 RCTs (19,211 patients) investigating the perioperative use of β-blockers in both cardiac and noncardiac surgical procedures showed, despite a significant reduction in the rate of AMI, myocardial ischemia and supraventricular arrhythmias, a potential increase in all-cause mortality rates and in cerebrovascular complications with the use of β-blockers in patients undergoing noncardiac surgical procedures that became significant (RR, 1.27; 95% CI, 1.01–1.59; and RR, 2.09; 95% CI, 1.14–3.82, respectively) after restricting the analysis to trials with a low risk of bias. Hypotension and bradycardia were significantly more common in patients receiving β-blockers. Finally, another meta-analysis also published in 2014 found increased risks of hypotension, bradycardia, and nonfatal stroke with perioperative β-blockade, regardless of the inclusion or exclusion of both the POISE and the DECREASE trials. Moreover, this meta-analysis showed a significantly increased overall mortality rate (RR, 1.30; 95% CI, 1.03–1.64), after exclusion of the DECREASE studies, in patients in whom β-blockers were started within 1 day before the surgical procedure.

It is likely that the proper β-blocking agent, started early enough preoperatively (to allow adequate dose titration) and administered to the appropriate subset of patients, would effectively and safely prevent adverse cardiac events in high-risk noncardiac surgical patients. This approach may not be easy to apply, however, in several clinical contexts. The role of intraoperative administration of the short-acting cardioselective β-blocker esmolol in preventing MACE with fewer adverse effects as compared with other β-blockers, with a potential favorable effect on mortality, should be investigated in the near future.

FURTHER STRATEGIES TO POSSIBLY REDUCE MORTALITY RATES IN NONCARDIAC SURGICAL PROCEDURES: EVIDENCE FROM OTHER CLINICAL SETTINGS

Volatile Anesthetic Agents

According to two meta-analyses and one Bayesian network meta-analysis of RCTs, the use of modern halogenated anesthetic agents (isoflurane, desflurane, or sevoflurane), compared with total IV anesthesia (TIVA), may reduce mortality rates in patients undergoing cardiac surgical procedures, seemingly because of a cardioprotective action whose mechanism is similar to that of ischemic preconditioning. However, some investigations failed to confirm any beneficial effect of volatile anesthetic agents on troponin release or mortality rates after cardiac surgical procedures. Moreover, a cardioprotective action was not observed in patients undergoing coronary stenting procedures.

The largest multicenter RCT comparing the use of volatile anesthetic agents with TIVA in patients undergoing cardiac surgical procedures is currently ongoing (http://clinicaltrials.gov/show/NCT02105610: Volatile Anesthetics to Reduce Mortality in Cardiac Surgery [MYRIAD]), and it will probably make a significant contribution to the definition of the role of volatile anesthetic agents in reducing myocardial injury and mortality rates.

If confirmed, such an effect might be used to prevent MACE and to improve survival in noncardiac surgical patients. However, the available evidence in this setting is currently scarce and somewhat conflicting. For example, although a large prospective observational study recently found a reduction in 30-day mortality with high inhalation anesthetic doses in a cohort of 124,497 patients undergoing noncardiac surgery (because of a reduction in postoperative respiratory complications), a retrospective analysis including 11,395 patients undergoing cancer surgery between 2010 and 2013 showed an increased mortality with the use of volatile anesthetics as compared with TIVA, possibly caused by an increased risk of cancer recurrence or metastasis (as suggested by several in vitro studies). A large multicenter RCT is ongoing to investigate the beneficial effect of a propofol-based anesthesia and the detrimental effect of a volatile-based anesthesia in cancer surgery procedures (http://clinicaltrials.gov/show/NCT01975064: Cancer and Anesthesia: Survival After Radical Surgery—A Comparison Between Propofol and Sevoflurane Anesthesia [CAN]). Large, multicenter studies are needed to assess the potential advantages of volatile anesthetic agents in patients at risk for perioperative myocardial injury or MI and to further investigate their role in reducing both cardiac and respiratory complications and mortality in patients undergoing noncardiac surgery. It cannot be excluded that volatile anesthetics could affect mortality in opposite directions in cancer and noncancer surgery.

Leukocyte Depletion of Transfused Blood

Removing leukocytes from blood to be transfused is thought to prevent transfusion-related immunomodulation, probably leading to a reduced risk of infections. In cardiac surgical patients, cardiopulmonary bypass may magnify the inflammatory mechanisms through which blood transfusions may lead to increased susceptibility to infections or to multiorgan dysfunction. Two large RCTs found a reduced mortality rate with transfusion of leukodepleted RBCs compared with standard buffy coat–depleted RBCs. Whether this favorable effect is restricted to the cardiac surgical population or whether it may also occur in other surgical settings is not clear. However, leukodepletion of blood products is regarded as best practice in most Western countries.

Insulin for Tight Glycemic Control

In a landmark investigation (Van den Berghe et al., 2001), maintaining blood glucose levels between 80 and 110 mg/dL through continuous infusion of insulin was found to reduce the mortality rate in patients admitted to the ICU after cardiac or noncardiac surgical procedures. Improved survival with intensive glycemic control also was shown in a subsequent meta-analysis of RCTs, as well as in an RCT in patients undergoing cardiac surgical procedures, although with fewer "tight" targets of blood glucose control (<180 mg/dL and 120–160 mg/dL, respectively). However, a meta-analysis including 29 RCTs performed in both medical and surgical ICU patients failed to show any survival benefit with intensive glucose control. Conversely, a higher risk of hypoglycemia was found. The large Normoglycaemia in Intensive Care Evaluation and Survival Using Glucose Algorithm Regulation (NICE-SUGAR) multicenter investigation also raised important concerns about tight glycemic control. An increase in mortality rates was found in ICU patients in whom blood glucose was maintained between 81 and 108 mg/dL compared with a higher blood glucose target (<180 mg/dL). Accordingly, caution should be used when adjusting glycemic levels in ICU patients to avoid dangerous hypoglycemic episodes. Further studies are desirable in the perioperative setting in which hypoglycemia (and relative hypoglycemia in the patients with diabetes) avoidance is extremely important.

Lung-Protective Ventilation

Protective ventilation, involving the use of low tidal volumes and moderate to high levels of positive end-expiratory pressure (with or without recruitment maneuvers), is one of the interventions shown to improve survival in critically ill patients. Three multicenter RCTs found a reduction in mortality rates with protective ventilation in patients with acute respiratory distress syndrome (ARDS). Data are accumulating to support the *prophylactic* use of protective ventilation to prevent ARDS in patients without lung injury. Accordingly, *intraoperative* lung-protective ventilation is becoming a standard of care in patients undergoing both cardiac and noncardiac surgery (e.g., major abdominal procedures). This topic is very attractive and deserves further large investigations.

Preoperative Intraaortic Balloon Pump Counterpulsation

In high-risk patients undergoing coronary artery bypass graft operations, preoperative mechanical cardiocirculatory support with IABP can reduce perioperative and 30-day mortality rates, as shown by a small RCT and four meta-analyses of RCTs. Although IABP placement may potentially lead to serious vascular or infectious complications, the rates of lower limb ischemia and local infection were shown to be relatively low (0.94% and 0.47%, respectively) in a retrospective study including 423 cardiac surgical patients receiving perioperative IABP. Whether this strategy may confer a survival advantage in carefully selected patients with high-risk CAD who are undergoing noncardiac surgical procedures should be investigated.

Vacuum-Assisted Closure

Although only a meta-analysis of 22 retrospective studies reported an improved survival in patients with deep sternal wound infection with the use of vacuum-assisted closure (VAC) therapy, this strategy was one of the most agreed-on among those included in the recently updated Democracy-Based Consensus Conference on mortality reduction in cardiac surgery. A reduced 90-day mortality rate with VAC therapy was also recently found in a small RCT in which 45 patients with abdominal injury or intraabdominal sepsis undergoing abbreviated laparotomy were randomized to temporary abdomen closure with or without a negative-pressure device (ABThera; Kinetic Concepts). This is a promising topic that deserves further research in both the cardiac and noncardiac surgery settings.

Levosimendan

Levosimendan, an inodilating (and antiinflammatory) calcium sensitizer, showed cardioprotective properties in patients with heart failure. Most remarkably, it has been shown to reduce mortality rates in patients undergoing cardiac surgical procedures, according to a small RCT and five meta-analyses. A Bayesian network meta-analysis found that levosimendan was the only inodilator drug associated with a reduction in mortality rates, compared with placebo, in patients undergoing cardiac surgery. Although no evidence exists in patients undergoing noncardiac surgery, it could be assumed that a similar favorable effect may apply in this setting, especially in patients with perioperative low CO syndrome. Unfortunately, three large RCTs, all published in 2017, found no effects on important clinical outcomes (including mortality rate) when levosimendan was administered in the cardiac surgery setting either preoperatively in patients with left ventricular dysfunction (LEVO-CTS and LICORN trials) or postoperatively in patients requiring hemodynamic support (CHEETAH trial). Although, in light of this new evidence, it is hard to keep believing in some favorable survival effect (at least in cardiac surgery). Future research could be addressed to the identification of specific dose regimens, timing of administration, subsets of patients, and clinical settings that might be associated with a significant impact on outcomes of levosimendan.

Remote Ischemic Preconditioning

Repeated short episodes of ischemia and reperfusion in a remote vascular territory (e.g., by applying a blood pressure cuff on an upper limb and inflating or deflating it every 5 minutes for three cycles) may protect the heart from ischemia or reperfusion injury. This effect is possibly caused by the release of one or more substances that reach the heart and activate cell-signaling pathways, probably involving mitochondria, this resulting in greater resistance to ischemic insults. An RCT of 329 patients undergoing coronary artery bypass graft operations found a reduced postoperative release of cTn (cTnI: AUC, 0.83; 95% CI, 0.70–0.97; $P = .022$) and a reduced all-cause mortality rate (HR, 0.27; 95% CI, 0.08–0.98; $P = .046$) with remote ischemic preconditioning (RIPC). Until recently, it seemed reasonable to assume that RIPC could have possible applications in noncardiac surgical patients at risk for perioperative myocardial ischemia. However, two subsequent high-quality multicenter RCTs (including 1612 and 1385 patients, respectively) found no effects of RIPC on clinically relevant outcomes in patients undergoing cardiac surgery. Despite the possibility that propofol anesthesia may have counteracted the beneficial effects of RIPC, current evidence no longer supports this strategy for either myocardial protection or mortality reduction.

FUTURE PERSPECTIVES

Further strategies, mostly not yet investigated in the perioperative setting and without a well-defined consensus about their clinical role, showed at least a signal of a potential effect on patient survival and deserve future high-quality research to either confirm the observed benefits or detrimental effects or evaluate the hypothesis that a similar effect could be extended to the surgical population.

In addition, other strategies that may potentially affect mortality in the perioperative period and, accordingly, should be adequately investigated in the near future, include the use of POC coagulation monitoring, the early institution of renal replacement therapy in strictly selected patients, and extracorporeal mechanical circulatory support in very high-risk patients.

Nutritional Support and Supplementation

Many studies addressed the role of nutritional, vitamin, and oligoelement supplementation in ICU patients. According to two relatively recent RCTs, a restricted caloric intake has been found to reduce mortality rates in critically ill patients. Consistently, another RCT recently showed an increased mortality rate in ICU patients receiving an "intensive medical nutritional intervention." The effects of glutamine and antioxidant supplementation are controversial: despite three RCTs that found a survival benefit in ICU patients receiving parenteral glutamine in addition to enteral or parenteral nutrition and one RCT that showed a reduced mortality rate in ICU patients receiving an enteral antioxidant supplementation, a subsequent large multicenter RCT found no improvements in clinical outcomes with the administration of antioxidants, and an increased mortality rate in patients who received glutamine. Similarly, the strategies involving the addition of various associations of immune-modulating supplements (e.g., omega-3 fatty acids, vitamins, selenium, and glutamine and antioxidants themselves) to artificial nutrition have been reported to increase mortality in randomized investigations. However, one multicenter RCT and one small RCT found a reduced mortality rate with selenium supplementation in patients with sepsis or septic shock and with the administration of ascorbic acid in postsurgical ICU patients with sepsis, respectively. The role of nutritional support in affecting important outcomes in critically ill patients (possibly including the perioperative scenario) is very intriguing but also not easy to investigate.

Synthetic Colloids

Another controversial topic, still not fully addressed by high-quality research in the perioperative setting, is the choice between crystalloids and synthetic colloids for fluid resuscitation. Although, in the authors' opinion, the evidences of increased risk of bleeding, kidney injury, and death coming from the critical care setting are sufficient to discourage the use of synthetic colloids also in the operating room, many colleagues worldwide disagree.

Sedation

Literature suggests that both the duration and depth of sedation may affect patient survival. In particular, two RCTs in the ICU setting found a reduction in mortality rate with daily interruption of sedatives and with a protocolized approach to pain, agitation, and delirium (leading to significantly lower doses of fentanyl and propofol), respectively. More recently, a post hoc analysis of a relatively small RCT showed a reduced 1-year mortality rate in patients younger than 65 years old with a high grade of comorbidity who received light sedation during hip fracture repair under spinal anesthesia compared to those who received deep sedation. The potential effects of deep or prolonged sedation on clinically relevant outcomes should be adequately investigated in different perioperative settings (it cannot be excluded, for example, that cardiac patients could benefit from deeper sedation). Moreover, future research should address the perioperative use, as a sedative agent, of dexmedetomidine, which has been suggested to reduce mortality rates in both septic ICU patients (compared with use of lorazepam) and cardiac surgery patients.

Inspired Oxygen Fraction

The inspiratory oxygen fraction (F_IO_2) administered intraoperatively varies widely, ranging from 0.3 to 1.0, with many clinicians (especially in the United States) indiscriminately administering 100% oxygen regardless of the clinical situation. However, there is some evidence that hyperoxia may have detrimental effects. In particular, an RCT of 480 ICU patients found a reduced mortality rate in patients in whom the partial pressure of oxygen (pO_2) was maintained between 70 and 100 mm Hg compared with standard practice (pO_2 up to 150 mm Hg). Although no similar studies have been performed in the surgical setting, a follow-up of an RCT in which 1386 patients undergoing abdominal surgery were randomized to receive a F_IO_2 of either 0.3 or 0.8 intraoperatively and postoperatively found a reduced long-term mortality rate among cancer patients (but not in noncancer patients) who received the lower F_IO_2. Even though there are no clear mechanisms that can explain these findings, the hypothesis that a restrictive perioperative oxygen administration may improve survival is interesting and merits further research.

High-Flow Nasal Cannula Oxygen

According to a multicenter RCT of 310 patients with acute hypoxemic respiratory failure, the administration of high-flow oxygen through a nasal cannula (HFNC) may improve 90-day survival compared with both conventional oxygen therapy and NIV. A subsequent meta-analysis of 11 RCTs (3459 patients overall) suggested that HFNC is superior to conventional oxygen therapy but similar to NIV in terms of respiratory outcomes. However, it failed to show any difference in mortality rate among the three techniques. Considering the abovementioned evidence about NIV, HFNC appears to be a promising technique that is worth investigating in the perioperative setting.

SUGGESTED READING

Berwanger O, de Barros E Silva PG, Barbosa RR, et al. Atorvastatin for high-risk statin-naïve patients undergoing noncardiac surgery: the lowering the risk of operative complications using atorvastatin loading dose (LOAD) randomized trial. *Am Heart J*. 2017;184:88–96.

Billings FT 4th, Hendricks PA, Schildcrout JS, et al. High-dose perioperative atorvastatin and acute kidney injury following cardiac surgery: A randomized clinical trial. *JAMA*. 2016;315:877–888.

Cholley B, Caruba T, Grosjean S, et al. Effect of levosimendan on low cardiac output syndrome in patients with low ejection fraction undergoing coronary artery bypass grafting with cardiopulmonary bypass: the LICORN randomized clinical trial. *JAMA*. 2017;318(6):548–556.

Devereaux PJ, Biccard BM, Sigamani A, et al. Association of postoperative high-sensitivity troponin levels with myocardial injury and 30-day mortality among patients undergoing non cardiac surgery. *JAMA*. 2017;317(16):1642–1651.

Gorka J, Polok K, Iwaniec T, et al. Altered preoperative coagulation and fibrinolysis are associated with myocardial injury after non-cardiac surgery. *Br J Anaest*. 2017;118:713–719.

Landoni G, Lomivorotov V, Pisano A, et al. MortalitY in caRdIAc surgery (MYRIAD): a randomized controlled trial of volatile anesthetics. Rationale and design. *Contemp Clin Trials*. 2017;59:38–43.

Landoni G, Lomivorotov V, Silvietti S, et al. Nonsurgical strategies to reduce mortality in patients undergoing cardiac surgery: an updated consensus process. *J Cardiothorac Vasc Anesth*. 2017;32:225–235.

Landoni G, Lomivorotov VV, Alvaro G, et al. Levosimendan for hemodynamic support after cardiac surgery. *N Engl J Med*. 2017;376(21):2021–2031.

Landoni G, Pisano A, Lomivorotov V, et al. Randomized evidence for reduction of perioperative mortality: an updated consensus process. *J Cardiothorac Vasc Anesth*. 2017;31(2):719–730.

Mehta RH, Leimberger JD, van Diepen S, et al. Levosimendan in patients with left ventricular dysfunction undergoing cardiac surgery. *N Engl J Med*. 2017;376(21):2032–2042.

Myles PS, Smith JA, Forbes A, et al. Tranexamic acid in patients undergoing coronary-artery surgery. *N Engl J Med*. 2017;376(2):136–148.

Parashar A, Agarwal S, Krishnaswamy A, et al. Percutaneous intervention for myocardial infarction after noncardiac surgery: patient characteristics and outcomes. *J Am Coll Cardiol*. 2016;68(4):329–338.

Pisano A, Landoni G, Bellomo R. The risk of infusing gelatin? Die-hard misconceptions and forgotten (or ignored) truths. *Minerva Anestesiol*. 2016;82(10):1107–1114.

Reed GW, Horr S, Young L, et al. Associations between cardiac troponin, mechanism of myocardial injury and long term mortality after non cardiac vascular surgery. *JAHA*. 2017;6(6):72–78.

Rossini R, Musumeci G, Capodanno D, et al. Perioperative management of oral antiplatelet therapy and clinical outcomes in coronary stent patients undergoing surgery. Results of a multicentre registry. *Thromb Haemost*. 2015;113:272–282.

Simon GI, Craswell A, Thom O, Fung YL. Outcomes of restrictive versus liberal transfusion strategies in older adults from nine randomised controlled trials: a systematic review and meta-analysis. *Lancet Haematol*. 2017;4(10):e465–e474.

Smilowitz NR, Gupta N, Guo Y, et al. Perioperative acute myocardial infarction associated with non-cardiac surgery. *Eur Heart J*. 2017;38(31):2409–2417.

Stens J, Hering JP, van der Hoeven CWP, et al. The added value of cardiac index and pulse pressure variation monitoring to mean arterial pressure-guided volume therapy in moderate-risk abdominal surgery (COGUIDE): a pragmatic multicentre randomised controlled trial. *Anaesthesia*. 2017;72(9):1078–1087.

Van den Berghe G, Wouters P, Weekers F, et al. Intensive insulin therapy in the critically ill patients. *N Engl J Med*. 2001;345:1359–1367.

Xu XP, Zhang XC, Hu SL, et al. Noninvasive ventilation in acute hypoxemic nonhypercapnic respiratory failure: a systematic review and meta-analysis. *Crit Care Med*. 2017;45(7):e727–e733.

Zheng Z, Jayaram R, Jiang L, et al. Perioperative rosuvastatin in cardiac surgery. *N Engl J Med*. 2016;374:1744–1753.

579

K

Ketamine, 309, 506
  for emergent noncardiac surgery, 411*t*
  for pulmonary hypertension, 346–347
Knowledgeable VAD personnel, in postanesthetic considerations for ventricular assist device, 117*t*–118*t*
Kommerell diverticulum, 374–376, 376*f*–377*f*

L

LAA. *see* Left atrial appendage
Label form, of NBD code, 81, 82*t*
Labetalol, 260*t*–261*t*, 266
Laparoscopic surgery, in pregnancy, 483
Lariat Suture Delivery Device (SentreHEART International), 399
Leadless pacemaker, 392
Leadless transcatheter-deployed intracardiac pacemakers, 77–78
Leads, pacemaker, 72–73
  bipolar, 72
  coronary sinus, 75
  passive fixation, 72–73, 73*f*
  removal of, 72–73
  right atrial, 72, 73*f*
  unipolar, 72
Left atrial ablations, and atrial fibrillation, 395–396
Left atrial appendage (LAA), 380*t*
  closure, 398–399
    anesthetic considerations for, 399
    endovascularly delivered closure, 398–399
    percutaneous closure, 399
Left bundle branch block
  cardiac electrical abnormalities, 202*t*–203*t*
  ECG abnormalities, 203*f*, 203*t*–204*t*
Left heart disease, pulmonary hypertension caused by, 344–345, 345*b*
Left subclavian and pedal arteries, in CHD, 170*t*
Left ventricular assist device (LVAD), 100–119
  current frequency of, 101*t*
  explanations of, 101*t*
  goal of, 100–101
  indication for, 101–102, 101*t*
  intraoperative anesthetic management for, 111–116
    Anrep effect as, 113
    Bowditch effect as, 113
    Frank-Sterling mechanisms as, 113
    key points of physiology as, 112
    series circulatory effects as, 112
    specific actions, 113–116, 114*t*
    ventricular interdependence as, 112
    ventriculoarterial coupling as, 112
  optimization during intraoperative period, 116–117
  perioperative management for, 104–111
    preoperative anticoagulation as, 108–109
    preoperative assessment as, 104–108
  postoperative considerations, 117, 117*t*–118*t*
  success rates of, 101*t*
  type of, in preanesthetic inquiry for ventricular assist device, 109*t*

Left ventricular hypocontractility, 225–226
  and left ventricular outflow tract obstruction, 226–227
Left ventricular outflow tract obstruction, 227*f*–228*f*
  left ventricular hypocontractility and, 226–227
  mechanism of, 226–227
Leukocyte depletion, of transfused blood, 572
Leukocytosis, 154
Level of evidence (LOE), 8–11, 10*f*
Levosimendan, 161, 258
  for heart failure, 574
  for heart transplantation, 135–136
Levo-transposition of the great vessels (L-TGV), 178–179, 178*f*
Liberal fluid management, 494–495
LiDCO Rapid device, 201–204
Lidocaine, 271–272
  intravenous, 506
  as local anesthetics, 297*t*
Light transmission aggregometry, test to measure platelet function, 54*t*
Lithotripsy, 96
Liver disease, cardiac condition in, 453–458
  circulatory syndrome and, 454–458
  preoperative cardiac assessment for, 453–454, 454*t*
  pulmonary hypertension and, 454–458, 455*b*, 456*t*
Liver transplantation, orthotopic, 453–465
  cardiac condition in, 453–458
    preoperative cardiac assessment for, 453–454
  comorbidities present in, 454, 454*t*
  complication of, 464
  hepatic coagulopathy and thromboses in, 462–463
  intraoperative hemodynamics for, 461–462
    anhepatic phase, 461
    neohepatic phase, 461–462
    postanhepatic phase, 462*b*
    pre-anhepatic phase, 461
  intraoperative monitoring for, 459–461
    arterial catheters, 459
    central venous pressure, 460
    continuous cardiac output, 460–461
    pulmonary artery catheter, 460
    transesophageal echocardiography, 459, 460*f*
  postoperative management of, 463–464
  preoperative testing for, 458–459
    cardiac catheterization, 459
    echocardiography, 459
    stress test, 458
Local anesthesia, 290, 296–300, 297*t*–298*t*, 298*b*
  for carotid endarterectomy, 321–322
Local anesthetic systemic toxicity, 298–300, 299*b*
Locoregional anesthesia, 326
LOE. *see* Level of evidence
Long-standing hypoxemia, 168
Lower extremity arterial disease, 335–338
  intervention, considerations for, 337
  intraoperative anesthetic considerations and management, 337–338